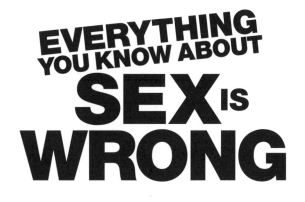

EVERYTHING YOU KNOW ABOUT SEX IS WRONG

Published by The Disinformation Company Ltd.
163 Third Avenue, Suite 108
New York, NY 10003
Tel.: +1.212.691.1605
Fax: +1.212.691.1606
www.disinfo.com

Design and Layout: raisedBarb Graphics

Library of Congress Control Number: 2005930394

ISBN-10: 1-932857-17-6
ISBN-13: 978-1-932857-17-7

Printed in USA

10 9 8 7 6 5 4 3 2 1

Distributed in the USA and Canada by:
Consortium Book Sales and Distribution
1045 Westgate Drive, Suite 90
St Paul, MN 55114
Toll Free: +1.800.283.3572
Local: +1.651.221.9035
Fax: +1.651.221.0124
www.cbsd.com

Attention colleges and universities, corporations and other organizations: Quantity discounts are available on bulk purchases of this book for educational training purposes, fund-raising, or gift giving. Special books, booklets, or book excerpts can also be created to fit your specific needs. For information contact Marketing Department of The Disinformation Company Ltd.

Disinformation is a registered trademark of The Disinformation Company Ltd.

The opinions and statements made in this book are those of the authors concerned. The Disinformation Company Ltd. has not verified and neither confirms nor denies any of the foregoing and no warranty or fitness is implied. The reader is encouraged to keep an open mind and to independently judge the contents

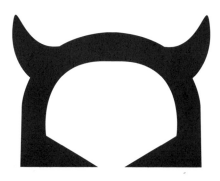

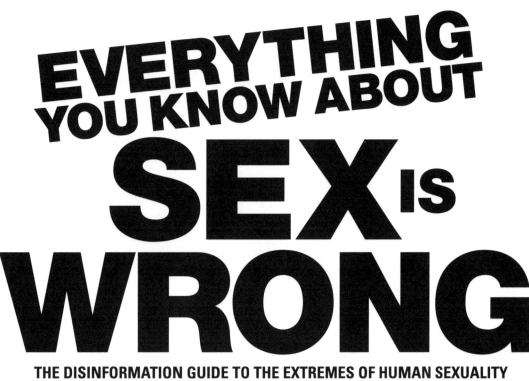

EVERYTHING YOU KNOW ABOUT SEX IS WRONG

THE DISINFORMATION GUIDE TO THE EXTREMES OF HUMAN SEXUALITY
(and everything in between)

EDITED BY RUSS KICK

Table of Contents

WORKING HARD FOR THE MONEY

SEX ON PAPER

OUR BODIES ARE A WONDERLAND

THE SEXUAL IS POLITICAL

HOLY SEX

CATEGORIES SUCK

EVERYTHING YOU KNOW ABOUT SEX IS WRONG

Editor's Introduction

Everything you know about sex is wrong? Well, maybe not *everything*, but I hope you'll allow for a little poetic license. Besides, when you start seriously digging into the vast, wild, largely uncharted world of sex, it can start to feel that way.

Masturbation is always a solitary activity. Nope.

Hardcore porn has only been around for a few decades. Uh-uh.

There are only two genders. Wrong.

Women's sex drives shut down when they're pregnant. Not hardly.

Everyone gets laid at an orgy. Porn is inherently degrading. Prostitutes and strippers are victims. Writing good sex scenes is easy. You must have sensation in your genitals in order to orgasm. Circumcision doesn't affect your sex life. There's nothing sexy about chess. Or blood. All myths.

But this book is about much more than knocking down false beliefs. The contributors tackle things you may not even have considered. Who knew that being cold could be a turn-on? Or that a woman in her seventies and a man in his twenties could have a great relationship? What's sex like when you're tripping on LSD? What goes on inside one of the world's largest dildo factories? Do erotic dancers ever get turned on by their customers? Who is the "Miller" in the Supreme Court's famous Miller standard for obscenity? And—perhaps the least obvious question of them all—is the rectum an Easter basket?

Still other writers in these pages are rescuing sexual knowledge in danger of disappearing: The goings-on in the infamous but now extinct porno theaters of Times Square. The legendary powers of the vagina. The work of the greatest erotic folklorist of all time. Japan's disappearing sex museums. The world's biggest collection of pornographic material. The most famous swingers' club, long defunct. The forgotten sex books published by bodybuilder Charles Atlas. The photo of Jesus and the adulteress that *Hustler* wouldn't run.

Maybe by reading some of these articles and essays, you'll realize that you're not the only one who has experienced altered states of consciousness during sex, that other people name their sexy bits, that at least one other person in the world gets an erotic charge from popping pimples.

The subject of sex is practically infinite, and it touches on almost every other aspect of existence—religion, language, politics, law, health, death, art, literature, humor, history, love, violence, psychology, money, lies, truth.... Everything we know about it may not be wrong, but we sure don't know much.

–Russ Kick
Tucson, Arizona

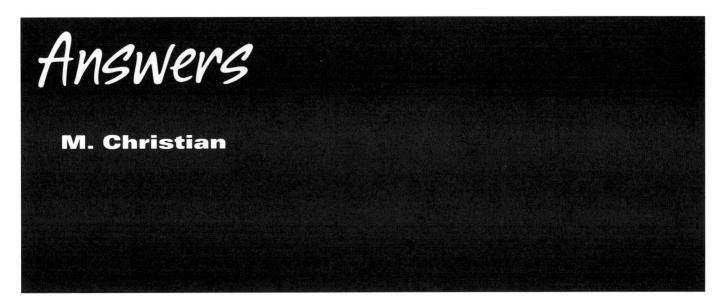

Answers

M. Christian

"San Francisco Sex Information, can I help you?"

If you've been on the phones, like me, you've heard a lot, and even if they sometimes fall into obvious categories, you really don't have any idea who the next caller will be: a woman who has never had an orgasm, a little boy who wants to know what a blowjob is, an older man who wants to step out of the closet and meet other men, a fetish dresser who wants someplace to buy shoes, someone who wants to learn how to have anal sex, or someone else who wants to know how to find his prostate.

San Francisco Sex Information is where those who don't know can call to talk to people who do. How do SFSI workers know so much about sex? We're not thrown onto the phones cold. To be an SFSI volunteer, you have to complete 52 hours of sex training (not hands-on), including panel discussions on aging and sex, sex and drugs, the law, sex work (you'll find me teaching that—I've written a lot of porn), consent, S/M, homosexuality, bisexuality, heterosexuality, crossdressing, and just about everything else out there.

And if we still don't know the answers, we can usually find the number or address of someone who does. The switchboard room is packed with reference materials and a wonderful computerized reference file of therapists, hotlines, stores, mail-order companies, social clubs, organizations, support groups, and much, much more.

This day, today, we start off with a question about VD—or, at least someone who thinks it might be.

⚊

"San Francisco Sex Information, can I help you?"

His accent is thick (Asian, Middle Eastern?) and his English

isn't all that great, but I manage to put together a rough picture: "My wife says she is sick. Says she has something wrong with her—infection?"

"A yeast infection?"

Silence for a moment. Consulting. "Yes, that is what she has." I run down the facts, calmly and slowly, telling him that lots of women get them, that they can be very painful, and that she should probably go to the doctor. As I tell him, another of the volunteers has pulled down a book on symptoms and complications for me to refer to. I nod my thanks.

"She has gone to a doctor," he says, dismissing. "I want to know, did she get from other men? From sleeping with other man?"

We are not doctors or therapists. That's one thing the trainers are very clear about. It's not mainly, as you'd think, because of legal issues—rather, we are told that it's because it's better to say you don't know and suggest the caller consult a professional than give them wrong information.

If she had called, we would have told her that her symptoms appeared to match that of a yeast infection but that she should go back to her doctor, who could answer more of her questions. But this isn't really a medical question at its heart; it's a question about fear and possessiveness: He's frightened that his wife has committed adultery (and the disease is the sign).

"From sleeping with other man?" The cultural wall is thick and well-fortified; still, I hope I can make their lives a bit easier: "Lots of women get yeast infections. They can happen all on their own—not from sleeping with another man."

We go on like this for a while: his fear and anger at his wife's supposed adultery and my insistence that a yeast infection is not what you'd normally consider a sexually transmitted condition (though some women can get one from a condom reaction). I finally convince him that his wife (probably) hasn't been sleeping with other men and he hangs up, relieved.

My shift is on Tuesday evening, 6:00 to 9:00 PM. Me, two to five other volunteers (rookies just off training and older volunteers who happened to drop by), and a supervisor, who has watched me with the call to make sure I didn't pass along inappropriate, insensitive, or Just Plain Wrong information. Sometimes, if a call is a rough one, the supervisor can plug in and listen along. Afterwards it's common for us all to talk

You really don't have any idea who the next caller will be.

about a call and share our take on the situation, what we should've said.

⌒

"San Francisco Sex Information, can I help you?"

His voice is rough and slightly hostile. It's hard to hear him over the static-laced payphone: "I have this girlfriend and she's really good in bed but I really like this guy I met on the way home last night and he was really good, you know, and it was really hot and he—"

"Do you have a question?"

"Well, I really liked what he did, you know when he—" He goes on for quite a while, giving me the play-by-play about his encounter with this other man.

Sometimes we let them run if we figure that they're just nervous. But if they're bragging or trying to get a rise out of us (for whatever reason), we cut them short.

The road traveled might be different for a lot of the callers (a single homosexual experience, being attracted to another person of the same sex, liking a certain movie star a lot), but the question is always the same: "Am I gay?" he finally gets out.

Some of them are disappointed in the response: "I don't know. Only you can really answer that. A lot of heterosexual people have homosexual experiences and vice versa. A lot of people call themselves gay and have sex with the opposite sex. The same goes for straight people. You don't have to be 'gay'; you could just like same-sex sex all or some of the time."

We talk for a few minutes, me trying to tell him that he doesn't have to label himself or let others do it for him. He is what he

wants to be, however he defines it. He really does want to listen, to hear what I have to tell him. After a point he calms down, says he might call again, and hangs up.

It's surprising, though, the number of people who demand negative information—who are actually disappointed when we don't back up their fears by telling them they're gay, sick, perverted: to validate their own crushed egos ("I know I'm a freak—I feel like one!"). They won't hear that from SFSI; we answer questions, talk, and refer callers to other resources. We try never to pass judgments—we let people say who they are, negative or positive.

Founded in 1972, SFSI is "a non-profit, free, non-judgmental sexual information and referral service." At various points we've been the only free sex-information service out there. We get calls from all across the country and around the world. The details of the SFSI training are kept a closely guarded secret, but one of the main points of it is to push the buttons of the trainees and get them to deal with their own prejudices and biased viewpoints before they get on the phones. The one thing we don't want a phone volunteer saying to a caller is, "Yech, you're sick!"

৪৪

"San Francisco Sex Information, can I help you?"

The heart-wrencher. He is either softly crying or has been crying heavily recently. His voice is two parts fear and one part anger. The cause could be any number of things: It just happened; I thought we were being safe; I didn't think it was going to happen; the condom broke; I did something and I don't know if it was safe. The list goes on. The real question, no matter how they frame it, is the same: "Am I infected?"

I take a deep breath. The first order of business with a call like his is to calm him down—then talk. Sometimes, if they don't ask, we'll suggest: "Would talking to a woman help?" (if the caller is a woman) or, "Would talking to a gay man help?" in his case. It doesn't really matter, because we all receive the same training, but it can make a crisis caller more comfortable, more at ease.

"I hear that you're upset."

"Yes, I'm upset. I'm really scared."

"What can you tell me about being scared?"

"I don't know if I've caught it, you know? I don't know if he's got it. It was just so quick and I didn't think about it at the time, and now I'm scared. Do you think I've got it?"

The technique is called reflective listening—we're trained to use it to help focus or defuse some of the callers. After a few minutes of listening to what he's saying and bouncing it back to him, he's calmed down enough and is breathing deeply. It's always hard, these kinds of calls. I've been down that frightening stretch of dark road myself when a condom broke.

I tell him that yes, he is at risk, but from what he says (it was unprotected oral sex), it is a relatively low risk—though not impossible. I reassure him and calm him, soothing him till he can listen. There's no reason to panic till he knows. I give him the information that oral sex is still debatable, but he's still bargaining for his life—especially after the new study that suggests that unprotected oral sex may be just as risky as intercourse—so why take a risk on your life? I tell him that the only way to be sure is to have himself and his partner tested as soon as possible to find out their status. Then, after either abstinence or good safe(r) sex for six months, get tested again.

Besides, I remind him, there are other things out there that are sometimes as bad or worse than HIV: the clap (gonorrhea), syphilis, herpes, hepatitis (which can kill faster than HIV), PID (Pelvic Inflammatory Disease), genital warts—the list is long and scary.

Afterwards, I'm shaking. I let the other volunteers take some calls while I sit and decompress. Sometimes we get hard calls, scary ones—I was abused; I was raped (those we talk down and try to get them to call the police or a rape crisis line); I was hurt. One of the things SFSI trains us for is a sex-positive attitude, but these kinds of calls remind us that while sex can be beautiful, it can also be frightening and dangerous.

By now the night is getting late. Outside, a street I can't name (because the switchboard is a secret) hums with late-night travelers. Next to me one of the phones chirps, and I pick it up.

✕✕

"San Francisco Sex Information, can I help you?"

"How can I get my girlfriend to go down on me?" he says without preamble.

Consent. SFSI is big on consent. In a world that frequently acts without asking, San Francisco Sex Information is a bastion of asking permission, of communication. "Have you talked to her about it?"

"Yeah, but she says she doesn't like doing it."

"Does she say what she doesn't like about it? Does she choke? Doesn't like the taste?"

"Yeah, she says she chokes on it."

I take a deep breath. "You can't get anyone to do anything they don't want to do, but you can talk to her. Tell her how much you like it and how much it would mean to you. If she's scared or nervous, take it real slow and at her pace."

He listens. I'll give him that at least. Sometimes the callers, mainly male callers, are angry at not getting their idealized lovers. We try our best to get them information about consent, safe(r) sex, and communication: Ask, be safe, and talk about it. I hope I get some of it across to him and wish him the best—and tell him he might want to have her call us, too.

Meanwhile, one of our female volunteers is having trouble with a caller. I can hear her voice, angry but level, disengaging from the call. I hear only one side of it, but it's enough to know most of what's going on: "Do you have a question? If you don't have a legitimate question, I'm going to hang up. If you don't stop, I'm going to hang up. I'm hanging up."

She clicks him off (I know it's a him) and looks at the phone with frustration and disgust.

I take the next few calls, along with the other male volunteers. We get nothing but hang-ups for about fifteen minutes.

It's a sad, but realistic, fact of life for any kind of switchboard (suicide, AIDS info, or whatever) that you have those callers.

"How can I get my girlfriend to go down on me?" he says without preamble.

They can get to you sometimes, the angry men, the mentally ill (men and women), the just plain lonely (who just want to talk about sex—of any kind), and the self-righteously religious. But then the phone rings again, and it's someone we can help, someone with a question we can really answer.

♡

"San Francisco Sex Information, can I help you?"

"I have, um, a question..." He sounds young, maybe midtwenties. His voice, while nervous, is laced with strength—I bet he's just trying to frame his question and isn't paralyzed by calling.

"Sure, that's what we're here for. Go ahead."

"I like to, um, ah, wear my girlfriend's panties...."

Reflexive listening: "And how does that make you feel?" I say back, getting comfortable—sometimes it can take a while to coax out the real question.

"Good—I mean, it turns me on and all."

For many calls, the bottom line, again, is, "Am I normal?"

One of the things the training teaches us is the myth of normal. We are who we feel we are, how we feel about ourselves—no one is "normal."

"How do you feel about that?"

"Okay, I guess."

I take a deep breath and start down a familiar road. He could have been calling about any kind of thing: I like to spank my girlfriend or boyfriend. "Just as long as he or she likes it, as well," we'd tell them. I like to masturbate—a lot. "Just as long as it doesn't interfere with your life," we'd say. I like to spy on the couple across the street having sex. "Do you think they'd like you to? They aren't consenting to have you watch. Find a couple who want to have you watch, who consent to have you watching." I like to get tied up. "Here's some addresses and numbers of where to learn to do it safely." But there's always the hidden, "Am I normal?"

"Lots of people like to dress in another gender's clothing. Some do it because it feels nice or different, others because it feels nasty and forbidden. Some go as far as to dress completely, from shoes to hair, while others just wear women's or men's underwear. Lots of women as well as men crossdress. It doesn't have anything to do with your orientation or preference in sexual partners—many heterosexual men as well as women like to dress like the other sex. There's also a strong tradition of it in the gay male and lesbian communities (drag and doing butch). It's a perfectly acceptable turn-on for many, many people."

I go on for quite a while, responding to his uh-huhs and okays to reassure him and let him know that he's just one of a whole global community of people who like to dress in their partner's underwear—or do full drag. More than anything, though, I tell him that it's only bad if what he does hurts someone ("How would your girlfriend feel about you wearing her panties? Maybe you should talk to her or get some girl's clothes of your own—") or if he feels bad about it himself.

He clears his throat and says with a smile in his voice: "Oh, she knows. She gives me hers all the time. It's just that, um, she's small and I'm big—where can I get some that fit?"

I smile and try to keep from laughing: *touché*! His voice is strong. This is a fellow with no problems about what he does; he just needs help finding some clothes that fit. I dig up a phonebook and tell him about large-size ladies' shops that wouldn't mind a guy walking in and certain dress shops (if he wants some fancy underwear) that cater to crossdressers. By the time he hangs up, we both have smiles in our voices.

"San Francisco Sex Information, can I help you?"

"Um, ah, hello?" She echoes, shy, embarrassed. She sounds older, maybe in her late to middle sixties, and her voice cracks now and again with fear and embarrassment. It takes a few minutes of casual banter for me to ease out the issue: She wants to orgasm.

Carefully, patiently, I explain the groundwork: knowing her body and what pleases her, how to fantasize (and that there is no reason to feel guilty about any fantasy), relaxation, and even some proper devices she might try (lubrication, a vibrator, and so on). After a point, I get worried that her nervousness and fear might keep her from relaxing enough to get the info, so I ask if she'd like a female volunteer.

"No, you're doing just fine. What else should I try?"

It's an incredible compliment, to have her reach out such a long way to a stranger, to me, and ask such a deceptively simple thing. We talk for many minutes, she telling me that she never felt this way about her body before, never felt the need to really try out her own sexuality. She tells me of her husband and how he used to just roll off and sleep and how she thought that was all there was to it. She remembered masturbating as a child and how good that felt but always thought that kind of thing was for children—and how she certainly wasn't that anymore and didn't know where to even start.

She rambles a bit, but still I'm incredibly touched. When she finally hangs up, it's with a sense of purpose and release. Yes, she deserves to have a happy sex life—even if it is with herself. No, there's nothing wrong with masturbation. Yes, this kind of thing isn't all that rare.

I sit and stare at the phone for a few minutes, thinking about her, somewhere out there, and the fear that had been in her voice when we started and how that fear had slowly ebbed to relief and laughing hope.

You get many kinds of calls on the San Francisco Sex Information switchboard. All kinds. All of them, in one way or another, are important.

And some of them are just plain special.

You can call the SFSI hotline at 415-989-SFSI (7374) from 3:00 to 9:00 PM (PST) Mondays through Thursdays, 3:00 to 7:00 PM Fridays, and 2:00 to 6:00 PM Saturdays.
San Francisco Sex Information
PO Box 190063
San Francisco CA 94119-0063
ask-us@sfsi.org
www.sfsi.org

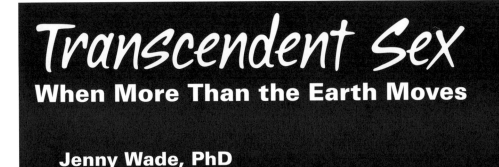

Transcendent Sex
When More Than the Earth Moves

Jenny Wade, PhD

A funny thing happened on the way to orgasm. The bedroom I was in began dissolving. Without having imbibed even a glass of wine at lunch, I watched in amazement as the white walls of the familiar room transformed into those of a round pink chamber with a silver Greek key border near the ceiling. Was this just some weird fantasy or daydream? My eyes were open, and I knew intellectually that I was in the same room, but visually I was seeing another place entirely.

I was suddenly no longer in any room with my lover at all, no longer sheltered in his house from the snow blanketing the wintry Northeast, but standing on the sun-bright shores of a sandy beach, squinting at the glittering waves. I was surrounded by vivid sea creatures, fish and octopi. Bemused, I wondered if I had somehow been swept into the water from the beach, but gradually I realized the sea creatures were not real, but images. Images painted in the unmistakable style of frescoes from the ancient civilization of Crete, a culture about which I knew practically nothing. It didn't matter. I was filled with the most exquisite rapture and bliss I had ever experienced.

Eventually, I found myself back in the familiar bedroom, still making love. My lover had apparently noticed nothing. Had I lost my mind? How long had I been "away"? I had never inadvertently slipped out of reality before. I didn't say anything about it, rather ashamed to let my lover know I had strayed so far from his attentions and feeling pretty crazy about it, to boot. But I never forgot it, either.

Later, on other occasions during sex, more strange things happened. I was filled with ecstasies a thousand times larger and more compelling than even the most intense orgasm. One day, I couldn't contain it anymore and began laughing; I embraced my lover and excitedly told him what had happened.

He looked at me oddly, then confessed that he, too, after a lifetime of sex, had been having some strange things happen when he was in bed with me. His experiences were nothing like mine. We both had been afraid we were crazy, but if so, it was the most glorious experience in all the world, one that opened each of us to ecstatic realms we had never dreamed existed, experiences beyond those offered by psychedelics or a meditation practice.

Both of us were experienced in other types of altered states, and, in fact, we're professional researchers of unusual states of consciousness. I decided to investigate what was going on in a more serious way, so I conducted a research study of 91 people who have had such experiences to learn more about them (the results have been published as academic articles and a popular book called *Transcendent Sex: When Lovemaking Opens the Veil*).

The fact is, the ordinary act of lovemaking can be the most widely available path to higher consciousness for most people. People who have experienced a transcendent episode during sex usually believe they have tapped into divine forces, even if they are atheists or agnostics. These experiences are so extreme, they change people's views of sex and spirituality. They have literally changed people's lives.

This research provides an explanation for the sexual-spiritual basis of most ancient religions by showing that mystical experiences happen every day in the bedroom to a significant portion of the population. Sacred sex is still going on. In fact, it seems to be irrepressible. Most large studies of sex turn up spiritual experiences, and most large studies of spirituality turn up sex. But this linkage has been hidden from the public eye, just as near-death experiences happened but were not talked about until they were recently "discovered."

It seems likely that one in every eight to twelve people will have at least one transcendent experience during sex in a lifetime, but most people are reluctant to talk about them for the same reasons my partner and I were. Most of the people I interviewed said they had never told anyone else about what happened to them in the bedroom—not even their lovers—because they were afraid of being called crazy or of having a deeply meaningful spiritual experience mocked or made fun of by others. That was what kept a lot of people from talking about near-death experiences, too, before they became part of the public conversation.

The act of lovemaking can trigger intense episodes that feature the identical characteristics found in the highest spiritual states documented in such diverse religions as Buddhism, Christianity, Judaism, and Islam, as well as those cited in the annals of yoga and recent research on shamanism. The controversy surrounding the combination of sex and spirit has kept one of the most powerful forces for ecstasy and personal transformation in the closet for centuries.

What about Tantric Yoga and Taoism, spiritual traditions that have been adapted to Western culture as a way of working with sexual energy? Those paths have always acknowledged the sacredness and transformational power of sex, but they usually involve special techniques and training, and the modern versions often focus just on more and better orgasms or relating to your partner better.

In reality, you don't need to believe or practice anything special to have a mystical experience during sex. You certainly don't have to be a sex god or goddess. It can happen to anyone at any time, and the experiences aren't necessarily what you'd think. They don't have anything to do with your conscious beliefs about religion, sex, or anything else!

Regular folks, the kind we pass on the street every day—hairdressers, lawyers, sales clerks, shop owners, who had grown up in average American homes, most of them with some kind of fairly traditional Judeo-Christian beliefs—report being transported to other realms during lovemaking. Some were very conflicted about sex, and a lot of them didn't believe in God any more. And then, boom! One day they got ambushed in the bedroom by something they never expected. Baptists had Zen experiences of nirvana during sex. Catholics went on shamanic journeys to other worlds. Jews felt the presence of the Holy Ghost. Atheists were possessed by ancient fertility gods or sucked into past lives. You never know what's going to happen, but it can change your life and change your attitude about sex and spirituality for good.

Transcendent sex is distinguishable from ordinary sex because people's normal sense of reality changes: They no longer feel like themselves, or their lovers may no longer be recognizable; the "rules" of how the world works may be changed, or they are no longer in the here and now but in another time and place. Sometimes all of these categories break down. Transcendent episodes during sex resemble the altered states associated with high levels of attainment in various spiritual traditions, including:

Seeing visions
Feeling transported to other locations
Experiencing waves of heat, energy, and light
Participating directly in the animal and plant life
   of the earth or in other natural forces
Reliving past lives
Being visited by gods and other avatars
Being possessed by spirits
Embodying spiritual forces, such as speaking in
   tongues
Dissolving into the primordial Void, such as
   nirvana or Samadhi
Dissolving into God or the great I AM

A good example is Chester, a student who had taken a graduate class on my research into sex, gender, and spirituality, and who called me up one day demanding to talk. I was afraid he wanted to dispute his grade, because he hadn't seemed particularly receptive to the material in class, but he wanted me to talk with his girlfriend, Alice, who needed help. She'd had a frightening transcendent episode while they were making love, which he was able to recognize and facilitate, although he had never experienced such a thing himself.

Alice had begun trembling violently in his arms as her soul seemed to leave her body, accelerating faster and faster the farther away it went. She had never had an out-of-body experience, and she thought she was dying.

Chester, unaware of exactly what she was experiencing, remembered what he'd learned from the class and had the presence of mind to encourage her to relax within the safety of his arms and to trust herself to the experience rather than to fight it. He watched her trembling subside, then saw her go into a "superdreaming" state in which her eyes were moving extremely rapidly behind her closed lids. As he stroked her soothingly, Chester felt what he described as waves of energy radiating from her body, discernible even when his hand was suspended a few inches above her skin.

Once she had calmed down, Alice said that she had permitted herself to go back into the experience, as if she had been willing to "go through a doorway." This time, instead of rushing through space away from her body, she found herself surrounded by the presence of God. At once she could feel throughout her entire being how totally precious and beloved she is—and everyone is—and that all the things she regretted in her life made absolutely no difference in this flood of unconditional love and light. God was nothing like she expected. Instead of learning how she didn't measure up or being given an assignment for what she was to accomplish in life, she realized that she was perfectly loved just as she was, regardless of what she had done or would do.

When she came back to the ordinary world, Alice was euphoric—and violently ill for some hours. The terrible nausea did nothing to dampen her ecstasy. She and Chester had eaten exactly the same meal, so they knew there was no physical reason for her sickness, and that was part of why they were frightened and sought my counsel.

Alice and Chester wanted to know if anyone else had ever gotten sick after a transcendent episode during sex, but this was a first. However, Alice gave me some important clues when she was telling me her story. The expressions she used for feeling remorse and shame was that she always "swallowed her guilt" and "pushed the guilt down into her stomach." Recently that guilt had become overwhelming, since Alice felt she had failed in a God-given mission to work with orphaned refugees overseas and had had to come back to the United States.

Now with her new understanding, there was no reason to retain the guilt. Alice said she recovered completely in a few hours and was still ecstatic when I met her weeks later. Of course, I had no expertise she needed beyond the truth of her own experience, but I could tell her that her experience was not unique. Chester's knowing what to do had provided the ground for her transformative episode to occur, and it deepened their love and faith so that both of them were changed.

✕✕

Alice and Chester's story illustrates another point: Since otherworldly sexual experiences can come upon people unawares, lovers may be far more vulnerable than meditators or others who are deliberately cultivating altered states. People who are unprepared—especially whose worldviews don't include spiritual or supernatural events—can be frightened and even destabilized by such a "break" in their normal reality. Some underwent several years of psychotherapy or other professional intervention to come to terms with their experiences.

It's important to understand how powerful these sexual events can be. Their dark side can lead to an addictive need to be in a relationship, delusions concerning the partner and "rightness" of the relationship, and have a negative effect on the person's ability to function.

In a mild example, a young man I'll call Cameron came to

me. He was in almost suicidal despair, which had lasted for several months. He worked in a high-tech industry and had no religious beliefs at all. In fact, he didn't believe in the supernatural. As he was making love with his girlfriend of over a year, he was suddenly swept into an ecstasy he could only describe as spiritual. The experience was so powerful and profound, it completely changed his understanding of the world, and it also seemed to convey to him that his relationship with this woman was "meant to be." The net result was that Cameron felt he was "a thousand times more in love with her" than ever and that there must be a meaning and purpose to his life of which he previously had been unaware.

Unfortunately, Cameron's girlfriend, who had not had the

The fact is, the ordinary act of lovemaking can be the most widely available path to higher consciousness for most people.

experience and was not inclined to a spiritual point of view, couldn't come to terms with the change in him, and she broke off the relationship. He was devastated. He searched vainly for support from therapists and even joined several religious groups to see if anyone could help him understand what had happened—and help restore his relationship.

Eventually, Cameron did receive help and understanding, but he is still afraid that he'll never fall as deeply in love again as he did with the woman he now believes must be his "soulmate," even though she quickly became involved with a series of other partners. He is afraid he'll never be able to enjoy sex again or even desire to have it with another.

Cameron's case is hardly an isolated one, and it serves to point out the difficulties people can have coming to terms with these experiences and what they mean, just as people who have had other nonordinary "openings" involuntarily (such as near-death experiences or "alien abduction" experiences) are often seriously destabilized. There are steps people can take to prepare themselves for this eventuality and to avoid putting themselves in harm's way in potentially dangerous liaisons with powerful partners, such as exploitative gurus or sexual predators who may use their capacity to induce paranormal states to influence the unsuspecting.

♡

For the most part, though, people reported very positive impacts from these sexual episodes, like those of other spiritual openings. Two stories, one from a woman and the other from a man, show how powerfully ecstatic they can be and how they come about. The woman describes a state similar to the experience of the Void in Buddhism or Hinduism. Similar descriptions are found in much of the Zen literature. She says:

The sense of him and my connectedness with him fills my awareness as the physical pleasure of my body begins to shade from foreground into background. What we are doing physically maintains and sustains this state, but awareness of our bodies, of my orgasm is no longer a focus. It becomes the ground, almost subliminal, for a more transcendent state. Our merged selves, our we-ness drops away into nothingness. It is the purest bliss without content, without the flow of time, without even desire because in that moment everything both is and is not. Nothing is there, just a void that has a feeling of whiteness.

On some occasions, this whiteness or void has then disappeared like a flood receding from the landscape to reveal what was always there, say, the furniture in the bedroom, the light coming through the window, the shadows on the walls, my lover's transfigured face. But when this happens,

"I am pulsating with divine energies that build and build until I feel that I will be annihilated by a shattering explosion."

all relationships among these objects and me are changed. The objects seem no more whole or solid than the space around them, so everything seems part of a single web, a continuum in which everything is the same, either three-dimensional or not.

If I move or change, the world moves or changes with me. I am everything, and everything is me, and nothing has a greater or more special value than anything else, not my lover, not me, not anything. There is no me here, there is nothing separate and no time flowing by. I can't say how it is here except that it is being one with God, not even that. It's being God because there is nothing there and nothing you are not.

I never know how long I'm there, how long any of it takes to happen. What changes my awareness finally is either my lover's coming or his withdrawing from my body. It depends upon whether I'm still in the whiteness or in that state of what seems like nonduality with everything. In both, I am still at some level so attuned to him that I know instantly when he is coming, but in

the whiteness, somehow some of my sensory channels seem absent and my knowing is at an inchoate, conceptless body level that is cellular. It is somehow without the symbolism of seeing his face or hearing his voice or feeling a difference in his movement. In the nonduality place where I am everything, it is just part of everything with me, but since there is no "me" and no "everything" and no "coming," it is only somehow a different way of The Way It Is.

However it happens, his climax or withdrawal gradually brings me back to myself.... I'm usually aware of my overall body condition first, racing heart and high body heat, then the breathing. Everything about being so much back in my body and aware of it seems effortful. It's hard to open my eyes, hard to move especially, even if I find myself in an uncomfortable position.... Taking up normal life again, normal separateness is hard, but it's still shot through with love and glory, a radiant softness.

Just as this woman's story represents what is associated with the highest levels of attainment in Eastern traditions, this particular man's narrative contains elements associated with *unio mystica*, the dissolving into God associated with the highest levels of attainment in the Western traditions of mystical Judaism, Christianity, and Islam. He reports moving from a state of "continuous rapture," in which love is flowing effortlessly from himself into his lover, to one where he starts to transcend his awareness of his partner altogether:

My awareness of her, though, is intermittent at that point. Where I begin to lose her is after I remember her, after I remember the feeling because it takes over, and it's as though I'm moving through her to something beyond her, beyond me. That's the religious part. She's a conduit, but then in that state, bodies become irrelevant, and in a way she does, too, I'm embarrassed to say. I'm actually opening myself to God and surrendering to God and feeling God entering into me.

The energies are so strong. I can have this experience without coming to orgasm, but it represents, not just physically but in some spiritual way, a climactic point where I break apart, where I fall into the Light. It's everything. Everything is sacred, and I am pulsating with divine energies that build and build until I feel that I will be annihilated by a shattering explosion at the same time I—no longer any "I" there—will have completely merged into the fires of God like a planet plunging into the furnace of the Sun. It's every possible good feeling, and it lasts just a second, but there's no sense of time. There is Joy flooding everywhere, light everywhere, and then wave after wave of slowly subsiding rapture.

Orgasm is the moment of supreme pleasure and regret all in one because the moment you come, you know it's going to end. It's like suffering is built into any pleasure, and as soon as you have the consummation, you begin to feel the regret because you know this is the beginning of the end. You're going to have to leave God's bosom. It's a real wrenching, moving away, knowing you're coming back to the world, coming back to your body, coming back to look at her. I still feel like I'm part way in that state, but I know I'm coming back from it....

When I can open my eyes and look at my lover again, she is still holy to me, and I know we have experienced this divinity and ours—together. I become more focused on her again and lose the focus on me, the way it was before.... But now I know we are two again and back to living in our separate bodies, which for a time had been discarded like pieces of scaffolding that had served their purpose and then been completely transcended. In that moment, there is an unbearable ache that arises in the heart.

In addition to suffusing love relationships (where they exist—many people had these transcendent experiences during one-night stands, casual affairs, or even with people they didn't like) with a sense of deeper connection, transcendent sexual episodes had other profound effects on people. Former atheists and agnostics became spiritual seekers; people developed more loving relationships, not only with their partners, but with others; still others determined to change dysfunctional life patterns and let go of self-limiting beliefs. Remarkably, a number of participants who had suffered childhood sexual abuse became able to remain present and enjoy sex, even becoming orgasmic. Their own words are convincing of how powerful such experiences are and how transformative they can be.

For instance, "Richard" says:

Having been a Catholic seminarian, sex was very taboo, and I'd grown up in a home with parents who were forbidding and repressed. These

experiences have really helped me rehabilitate sex from this cesspool of moral judgment. I realized for the first time that sex really could be a vehicle for transcendence. That seemed to be the whole point of my experience. It's really deepened [my relationship]. The problems don't matter, because all that matters is our closeness. It has that feeling of a Spirit-guided state, where the point of power is in the present. It's a physical manifestation of my spiritual practice, and I see it as one of the highest forms.

A woman, speaking for many, mentions how much easier it is for her to act with compassion: "It transformed my life, my outlook. I have these feelings for my partner now, seeing the hairs in his ears or something that would maybe be ugly or whatever, and I just feel so good for him. It's wonderful. And it translates to other people. It does translate."

Elaine, a woman who lives in a spiritual community and has been a practicing Buddhist for decades, says of her sexual spiritual openings:

I suppose when I describe it, it will sound like a form of psychosis.... Of course, you know this is not a psychotic experience by its results. Once time is no longer still...and normal life resumes, you are changed, but in a good way. Your other relationships are enhanced by the experience also because you have changed. Somehow a string of that love experience is woven throughout your other relationships, career, etc. [You gain] tolerance for others who are not so knowing...and a great compassion for them, as well as others.... The impact of such an experience is immense.

But the variety of experiences people can have is vast, and their background, psychological maturity, and beliefs, as well as the circumstances under which transcendent sex occurs, are infinite. Anything can happen—and whatever happens can have unpredictable results, depending upon the participants.

One woman probably summed up the myriad possibilities best by saying:

A low form of sex makes for a low form of spirituality, and a low form of spirituality may make for a low form of sex. The quality of the sexual experience relates to the capacity of the individual to hold it in a spiritual place. Spiritual sexuality is a very precious thing.... That doesn't mean that it's going to make life easy; it will make it rich.

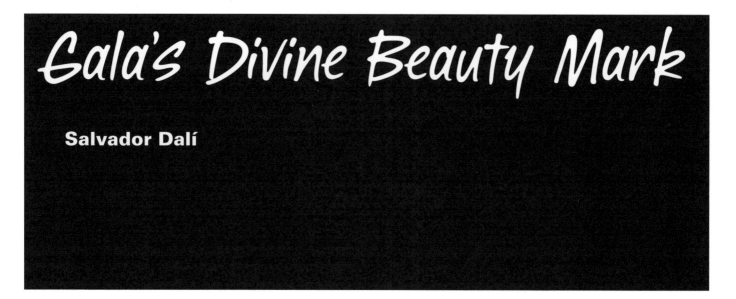

Gala's Divine Beauty Mark

Salvador Dalí

Editor's Note: When Surrealist painter Salvador Dalí met Russian intellectual Gala in 1929, she had already served as a muse for several members of the movement, including her then-husband, poet Paul Eluard. She eventually became Dalí's muse, wife, agent, and reason for living. "She calms me. She reveals me. She makes me," he wrote. In this worshipful excerpt from his 1973 autobiography, Comme on Devient Dalí *(published in English as* Maniac Eyeball*), the master writes about their early two-month sexathon and the part of Gala's body that gave him the most pleasure.*

Had Dalí Already Made Love To Another Woman?

Dalí cannot come with any other woman. It is impossible. You cannot be unfaithful to your shadow, and to lose it is to lose your soul. That is quite enough for me, and I do not think either of having children. Those embryos disgust me. Their fetal aspect bothers me wildly. Nor could I ever, like any genius, give birth to anything but an idiot.

I kneaded them in my hands, smelled them with delight, trying to recapture a bit of her presence and her life.

I also do not want to face up to the reality of Gala's death. My mind would need to call on all of its resources to survive that. But with the training she has put me through I am certain I could maintain my intelligence at the level of my love of life. Though henceforth I could overcome the most abysmal of misfortunes, she would remain irreplaceable. I have moreover so often thought of her death, from the very first day of our love, that I am as if prepared for that tragedy. Gala today, as on that first day, goes on saying that her death would be the finest day of her life. Perhaps I would say, despite my immense sorrow, as I did the day after our first coming-together, in Figueras when I saw her to the train as she was departing for Paris, despite my love and my sorrow at seeing her leave, "Alone at last." For nothing is greater than to discover one's true dimensions and put up with one's solitude. Gala taught that to me, so it would be one more way of paying deep tribute to her by going on living as she had wanted.

At that time, I was hardly inured despite my pride, and like one obsessed I had to look for my strength and courage among the things she had imprinted with her mark, her odors, her memory: an old pair of rope sandals, a swimsuit, a pebble. I kneaded them in my hands, smelled them with delight, trying to recapture a bit of her presence and her life, and warming my heart with the magnetism they still radiated.

I had my work. I locked myself in my Figueras studio for a month. I finished *The Great Masturbator* and *Portrait of Paul Eluard*. I felt it incumbent on me to fix forever the face of the poet from whose Olympus I had stolen one of the muses.

I left for Paris at the end of the summer, to arrange for my first show, which was to open in November at the Galerie Goëmans. That period remains for me a series of strong images that embody the voluptuousness of deliberate defeat.

I am in a florist's shop and do not have enough money to pay for the hundred roses I have just ordered for Gala.

I wait until the very last moment before going to see Gala, whom I am dying to see again.

On our honeymoon at Sitges and Barcelona, I let Gala go back to Paris alone, so as to go and see my father, who tells me it is unthinkable that I should marry a Russian woman. Despite my denials, he believes Gala is a drug addict and has turned me into a narcotics dealer, which alone in his eyes would explain the unlikely sums of money I have been making.

He was to write me that he disowned me. Out of pain, I decided to shave my head completely and, before leaving Cadaqués, went and buried my hair on the beach with a batch of sea-urchin shells fragrant of cunt.

I am on the highest hill overlooking Cadaqués and stare at my village for a last farewell. With my bald scalp, I leave for Paris, a picture of the anguish, pain, and sorrow that indicate the passage to maturity and the landmarks of the Galactite ordeals.

In Paris, all the paintings in the show have been sold and my success is enormous. Gala has just finished transcribing my notes that I plan to publish as *La Femme Visible* (*The Visible Woman*). Buñuel wants us to start work without delay on the scenario for *L'Age d'Or*, a new film that has just been commissioned from him by the Vicomte de Noailles, who put up a million francs, a fantastic budget for those days. A leaf of my life is being turned; I am emerging from the shadow to the light.

To live with Gala became an obsession to me. To digest her, possess her, assimilate her, melt into her. With my shaven skull and fiery eye I looked exactly like a Grand Inquisitor, but one consumed with love. Gala understood that we had to flee the world so as to temper ourselves as a couple in the crucible of life alone together.

A small hotel on the Riviera, at Carry-le-Rouet, took us in. We rented two rooms. In one, my easel, my canvas of *L'Homme Invisible* (*The Invisible Man*), inspired by the research of Archimboldo, on whom I had meditated for so long, my books, and my brushes; in the other, the bed. They brought our meals up to us. We opened the door a crack only to let in the valet or chambermaid.

I was methodically exploring Gala with the detailed care of a physicist or archaeologist exalted to high pitch by delirious love. I fixed in my memory the value of every grain of her skin so as to apprehend the shadings of their consistency and color; so as to find the right attentive caress for each. I could have drawn up a map of her body with a perfect geography of the zones of beauty and fineness of her fleshly coil and the pleasures to be derived and evoked. I spent hours looking at her breasts, their curve, the design of the nipples, the shadings of pink to their tips, the detail of the bluish veinlets running beneath their gossamer transparency; her back ravished me with the delicacy of the joints, the strength of the rump muscles, beauty and the beast conjoined. Her neck had pure grace in its slimness; her hair, her intimate hairs, her odors intoxicated me; her mouth, teeth, gums, tongue overpowered me with a pleasure I had never even suspected. I became a sex freak. I wallowed in it to the very paroxysm of cockcunt, voraciously gobbling, frenzied in the unleashing of my finally sated instincts.

Even today, from those passionate hours of our isolation in sex, my memory retains the images of our orgiastic comings-together—animal but perfect and beautiful in their wildness. We were like two monks of sex, at every hour of the day celebrating the adoration of their god. [...]

How Dalí's Love For Gala Expressed Itself

During these two months devoted to *l'amour* and the adoration of Gala, I had gone down to the very sources of the pleasure of living in the abyssal depths of being. It was a kind of journey to the center of being I had made, going back to my intra-uterine memories, to the very nourishment of the birth-

> **I could have drawn up a map of her body with a perfect geography of the zones of beauty and fineness of her fleshly coil and the pleasures to be derived and evoked.**

ing placenta, and in my wild mind seeing Gala's cunt and my mother's belly as one. A philter sweeter than honey flowed within me. Gala's senses, Gala's belly, Gala's back exalted my dreams, their shapes mixed together, merged, compounded as the lines and rhythms of the waves of joy that rocked me and carried me over an ocean of felicity. My paranoia knew no bounds. My delirium rose to perfection, and Gala's super-intelligent complicity allowed me to attain the omega point of my inventions. All I had to do was touch the beauty mark on Gala's left earlobe to be carried away on the flying carpet of my wild love.

This wonderful spot seemed to me to be the proton of my beloved's divine energy, the sun of her heart, the geometrical locus of our passion for each other, the very point at which any contradiction between our two beings ceased to be. All I had to do was rub it with my finger to be flooded with strength and faith in my own destiny. This divine beauty mark to me was the proof of the definitive death of my brother Salvador, his mystical tomb; stroking it, I was rubbing against his gravestone. I thus took blanket possession of my existence in one stroke and had the intoxicating feeling of erasing the memory of this dead brother at the same time that I possessed the whole of the woman I loved, capturing all the

This wonderful spot seemed to me to be the proton of my beloved's divine energy, the sun of her heart, the geometrical locus of our passion for each other.

beauty of the world and even living and making love to my own life. Even my father was not immune to being symbolically gobbled when I took Gala's earlobe between my lips and let it slowly give me suck.

Later, Picasso capped my great happiness by showing me he had the same beauty mark as Gala in exactly the same place. That day, he even made her a present of a Cubist painting—showing that even that awesome personage's possessive genius could not resist Gala's radiation. It is true that Gala selected the smallest among the paintings he let her choose from. A fulcrum is all you need to raise the globe, and with Gala's beauty mark I can reconstruct the geometry of Dalínian intelligence. Her sacred ear sucked away all the dizzinesses of my soul to allow me to be reborn lucid, complete within unity, the master of the genius of my twin's personality, capable of overcoming my father's curse, the virile son of my mother. My entire unconscious found stability around that axis, like a planet around its sun, a believer taking his Host. Magical beauty mark, alpha and omega of Dalí!

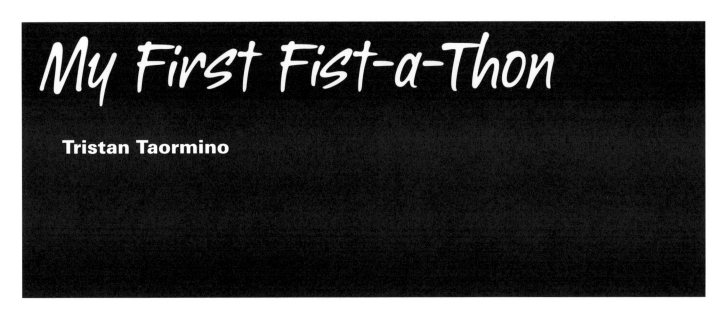

My First Fist-a-Thon

Tristan Taormino

In 2002, I went to my first kinky summer camp and had a ball. Two years later, the organizers invited me back to the seventh annual event, now relocated to a more adult-friendly retreat on 200 acres of secluded land. In addition to teaching classes, I was asked to host a special event. Their suggestion: Tristan's Fist-a-Thon. Since fisting, and in particular, deflowering anal-fisting virgins, is one of my passions, I wasn't hard to convince. The premise was that we'd see how many people I could fist both vaginally and anally, plus how many could be fisted by others, in the span of two hours. We weren't raising money like a typical 'thon, more like raising consciousness in a did-you-know-I-could-expand-you-and-your-orifice-like-this? kind of way.

In an old barn converted into a dungeon, we set up a row of massage tables and spanking benches draped in disposable, absorbent bed-sheets. Next to each one sat a folding chair with paper towels, gloves, lube, and baby wipes. There were thick black mats on the floor for the overflow of fistees. On the stage, I laid out an assortment of toys, including a purple-and-white-swirled buttplug that looked like a candy cruller, a red rubber, teardrop-shaped plug, and a black vinyl plug I nicknamed "Superstar" for its ability to help me get people's asses to go where they'd never gone before.

I welcomed everyone and reviewed the ground rules:

Fistees, please warm up *before* I get to you. Play with your ass or have someone else do it, so by the time I get to you, you're already on your way. Feel free to use any of the toys, but cover them with condoms. I can only fist one person at a time, so please be patient. General orgy rules apply: Don't touch anyone without permission! Once I have gotten my entire hand inside you, the fisting will be added to the list by the official tally master; then, unfortunately, I must move on. But I encourage you to keep going with a partner, ask a friend to take over for me, or finish yourself off.

First up was one of my camp cabinmates, a gorgeous, curvy blonde woman who'd never been vaginally fisted before. Her fiancé licked her pussy during my announcements, and when I made my way over, he moved to kiss her and play with her nipples. I snapped on a purple nitrile glove, and she moaned as I worked my way inside her pussy. She was wet and open.

The premise was that we'd see how many people I could fist both vaginally and anally, plus how many could be fisted by others, in the span of two hours.

I played with her for a while, eventually getting all five fingers in, but when it came to that point where my hand's diameter is thickest, it felt like too much for her. She was disappointed when she decided to stop, but her man stroked her face, and I knew she'd be okay.

I moved over to a fiftysomething guy I recognized from the audience at one of my classes earlier that day. He had one of my favorite toys in his ass—a clear acrylic plug with a convex base that acts as a magnifying glass; I often use it in demonstrations during workshops to give people a chance to see all the way inside someone's butt. We worked together for a while, and when I slipped in him all the way, I heard faint clapping in the background. Two down, a roomful to go.

I moved onto the stage, where another guy had been warming himself up with a colorful, corkscrew-shaped dildo. As I slipped four fingers inside his ass, with my peripheral vision I saw a woman in a corset with her hand in another woman's ass. A few minutes later, I followed suit and buried my right paw in this man's butt. I realized I had forgotten his name. I heard moans all over the room and saw the tally master busily making notes on his clipboard.

One woman named D. was sprawled on a mat, surrounded by four or five people and howling in ecstasy. They beckoned me over, announcing that she had already been vaginally fisted several times by different people.

"Does it count more than once if it's by someone else?" a fister cheerily inquired.

"Yes, absolutely!" I exclaimed, and the tally master nodded. Then I got down on my knees between her legs, and it took me all of one minute to slide inside her up to my wrist.

"She's already warmed up for you," one of her gang of pals said.

"You've got small hands," the woman whose pussy surrounded my fist said. "Can you fit them both in there?" The answer was yes.

I moved on to a guy from the Midwest who'd introduced himself the first day of camp; his wife said she was shy and didn't want to be in the midst of the action, but I encouraged her to watch so she could practice doing it when they got home. We managed an impressive five fingers but just couldn't get past that widest part of the hand. We decided to call it a suc-

cess at *almost*, and I took a deep breath.

My next fistee was a sweet guy I'd done a demonstration on earlier in the day, when I slipped a Lucite plug in his ass and told him to return it to me whenever he wanted. His partner was a redhead whom I'd seen naked in the striptease contest the night before. I came over, excited to see the progress they'd made. She had gotten in for a second, but it was un-

Then I got down on my knees between her legs, and it took me all of one minute to slide inside her up to my wrist.

comfortable, she said. I concentrated, and we all took some deep breaths in unison. I was suddenly channeling all the energy of everyone before him; the intensity deepened, and he opened up around my hand. I felt like I stayed inside him for hours, although I know it was only a few minutes before I came out. I was high. I was exhausted. It was five minutes to 11:00.

My total came in at eight fistings of six people: three anal, one vaginal, one double-vaginal (which we decided counts twice), and two people who took five fingers up to the knuckles, which deserves recognition. The grand total was twenty-two fistings of seven different people: D. was fisted fifteen times (including two double-fistings) by eleven different people, and one man was fisted twice by two different people. D. deserves the Miss Congeniality Award, and others should be singled out for their willingness, bravery, and enthusiasm. Next time, there will be sashes and trophies for sure!

Blood

Jennifer Bennett

I have never let anyone else enter my body like this. Blood has been a pleasure, a torture that I have reserved for myself. But now I hand you the blade, tell you that there is one last task I have for you tonight. You have been wonderfully submissive, and a certain power and mystery (I am loathe to call it magic) charges the air. I want to give of myself with the trusting, need-filled hunger that you show, but I can't. I don't understand submission in the same way, and fear I can't ever bridge that gap. Submitting to a man doesn't feel like a choice I can make for myself but the fulfillment of an external expectation. But understand this: I appreciate your gift of yourself to me. I feel that you do belong to me, preposterous as that notion is; right now it is the truth.

I hand you the blade and tell you to cut me. I point to the spot on my left forearm where I want the mark.

I've been waiting for the right time to open my flesh to you. Wanting my own mark to match the small cross I gave you a month or so ago, now a small, light scar. I've been planning on recutting it to thicken the white keloid lines. It was only the second or third time I'd cut you and the first time that I really let myself give in to my excitement. My sudden sense of arousal surprised me and, I think, frightened you.

I'd slowly cleaned the blade with precut alcohol swabs, savoring the sharp, stinging smell as it swelled and then evaporated. I used maybe ten packets between the blade and your flesh, more than enough to prep your arm physically. Enjoying the psychological preparation and ritual sense of cleaning you, the heightened impact on all your senses that the alcohol effected. Smooth and cool on your arm, the smell hit your nose, and you closed your eyes, then opened them again. You wondered if I was ready and raised your head, no fear in your eyes as they met mine. You held out your arm, aware that it was a sacrifice, a holy act and not just kinky sex that I wanted.

I picked up the clean blade, suddenly shaking with excitement. I cut you, not too deeply. Tension flowed from my body through the blade with the force to part flesh. Your skin opened, blood welled up at the apex of the cross. I bent to lick it delicately but couldn't bring my mouth away. I sucked wistfully, body writhing around the slit in your arm. Sucking and swallowing. My tongue moved into the wound, you pulled away slightly at the pain. I looked up at your face, aware that my eyes must look slightly mad, pupils dilated and burning into yours with my plea for more blood. You worked your arm, massaged the skin, made a fist to bring it to the surface for me. It was so dark against your pale arm. I wanted to cry, drip salty, stinging drops on the wound and lick up the small river that would course toward the fold in your elbow. I was done sucking. I opened more foil packets, quickly cleaned the

I hand you the blade and tell you to cut me.

blade and wiped up the wet streaks from your arm.

But tonight I hand the blade over and ask you to cut me. I'd told you before that this is off-limits behavior, and you are confused, unsure if I really want this or if I'm responding to the energy in the air or some darker force within myself of which you're still unaware. Probably both of these are true, but I know that my feelings won't shift back now that the boundary has broken open.

"Tell me how," you whisper. "You're the expert."

I am. In the decade of my life in which I was most unhappy, I cut myself with changing degrees of frequency, intensity, and depth. From fifteen to twenty-five, I could always depend on the blade of a knife to calm me.

I still have scars on the backs of my hands and wrists that I scratched into myself during eleventh-grade biology class. I, too squeamish to pin a worm to the tray and slit lengthwise, had no compunction about using that same pin or blade to slice into myself. I still have vague, wide scars on my breasts, cut vertically down toward the nipple. And the thin line across my cheek that I cut with a piece of glass I'd hidden in my pocket one January between semesters. This was in college when my girlfriend and I were fighting all the time, and the

My scars aren't just mute white lines; they're a roadmap.

only way I could think to make it stop was to slap her across the face, slicing my cheek open in the next moment. The two actions parallel in my mind: the smooth, clean arc of my palm slicing through the air to connect with her heated, red-spotted cheek and the twin motion of my hand moving from pocket to ear, dragging the glass forward and bringing the blood and heat to the surface. It stopped the fight and began the unraveling of our life together.

I would repeat this act one more time with another woman, pushing her out of my way and into the hallway wall on my way into the bathroom, where I locked the door and opened a razor, freeing the blade. Severing her responsibility for the relationship going bad. Giving her the reasons to begin to retreat.

I've only brought others into my cutting against their will, irrevocably showing them my anger and violence. But you, you invite yourself into the anger and violence, S/M the midwife that sees you through the pain and lets you share in the passion. You like my scars; I think they're proof to you that I'm a serious person. You trust that, like you, I know what it means to be unhappy.

My lack of interest in drugs and alcohol could have worked against me, making me seem too straightlaced and boring for you. But eight years of being queer and over a decade of self-loathing under my belt seem to guarantee that there is a genuine fuck-up under the flesh. You get to peel that open. My scars speak more to you about the person that I was than my pictures and portfolio or my scrapbooks and stories ever could. Because you know that whatever was going on around me, I still kept my secrets intact, kept the depraved, sick girl alive with every slice. This you like; this you can relate to.

But there is so much that you don't know. I can never just tell the story of my past, never make the words translate the experience. My scars aren't just mute white lines; they're a roadmap. Only the story has a different ending now: not suicidal expectations but the possibility of traveling with someone else. Experiencing such exuberance in cutting you is new to me. Though I'd cut one person before, I never experienced the vicarious high, all the beauty and satisfaction of cutting with none of the bad aftereffects—disconnectedness and limp, hopeless depression. It's safe to cut you. I hope it's safe to let you cut me. I know it's still not safe for me to cut myself.

I hand you the blade and a fistful of alcohol packets. I breathe the odor in slowly as it seeps out and fills the room, preparing for you.

"Any words of wisdom?" you ask. Of course, I smile. I am the expert. I instruct you: Cut hard. It will be much harder to cut deeply than you think it will. It's no scalpel, for godsakes, but a utility blade. That means it's serrated, and you will have to drag it hard down my arm. Trust me; it will hurt much more to recut over a small scratch. Do it once, using firm pressure. Remember, you can't cut too deeply, not here on my arm, not with this blade. Don't be afraid. I look into you, see that you are nervous and shaky.

"You know why I want you to do this, don't you?" I ask. Not sure if the motion of your head is a response of yes or if you are just trembling. I want to belong to you, too.

❦

I don't think that anyone else has cut me before, though one would think that I'd remember that, even fifteen years later. I've forgotten more traumatic incidents, though, and suffered through recovering them, so I know how powerfully the brain and body can work together to reweave the past, leaving small creases in which the truth lies.

My first high-school boyfriend introduced me to S/M all those years ago, and I'd forgotten that until this year when you and I started playing. Back in high school I didn't have the vocabulary of S/M. Without an intellectual context, the experiences he led me to couldn't take hold inside me or gain meaning. They just sat, abstracted and forgotten until I needed access to them.

He may have cut me. I know he cut himself. And I cut him at least once, making thin ribbons of blood pop up on his chest with the blade I held between my teeth. I did this at his instruction with no thought or feeling about it. I was his sexual *tabula rasa*, always saying yes. He must have culled these images from somewhere, tried to dress me up and bring them to life. The scenes seemed overwrought, too self-consciously devised to be genuinely sexy. I don't know if they were real fantasies for him or merely extreme scenes copied from pornography onto my flesh.

He used to scratch me hard and tease me, his long, black-painted pinky nail digging into me. I bled for him in other ways, though. I bled every time we had sex for one year, always so embarrassed and ashamed, taking my blood as a sign that I still wasn't used to it, that I was too tight, that it hurt, that I didn't enjoy it. Letting him fuck me was the only way I did begin to bleed on a regular basis, my post-coital spotting a thin substitute for menstruation.

You, too, seem to possess this magic of making me bleed. I have quasi-regular periods now, though at times it is hard to attribute the cause of the bleeding. I've never felt embarrassed or ashamed or inadequate with you, though. You take my blood as a testament to how much I like it, how open I am, how deeply you touch me, affect my body.

You roll your eyes at the squeamish and vulgar attitude of most men upon encountering blood in a woman's vagina, always remaining calm when I expected you to freak out. Even when the sheets were so soaked that they had to go into the wash immediately, along with the mattress pad, while I scrubbed the mattress, legs streaked with drying blood. Your cheeks still sticky with my blood, a random smear of it on your forehead distilled by sweat, and a darkening crust in the corners of your mouth. Or when we left a fine blood-spray pattern on the sheets from the force of our fucking, a mist showering down each time your body impacted against my upturned ass. Your own hand stained from opening me up, small jelly-like clots stubbornly sticking further up your arm.

Or when I've masturbated with your cock still inside me, lubricated with my own blood, coating my hand and cunt. Later finding random, bloody fingerprints on the sheet or wall, scrubbing my nails and still picking crusted crescents of blood out of my cuticles later at dinner. Sucking the blood off of your cock has almost sent me into sensory overload, the creamy, coppery taste mingling with the smoky, fecund taste of you. Or when your mouth has been latched tight to me while standing over you, hot ochre drops of blood dripping onto your chest and running down to stain your cock and hand.

But tonight we've showered after fucking, washing away blood and cum and lube, and I'm clean and pure and offering myself to you. Take blood from me and make me yours. I breathe deeply, open my eyes, and look at you with no fear.

⤫⤫

You make the first cut down my arm. It's deep, it hurts, and I feel it like a regular person. I worry for a second that you'll go too deep, but you don't, of course. There's a half-inch opening in my arm. You reposition the blade and push in; I feel the pop as the point breaks into my flesh, and the slow, dragging scrape as you cut crosswise. It catches slightly as it crosses the center of the other cut, and you compensate by pushing in deeper, startling both of us. The half-inch cut is now a deep, slightly uneven cross from which blood is starting to drip. I'm transfixed by the path it is wending down my arm. You're crying a bit; a few tears drip off your cheek.

You bend in to suck, not ravenous as I am, but licking lightly, the way you first do when you encounter my clit. Then slowly and methodically, careful to catch each rivulet with the wet upsweep of your tongue. It's exhausting and breathtaking. You can't believe that you've done it. You're amazed, shaky, a little disgusted, but also somewhat proud, savoring the moment in a kind of triumph over your fear.

"It's wrong," you say. "But you like it," you whisper, curling my hair between your fingers that knot into a fist. I nod yes, supremely calm and centered. I feel I'm at the center of creation, sitting still while everything else spins around me. You clean my arm and the blade, insist on putting the Band-Aid on, playing nursemaid all the way. It feels so normal, yet I'm slowly remembering that others would be horrified by this. Even you say, "It's wrong." You're crying and shaking, so I pull your head close to my chest, a mother's gesture bringing you into the center of my calmness. I feel as if someone should be filming us, like we're specimens about to be analyzed. I shake my head to clear the negative thoughts, concentrate on the alchemy we've performed.

Sucking the blood off of your cock has almost sent me into sensory overload, the creamy, coppery taste mingling with the smoky, fecund taste of you.

Is this what they mean by "blood sports"? Blood sports are always defined as edge play, even among experienced players. It's not just the risk that the fluid brings with it, the possibilities of HIV and hepatitis. Blood play is generally not allowed in public play spaces, even when universal precautions are used and biohazard bags are available. It's an automatic stop in action.

I bled at the first big play party I attended. I was face-down on a wooden table, full-length black silk skirt pulled up over my ass, which was getting worked over with a variety of paddles and brushes. A small dot of blood appeared on my ass; everything stopped abruptly while the dungeon monitor was called over. He inspected it and slapped a Band-Aid on, giving us the okay to continue. Later in the evening I went to the bathroom and discovered I was bleeding, my vagina making a way for the blood to leave my body. I vaguely remembered reading that tampons were a necessary item to bring to play parties. I was without, so I stuffed my underwear in my purse, my ass still too hot to tolerate them, and left early.

We've shared the most intimate of fluids.

I wonder how we would manage if we weren't fluid-bonded. The barrier of a condom or glove wouldn't be effective. Blood seeps into our sex incidentally; we can hardly ignore it. To bring it about purposefully seems safer. Cutting without tasting seems wasteful, decadent, like smashing champagne bottles against a boat.

Bloodletting doesn't feel that risky. It feels extreme to me only when I view it from outside. I joke that in the pervert world we're married now. But we are in some way. We've shared the most intimate of fluids, bonded in a way that none of our other current lovers can access while we're still together. We've taken the step into fluid-bonded polyamory that precludes plastic or emotional barriers. Married by similar mars in our flesh, like-marked left arms with small, pink, cross-shaped cuts that will heal smooth and white, tiny beacons of the body inviting you to come here, look closer, see what's inside. Taste of my body. Taste of my blood.

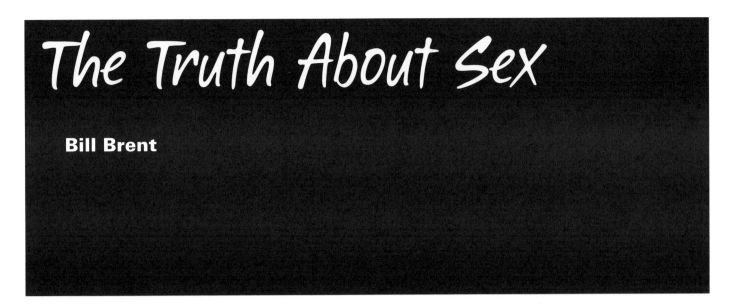

The Truth About Sex

Bill Brent

The TRUTH?
You want THE TRUTH?

Fuck you. But here's one version, anyway:

My parents were the first people to radicalize me about sex. They would not like to read this (one reason I changed my last name at age 25 is because I was starting to sound off in public, and I knew it would embarrass them less), but I used to sneak into their room when I was twelve, thirteen, and read all their stashed porn. Some of it was kinky; some of it was educational (*The Joy of Sex* was the sex-ed book that classrooms *should* have had); and some was ragingly sexist and grotesquely homophobic.

The first man I ever felt an erotic crush on was my father. He always walked around in nothing but those revealing, white BVD briefs; he always smelled like a man. How could I not? No one else was within close range. The junior-high locker room was too harsh and threatening, so I took advantage of an alarmist quack's diagnosis of my heart's condition to escape the horrors of P.E. at the first possible leap.

My parents kept a large, smelly, greasy dildo under their bed. I liked that. Their sheets always smelled of sex, rank sex. I liked that, too.

I have always liked that which offends nice people, because it is usually honest.

My parents were not nice people, which is why I loved them so much. They were petty, bitchy, loud, secretive, drunk, dramatic, stingy, generous, friendly, aloof, stoned, obvious, inscrutable, insufferable, and absent all at once.

To this day, I still like myself better when I look ugly than when I look nice.

The nice-looking kids at school snatched my lunch bag from under my desk and tossed it around the classroom while the school's least competent, most out-of-touch teacher was writing equations on the blackboard. Then they stopped their little circus and acted nice when he turned back to us, and later resumed their game until my lunch lay in trashed, tattered pieces across the floor, and I ran screaming from the room—*they're* the ones I still want to disembowel and carve up into ragged, little finger-sandwich pieces. Yeah. Let's see how nice they'd look as *empanadas de cojones*.

Oh, and I like my balls more when I scratch them and my fingertips come up smelling like vinegar. It's more human.

Even though my parents hid their porno stash and their sex toys, I never felt guilty enough about checking them out to stop, because I figured that if they really meant to keep us kids out, they would have locked their bedroom door, right? (They only did that when they smoked pot, which all of us

I have always liked that which offends nice people, because it is usually honest.

could smell anyway.) But that glimpse into the patchy world of fucked-up adults warped me with the notion that sex was best when it was edgy and predatory and fraught with the peril of getting caught.

Kind of like art.

My parents never abused me, though, unlike the cretins I went to school with, who seemed to have an eerie sixth sense about my impending queerness. I wish they'd let me in on their secret. Or maybe they were just vicious that way to anyone who was "too" fat, "too" brainy, "too" shy, "too" uncoordinated, or just too easy to frighten. "Faggot" was the cruelest thing you could call any kid with an obvious social deformity. I still wonder how much of my emergent sexuality was informed by those vultures. A story that repeats, over and over, throughout the not-so-monitored halls of American schooldom. Welcome to the food chain, kid.

That glimpse into the patchy world of fucked-up adults warped me with the notion that sex was best when it was edgy and predatory and fraught with the peril of getting caught.

So, yeah, I like grim. I like bitter. I like coffee that hurts when you drink it. And I like staying pissed off. It helps the words keep flowing like blood from the wound.

I was raped—if not rectally, then verbally, psychically, socially, emotionally—and I've watched everyone deny the blame for that. I've been the repository for so much misdirected vitriol that I've practically achieved sainthood. It's ironic that I internalized that hatred so long I became one of the most sold-out acts of sluttery ever to emerge from the hallowed halls of suburbia—the hollowed walls of disturbia—the shallow malls of slummerbia—only to bottom out on crystal meth and finally renounce it all: the promiscuous sex, the race of drugs, the bland intrigues of the quest for love. It's my way of stealing back time. More hours to think and write. I sleep better, I feel happier, and I have no complications to my life. I've finally become the kid I always wanted to be.

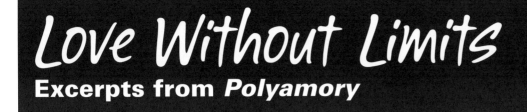

Love Without Limits
Excerpts from *Polyamory*

Deborah Taj Anapol

What Is Polyamory?

"Most of you are jealous and possessive in your love. When your love turns to possessiveness it makes demands. The demands then alienate the loved one and you incorporate anger and fear into the relationship. With these come bitterness and aggression, and whether we speak of individual love relationships or global interactions, what you call love, but is in fact ownership and manipulation, takes over and the problems then flow."

—Wayne Dyer, *Gifts from Eykis*

Our culture puts so much emphasis on monogamy that few people realize they have a choice about how many sexualoving partners they can have at one time. Even harder to grasp is the idea that multi-partner relationships can be stable, responsible, consensual, nurturing, and long-term. Polyamory is not a synonym for promiscuity!

I myself didn't realize that polyamory was really a possibility until I'd failed several times at the usual possessive and dependent arrangement that commonly passes for love. As time went on, I began to realize that, for me, monogamous marriage was profoundly isolating and intolerably lonely, partly because of the strict limits on whom I could love. My husband at the time was only willing to love and accept me if he could be sure that I loved and desired no one else.

In truth, however, I still cared deeply for all my past lovers and sometimes encountered others to whom I felt strongly attracted. Sure, I could suppress these feelings, but the bottom line was that in order to maintain my monogamous commitment I had to pretend to be someone other than who I really was. If I acknowledged being attracted to other men, my husband quickly let me know that I was out of line. Worse yet, as a trained observer of human behavior, he could easily detect any signs of attraction unless I was careful to cover them up. Our relationship didn't feel very intimate because it wasn't!

Another pattern I began to notice was that, after about four years of exclusive commitment to one partner, I would grow increasingly restless and dissatisfied. At first I thought the solution was to find a new and better partner. After several of these four-year cycles, I realized I was just repeating the first stages of relationship over and over. Most of the long-term marriages I'd observed in my parents' generation seemed to go on automatic pilot after a few years, an alternative that didn't appeal at all. Nevertheless, I suspected that genuine intimacy could continue to unfold over many decades. In order to find out what was possible *later on* in a partnership, I realized I would have to find a way to *sustain* intimate relationships over time.

I knew that my real self wanted to give and receive unconditional love. I'd experienced this kind of total acceptance only

As time went on, I began to realize that, for me, monogamous marriage was profoundly isolating and intolerably lonely, partly because of the strict limits on whom I could love.

outside the arena of marriage, in a few special friendships and in the contexts of psychotherapy and spiritual teaching. Next to this kind of genuine intimacy, most romantic liaisons seemed like protection rackets. I knew I was capable of loving more than one person at a time, so I assumed others must be, too. But, strangely enough, it never occurred to me that polyamory could coincide with marriage. So I decided that I was through with marriage and set off on a quest for sustainable intimacy.

It's been quite an amazing journey! It took me many years and one more marriage and divorce to realize that the secret to keeping any intimate connection alive is simply to be wholly authentic in every moment and to practice radical honesty. I've learned that relationships based on truth, self responsibility, and unconditional love can take many forms, but even small withholds will gradually erode any relationship. I've learned that it is indeed possible to love more than one person over many years. I call this lovestyle *responsible nonmonogamy* or *polyamory*.

The Facts

Most of us are not monogamous in the strict sense of the word. That is, we do not limit ourselves to one sexual partner for an entire lifetime. Census data reveal a global tendency for couples to divorce after four years of marriage.[1] And while many aspire to serial monogamy, or one partner at a time, national surveys repeatedly reveal that most Americans do not observe this rule very scrupulously, either. Statistics for

I use *polyamory* to describe the whole range of lovestyles which arise from an understanding that love cannot be forced to flow, or not flow, in any particular direction.

married men and women reporting extramarital affairs range from 37% to 70% for men and from 29% to 50% for women. And these proportions, particularly for women, increase as time goes on since more and more married women are working outside the home and consequently have more opportunities to encounter potential lovers. For single, unattached men and women, the incidence of multiple, simultaneous relationships is undoubtedly even higher.

Unfortunately, the vast majority of multi-partner relationships are neither ethical nor responsible. Lies, deceit, guilt, unilateral decisions, and broken commitments are so commonplace in classic American-style nonmonogamy that responsible nonmonogamy may sound like an oxymoron.

When words like *cheating*, *unfaithfulness*, or *adultery* are used to represent a breakdown in sexual fidelity, divorce is likely to be the outcome.

Because so many of us have been raised to believe that it's simply not okay—with God, our parents, or our partners—to

be polyamorous, we fail to realize that we actually can include more than one sexualoving partner in our lives in an ethical and trustworthy fashion. We never realize the joy we can find in willingly sharing a lover. We never realize that we can design a lovestyle which is both nonmonogamous and responsible—one which can be positive for us, our loved ones, and the rest of the world—one which is also consistent with basic spiritual principles.

The bad news is that it won't necessarily be easy. But few people find monogamous relationships easy, either. Still, there is no denying that polyamory demands a good measure of maturity, self-esteem, skill, and commitment. If you're not willing to undertake the necessary preparation, polyamory is not for you. But if you value the depth, richness, excitement, and evolutionary opportunities found here—enough to give it everything you've got—polyamory can be a very rewarding choice.

Definitions

So what is polyamory? The word *polyamory* comes from Greek and Latin roots meaning "many loves." I use it to describe the whole range of lovestyles which arise from an understanding that love cannot be forced to flow, or not flow, in any particular direction. Love that is allowed to expand often grows to include a number of people. But to me, polyamory has more to do with an internal attitude of letting love evolve without expectations and demands than it does with the number of partners involved.

The term *polyamory* was first proposed by Church of All Worlds founders Oberon and Morning Glory Zell to replace the awkward expression *responsible nonmonogamy*. Cyberspace conversations via the Internet popularized its use all around the world and helped bring it into general usage. However, we can better understand the meaning of polyamory by taking a look at the more descriptive words *responsible nonmonogamy*.

The *nonmonogamy* part of the equation, while difficult to say swiftly, is far easier to describe than the *responsible* part. Nonmonogamy used to mean having more than one spouse during your lifetime. Now it means having more than one sexual partner during the same time period. Whether the partners are married, legally or spiritually, and even how they interact sexually, is not particularly relevant to our definition of nonmonogamy. We're simply speaking of all sexualoving relationships other than those limited to two people.

Singles who are dating more than one person are nonmonogamous, and couples who are sexual with others with or without the knowledge and consent of their primary partners are nonmonogamous. Three or more people who consider themselves to be married are nonmonogamous. Anyone with a circle of sexual friends is nonmonogamous. People who resume a sexual relationship with an ex-spouse or ex-lover after finding a new partner are nonmonogamous. Even people who choose to have no sexualoving partners at all and remain celibate may be nonmonogamous.

Over the last several decades a number of words and phrases have been used to describe specific forms of responsibly nonmonogamous relationships. Some of these are *polyfidelity, open marriage, open relationship, group marriage, multilateral marriage, intimate network*, and *triad*. Other less specific terms include *expanded family, nonexclusive relationship, intimate friendship*, and *inclusive relationship*.

Polyamory can include all of these, and it is not limited to any one of them. In fact, polyamory even includes couples who are currently monogamous but who do not necessarily intend to remain exclusive forever. One thing that all these types of relationships have in common is that they are both sexual *and* loving or *sexualoving*, with *no separation between the sex and the love*. In other words, we're not talking about casual, indiscriminate sport-sex.

Another thing that polyamorous relationships have in common is that they involve *consciously choosing* a particular lovestyle, rather than simply accepting the type of relationship which is most common in any given time and place. In polyamory you can design a relationship to fit your individual needs rather than automatically doing the same thing that everybody else does.

Polyamorous relationships may differ, however, in their basic intentions and approaches. Some polyamorous relationships resemble traditional monogamous marriage in their emphasis on creating an impermeable boundary around the group, operating according to a well-defined set of rules (sometimes called a social contract), and expecting family members to replace individual desires with group agendas. I call this type of relationship *old paradigm* regardless of whether it is polyamorous or monogamous.

Other polyamorous relationships have a primary focus on using the relationship to further the psychological and spiritual development of the partners. These relationships tend to put more emphasis on responding authentically in the present moment, allowing for individual autonomy, and seeing loved ones as mirrors or reflections of oneself. These *new paradigm* relationships also may be either monogamous or polyamorous. Of course, many people these days are in transition and find themselves attempting to blend elements of old and new paradigms, as well as monogamous and polyamorous lovestyles, but these distinctions are useful in clarifying the direction in which we wish to move.

Another dimension we must consider is the diversity of forms polyamory can take. In order to do this we need to have at our disposal language that enables us to communicate without resorting to conventional words that are judgmental, value-laden, or ambiguous. To that end, we propose the following terms.

Next to this kind of genuine intimacy, most romantic liaisons seemed like protection rackets.

Primary relationship. Lovers who are in a long-term, committed, marriage-type relationship are *primary partners*. Usually primary partners live together and share finances, parenting, and decision-making. Primary partners are not necessarily legally married, but they *are* bonded together as a family.

Secondary relationship. Secondary partners may also have a long-term, committed sexualoving relationship. But usually they live separately, have separate finances, and see themselves as close friends rather than immediate family. Secondary partners may take on roles in each other's families similar to those of cousins, aunts, and uncles in an extended family of blood relations.

Tertiary relationship. Lovers who spend time together only once in a while or for a brief time are *tertiary partners*. Their contact may be very intimate, but they are not an important part of each other's day-to-day life.

Polyamory can be practiced by any number of partners in any combination of primary, secondary, and tertiary relationships. While some polyamorous people object to the whole concept of hierarchies of commitment and rankings of love (as in the old Chinese practice of "number-one wife"), varying levels of affinity can occur naturally. This diversity of form, along with the realization that identical forms may result from radically different dynamics, automatically creates a social environment different from our familiar homogeneous, avowedly monogamous culture. And this diversity challenges us to develop ethical guidelines which apply to the *quality* rather than the *form* of the relationship.

What Forms Can Polyamory Take?

Open marriage or open relationship. These are both nonexclusive couple relationships, the main difference being whether the couple is married or not. In this scenario the partners have agreed that each can independently have outside sexualoving partners. A wide variety of ground rules and restrictions may apply.

Intimate network. This is a lovestyle in which several ongoing secondary relationships coexist. Sometimes all members of the group eventually become lovers. Sometimes individuals have only two or three partners within the group. The group can include singles only, couples only, or a mixture of both. Another way to describe it would be as a circle of sexualoving friends.

Group marriage or multilateral marriage. These are both committed, long-term, primary relationships which include three

We're simply speaking of all sexualoving relationships other than those limited to two people.

or more adults in a marriage-like relationship. A group marriage can be open or closed to outside sexual partners.

Polyfidelity. A lovestyle in which three or more primary partners agree to be sexual only within their family. Additional partners can be added to the marriage with everyone's consent.

Triad. Three sexualoving partners who may all be secondary, all primary, or two may be primary with the third secondary. It can be open or closed. A triad can be heterosexual or homosexual but is often the choice of two same-sex bisexuals and an opposite-sex heterosexual.

What Polyamory Is Not

Perhaps you are wondering whether polyamory includes swinging? Superficially, polyamory and swinging may appear to be the same. Admittedly, there is some overlap. But while swinging is generally consensual and honest, the emphasis is usually on recreational sex rather than love and intimacy. My perception is that in swinging, people tend to have sex first, although they may become friends over time. In polyamory, people are more apt to become friends first, although they may later get involved sexually. Swinging offers a maximum of sexual experience with a minimum of emotional involvement. In fact, many swinging couples make it a rule *not to fall in love* with their swinging partners. Consequently, I view swinging as a hybrid—monogamous on the love dimension while allowing specific nonmonogamous sexual experiences. Some people start out experimenting with swinging but end up realizing they prefer polyamory—and vice versa.

Swinging and polyamory also differ in that swinging has more of a commercial aspect. Large conventions, glossy

magazines, tropical vacation tours, and a national network of swing clubs provide happy hunting grounds for those seeking sexual adventures. Polyamory is less a recreational activity than an alternative way of life which often encompasses economic, nutritional, and political alternatives. It is more likely than swinging to be inclusive of different sexual orientations. Grass roots polyamory support groups are more likely to focus on discussions and potluck dinners than sexy lingerie and the latest in dildos.

Polyamory is not philandering, and it is not a way to justify an uncontrollable urge to continually seek out new partners. Polyamory has nothing to do with proving that you're a real man or a real woman. It's not an excuse for having secret affairs or a means of establishing your independence. It is not simply sex for sex's sake, but an expression of your heart and soul.

My Own Story

For over two decades I have been working in the laboratory of my own life to discover how I can love and be loved more fully, more freely, and more consciously. Having always been a highly erotic person, I've struggled for many years to fully integrate my sexuality with my emotional, spiritual, and intellectual life. Part of my path has been to discover how to open deeply to others without the props of exclusivity and ownership. Part of my path has been to discover how to catalyze group energies into viable communities of intimate equals, groups that do not rely on the presence of a guru for inspiration or leadership. It's been a long journey, full of surprises and flavored by both ecstasy and pain.

Sometimes it seems that I'm finally coming home. Sometimes it seems that I've gotten nowhere. But through it all I find that my most important ally is my faith in the truth of my own experience. The more I can allow myself to know that truth—regardless of its political correctness—and express it, the more I find myself on solid ground. Some of my ideas about love and relationships have changed since the first edition of my book was published, and I want you to know that they are still changing. At the same time, my deepest values, my dearest dreams, and my most magnetic attractions seem to stay the same over time. But as I grow in understanding, the expression of my core self does take different forms.

As I look back, I realize that I have been building an intimate network over the last twenty-some years. This process started in 1975, about a year after I separated from my first husband and fell head over heels in love with Jack. When he first made love to me, I sensed he was worshipping the Divine. I literally saw stars. This was my first Tantric initiation, and it changed my life forever. Alas, it quickly became apparent that Jack and I were not going to get married and live happily ever after. For one thing, I was about to leave the state to go to graduate school, and for another he'd informed me that he was nonmonogamous and had several girlfriends. Besides, we pushed each other's buttons so intensely, we really couldn't spend much time together. I was still very young and understood little about relating. At the same time, I knew that Jack had touched my soul so deeply that I wanted him to stay in my life forever.

I realized I had a choice. I could transcend my jealousy and expectations and love him unconditionally, or I could try to shut him out of my heart and forget about him. I chose to keep loving him, not knowing at the time where this would lead me. Several years later I married for the second time, trying to fit myself into the traditional mold with an ambitious, personable husband and a house with a white picket fence. He too had unfinished business with an old lover, but while continued friendships were acceptable to him, extramarital love affairs were not. I was researching domestic violence for my doctoral dissertation at the time and was horrified to realize that the dynamics of domination, control, jealousy, and dependency that I'd observed in the abusive marriages I was studying also existed, at a more moderate level, in my own marriage. Determined to find a way to love in alignment with my beliefs and life purpose, but still not knowing how it would look, I divorced again.

I soon became part of a group of renegade psychotherapists who met every two weeks for a couple of years. We would take turns leading the group, facilitating others, working on our own stuff, exploring the group mind, and creating innovative tools and combinations of tools to take us into new psychospiritual territory. We also fantasized about developing a more cooperative, communal lifestyle, but this aspect never went as far as I'd hoped it would. Although many of us were in open relationships and some of us had partners within the group and exchanged or shared partners over time, we did not think of ourselves as polyamorous. In fact, my participation in this group predated my "coming out poly" by several years.

Nonetheless, Aaron, my primary lover at the time, and I were fascinated by the dynamics of triangular relationships of all kinds. We made it a point to experiment with them whenever possible, both in the group I just described and in other situations. Aaron introduced me to Damian, an acquaintance of his who was well-versed in both pagan and Tantric practices. I asked Damian to teach me Tantra, and he readily agreed. For the first time I began to see that the play of energy that spontaneously arose between me and some of my lovers could be deliberately invoked and channeled. Damian shared our passion for triangles, and soon Aaron, Damian, and I found ourselves exploring three-way sexual interactions. We also found ourselves tripped up time and again by our gender roles. None of us had firm enough boundaries, none of us had done enough sexual healing, and even though we were relatively free of jealousy, none of us were free enough from our other conditioning to really connect with each other.

Toward the end of this period, I met another man who, along with Jack, would eventually become part of my present intimate network. But it would still be many years before the seeds I planted way back then would bear fruit. Now, after many seasons of patiently—or often impatiently—waiting for individual relationships to deepen and for different parts of my network to come together, it truly feels like a miracle every time old and new friends and lovers finally meet and connect with each other with a shared understanding of the possibility

Polyamory is not philandering, and it is not a way to justify an uncontrollable urge to continually seek out new partners.

we have to weave our lives together. Of course, not everyone loves each other at first sight—though some do—but all are curious and excited about the journey we are taking.

Meanwhile, discouraged both by my inability to succeed at traditional marriage and my inability to do much more than apply psychological Band-Aids to the battered women and children who were casualties of our family institutions, I began to research alternatives to monogamy and the nuclear family. As luck would have it, practically the first people I encountered were the group whose beginnings are described in my book, *Polyamory*. By this time they had been together for over ten years and had grown to a core group of four with two more in the process of joining them full-time. I learned a great deal by becoming part of this extended family, including all the basic principles of new paradigm relating. They reached out to me with such love and support, it would have been easy to let my quest end there, but I seemed to have a need to blaze my own trail, so I continued building my network from scratch.

Richard was one of many intimate friends I made in the next few years and was also an important teacher for me. He came into my life at a time when I was relating to several different men who each brought out different parts of me. You might say that I had a lover for each chakra. For the first time in my life, I was fully engaged on every level, and as a result, I attracted a man who could meet me on every level.

Richard had been in an open marriage for about 20 years and soon told me he was looking for a number-two wife. Our sexual, emotional, and intellectual chemistry was extraordinary, and he was very skilled at making me feel special while clearly giving priority to his wife and children. We were all professional psychotherapists, so we were very conscious of the subtleties of our group dynamics. My position was similar to that of "the other woman," except that he didn't keep me secret from his wife. The three of us would sometimes hang out at their home or go out together, but she didn't seem open to developing much of a relationship with me. She told me once she'd seen too many of my counterparts come and go over the years to think I'd be around for long. Indeed, this was a passionate but stormy relationship which taught me a tremendous amount about open relating, but which ultimately proved to be an obstacle to creating an intimate network for myself.

Both Richard and David fit the profile for dominant or alpha males. They were mature, powerful men who knew their strengths and found it natural to take a leadership role. I enjoyed relating to this kind of man but found that my other lov-

I knew deep in my bones that choosing monogamy out of fear and a desire for security wouldn't get us very far.

ers felt competitive and overshadowed by them. While I felt blessed by the presence of sister-wives and wanted to further explore my bisexual nature, I knew that a situation where one man was being shared by a group of women wasn't going to mesh well with my sexual appetites.

At this point I'd been single for about seven years, and, while I enjoyed my intimate network, I was feeling the urge to bond more deeply and create a primary, live-in relationship for myself. I pictured a loving, gender-balanced family of four to six adults and several children (my daughter from my first marriage was now a teenager). I decided to begin by pairing up with a man who also wanted a group marriage and who expressed a strong desire for cooperative living. Perhaps the two of us could form the core for a larger group. For six years we thrived in our open marriage but never succeeded in growing beyond the dyad. This marriage lasted longer and was generally an improvement on my monogamous marriages. Unfortunately, my partner and I frequently were attracted to and found attractive by very different people. So even though we were aligned on many important life goals, building family together began to seem unrealistic.

Eventually, I realized that whatever we might say or think to the contrary, the institution of marriage had had its way with us. I simply could not stay conscious enough to avoid being sucked into the old Dominator stereotypes, even if monoga-

my was not an issue. Finally, I came to realize that polyamory is not enough to serve as a basis for marriage.

When I ended this marriage a few years ago, I was determined that I would not repeat my pattern of seeking refuge in a couple relationship of any description because I'd failed to create a viable expanded family. Luckily, I discovered that many former lovers who had drifted out of my life during my open marriage were still there for me in significant ways and ready to renew our connections. But once again, I found myself challenged to maintain my intimate network in the face of jealousy from first one, then another new lover.

These were men who'd initially been attracted to me because I was polyamorous but who then "fell in love" and wanted the safety of an exclusive relationship, at least temporarily while their newly-in-love brain chemistry was engaged. If you want a monogamous commitment, find somebody else, I told them, knowing full well that they themselves had had plenty of negative experiences with serial monogamy. I knew deep in my bones that choosing monogamy out of fear and a desire for security wouldn't get us very far. I knew, even if they didn't, that couple entanglements only made the whole process of family-building more drawn out and difficult, and I wasn't about to go down that road again.

It's uncomfortable to be on either side of this struggle. The truth is that we all have conflicting desires for inclusivity and exclusivity. When we become polarized on the monogamy issue, we find ourselves distorting the reality of our complex emotions for the sake of a purist mentality. Knowing that my reputation might lead people to believe that I was rigidly polyamorous, I worked hard at keeping an open mind about monogamy. I've never met anyone I found totally fulfilling on every level, I would say, and I doubt that such a one exists. Don't take it personally. I'm a multidimensional person and I'm attracted to different qualities in different people. The more my heart opens, the more people I feel love for. If I ever feel moved to choose to be monogamous, I will, but not because someone insists upon it.

So why was I attracting lovers who ended up demanding monogamy? I didn't know, but I knew I'd better find out because the whole process was very painful and certainly took all the fun out of polyamory. I began to ask myself hard questions. Was my own deeply conditioned desire for a white knight who would solve all my problems and take care of me forever sending out mating calls? At one of my own workshops I vowed to let go of this complex. Was I getting involved with too many lovers and needing some external constraints to narrow my focus? I decided to pay more attention to my own priorities. Was I simply coming up against cultural patterns that wouldn't disappear just because I challenged them? If so, how could I expect anyone else to break through centuries of conditioning when I couldn't do it myself? Without the support of my intimate network and the larger polyamorous community I've been building over the years, I'm sure I would have given up at this point. Instead, I realized that I needed to once again let go and allow the process to unfold in its own way.

And so began another cycle of deeper connections with old intimate friends and the appearance of delightful new additions to my ever growing family. I continue to pray for the strength, wisdom, humor, and clarity to take up permanent residence in the space of love, which is really what my life is all about.

Patterns

We don't have information yet on sufficient numbers of people to say with certainty how most people build their families, but these are some of the patterns we've observed. I offer them to you as suggestions, not as absolutes.

Two plus two equals three. It's very rare for three or more single people to bond with each other all at the same time. And a single person is often reluctant to become the odd-one-out with a couple. But many stable triads that we know of, like the one described above, formed when two couples got together and then one couple broke up, with one person going off separately.

Twelve divided by two equals two. Another common occurrence is for an intimate network of mixed couples and singles to end up with many of the singles coupled with each other and some of the couples uncoupled. We don't know of any intimate networks that have transformed into group marriages, but it is common for people to end up trading partners.

Three plus one equals three. Threesomes just don't seem to want to expand into foursomes. This holds true especially when adding a baby to a triad. This is not to say you can't do it, but it can be rocky, especially if there are unresolved issues about biological parentage.

Into the bed and out of the relationship. Leaping into bed with prospective family or network members may seem like a good way to get things started, but it usually isn't if you're interested in a long-term relationship. The reason is that in a group of people you're likely to find some bonds heating up before others. If you wait until everyone feels ready to proceed, you're much more likely to stay in balance.

Threesomes just don't seem to want to expand into foursomes.

Out of the bed and out of the relationship. It's also possible to err on the side of caution and be so hesitant about getting sexual prematurely that the natural flow of intimacy is effectively squashed. Once this happens, it can be very hard to overcome the aura of celibacy or disinterest.

Shopping lists are toilet paper. It's become popular in some circles to compare shopping lists or social contracts as a way of screening potential partners. While comparing values and lifestyles is undoubtedly important, the reality is that most of us aren't totally conscious about who we are and what we want and need—especially in the unfamiliar territory of responsible nonmonogamy. This is why so many matches work only on paper and not in person. It's not unusual for people to end up with partners who are the exact opposite of what they said they wanted.

If A=B and A=C, B does not necessarily equal C. This is another case of real life refusing to conform to theory. As much as we would like the people we love to love each other, often they do not. You may choose to expect a miracle, but don't count on all your lovers understanding what you see in the others.

Same-gender relationships are all-powerful. Whether you are gay, straight, bisexual, or don't know, you need to recognize that the quality of your family life will be determined by the quality of the same-gender bonding. This bonding can express itself in many ways, so long as it occurs. If homophobia is allowed to remain an unexamined shadow issue, it may well sabotage your best efforts. Even where homophobia is not an issue, same-gender bonding can be very delicate and needs sensitive care and nurturing.

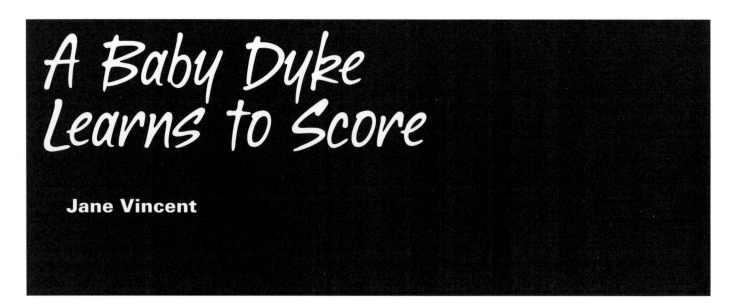

A Baby Dyke Learns to Score

Jane Vincent

Disclaimers: *I am a bi-dyke. I sleep with women and men. I am queer in my sexual partners and practices. Although I would not describe myself as a lesbian, I identify as a dyke sexually and politically.*

Additionally, I am a slut. I am a slut not because I'm bisexual. And I'm not bisexual because I'm a slut. I'm a slut because I like to fuck. This essay is not about a quest for love. It is about sex, specifically sex with women.

"A woman has to know how to please herself before she can pleasure another woman." I received my first piece of advice from a lesbian poet who wrote of peanut butter earth. We were skipping assembly, hiding behind the curtain of the cafeteria stage. Kit was one of four "out" kids in my high school of 2,800 and the only girl. She was inspirational. My crush on her cemented my suspicions that I was not straight. However, her words amplified my inadequacy. If I couldn't get myself off, how was I supposed to get another woman off?

Our open relationship allowed me to embrace my new identity as her girlfriend while fucking half a dozen random guys.

When I was twelve, I learned that boys are easy. But for a young bi girl, boys can only go so far. I fantasized about women, but my fantasies were very vague. I had no idea how to meet queer girls. And what was I supposed to do with them?

Freshman year of college, I took a queer theory class, fell in love with academic sex, and began to come out. In an attempt to meet queer women, and learn a thing or two, I volunteered as an usher for the Mix Gay and Lesbian Experi-

mental Film Festival's lesbian erotica screening. There were scenes ranging from phone sex to fisting. But the image I could not escape was the black plastic cock. I was appalled by the dildos. I wanted to "be with women as women" and saw these masculine phalluses as intrusions in our (at that point imaginary) love life.

That spring I met Michelle. She asked me to audition for her play. I bought her baklava. We were girlfriends. It was that simple. Michelle introduced me to polyamory. Our open relationship allowed me to embrace my new identity as her girlfriend while fucking half a dozen random guys. It seemed the only person I wasn't fucking was Michelle.

I would go over to her house and make dinner. We would make out, shirts off, grinding, rolling, holding back wrists, no bras.... Then her hand would graze my panties, and I would freeze. I had no idea what to do. I kept thinking of Kit's advice and the fact that I had never had an orgasm. Even if she was a stone top like the women I had read about in my queer theory class, I assumed you couldn't fake an orgasm with another woman. She would know. So I got up to pee, fell asleep, or watched *Daria* on TiVo.

When I returned to the city after a summer in Texas, I renewed my pursuit of women. I needed to advertise that I was femme queer, not just another straight girl. I went to queer bars. I went to erotic readings and art shows with queer content. I started reading lesbian and bisexual erotica on the train. And I started getting numbers. But I still had no idea what to do.

So I researched. I read piles of books. I watched better and better porn. I made friends with other queer girls and subtly pumped their brains. I even did an ethnographic research paper on lesbian hedonism for a class. However, my greatest learning experience took the form of an apprenticeship.

I found myself dating two older women (28 and 32) who were also dating each other. One evening the three of us dressed up in fetish gear (my first time in a corset) and strolled to a queer fetish party. Afterwards we stumbled into the big bed of the loft I was subletting. We were too exhausted for any fun that night.

With the morning sun came snuggling, which lead to cuddling, which lead to stroking, which lead to making out, which lead to no-holds-barred three-way lesbian action (oh yeah, baby). Actually, it was more like a rotating two on one (you get her tits, I'll cover her cunt. Okay, now, switch!). The best part was I could watch Rita eat out Sarah or Sarah fingerfuck Rita, then I could try. It was like a kinky workshop.

About the same time, I got myself off. I did a lot of research, as I am prone to do. I knew penetration wasn't what I needed (I had had plenty and look where it had gotten me), so I focused on clitoral vibes. I wanted something small and non-threatening but strong and adjustable. I recruited a friend to escort me to Toys in Babeland. She hugged the wall by the books while I shyly ventured around the center table of vibrators. A staff person approached and asked if she could help. I pulled out my notes and said I was looking for the honey bear. She found it right away, his arms raised like a clit-hugging ballerina. The honey bear fit discreetly in my palm. The remote was also palm-length, the two connected by a white cord. I bought him without exploring the rest of the store. I took him home and named him Albert.

I had read enough Betty Dodson at this point to know not to pressure myself too much. For our first date, Albert and I got to know each other. I could feel something building stronger and stronger, as he gripped my clit, his body hugged by my labia. At the last minute I turned him off. I thought I was going to piss or scream or something to let the building know what I was doing.

On our second date, both of my roommates were out. First, I played with Albert on my breasts, pinching each nipple. I licked my left middle finger and started to stroke my clit. Then I moved Albert down. I settled him into place with the vibrations turned off. I stroked Albert as he pinched my clit, his body stimulating the legs of my clitoris and rubbing against my urethra.

Then I turned him on low. I made sure to breathe, watching my diaphragm rise and fall like theater vocal warm-ups. I started having little shivers and jumps. I turned him up higher. I was breathing fairly hard at this point. I remembered Betty

Dodson talking about Kegel exercises. I clenched my vaginal muscles, tight, tight, tight, in time with my quick, gasping inhalations. I could feel it building again. My right hand, raking my thigh, started moving towards the controls to turn it down. I moved it to my breast and squeezed full-palmed (in the same rough, awkward grasp of so many junior-high and high-school conquests).

When I came, I stopped breathing for two minutes. My body shook, and my neck froze, head thrust back like a seizure victim. My toes curled, and my fingers locked in double-jointed akimbo. Albert purred. I had made a new friend.

Now I knew what to do. I needed new women to play with. I started looking for chicks on the Internet. Craigslist had been my resource for casual dick and a new coffee table. However, their women-for-women forums regularly spouted against bisexuals; understandable, since the only other bi-women posting seemed to be looking for a third to join their boyfriend. No-strings-attached casual-encounters postings received more penis pictures than those looking for male dates.

I went to women-and-transgender-only sex parties and play parties. Everyone seemed to be talking, with an established couple doing a spanking, flogging, or piercing scene every now and then. Aside from the hot voyeurism, there didn't seem to be much mixing of strangers.

Finally, I went to a bisexual "date bait" with two friends. Date bait is a form of speed dating in which a group meets in a bar and everyone goes on eight or ten or twelve "mini-dates" of three to five minutes. Attractions are recorded on scorecards

The best part was I could watch Rita eat out Sarah or Sarah fingerfuck Rita, then I could try.

and matches are made by the organizers. Although I made several matches, only one resulted in a date.

Moira was a lighting designer with plugs in her ears and a wicked sense of humor (translation: She was from the Northeast and used *wicked* as the universal adjective). We interpreted our match as a future with dozens of babies. However, we quickly fell into a pattern of friendship. Of course, our friendship involved regular masturbation and toy-trading. We would turn on a porn and turn on our vibes. Occasionally, she would crawl over me to explore my toy box.

One evening, Moira's eyes grew large as she found my new double-header. "Ooh, can we play with this?" I flipped her on her back and had her hold her bullet against her clit. With a black latex glove (because I had been knuckle-deep in my own pussy moments before), I began to massage her G-spot.

She groaned as I inserted each new finger. With three fingers inside, I slipped the condomed dick along my palm and into her cunt (think of a shoehorn). I jerked off the second half of the cock, each stroke thrusting the dildo deeper. When Moira came, she soaked the bed. I had to change the sheets and put a towel beneath the new ones to create a dry spot for sleeping.

The final test of my lesbian prowess came when I began to date a lesbian sex expert (sexpert?). I had invited Rachel over to my apartment for sushi. When I walked down to pick her up from the train station, she was wearing fishnets with spar-

Craigslist had been my resource for casual dick and a new coffee table.

kly seams, open-toed, strappy, 1940s pin-up shoes, and a jacket that was only waist-length (she also had impressive cleavage, but that was under the coat). I remarked that she was too pretty to be standing on that corner (ah, sex worker humor) and flagged a gypsy cab to take us back to my apartment (only five avenue blocks, but it was snowing and I could see her toes).

We ordered sushi, and I let her have my miso soup. Then we decided to watch a movie, but we didn't watch the movie for

long (blush). Although the entire night and morning after was wonderful, there were a few highlights:

- Her face and little whimper/squirms as I nibbled her nipples. So hot!

- Struggling for access to her tender bits, I joked that I may have to rip off her fishnets. When they still weren't off a couple of minutes later, I said, "Seriously, do you plan on wearing these again? 'Cause I will rip them off you."

- At one point I was straddling her, riding her fingers while the back of her hand ground against her clit. Throwing my head down, my long, curly hair trailed across her face. I tried to swing it out of the way, but she resisted, draping my curls across her cheeks and forehead.

Needless to say, I passed the test with flying colors, and a handful of orgasms to boot.

At this point, I'm a girl with experience. It is not uncommon to find me demonstrating proper G-spot stimulation techniques to an audience of five or more. I find the time to enjoy frottage (hump and grind), G-spotting, female ejaculation, fingering, fisting, oral, anal, sex toys, strap-ons, BDSM, solo, partnered and group sex, and red, purple, turquoise, and black silicone cocks. This baby dyke is all grown up.

Egg Sex

Susie Bright

In 1966, when I was eight years old, my mother gave me a little pink book, *A Baby is Born*. In great detail, and with lots of close-ups and diagrams, it described exactly what a sperm and egg looked like and how they joined together, with subsequent portraits of the developing fetus.

How did the sperm meet the egg to begin with? The book said simply, "Mommy and Daddy love each other very much. They lie close together and, after performing intercourse, the sperm is on its way to fertilize the egg." There was no accompanying diagram, so I made what was probably my first earnest attempt to read between the lines of any piece of literature. I gleaned nothing.

Twenty-five years later, I was pregnant, and this time I went out and bought my own collection of pink and blue books bulging with instruction for prospective parents. Of course, there was a great deal to learn about fetal development and breast-feeding techniques, but I couldn't help but check each index under "Sexuality—during and after pregnancy." All the manuals, from Dr. Spock to the latest yuppie know-how, followed an almost identical script: "Mommy and Daddy love each other very much...." Following this vein, the paragraphs on sexuality gave advice that was inexplicit, vague, and almost threatening in their avoidance of the nitty-gritty.

Steeped in a romance-novel notion of marriage, sexual advice to pregnant moms, whether revealed in print or in the strange silences at the doctor's office, gives short shrift to the dramatic changes in women's sexual physiology and desires. Great emphasis is placed on how to cope with the ambivalent husband's feelings towards his wife's body and the burden pregnancy puts on their normal sexual routine.

None of these books were written in the 1960s. All of them glow with feminist and holistic approaches to mothering, sup-porting working moms, refuting the sexist prejudices against breast-feeding, and offering all manner of enlightened positive self-esteem for the mother-to-be. I began to wonder if anyone *knew* what went on in women's sexual lives during pregnancy. The most definitive statement the books managed was: Sometimes she's hot, sometimes she's not. This wouldn't be the first time that traditional medicine had nothing to contribute to an understanding of female sexuality.

Meanwhile, my clit started to grow. Everyone knows that a pregnant woman's breasts swell in accompaniment to her belly, but why had no one told me that my genitals would also grow? My vulva engorged with blood; my labia grew fatter; my clit pushed slightly out of its hood. I was reading absolutely everything on the subject of pregnant sex by this point, and, by picking out the fragments of pertinent information, I learned I was not peculiar in this regard.

It's a little embarrassing to be 31 years old and finally get the message that my primary and secondary sexual characteristics are not simply for display and petting. I was being physically and psychologically dominated by the life growing inside me, and of course I wanted both to escape and to submit. I was unusually sensual and amorous, and yet, 20 weeks into pregnancy, I found I could not successfully masturbate the way I had been doing since I was a kid. I was stunned and a little panicky. My engorged clitoris was different under my fingers; too sensitive to touch my usual way, and what other way was there?

That's when it hit me. The experts all say that it is a mystery why some women get more horny when they're pregnant, while others lose interest. I'll tell you something—no one loses interest. What happens is that your normal sexual patterns don't work the same way anymore. Unless you and your lover make the transition to new ways of getting excited and reaching orgasm, you are going to be very depressed about sex and start avoiding it all together.

It's not just a technique change, either. Feeling both desirable *and* protected are essential to a pregnant woman, and if protection is not forthcoming from the outside, she will build a fortress that cannot be penetrated.

I no longer believe that some women don't feel sexual during those long nine months. Some are frightened by the sexual changes their growing bodies demand. But so many others confided to me, "I was so hot, and I couldn't explain it to just anyone."

It's an awesome feat of American puritanism to convince us that sex and pregnancy do not mix. It's the ultimate virgin/whore distinction. For those nine months, please don't mention how we got this way—we're Mary now.

Your average Mary's physical transformation is quite different from an immaculate conception. A woman's vagina changes when she is pregnant, much like her vulva and clit. The lubrication increases; its smell and texture are different. Often exhibiting a pregnancy-type yeast infection, her genitals smell like a big cookie.

When I fucked during my pregnancy, I felt like I was participating in a slow elastic taffy pull. I was more passive sexually than ever before, with no ambition to strap one on, or get on top, or do much of anything besides take it all in and float. I was one gigantic egg cozy.

It's an awesome feat of American puritanism to convince us that sex and pregnancy do not mix.

Truthfully, you don't get gigantic for at least five or six months. The advice books make much controversy over positions for intercourse, but I didn't find positioning to be that big a deal. It's typical of mainstream sex books to focus on "positions" in the masculine way one might prepare a sports manual. You can fuck on your back for a long time if you like, as long as your partner doesn't insist on collapsing upon you. Flat on one's belly is of course impossible after six months, but slightly turned to the side works just fine. It is often recommended that the woman get on top, but as I said, I couldn't be bothered.

Sex is also a crucial way to prepare for childbirth. Start with the premise that birth is the biggest sex act you will ever take part in, and everything will flow from that. If you are smart and take childbirth preparation classes, you may even get a teacher who knows something about the sexual side of birth.

My teacher was very subtle. She gave us an almost unreadable handout in the fourth month, an instruction sheet for an exercise called "perineal massage." I thought of my perineum, the little inch of skin running between my vagina and my anus. How could rubbing something the size of a birthday candle help me in labor?

The flyer (which opened, of course, with the obligatory spiel: "Mommy and Daddy love each other very much....") said that Daddy should massage and finger the vaginal opening until he could put more and more of his fingers inside, relaxing the vaginal muscles through such caresses until he might be able to press a small orange or even his whole hand into Mommy's opening.

His whole hand! I called up one of my friends who has the breadth of experience as both a mother of two and a retired pornstar. "Is 'perineal massage' really fistfucking?" I asked her.

"Of course," she said, laughing, "and it really helps."

I could see why immediately. A hand going inside my pussy is a little like a baby's head trying to move outside into the world. How exciting! For the first time I felt a surge of confidence about my chances for a successful labor. Since I had practiced fisting, clearly I was in great shape for the real thing.

Perineal massage is not discussed in every hospital or prenatal setting. Most couples and their care providers are steeped in the dominance of penis-vagina intercourse. It requires a different sort of orientation to devote attention to the possibilities of fingers and hands. But with a little encouragement and a flyer with pictures and plain English, I think more parents would enjoy the intense relaxation and vulnerability that comes with fisting, or "oranging," if you prefer.

I pestered my teacher for three weeks about whether she thought using a vibrator during labor would be helpful for pain relief. She said each time that we would discuss it next week. She recommended all sorts of other distractions and exercises: going to the bathroom frequently, changing positions, getting in the bathtub, focusing on a special object, etc. Well, I decided on my own that my Hitachi Magic Wand was going to be my focus object. I believed that stimulating my clit would be a nice counterpoint to the contractions going on inside my belly.

I have a great photograph of me in the delivery room, dilated to six centimeters, with a blissful look on my face and my vibrator nestled against my pubic bone. I had no thought of climaxing, but the pleasure of the rhythm on my clit was like sweet icing on top of the deep, thick contractions in my womb. I would have been too tired and distracted to touch myself with my fingers at that point, and the power cord was just one of about ten that the doctors had coming from my bed. Due to my baby's unusual breech position, I had a complicated birth that finally ended in an emergency Cesarean. But I had a great labor.

My friend Barbara confessed to me after her first child that she had never been so turned on in her life. When the baby's head was crowning, she called out to her husband over and over, "I want to come, touch me, please touch me!"—and he thought she was hysterical.

We are utterly unaccustomed to seeing birthing as a sexual experience. A lot of us think of childbirth as something close to death; at least, that's what I was afraid of.

I heard women screaming in the rooms next to me at the hospital, and I knew those screams weren't exclusively from physical pain but from wild, wild fear. It's terribly frightening when you don't know what your body is doing and when your sexuality is divorced from this incredible process. Being afraid makes the pain much worse and makes your stamina unknowable.

There was a traffic jam of births at the city hospitals the week I had my daughter. It was about nine months after the big earthquake hit San Francisco, and apparently staying home had been a fertile pastime during that otherwise sobering period. The other women who had children the day and night I was in the hospital did not appear to have husbands at their sides. It was easy for me to imagine their stories: They were single; they were lesbian; they had husbands who didn't want to see them that way; they had husbands who had left them earlier in their pregnancies; they had husbands in the service and far away.

I didn't read a single parenting book that reflected any of these lives, although they are as commonplace as conception itself. The fractured fairy tale ("Mommy and Daddy love each other very much....") is only resonant in the sense that parents need to be loved and nurtured, because they are about to give of themselves in a way that they never dreamed possible before.

If the mother doesn't receive tenderness and passion during her nine months, the bitterness she develops lasts well beyond childbirth—her kids will know all about it. Perhaps I could encourage childbirth professionals to advocate good sex during pregnancy as a key to psychologically healthy children.

After the birth, you will get doctor's instructions to abstain from sex for the next six weeks. We've all heard the woman who says, "I don't care if I don't have sex for the next six years." But if her pussy is so sore, why can't she enjoy oral sex? Her breasts are leaking colostrum, ready to start ex-

pressing milk, and they need to be sucked by someone who knows about sucking breasts—babies don't always get the hang of it instantly, or at mom's command.

The truth is, this six-weeks rule is arbitrary, and it's based on the fear of an infection resulting from a man ejaculating inside the vagina. There is a lot more to "sex" than this. Nothing magic happens at the end of six weeks. Not everyone's os and vaginal passageway are in the same condition after birth. Having had a Cesarean, mine had not been through a full-blown vaginal birth. Without knowing exactly what risk I was taking, but knowing that the doctor didn't know what he was

I have a great photograph of me in the delivery room, dilated to six centimeters, with a blissful look on my face and my vibrator nestled against my pubic bone.

talking about either, I came home from the hospital and made love on the sixth day after my daughter was born.

I've spoken with many women who admitted the same. "My husband and I had waited so long for this child," said my nurse practitioner/midwife, who had a child after she was 40, "that we had to be intimate right away." I appreciated her using the word *intimate*, because I don't think it's the case that you just have this wild hare to get it on once the baby is born. You want a closeness, a release, and a celebration that you haven't necessarily experienced during labor.

My midwife also told me that she started asking her patients how soon after childbirth they had resumed intercourse. Lots of people break the rules, as you can imagine, and she found that women who had intercourse earlier on also resumed periods much sooner than those who waited. This little discovery—from a professional who wouldn't ordinarily tell me such things—reminded me again how little we know because no one shares taboo information.

Nursing is another source of mixed feelings, erotic and otherwise. One woman winces in pain from chapped and bleeding nipples, while another has orgasms from her baby's suckling. Again, if these things were brought out in the open, a lot of nipple soreness would disappear. Breast-feeding does not come instinctively, and it helps to have someone show you, as well as tell you, how to nurse comfortably.

I was satisfied just to nurse my baby competently. My erotic feelings came not so much from my baby's sucking as from feeling my breasts express themselves at other times. Sexual arousal will make your breasts leak when you're lactating, another important fact missing in most parent handbooks. As much as I have lectured on G-spot orgasms, I had never had anything come out of me when I was making love before, and this made my head swim with embarrassment at first and then arousal.

I've always been one of those women who could be secretive about her climax. I could come without crying out. I could be very sneaky. Having my nipples not just stiffen, but release milk like a faucet every time I was turned on took me for a very un-private loop. But I loved rubbing it on my lover's chest, or

When the baby's head was crowning, she called out to her husband over and over, "I want to come, touch me, please touch me!"

my own. I felt some feminine equivalent of virility, making the biggest wet spot of them all. This was the very opposite of being hooked up to the electric breast pump, which made me feel like a working cow. Handy, but totally unerotic.

It would be unfair to conclude the erotic disposition of pregnancy without talking about changes in sexual fantasies. Our fantasies often seem to be written in stone at an early age and are not too easily transformed in our adult years. But having a baby is the next big hormone explosion a woman can have after puberty, and she may surprise herself with what comes to mind at the moment of orgasm. I did.

In retrospect I see that my fantasy life during my pregnancy was cathartic. One of my biggest and most irrational reservations about having a child (besides fearing that I would die in childbirth) was that if I had a boy, I wouldn't know how to raise him. I would be a disaster, whether teaching him how to use the toilet or to fly a kite.

Petty sexual stereotypes aside, I didn't know what little boys were like. I have no brothers, was raised by my mom, and always preferred dresses.

I'm a single parent, but I had conversations with the father of my kid now and then during my pregnancy. He was concerned that I was planning a politically correct dress code for the young one. "If it's a girl, I suppose you'll always make her wear pants," he pouted.

"Oh no," I said. "If I have a little girl, I'm going to make sure she has the frilliest, laciest, puffiest dresses you ever saw," remembering the kind of dresses I always wanted.

"And if it's a little boy," he started.

"Of course," I interrupted, "He'll have the frilliest, laciest, puf-fiest..."

My teasing was just a cover. I really didn't know what little boys were supposed to wear.

One night, I was making love with my friend, John, and I imagined that he was my son. I came like a rocket, and I didn't have the nerve to tell him about it for weeks. In the meantime, I could not get this image off my mind. I recalled a really tacky porn movie I had seen years ago, *Taboo*, where beautiful mom Kay Parker has a son (in real life, a grown-up actor named Mike Ranger) who only has eyes for her. I wasn't aroused by the movie the first time I saw it, but now this scene could turn me on instantly. I couldn't masturbate or make love to anyone, man or woman, without conjuring up this incestuous exchange.

At the same time, while making my plans for the baby and talking to friends and family, I was noticeably more at ease about having a boy child. I didn't know what sex my baby was, and unlike so many other moms, I didn't want to know.

I started noticing mothers with their sons on the street, and I didn't panic; I smiled at them. Somebody gave me a book on how to be a "dad," with all sorts of fabulous hints on butch activities, from skipping stones to throwing a ball. I read the whole thing and thought it was a blast. I asked all my friends how many of them had fathers who did any of these things, and our answers shed a lot of light on our gender points of view.

When my team of doctors finally pulled Aretha from my womb, they were exuberant. "It's a girl!" somebody said. I was shaking very badly from the anesthesia, but this warm lit-tle yolk of feeling spilled in my head, and tears of relief came to my eyes. I was so pleased to have a daughter.

When I came home and had my first chance to fantasize (something sleep deprivation cut into quite a bit), I could not for the life of me conjure up my imaginary son! He had split. My incest fantasy had expressed my fear of having a boy, and when that possibility disappeared, the fantasy lost its magic. I don't know what would have happened to my fantasy if I had indeed come home with a son. I think I would have moved on, just as I did after Aretha's birth, to new sets of anxieties which became fresh erotic fodder.

Now I fantasize about being pregnant again—talk about kinky. In reality I have no desire to be eating soda crackers for a month and having to go to the bathroom every ten minutes for the next half-year. But I do have glowing memories of the sexual discoveries I made during pregnancy, and I'm grateful I had a sexually loving and inquisitive support system around me. If the whole process could be like that.... Well, maybe I'll have another one, I tell myself, when my daughter is old enough to change the diapers.

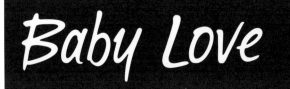

Baby Love

Christen Clifford

Before I became a mother, I believed that motherhood would change me: My maternal instinct would smooth me, balance me, make me patient, give me a nurturing generosity. I'd become a better person, but I wouldn't lose myself. I'd breastfeed exclusively but still find time to write. I'd make homemade baby food but still fuck. I had it all figured out.

I bought all the new books on mothering that I read about in the *New York Times* and the *New Yorker*—*Bitch in the House*, *The Mask of Motherhood*, *The Myth of Motherhood*, *The Price of Motherhood*, *A Life's Work*, *Fresh Milk*, and a book a friend recommended—*Fermentation*—the only erotic novel I could find that featured a pregnant woman. But no one else's narrative could prepare me for the next stage of my sexuality.

People always tell you that becoming a parent will change everything, but what I didn't count on was that it *wouldn't* change me. The problem is that I'm still the same person, a sex-obsessed neurotic facing a new reality: My husband and I love our son more than we love each other. It's like being in a permanent threesome, the kind where one person—not you—gets all the attention.

How do I summarize my sex life before the baby? Well, I had one. I lost my virginity at fifteen, had four partners by the time I was seventeen. I considered myself pansexual, theoretically as open to getting turned on by a coffee table as a person. I had boyfriends and a few girlfriends, some serial monogamy with lots of fucking around in between. I reveled in being provocative. Fueled by alcohol, I instigated group sex at parties. I tried everything I could think of: oral, anal, BDSM, and beyond.

I confused sex with love most of the time, and sometimes that was okay and sometimes it wasn't.

I met Ken when I was 25 and he was 34. What we had was probably typical: In the beginning it was all love and lust, fucking in bathrooms and trains, dancing all night, having sex all day, experimenting madly, and feeling like we couldn't get enough of each other. Eventually, of course, we did get enough of each other and slowed down. On weekend mornings, we did nothing but fuck and eat and read the paper. Then weekend mornings became more and more about reading the paper.

When I hit 30, we decided we were ready for a baby. Sex without birth control was hot. I hadn't fucked without a condom since I was eighteen, and the skin-on-skin friction was arousing, but so was the idea of sex as an extension of humanity, of something bigger than just us. I had one of those dream pregnancies—I exercised every day, felt great, and looked fabulous. It suited me, and I reveled in it. I had new tits that I absolutely adored. A certain type of man paid me a lot of attention. The hormones were like being on E all the time; my husband and I had sex every day. At parties I listen-ed politely to the horror stories of couples who didn't have sex for four months after their babies were born and was privately dismissive: "That'll never happen to us."

But we were, in fact, just like everyone else: Our sex life went down the toilet right away. It started with the birth, which didn't go as planned. Felix was premature, so I had him in a hospital with labor-inducing drugs, not in a hot tub with a midwife. Still, I refused painkillers because I had this fantasy that I was gonna be a rock star in there.

I wasn't. I was in diabolical pain and shat everywhere, including standing up on the bed while barking at the nurse, "No I'm not having the baby I'm just taking a shit put something underneath me now."

This essay originally appeared—in slightly different form—on Nerve.com.

The worst part: I ripped open, requiring more than 20 stitches.

I'd never had stitches anywhere before, had never broken a bone. It was quite a shock to be injured, and to be injured *there*. When I finally got the courage to look, it was a huge relief to see that my clitoris was still there, and in the same place. But I discovered a womb with a view. The rumblings I had heard from women, not in complete sentences even, just mumblings of "never the same again"—this is what they were talking about. A swollen mass of red flesh. A gaping hole where tightness had been. I swear I could see my cervix.

"You should try masturbating while breastfeeding. It's *amazing*."

I felt disfigured and damaged. I didn't cry; I shook. *This isn't happening*, I thought. *No one must know.* I blocked any thought or feeling below my waist, wore cleavage-revealing clothing, encasing my milky breasts in black lace bras under ripped-open tank tops. I became obsessed with Kegel exercises.

Eventually, I felt around and masturbated, tentatively. As I became aroused, my breasts squirted milk. That was cool. I felt like a teenage boy trying to see how far he could shoot. When I told this to one of my mommy friends, she said, "You should try masturbating while breastfeeding. It's *amazing*."

I didn't want to miss out. I went home, got out my mini-massager and settled into the Glider rocking chair with Felix at my breast. Then the doorbell rang.

It was the FedEx man. I buzzed him in, but he couldn't get through the second door, which sticks. So I went to the door in my bra and yoga pants and signed for the envelope with Felix still nursing. When the FedEx man turned to leave, I realized I still had the vibrator in my hand, not my keys, and the second door had closed behind me. I was now stuck in the vestibule with a vibrator and a baby. I rang the bells to my neighbors' apartments, and no one answered.

I started to cry hysterically. It was sleeting and below zero, and *I'm barefoot and practically naked with an infant and where can I go like that and what the fuck was I doing anyway? Only a sick person tries to masturbate with a baby, for God's sake. And I'm locked out of the house and everyone will know what I was doing and...*

Noticing my distress, the FedEx man rang the bell at the house next door. My neighbor—a blue-collar father of three fond of revving his motorcycle at eight in the morning—waved me over. I hid the vibrator under the rug and ran. He settled us on his couch with a blanket and asked if my kitchen window was locked. I whimpered "no," and he went to break into my apartment. I looked at his kids' Crayola drawings and hoped he didn't find the vibrator, or worse yet, step on it and break it.

He came back with one of my coats and asked if I wanted to finish feeding. I mumbled, "No, thank you, thank you," still crying. I ran home, retrieved the dastardly vibrator, threw it in the back of my drawer, and fed Felix tenderly from the other breast, apologizing to him the whole time. I vowed never to masturbate again.

But an hour later I was already thinking how hot that was of my neighbor—taking control and saving me, all knight-in-shining-armor-like, when I was so vulnerable.

That incident crystallized the whole Madonna/whore thing: the feeling that as a mother, I wasn't allowed to be sexual. My black bras and obvious cleavage were meant to counteract that notion, and they may have fooled other people, but I couldn't trick myself into feeling sexual, or even sexy. I desperately wanted to subvert the image, but I was just like everyone else.

When Felix was two months old, I decided that my husband and I absolutely had to have sex. I didn't feel like it, but I was so paranoid about us losing our sex life that I started something. We fooled around on the couch while Felix took a nap in the bedroom.

I was terrified that it would hurt, that I wouldn't get turned on, that I wouldn't be able to come, that it just wouldn't work. I was scared that he was so turned off by seeing a baby come out that he wouldn't want to go in. And he didn't. He found my clitoris and stayed there. We had a gentle session of mutual masturbation and regained some sense of intimacy.

But still, no intercourse. Despite my doctor's reassurance that I was healing well, I had convinced myself that sex would be unbearably painful. At the suggestion of my shrink, I gave myself a "sex hour" while the baby napped. The idea was to experience the pain I anticipated by myself, so I would know what to expect. While Felix gurgled in my arms, I got everything out and ready to go. I put a towel in my rocking chair. On the coffee table I lined up two dildos, a butt plug, some lesbian porn, three vibrators, and two bottles of lube. I was nothing if not prepared.

As soon as Felix was asleep and situated in his crib, I put in *Lez Be Friends*. But the close-ups just made me think of changing diapers. I used a lot of lubricant and inserted the narrowest dildo carefully. It didn't hurt as much as I thought it would. I was determined to get turned on, and when I did, it felt like it was happening to someone else. I came, but not in that supercalifragilistic-Prince-song-sex-relief way that I used to. My orgasm was almost in spite of itself.

At a yoga class a few weeks later, I felt my muscles, my bones, my skin, for the first time in months. I realized that I literally don't feel my body anymore. Before I gave birth, every bump and bruise would send me to the chiropractor. Now I was sure my back was screwed up from hunching while nursing and carrying car seats and strollers, but I didn't even notice. My body was no longer mine.

I knew that no one has sex for months after having a baby (except teenagers, my doctor told me). I knew most of my mommy friends weren't having sex. Felix demanded my attention day and night. So why was I still obsessing over it? I had used sex to fill every possible hole in my life up until the day I gave birth (actually, even on the day I gave birth—I gave Ken a blowjob right before we left to go to the hospital). Now I didn't have any room left; I was full of Felix. The constant motion of early motherhood actually decreased my neuroses. I didn't have the time to worry myself sick by cataloguing my humiliations. I was doing something important: keeping this tiny human alive with milk from my breasts. My body was doing what it was meant to do. I didn't need an orgasm to slam me out of myself.

Still, I missed my husband. One night in bed, I said, "I think you need a nonsexual tour of the region, so that when we do have sex again, you know what you're getting into. Literally." I spread my legs and directed the reading light between them. I opened my sex with my fingers and showed Ken the ridge of scar tissue that stretched diagonally from the right side of my vagina to the left side of my anus. I took his hand so he could feel the area just inside the right wall of my vagina. "This still hurts. That great move you have will have to wait."

He was tentative. "I saw a baby come out of there, " he said. "It's not for fun anymore."

It was understandable that *I* didn't want to have sex, but wasn't he supposed to? My mommy friends were starting to complain about their husbands' libidos. Gisele told me she kept Ernesto happy by giving him a blowjob every three days. I knew that Ken was as busy as I was, as tired and cranky, and in shock at being a father and responsible for our little family. But I hated feeling so undesirable. I hated that even talking about sex was suddenly uncomfortable.

✕✕

Seven months after Felix was born, the three of us came home from an afternoon walk. With Felix still asleep in his stroller, I said, "How about we take a chance he'll stay asleep?" We were both tentative. Ken undressed and got into bed while I went to the bathroom. I didn't want him to see my body, so I took off my jeans and socks, then got into bed and slipped off my underwear, T-shirt, and bra. We didn't look at each other, just hugged hard and tight for a long time, then loosened up and kissed. I took his ass in my hands and noticed it was

softer. I was glad that I wasn't the only one who was out of shape. I had forgotten that just the feeling of his cock in my hand could turn me on.

He put his hand on me, opened me, found the wetness inside, rubbed my clitoris until I told him to fuck me. He put on a condom and entered me gently, missionary position. I would have preferred the heat of his penis, but there was no way I was going to have sex without birth control. I kept asking him to look at me. I wanted not to be invisible.

It was a little uncomfortable, but not the body-wracking pain that I expected. I relaxed into the pleasure of being fucked. After awhile he came, looking in my eyes, then lay next to me and used his hand to get me off.

Afterward, I asked the million-dollar question. "Does it feel different inside?"

"Not really...maybe a little.... To tell you the truth, it's been so long...."

We laughed. I realized I missed the afterwards as much as the sex: the hormone high, the smell.

After that night, we had sex every week or two for a few months. Then it dwindled away again. Felix grew. He needed more; I had less. Our romantic little family was actually

"I saw a baby come out of there," he said. "It's not for fun anymore."

a small corporation. We were really tired. Familiarity breeds contempt. Resentment builds upon resentment. We lost our humor.

⌣

I love my son more than I love my husband. I didn't come to this realization; it was just there one day, and it always had been there, from the day Felix was born. I know Felix's body better than I know my own. Right now, his ear is exactly as long as my middle finger from knuckle to tip. He has a patch of dry skin on his left shin. His fingers still splay like starfish, hot against my skin. I lean in too close; I want to get a whiff of his breath. When I read him a book, I surreptitiously press my lips to his hair over and over, very lightly so he won't notice and bat my hand away. He knows I'm too into him. When I feed him, he pushes my face away. He wants the breast and the milk, not the mother. I'm terrified he'll grow up to be one of those boys in high school who only look at women's breasts, not their faces. I worry that I will be jealous of his girlfriends. I never thought I'd be the type to try to create a mama's boy, but I have a weak character.

Sometimes I'm afraid I go too far. I linger a little too long when I look at his little, dimpled ass. I enjoy it too much when I put lotion on after his bath. I know everybody loves a naked baby; I know children are inherently sexual; I know it's normal to be turned on by your infant. One fatherhood book has a sidebar that tells new dads not to get freaked out if they get a hard-on. But this is tricky territory. Is it wrong to encourage him to touch himself during his few diaper-free minutes? Is it okay to think of my baby when I masturbate? Is that just a manifestation of his all-consumingness? Babies are like a gas—they expand to fit all available space.

But I worry that I'll subtly cross the line, that the sexuality I share with Felix will fuck him up. My parents never talked to me about sex; my son may have the opposite problem. In my mind, I can fuzzily see the progression from innocent play to abuse. They are little; they are yours; you forget that they have their own wants and needs; you think you can do anything with them, for them, to them.

I would never abuse my child, but I understand a little those who do.

Sometimes when Felix takes his nap, I get out the Hitachi. I don't think about my husband. Nor do I think about Johnny Knoxville, or that butch dyke at the coffee shop, or being taken from behind by a faceless stranger. Right after the baby was born, I imagined mothers licking my wounds. Now I think about other men who are fathers. Sexy men, new men, but fathers. Tackily enough, my friends' husbands. They would understand the leaking breasts, the extra pounds around the hips, the moodiness.

But always, my thoughts turn to Felix. I have a hard time concentrating on my clitoris, even with all that roaring power on it. I start thinking of when his next doctor's appointment is, or how cute it is that *yellow* and *sausage* are his first multisyllabic words.

For someone who has, for better or worse, gotten strength and power from being desired, I am now operating unsuccessfully in two parallel universes. On one hand, I have never been so desired in my life. Felix ravages my breasts as no one else ever has. It's not sexual hunger—it's actual hunger. Even now, at a year and half, he runs from across the room at the sight of them, tackles me onto the floor or couch, climbs up my body until he's within reach, then draws back and takes a good look, grins and goes in for the attack. People always say of breastfeeding, "It's sensual, not sexual." But it *is* sexual. He nuzzles and paws at me, grunts, throws his head from side to side as he latches on, his pink mouth warm on my nipple. He tries to get as much as he can into his mouth as his whole body burrows into me, his little heels digging into my thighs and still-soft belly. He kneads the breast he's nursing from with his hand to get more milk, and uses his free hand

to tweak, twist, and pull on my other nipple. I wonder if he's holding onto it protectively, so no one else can get it.

Who would give up being desired like that? Not me. Because the opposite universe is the one in which no one wants me. I'm a mother; I have little to no value to the outside world.

In keeping with our Felix-centered life, two months ago my husband and I invited 32 babies and their parents to a Valentine's baby brunch. We bought cases of cheap champagne, and the parents we know from yoga and work and the playground ate quiche and bagels, got drunk, and pretended it was a kids' party. I started drinking at two. By 9:30, after the last guests left, I slurred to Ken, "I love Felix more than I love you."

It was the first time I'd said it out loud. I continued: "And you love Felix more than you love me. What's up with that? I want you to love me more than you love him, but I still want it to be okay for me to love him more than you."

Despite my drunkenness, he was patient. "It's different, that's all," he said. "It's a different kind of love."

"It doesn't matter," I said, then passed out. Happy Valentine's Day, honey.

My husband and I are fully in the cult of the kid. Our culture now rewards long-term breastfeeding and spending $800 on a stroller. We are supposed to sacrifice everything for our children: certainly sex, even romance. But I want to have a romantic life with my husband. I don't want to wake up when Felix is in school, or going off to college, and not know who Ken is. I want to be a model of erotic love for Felix to learn from.

I'd like to be able to say that by applying the golden rule of threesomes—play with everyone and take turns—I could come to some reckoning, but I can't. I can't resolve my sexuality changing, nor the placement of my erotic longing onto my son, nor my worries about psychologically damaging him. My husband gamely says, "It's okay; it's just all about you two for now." I try out the long view and understand that this is just a phase. I will stop breastfeeding Felix eventually; he'll get older and more independent; our physical attachment will decrease; he will probably not turn into an ax murderer as a result. I'm not sure where that leaves Ken and me. Maybe we'll wind up scheduling sex, like the advice columns tell you to. It sounds more businesslike than bold. But as I recall, a *ménage a trois* is difficult to negotiate: all those jangling limbs and sensitive egos, desires and expectations clashing up against one another, all that excitement and disappointment keeping each other in check.

A Middle-Age Manifesto

How I Stopped Worrying and Learned to Love the Lube

Debra Hyde

It hardly seems possible that years have passed since a movie made waves with its portrayal of older people having sex, but that's what *Something's Gotta Give* did in 2003. Granted, the thought of Jack Nicholson getting it on has a certain gross-out factor to it, but I felt the same way over 30 years ago when I saw a much younger Nicholson bed a very busty Sally Struthers in *Five Easy Pieces*. But that's a Jack Nicholson thing, not an old-people-sex thing.

The public response to the consummation of Nicholson's and Diane Keaton's characters was, however, revealing. It told us that we're far more inherently invested in our youth culture than we know. It showed we think more of a man seeking young trophies over engaging in a peer pairing. The movie spoke volumes about our attitudes towards sex and aging.

Certainly, the under-35 crowd reacted as if they'd seen their own parents going at it, and perhaps they did experience a generational culture shock when they saw that (gasp!) a body goes flabby before the sex drive does. But it also showed us that we have, on the whole, such little respect for and understanding of the human life cycle that we prefer denial and shock to awareness and acceptance. We remain too keen for bodies that are perky or taut in all the right places. Mothers I'd Love to Fuck (MILFs) count only if they're relatively young-looking, thin, and insatiably horny. Grandmothers remain off-limits, even if they're out looking for it.

However, Keaton's and Nicholson's aging bodies held forth a truth and reality: Most of the American population looks like them. Not like Pitt and Jolie. Or J-Lo and whomever. Most of America is growing older. Fact is, of those born during that post-War population bulge that made demographers bug-eyed, the eldest are now nearing 60. And most sport bodies akin to Keaton and Nicholson.

Yes, I know. We're all tired of "boomers this" and "boomers that," but the fact remains that there's a reason HBO's *Real Sex* doesn't always show lithe, svelte bodies. Most of America is flabby, fattening, and horny—and you're going to see it reflected in everything from documentaries about swinger events to commercials hyping erectile functioning.

I know; I'm among those aging boomers. Born smack-dab in the middle of boomerhood's near-20-year birth span, I was a child when the Beatles came ashore, a (now so-called) tween when the Monkees were over and Woodstock was happening, and a young woman when women's lib, the sexual revolution, and gay rights converged on my consciousness. I went through my teen years and into early adulthood loving sex and hating disco with the best of them.

But as the 1970s ebbed and college ended, I shrugged off drugs and shrugged on a corporate suit, then cast the career aside to become a suburban mom (perhaps of ill repute—I

A body goes flabby before the sex drive does.

never entirely gave up my contrary, iconoclastic ways). Today, I'm slouching towards a life event that a mere 20 years ago seemed implausible: menopause. More specifically, I have a front-row seat to that dazzling pre-show called peri-menopause.

Certainly, life has always presented bodily challenges. It wasn't a delight when my body began to shed its tautness as my twenties waned and when multiple childbirths hastened changes in physical appearances during my thirties, but it was another thing entirely when my first hot flash forced me to sit down to avoid fainting. Life smacked me upside the head when, to avoid a suffocating perspiration, I dropped a layer of clothing, only to sit confounded as the sweat evaporated and chills ensued.

Perimenopause is night sweats, aching ankles, and insomnia. It's the onset of bladder weakness and constipation, thanks to a drooping pelvic floor. It's puberty in reverse, where lessening hormones change the body almost as profoundly as the dictates of raging hormones did decades earlier.

Yet however flabby the flesh might be, it's still quite willing. Desire does not end when hot flashes commence. The urge to satisfy myself has not abated, nor has the need to share a moment's lust with my lover, and as long as the heat still rises from the pavement of my libido, I'm indulging.

However cliché it sounds, with age comes wisdom. My lover and I might well be older and uglier, but wisdom lets us cast off the last vestiges of youthful repression as we endeavor in what might be our last erotic hurrah, may it last a decade or longer. No longer ignoring our urges for the sake of the status quo, our fucking includes bondage and whips, dominance and submission, teasing and spanking. Sex includes erotic thrills that we were unaware of in our younger days and are now eager for in our latter years. It's an extended foreplay of the rough sort that culminates in clutching and coming and completion, the likes of which leave us slack-jawed and silly.

It's puberty in reverse, where lessening hormones change the body almost as profoundly as the dictates of raging hormones did decades earlier.

We also find ourselves expanding our repertoire by revisiting older practices that, in by-gone days, one abandoned the instant necking and petting gave way to fucking. At our age, running five miles might make one too tired to fuck, but one is never, it would seem, too tired for an orgasm, and we've acquired a whole new appreciation for the handjob. The erotic connection it provides is surprisingly exciting. Plus, really, just how tame is a handjob when my hands are bound by rope and his dick is aimed at my tits? When his climax involves my grip pulling his sac tight while he frantically jerks off?

All this hectic hedonism might make you think that we're making up for lost time, and I suppose an element of that did exist in the early days of our erotic union. But these days, we indulge because we're still mutually aroused by the sight of each other, we still rise to the thrill of sex (however we define it on any given day), and we absolutely delight in the languor of afterglow. Where the vagaries of modern life try to stress us apart, sex keeps us tightly unioned and mutually appreciative. It provides a consummate excitement, release, and closeness unmatched elsewhere in life.

However, aging hasn't been without its sexual pitfalls and limitations. My libido is depressed as often as it rages, and I'm ever aware of those "flat days" where my body feels like dead wood. Hormone depletion has left me susceptible to yeast infections, and that drooping pelvic floor of mine has made emptying my bladder before fucking a necessity.

But no one change has affected me more than the pinnacle I reached a few months ago: vaginal dryness.

Unlike other symptoms, vaginal dryness was proof undeniable that I was aging, and it represented a loss far more profound than I ever suspected possible. Getting wet was the agent provocateur to my personal eagerness. It symbolized spontaneity, and spontaneity, I suppose, is a thing of youth. Getting wet meant I wasn't really, noticeably aging. It was my form of delight and denial.

The lack of lubricant meant only one thing: My cunt was getting old.

Waning had truly commenced, and I mourned my loss of lubrication. I missed it intensely, especially because my lover could no longer penetrate me without leaving me sore, and readying for sex came to include logistics much like those condoms required in more promiscuous times. As well, I began to question my sex drive's life expectancy, wondering if my capacity to orgasm would soon evaporate. And if I failed to orgasm, would I be able to enjoy sex? If my sex drive failed first, how would that affect our couplehood?

But those were, it turns out, the worries of neurosis, not the realities of the body. I still come—often, in fact. I'm still intensely curious about sex and still long for it. I masturbate, and I still have dreams that, while they don't quite rise to the level of wet, they certainly wake me up, wanting. My concrete experiences didn't match my worries, and I told myself to stop worrying.

About the same time that I realized my drive had not abated, a quite unexpected and fortunate shift in perception occurred: I became aroused and expectant at the overt snap of a lube lid. It—and the more covert sound of him coating his cock in liquid assistance—reaches my lizard brain and makes its primal connections fire. These sounds mean I'm about to get fucked and, savoring sex, I await these new hints every time we get naked.

Other expectations also entered my erotic likings. I began to relish how easy and fierce penetration had become. I love how he sinks into me, and I marvel at how much harder he feels in that one initial push than he had in the several strokes it used to take to penetrate me.

However Pavlovian, I find myself responding to these new cues. I've learned to love the lube.

I have a new sense of sexual readiness, thanks to this subtle acclimation-turned-eroticism. I have a new mechanism on which to ping, and it has retooled the act of—and the art of—fucking for me. For now, those are enough new tricks to counter dwindling abilities.

Time will, of course, continue its onward march. I won't claim to know what will come to me as perimenopause slides into outright menopause or how I will react to it. But I am girding myself for battle. I'm filing away menopausal help tips—estrogen suppositories! vegetable laxatives!—and I aim to preserve my sex drive for as long as possible. I plan to be an activist consumer, pestering my OB/GYN to assist me in my crusade.

I know, too, that someday my middle will thicken, and my wrinkles will crease deeper. Time will someday render me older, then aged. But as long as I'm still capable of luring my

The lack of lubricant meant only one thing: My cunt was getting old.

partner into bed, as long as we consume each other in love and lust, I'll consider life a frolic. A big, phat, naked frolic.

And you know what? The rest of the world should just get over it.

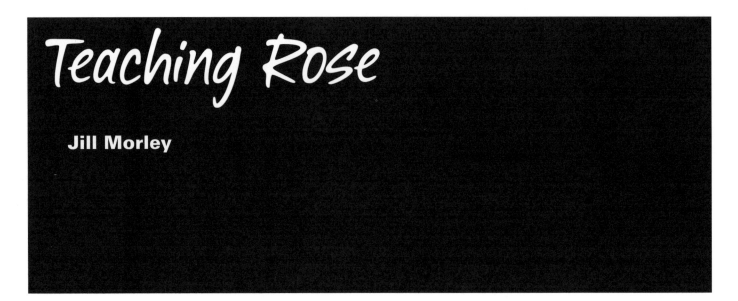

Teaching Rose

Jill Morley

She met me at the door in a black, sequined thong bikini and white feather boa. Not what I expected. Don't get me wrong, I knew she wanted to learn erotic dance, but at 71, you'd think she'd take it slow. Not Rose.

She had approached me after one of my shows. Said she liked the way I danced and asked if I taught stripping. She had been fascinated with it after going to a strip club a few years before with a male friend and had been looking for a teacher ever since. She was just now getting the courage to do it. A little late in life, she admitted, but she figured she could still dance for women, since men "probably wouldn't want to see an old bag like me" dance erotically. Even though she was in good shape and looked about 45, she knew men liked their

How could this woman of 71 get all giddy over getting half-naked in public the way I did at 23?

beer cold and their women young. But she wanted to make a statement. And she wanted to do it topless.

I never taught stripping before. The concept seemed ridiculous. I even told her the moves basically came from a feeling and it was a matter of connecting to that feeling. Not hours of learning endless choreography. In a way, I felt deceitful agreeing to teach her this trade for $40 an hour. For me and most strippers, it is strictly on-the-job training. Connecting to the female instinct, right there on the playing field. My definition of erotic dancing would be this: the ability to generate a magnetic sexual pull with one's hips.

The thought crossed my mind that she could be an old lesbian having her kinky little way with me, but I figured I had exploited my body in way worse situations. This would be a piece of

cake. Another notch in my G-string. Besides, I wanted to ask her what "fascinated" her about it. At 30, I'd quit actual go-go dancing two years ago, and I'm over it. The novelty played itself out. I do a one-woman show about my experience as a go-go girl, using dance to glue scenes together and to show how different characters strip, but I always look forward to the end when I can put my jeans and T-shirt back on. How could this woman of 71 get all giddy over getting half-naked in public the way I did at 23?

I barely remember the thrill of revealing some skin for the first time. It was at a sports go-go bar in Hackensack. A former tomboy, I've always had an athletic body. But the boys would rather have had me be their shortstop than their girlfriend. I always felt like a linebacker in a prom dress, but there on the peanut-shelled Hackensack stage, I was a half-naked prom queen, all eyes focused on me. I pictured my fair-skinned, bikini-clad body swinging around the pole in slow motion, my brown eyes shining mysteriously, long auburn hair flowing like a L'Oréal commercial. All the attention I never got as an awkward adolescent, I got in droves as a New Jersey stripper.

It didn't take long for that life to get old. The thrill was gone after a few years. When I stopped valuing that kind of attention, grew tired of it, even repulsed by it at times, I had to quit. I wrote my show about that journey, *True Confessions of a Go-Go Girl*, and performed it in New York City. Who knew it would ignite the spirit of Rose?

Rose had watched my show attentively in the front row, hands folded on her lap. Dressed in a black silk, button-down blouse and slacks, she looked like she could have been one of my mom's neighbors in suburban New Jersey. She had dark, wiry hair and wore big eyeglasses that took up much of her face. Despite her age, she was rapt, like a small child studying a bug on a flower.

I was slightly nervous riding my bike to her apartment on the day of our first lesson, but I laughed to myself. I had no idea what I would teach her. Just figured I would turn the music on and take it from there. For comfort, I wore sweats, sneakers, and put my long, greasy hair in a ponytail. Yes, I dress for comfort now, not to sexually arouse. Especially when I'm to teach erotic dancing to a septuagenarian. I paused just before knocking on the door.

Rose opened the door wide, exposing much of her body to any neighbor who might have been passing in the hall. "Hi, Jill, is this okay to work in?" she asked. Her choice of weaponry was a black, sequined bikini with fishnets.

"Uh, yeah, sure." I actually got a little self-conscious and hoped she didn't expect me to strip down the way she was. I totally thought she'd be in workout clothes, but God bless her. There she was.

"I got it at Patricia Fields on sale," she said proudly as she flipped her boa over her shoulder. Pat Fields was where all the strippers shopped. We even got discounts just for being strippers. I could tell Rose was working on being an insider.

Her body was surprisingly shapely and strong. She told me she had been doing yoga, weight lifting, and taking a Pilates class to increase her strength and flexibility. Her back and arms were powerful, her legs well-formed, and her figure hourglass. There was barely any sort of varicose vein action happening, or loose skin. She told me she'd had her breasts done six months before so they would look firm again for topless dancing. Her surgeon asked why she was getting them done at her age. When she told him, he thought she was nuts but wished her luck. One of her young gay male friends, Daryl, nursed her while she was in recovery. The breasts did look firm, but each had a scar going from the nipple to just under the curve of the breast. She planned on getting tattoos to cover up the scars. Maybe roses.

Already, she was experimenting with stick-on tattoos. Today, she had a dragon on her thigh and black nail polish on her toenails. No piercings yet, but the lady was hardcore. Beat-up combat boots stood in a corner of her living room. Most of her boyfriends, she said, were a lot younger, sometimes half her age. The men her age usually sat on park benches outside her building, feeding pigeons. She couldn't exactly relate to that. The black sheep of her family, she was always known for doing her own thing. Her family accepted her but thought her eccentric.

All her life, she said, she had a good body and would get catcalls when she walked down the street. She loved that. "Lived off" that. A natural exhibitionist, she likened herself to a peacock. Rose wanted to prove that it was never too late to learn something new, even if it was erotic dancing taken up by a senior citizen.

A real-estate broker, Rose also ran a bed and breakfast out of her apartment. She charged $75 a night.

"I thought we could work in the guest room because one of the walls is mirrored," she said excitedly. Her high heels plunged into the carpet with each step.

"Are these heels high enough?" Rose asked, kicking up a leg.

"They'll do," I said encouragingly. "Besides, we'll worry about costuming you later. Let's just get to the dancing."

Rose beamed as she pressed play on the box, giving us some Toni Braxton tunes. She told me how sexy Daryl was when he danced to this CD. He had made her a tape of it. We had to play it loudly because the battery on her hearing aid was getting weak.

Standing in the sparse, blue-carpeted room facing the mirror, I started the gyrations first. Shifting my weight from side to

Spreading her legs in a thong bikini in front of her guest-room mirror seemed to do the trick.

side in faded gray sweats, I showed her how to move her hips in figure eights, a staple move. She was a little off at first but eventually picked up the rhythm, arms dangling at her sides. I told her we'd get to arms later and not to feel odd about touching her body. Watching me in the mirror, she copied every move. Once in a while, her heels would get stuck in the carpet.

We did another move she calls "the wave," where you isolate your body much like a cobra. We did this and the figure eights in repetition for about an hour. She started to get the hang of it before I left, and she thanked me for my time. She said she was glad she could learn it that way instead of embarrassing herself somewhere. Then she showed me her breasts up close and told me of her tattoo endeavors.

As our weekly lessons progressed, Rose continued to improve, started using her arms more, and yes, we even got into floor work. At one point, both of us were lying on our backs facing the mirror, legs spread eagle, my feet clad in sneakers, hers in heels. She was loving it. She told me she was really into raunch. That this other woman had taught her burlesque moves but it didn't satisfy her. Spreading her legs in a thong bikini in front of her guest-room mirror seemed to do the trick.

She started experimenting with costumes—red evening gowns, pink spandex, and feather boas. She became an expert at taking off her top and tossing it effortlessly into the air, revealing her newly firm breasts. She'd smirk and a little spark in her eyes would go off whenever she did this maneuver, making it even more of an event.

◎♡

After four months, the time had come. I told Rose I was throwing a party and would like her to dance there. Other people were go-going and she was definitely ready. I knew my friends would love her. Flattered that I would invite her, she asked all kinds of questions, like what should she wear? Should she show up in costume or change when she got there? How many sets should she do? Was she to strip completely naked? Would people be tipping? All sensible stripper questions.

The affair was a glamorous one at a small club in Soho. A designer friend made metallic dresses for some of my girlfriends to wear. Some of the boys were wearing vinyl pants or suits. Many ladies, including Rose, arrived wearing boas.

Slithering sensuously, she held the wall and stuck her ass out, a move I never taught her, but it's a classic.

She came with Daryl, who was there to cheer her on. Girls were already shaking it on the platforms when she arrived. Rose picked a seat on a red velvet couch right next to the go-go girls and deliberately studied their moves.

"You can get changed in the back when you're ready," I said. "But first, you need a stripper name!" We decided to call her "The Rose."

An hour later, after careful observation, The Rose changed into this black lace catsuit with a black bra and thong underneath. When she emerged from the dressing room, a lot of men were staring. Not in a "who does that old broad think she is?" way, but in a "who *is* she?" way.

I guided The Rose to the platform and helped her up. Once she got her balance, she squinted at the colored lights for a millisecond before her exhibitionism kicked in, then she gyrated like nobody's business. Blue and red lights showered her body as she danced. Running her hands over her black lace catsuit, she did the wave. Slithering sensuously, she held the wall and stuck her ass out, a move I never taught her, but it's a classic. Several people gathered around to watch. She definitely looked like an older woman, but she was so sexy that it made me wish I had an army of older strippers dancing on platforms around the room, surrounding us in experience and sensuality. A few men and women went up to tip her.

"She is hot!" my friend Paul said.

"There's no way she's 71," my friend Val said.

"You go, girl!" her friend Daryl said.

She slid the catsuit down over her shoulders to her waist. Then she pulled her bra straps over her shoulders, holding the boa over her breasts. She popped the bra and threw it into the cheering crowd, eyes glinting mischief. With much finesse, she lifted the boa up in the air, revealing her toplessness and rose tattoos. More cheers, applause, and dollars thrown her way. The Rose was a hit.

After her dance, she covered her deflowered breasts and thanked me profusely for the opportunity. I could tell from the sweat on her brow and the glow from her face that she was buzzed from all the excitement. Several people asked her questions and complimented her bravery. When she got dressed, she thanked me again.

She later told me that before she got on the platform, she was in a state of terror. But she made herself do it anyway. A total stripper trait. The reaction from the crowd, she said, was unexpected but inspiring. She went home very satisfied and eager to do it again. She also told me that she had made $12 that night. Unfolded them on her living-room couch and stared at them for hours. Rose said she didn't think she could ever spend them. Not in a million years.

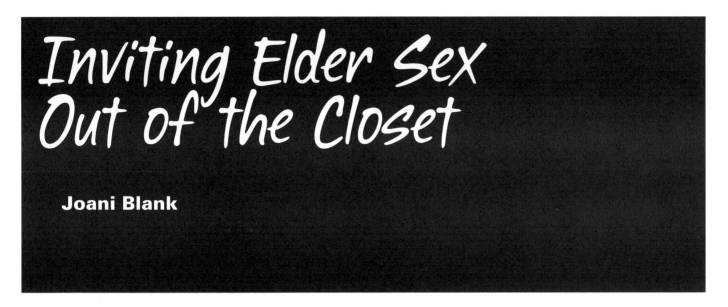

Inviting Elder Sex Out of the Closet

Joani Blank

In 1997, as I approached my sixtieth birthday, I started to wonder what people in their seventh, eighth, and ninth decades were doing sexually. Sex jokes, sarcasm, and cynical statements aside, just about the only words I'd ever heard older women speak about sex were, "I'm too old for all that." Men didn't say much either, but might occasionally suggest that they couldn't "get it up anymore" and therefore were no longer "able" to have sex, even if they wanted to. At the same time, heterosexual men in monogamous marriages or other committed relationships often implied that they'd like to continue being sexual but that their wives or partners were no longer interested or willing.

Nonetheless, there were occasional intimations that an oldster was "still doing it." And I suspected that more older folks were still doing "it" in one variety or another than the dearth of frank talk about sex suggested. I've been in the sex field long enough to know that very few people of any age, and virtually no one over 60, talks openly and honestly about their sex lives—even, in many cases, to their beloved partners. But there is value in helping people to begin talking about sex. And my experience suggests another truth: Once people get started talking, there's often no stopping them.

As I flipped through the few books available on the subject of elder sex, I found that for the most part the content consisted of how to overcome the physical limitations resulting from specific medical problems, as well as those associated with healthy though aging bodies. Societal norms dictate that older people, especially really old people, are not sexual creatures. None of the existing books asked older people to simply tell us what they do and how it feels. In fact, the tone of many of these books is one of grim determination, exhorting the elderly to keep going or to start again.

I thought we needed something better.

I began to solicit stories for an anthology that would recount the great sexual variety and whole-hearted erotic appetite of real older women and men. That anthology, *Still Doing It*, was published in 2000, with a foreword by the legendary sex educator Eleanor "Ranger" Hamilton, my own introduction, and 34 uncensored and exuberant first-person accounts of sex after 60. I was surprised and delighted as the submissions came in by how many of the accounts were not just sexually open but frankly funny, even to the point of being flip. Here's Steve Hamilton, in his seventies, who lives and volunteers in senior housing: "It can be even more fun when your arthritis acts up. Wow! It took us two hours just to get our clothes off! Or, we had to do it twice when we couldn't get out of the tub!"

Throughout my career, when I've recommended that an older person try to start talking a little about sex, I've repeatedly heard the lament: "Nobody in my family talked about sex

Nonetheless, there were occasional intimations that an oldster was "still doing it."

when I was growing up." I usually respond that hardly any of us grew up in a household where family members talked about sex, no matter how liberal or conservative the family, no matter which decade witnessed their growing up.

Why is this? Although our culture has generally moved beyond the narrow moral strictures of sex-for-procreation-only, a significant portion of our population still looks askance at sexual couplings between people who are beyond their reproductive years and casts an even more critical eye on solo sexuality in later years. Those who talk about sex risk the criticism of those around them for going against societal norms.

Another cultural bias that limits elders' sexual options is our idea that sex equals intercourse, that only intercourse really counts as sex. Far too many men and women are still constrained by that idea. If their bodies no longer cooperate in producing the physiological changes required for penis-in-vagina intercourse, they decide that all sexual activity should cease.

Happily, *Still Doing It* is still in print and readily available. What are my ambitions for it as it nears the decade mark?

"Sex is the real reason I jog, work out, gulp down vitamins; all this I do to remain, pardon the expression, fuckable."

I don't expect the stories in *Still Doing It* to convince huge numbers of older readers who are not currently sexually active to suddenly get busy in the bedroom, especially if they have not masturbated or had partner-sex for many years—though I would be delighted if they did! Rather, I'm hoping that the book and its honest experiences help oldsters who are still sexually active to realize that they are far from alone and that their peers engage in as great a range of sexual practices as their younger counterparts. Here's a sampling:

At 70, I'm slowing down to a sprint. I need new glasses (the better to see you with, my dear) and I have more wrinkles, but I have never given up masturbating and fantasizing.

~

She lowered herself and began a gentle, rhythmic thrusting, eyes locked with mine. We shared two bodies, one pleasure, one sure chord between us.

~

We get together about once a month with our two favorite couples, who are both in their fifties. [That from a couple in their seventies.]

~

She has no problem using a dildo/harness [on me]…and she likes me best on my back.

~

This is the best I have ever felt about my sexuality. I no longer fear that people will find out I like being submissive to women.

~

Sex is heaven on Earth, God's reward for the difficult things in our lives. Sex is the real reason I jog, work out, gulp down vitamins; all this I do to

remain, pardon the expression, fuckable.

In fact, many of my contributors are "doing it" more, doing different things, and enjoying it all more—in some cases a great deal more—than they did in their younger years.

I'm also eager that those of us in our twenties, thirties, and forties, whose experience of elderhood is still a few decades away, become more accepting of the sexuality of our parents' generation. In particular I'd love to see a greater openness on the part of younger people toward the sexuality of their own parents, grandparents, and other older family members.

Almost no one can imagine his or her parents being sexual at any age, but it is important that younger adults respect their parents' desire for privacy, excitement about a new boyfriend or girlfriend, or decision to remarry or to live with a lover. Older parents don't want their adult kids meddling in their love lives any more than teenagers want their parents interfering in theirs.

Most of all, I hope *Still Doing It* continues to encourage people in their forties and fifties who may be acutely sensitive to diminishing sexual interest. This group includes those separated or divorced after sometimes lengthy marriages or relationships, those whose sexual problems have been getting worse so gradually they didn't realize it was happening, men who used to be able to take an occasional erectile failure in stride but can no longer do so, women whose desire and sexual interest haven't returned as they had hoped after their children grew up, and those so stressed by busy careers and lives that sex has all but disappeared from their daily lives. I also hope my book still speaks to middle-aged readers who see their current sex lives as happy, to assure them that things don't inevitably get worse with age—and that, indeed, sex may get a whole lot better.

In the original call for submissions for *Still Doing It*, I told potential contributors that they might wish to write about how they had overcome obstacles to fully enjoying their sexuality. Several of the men wrote about specific physical limitations, medical problems, and erection failures. Both men and women wrote in some of these stories about overcoming years of loveless and/or sexless marriages or involuntary celibacy. But mostly their stories describe what does work, not what doesn't, even in the most unusual circumstances—as in this delightful passage from an author who was hospitalized:

With soft sounds he licks and sucks my nipple, drawing the flesh around it up so deftly that I become young and ageless. Sighing, I arch my back and press all of me against him. Just as Peter's

hands slide farther down, a startled nurse crashes into the room. "Are you all right?" she cries. "The monitor at the nurses' station went crazy. Your heartbeat seemed totally out of control."

Flushed and hot from kissing, I smile innocently and say I feel fine. "Could something be wrong with the monitor?" I inquire coyly. [From "Vintage Sex" by Lin Stevens.]

As we age, we all face natural changes in our bodies, ageist anti-sexual attitudes in the world around us, and the deterioration of sexual self-confidence that can result from these attitudes. The people who wrote for *Still Doing It* managed to have a good time despite these obstacles. Some, who were over 60 when the book was published, had the good fortune to be younger adults during the sexual opening that we experienced in the late 1960s and 1970s, and they have no intention of stopping or even slowing down. Even for those who were older at the dawn of the 1970s, more relaxed attitudes toward sex have been beneficial.

During my 30-plus years in the field of human sexuality, and even more, looking back further to the 1950s and my high-school and college years, I've seen significant improvement in our attitudes toward sexuality, specifically as they relate to older people. First, as older people become more independent, they're more willing to engage in sexual activity, with or without the approval of their adult children. Older parents are increasingly less likely to live in the same house, neighborhood, city, or even state as their children or other younger relatives, so they can more readily do as they please away from their children's watchful eyes.

Second, there has been a slight but noticeable improvement in the way the media treat the sexuality of older persons. Sure, jokes about elder sex, some of them quite cruel, still abound. But once in a while a film, TV drama, or sitcom acknowledges the sexuality of older characters in a fairly matter-of-fact way. It's always a pleasant surprise when it is at least implied (though never depicted) that an older couple's sexual activity isn't limited to affectionate glances, embraces, and snuggling.

Third, the overall health of older people continues to improve. We are more attentive to our diets; we exercise more; we stay better informed about the world around us. In sum, we take care of ourselves altogether better than seniors did even a generation ago. Being healthy increases the likelihood that we will be having sex in our older years, and being sexually active undoubtedly helps us live longer in good health.

Physicians and other health professionals are slowly but surely becoming more aware of the sexual issues that may be raised by their patients, as well as being more informed about the sexual effects of medical conditions and medications. Even if they don't ask their patients questions about sexual changes associated with health problems, they may at least offer information, for instance about sexual side effects of medications or about when it is safe to resume sexual activity after surgery or illness. Drug testing is now more likely than in past decades to include consideration of the sexual side effects of new treatments.

Where health professionals fail to volunteer information about sexuality, which still happens far too often, I fervently wish that they would at least be receptive to direct questions from their older patients (as well as those who are younger). Of all helping professionals, physicians are the most likely to be asked questions about sex and the least likely to know the answers. In the 1970s there was a slight increase in the number of medical schools that offered some, but limited, sex education to their students, but now many of these courses are no longer taught.

It has long been known that many people who become clinically depressed lose interest in sex. In fact, depression of any severity takes its toll on libido, in both men and women. Unfortunately, one prevalent side effect of most antidepressants is the inhibition of arousal and/or orgasm. So, ironically, at the same time that anxiety and sadness decrease and the heart and mind open to new sexual possibilities, the body often becomes less responsive. Many people who are taking these medications while in ongoing sexual relationships, however, are happy to trade off some of the sexual heat they remember from past years for the relief from the debilitating

> **I'd love to see a greater openness on the part of younger people toward the sexuality of their own parents, grandparents, and other older family members.**

depressions that had made it virtually impossible for them to connect intimately with their loved ones.

No story in *Still Doing It* mentions Viagra or the other erectile-dysfunction drugs, because they were collected before the blue pill became an overnight sensation. As valuable as Viagra has proven for many men with serious erectile dysfunction, its widespread popularity suggests that both men and women are still firmly in the grip of the intercourse bias. The public's passion for this "wonder drug" implies that it's more important to be able to "perform" than it is to give and receive sexual pleasure. Some of the male contributors to *Still Doing It* may well now use Viagra, but their essays tell happy pre-Viagra stories of fulfilling sex that is only rarely dependent on firm and 100% reliable erections.

✕✕

I'd like to share a passage from the opening story in the book, a remarkable piece by Louise Meadows called "Twilight with Leo," about a couple reunited more than four decades after their high-school romance. Much of the story is gloriously

Of all helping professionals, physicians are the most likely to be asked questions about sex and the least likely to know the answers.

explicit, but this passage sums up, for me, the potentials of senior sexuality:

> Reuniting with Leo after all this time means that I have finally realized my sexuality…. At first, we both suffered profound feelings of regret and remorse that we had endured forty-three years of unpleasant marriages before getting together again. But now we have simply accepted what happened to us and we cherish our bliss. The insights about sex and emotional relationships that I've gained have been phenomenal…. My orgasm lasts longer than Leo's and I experience hours of afterglow following the sex act, during which I love to fondle Leo's body. Ironically, even though we're not legally married (for financial reasons), I now know the meaning of "married love."

A wonderful range of playfulness and heat, connection and love displays itself in the stories of the *Still Doing It* authors. I hope that those virtues are—and remain—a part of your life, and mine.

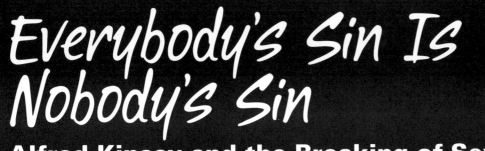

Everybody's Sin Is Nobody's Sin

Alfred Kinsey and the Breaking of Sexual Silence

David Steinberg

In the late 1930s, Alfred Kinsey had what he thought was a rather simple idea: Given that no one had the slightest idea what people really did and did not do sexually, and given—as he discovered from a questionnaire he distributed to his students—that a lack of simple information about sex was causing massive confusion and heartache, why not do a survey that would provide some hard information about people's sexual practices? Why not talk about the unmentionable (sex) and replace sexual ignorance and myth with sexual information and education?

A simple idea, perhaps, but hardly a simple task. How could a group of researchers hope to get people to talk truthfully about their sexuality—about what they did sexually, what they fantasized about, how they felt about it all—when hardly anyone felt free to talk to anyone about sex in the first place?

Kinsey, a dedicated rationalist with precious little understanding of social graces but a disarmingly straightforward way of talking openly about sexual matters, believed that with sincerity and obvious scientific objectivity people could be put sufficiently at ease that they would disclose their sexual histories, their sexual feelings, their innermost sexual secrets. Kinsey's basic method—a contribution to sexual science as profound and long-lasting as the data he produced—was to transcend socially enforced sexual silence so directly and unapologetically that the very act created a bubble of sexual sanity inside a sexually crazy world, a bubble in which speaking honestly and openly about sex was not only permitted but even highly valued and encouraged.

If one wanted to hear people's sexual truths, Kinsey understood, the most important thing was to leave both moral and psychological judgment behind, since it is the fear of being morally or psychologically judged that causes people to keep sexual secrets in the first place.

Engage subjects personally and directly, Kinsey explained to his staff. Make clear that their information is to be used entirely for science, not for prurience, and that anything they confide will be held in strictest confidence. Most of all, demonstrate to subjects—by the nature of the questions asked, by your own demeanor, tone of voice, body posture, facial expressions—that whatever they reveal about their sexuality will be received sympathetically and respectfully, without judgment, without scorn, in the spirit of objectivity and scientific neutrality.

Even if interviewers could make their subjects comfortable and trusting, there was a second problem Kinsey needed to address. What about representative sampling? How could Kinsey get anything like a representative sample of all Americans when he would be lucky to get a significant number of

> **Kinsey's basic method was to transcend socially enforced sexual silence so directly and unapologetically that the very act created a bubble of sexual sanity inside a sexually crazy world.**

people to talk to him at all? Obviously, whoever chose to give Kinsey's researchers their sexual histories would be a self-selected, statistically skewed group.

Kinsey's response—a response acknowledged today to be only partly helpful—was to make his sample as large as possible, since the larger the sample, the less relevant sample skews become. His goal was to take sexual histories from as many as 100,000 people, from hundreds of cultural subgroups he identified, throughout the United States. He managed to interview just under 12,000 before the Rockefeller Foundation pulled the plug on his funding and brought his research to a skidding halt in 1954.

When the first report of Kinsey's findings, *Sexual Behavior in the Human Male*—an 800-page compendium heavy with statistical tables and graphs—was published in 1948, it unexpectedly shot to the top of bestseller lists across the nation, instantly changing the American sex-informational landscape forever. His parallel report on women, *Sexual Behavior in the Human Female*, published in 1953, was also a huge hit with the public. Not surprisingly, the two studies were immediately as controversial as they were popular.

What Kinsey found was that American men and—worse, much worse—American women were more sexually active,

The publication of Kinsey's study in 1948 was the opening salvo of a monumental battle that has been raging ever since—between science (factual information) and religion (moral judgment) on the subject of sex.

more sexually adventurous, more diverse in their sexual desires and activities, more sexually exploratory, more likely to step outside the box of socially approved sexual behavior, than anyone would ever have imagined. Much more.

Even adjusting for Kinsey's potentially skewed samples, his studies made painfully (or excitedly, depending on your point of view) clear that what Americans actually did sexually was completely unrelated to what people previously thought Americans did. The national wall of sexual silence had been breached; the cat was out of the bag. Homosexuality, bisexuality, premarital sex, extramarital sex, postmarital sex, oral sex, anal sex, masturbation, sadomasochism, sex with animals, sex with and among preadolescents and children, sex among older people, sex with prostitutes—all of these were common practices among the grand American populace.

The core assumption of post-war, proscriptive American sexual "normalcy"—that the overwhelming majority of people confined sex to heterosexual intercourse within marriage, generally in the "male-superior" position, and that only rare and occasional deviants would ever so much as think excitedly about transgressing those sexual boundaries—was revealed to be utterly, categorically, devastatingly false. While

the precision of Kinsey's statistics on how many people engaged in various forms of "deviant" sex might be challenged, there were—without question—millions, tens of millions, of Americans whose sexuality ranged all over the forbidden map, and they weren't all going crazy, committing suicide, having their lives turn to ruin, getting pregnant, and dying of grossly disfiguring sexually transmitted diseases, as the popular sex mythology of the day would have predicted.

"Everybody's sin is nobody's sin," Kinsey proclaimed, triumphantly throwing open the doors to what has become a fifty-year-long era of sexual expansion and creativity that half of this strange country welcomes with joy and celebration, and the other half blames for just about everything wrong with the world today.

✕✕

The publication of Kinsey's study in 1948 was the opening salvo of a monumental battle that has been raging ever since—between science (factual information) and religion (moral judgment) on the subject of sex. This ongoing conflict between secular and theological forces for control of sexual desire and behavior in America—a cultural collision as cataclysmic in 2004 as it was in 1948—forms the core of *Kinsey*, Bill Condon's brilliant, complex, and thoughtful film about Alfred Kinsey, his family, his colleagues, and his work.

The film—enthusiastically received by just about everyone in the sexology community (sex educators, researchers, therapists, and counselors) and condemned with equal fervor by a broad spectrum of stalwarts of the religious right, is the latest artistic endeavor to bring into stark relief the core differences in sexual values that continue to split this country right down the middle. It all comes down to whether you believe that Kinsey's phenomenological, fact-based, morally neutral approach to sex, and the information that this approach revealed about the sexual practices of American men and women, was a great leap forward or a great leap backward into an abyss of fire, brimstone, and social dissolution.

A quick survey of mainstream film reviews shows that there is little question that, politics aside, *Kinsey* is a beautifully crafted, brilliantly acted, subtle, nuanced work of art. Aside from publications of the religious right, reviewers have been close to unanimous in their praise of the film, of its director, Bill Condon (*Gods and Monsters*), and of its lead actors, Liam Neeson and Laura Linney. Many reviewers were quick to whisper "Oscar" for Neeson's moving portrayal of Kinsey as a dedicated, somewhat dictatorial, socially awkward researcher, committed to discovering and publicizing the truth about American sexual behavior and desire, regardless of political and social consequences. Linney is stunning as Clara McMillen, Kinsey's freethinking, outspoken, appreciative (though in many ways long-suffering) wife. And John Lithgow brings real depth to the character of Kinsey's Bible-thumping, antisexual father ("Lust has a thousand avenues—the dance hall, the ice cream parlor, the tenement salon, the Turkish bath.... Some speculate that rampant adultery is the cause of earthquakes."), who might easily have been reduced to caricature by a less talented performer.

One of the greatest achievements of *Kinsey* is the subtlety with which it examines the emerging sexual subculture of Kinsey's associates and researchers—what develops, sexually and socially, among a group of people whose personal and professional lives fall decidedly outside of society's sexual norms. The film shows Kinsey, McMillen, and most of their inner circle enthusiastically acting out their belief in sexual openness between consenting partners, but then having to deal with the complicated emotional consequences of their multiple involvements—a task that takes them well outside the comfortable realm of scientific objectivity. To its credit, *Kinsey* depicts their nonmonogamous pathfinding as neither a lighthearted romp through fields of unlimited sexual pleasure nor a foolhardy error of sexual excess, offering instead a sympathetic look at a group of people committed to bringing the radicalism of their sexual politics into their personal lives, and struggling—successfully, for the most part—with the sometimes painful, potentially destructive emotional and relational issues that their actions call into play.

Kinsey paints an amusing (and horrifying) picture of the predominant sexual culture of the 1930s, offering a collage of the sorts of sexual misunderstandings that spurred one young zoology professor to undertake a huge sexual survey that would change the belief system of the nation. Cunnilingus, it was commonly believed, would result in a woman becoming infertile. Sexual intercourse was the only form of sex worth pursuing, once available (in marriage). A boy who masturbates is likely to be "sexually dead" as an adult. As for manually stimulating women for arousal, *Kinsey* offers this quote from *The Ideal Marriage*, the leading sexual guide of the day: "There is but one finger of love to approach the female genitalia and that is the male penis."

The film shows that it was Kinsey's desire to debunk these sorts of sexually destructive myths that inspired him to undertake his monumental work. "The lack of information on what people do sexually leaves most of us feeling anxious or guilty," he instructs students in his popular course on human sexuality (available only to those who were married, engaged, or could pretend as much). "The gap between what we assume people do and what they actually do is enormous."

As Kinsey states in his introduction to *Sexual Behavior in the Human Male*, his purpose was to obtain "an accumulation of scientific fact [about sexual behavior] completely divorced from questions of moral value and social custom." This is Kinsey's Great Heresy—daring to separate scientific information about sex from the mediating influences of morality and social convention. But to Kinsey, issues of morality and convention only muddy the waters, only act to prevent people from telling the truth about sex—to themselves as well as to others. "The only way to study sex with scientific accuracy is to strip away everything but physiology," Kinsey says. As for love: "It's impossible to measure love, and without measurement there can be no science. When it comes to love, we're all in the dark."

Condon's main purpose with this film is clearly to tell the Kinsey story as history, but he is obviously aware of the allegorical parallels between what Kinsey faced in 1948 and what advocates of sexual truth, information, openness, and diversity face in the US today, and he effectively uses the film as a forum for the importance of all of the above.

The film is a virtual paean to diversity in all its forms, sexual and otherwise, a diversity Kinsey discovered while studying the gall wasp long before he became interested in human sexual behavior. Kinsey collected and catalogued over one million (!) gall wasps, intrigued that no two of them were ever alike. "If every single living thing is different from every other living thing," Kinsey exults, "then diversity becomes life's one irreducible fact." As for humans, "Everyone is different," he proclaims. "The problem is that everyone wants to be the

"The gap between what we assume people do and what they actually do is enormous."

same. They're so eager to be part of the group that they're willing to betray their inner nature to get there."

Kinsey is full of references and scenes that, on one hand, are about the misunderstandings and political backlash that Kinsey faced in the 1950s, but at a second level speak equally strongly to the sexual political struggles we face today. "In a puritan culture, sex remains a dirty secret," Kinsey says, for then and for now, adding: "Sexual morality needs to be reformed, and science will show the way."

Challenged by a political movement that seeks to discredit and undermine his work, Kinsey angrily responds, "The forces of chastity are mobilizing once again to challenge the scientist, intimidate him, convince him to cease his research." Again, words that are as timely today as they were when Kinsey uttered them fifty years ago.

As conservative outrage mounted over his studies, Kinsey was accused in Congress of being part of the Communist conspiracy to undermine American morals, and pressure was brought on his financial benefactor, the Rockefeller Foundation, to disassociate itself from his work. Fearing political backlash, the Foundation agreed to back out of "the business of sex research," offering the sorry excuse that Kinsey was now in a position to get funding from other sources. That proved not to be the case. Attempts to find other sources of funds—Indiana University, the Huntington Hartford Foundation—all failed. In 1954, no one wanted to jump into the sexual fires that Kinsey's books had ignited.

"[A grant] might be misunderstood as an endorsement of sex," Huntington Hartford explains to Kinsey, apologetically, at the end of a dinner party awash in chic sexual conversation and innuendo. "I can't afford that kind of exposure."

Nine additional books that Kinsey hoped to publish never came into existence. His dream of expanding his 12,000 sex histories to a larger sample of 100,000 also never came to pass. Lost in a sea of defeat, Kinsey grew increasingly depressed. He died of a heart ailment and pneumonia in 1956, just two years after losing his Rockefeller funding.

Is sex most fundamentally a moral issue or a psychological one? Does one arrive at a sense of sexual ethics from a preordained list of proper and improper acts and partners or by paying respectful attention to the dynamics of intimate interconnectedness, pursuit of pleasure, and possibilities of mutual personal discovery? Is sex, most basically, something to be studied, observed, and explored, or something to be controlled, limited, and feared?

Having failed to pressure Liam Neeson to back away from starring in the film, conservative Christian groups mounted a national campaign to discredit both *Kinsey* the film and Kinsey the man.

Do we seek to understand sex from the standpoint of rational, scientific study, or from the perspective of undocumented myths and rigid moral beliefs? Do we address sex from a fact-based or from a belief-based point of view?

These issues, the ones that made Kinsey's work so controversial in 1948, are very much the subject of intense national debate today. So it's not surprising that the release of *Kinsey* stirred up yet another storm of antisexual protest. The idea of a film—especially a strong, well-produced, well-received film—that honors Kinsey for his contribution to moving the US out of the sexual dark ages infuriates sexual conservatives. Having failed to pressure Liam Neeson to back away from starring in the film, conservative Christian groups mounted a national campaign to discredit both *Kinsey* the film and Kinsey the man.

Generation Life, a collegiate anti-abortion group, planned to picket theaters showing the film nationwide, objecting to Kinsey's "pseudo-scientific defense of sexual perversions" and his responsibility "for my generation being forced to deal face-to-face with the devastating consequences of sexually transmitted diseases, pornography, and abortion," according to Generation Life spokesperson Brandi Swindell. Morality in Media president Robert Peters dismissed *Kinsey* as "an effort to rehabilitate a father of the hellish sexual revolution."

In the words of Arlen Williams, a conservative Illinois columnist, "A movie is now being shown that promotes one of the most evil and destructive figures in the 20th Century"—Alfred Kinsey, "Darwinist zoologist, sex researcher, sex research defrauder, sexual anti-moralist, sexual abuse enabler, personally sexual pervert [sic], and pseudo-scientific high priest of the Sexual Revolution." The issue, to Williams, is straightforward enough—the divide between those who remember "the harmful practices of sin" and "those who uphold [the idea that] life may be enjoyed from beginning through end."

Robert Knight, director of the Culture and Family Institute, and spokesperson for Concerned Women for America, similarly bemoaned Kinsey's contribution to the changing sex culture of the last sixty years. "Kinsey's conclusions paved the way for condom-based sex education in...schools," he said, "and furthered the agenda of pro-abortion groups.... From abortion to homosexuality to pornography, Kinsey's research has been cited as proof [that] science has done away with societal [sexual] restraints based on religious beliefs."

Knight, who says that "Kinsey's proper place is with Nazi doctor Josef Mengele," called Kinsey "a sexual revolutionary masquerading as an objective scientist."

What Knight fails to realize is the sad fact that, in a culture as irrationally antisexual as ours, just being an objective scientist who dares to study sex itself makes a person a sexual revolutionary of the highest order. In a social system based on sexual ignorance and misinformation, the very idea of sexual science, sexual knowledge, and sexual understanding is subversive.

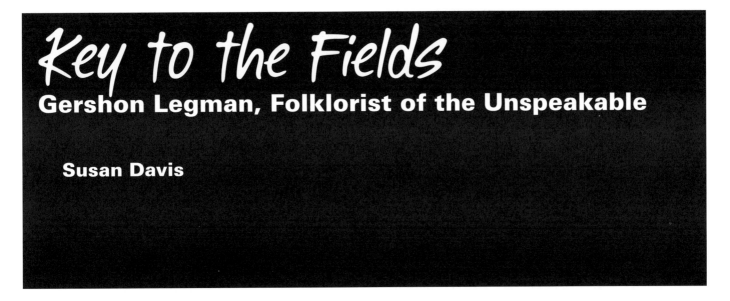

Key to the Fields
Gershon Legman, Folklorist of the Unspeakable

Susan Davis

To take the key to the fields—*prendre la clé des champs*—means to take one's freedom, to walk out and away from the town or farm. Gershon Legman—folklorist, sexologist, and social critic—chose this old French saying to name the homestead he made for himself in the south of France. It carried for him those senses of radical personal freedom: away from the city, away from old ties, and especially away from the censorship of Cold War America.

Born in 1917, Legman made an unprecedented career for himself as he struggled to write the unspeakable and publish the unprintable. He constructed an intellectual life off the radar of official culture, embodying and prefiguring radical ways of writing about sex. Uncharted lives are often worth knowing about, and to look closely at the work and life of this energetic and learned man is to see the price and prizes of intellectual freedom.

As Legman tells us in his unpublished autobiography, "sex was always very important" to him. From an early age, he was absorbed in "a million dreamlike projects, all invariably and very intimately connected with sex, sex technique, sexual folklore, its language, its literature and its immemorially practical and beautiful art." He collected, documented, and analyzed sex practices, dedicating himself to making anyone within earshot admit what could not be admitted about sex and culture. Prophetic, he was unassimilable.

By the early 1950s, it had become impossible for Legman to publish and distribute his own books and magazines in the United States. He had been spied on by the FBI, threatened with arrest by the State of New York, and he lost his mail-based magazine-publishing business to Post Office censors.

He'd seen publishing friends jailed for distributing erotica, seen those friends knuckle under. Perhaps worse, his books had been confiscated, which meant no one could read them. His work risked invisibility. In 1953, Legman did something sensible and radical. He left his home in the Bronx and moved to Paris to work for West 57th Street publisher and bookseller Seymour Hacker.

Hacker wanted to bring out books in Paris that could not legally be printed in the United States. From France they would trickle out to an English-speaking readership, even make their way to North America, not incidentally enriching Hacker. Legman's widow, Judith, writes that the publisher needed "somebody who would be willing to be on the spot for a period of several weeks to read proof for the French printers…someone who knew something about printing, to watch over the process and make sure the books were bound up in the right order.… Hacker may have bought the ticket that took Gershon to Paris to do this work for him."

He had been spied on by the FBI, threatened with arrest by the State of New York, and he lost his mail-based magazine-publishing business to Post Office censors.

In France, Legman could continue writing on sex in a lively expatriate atmosphere, and it was a lot cheaper than New York, where there was a housing shortage and a postwar slump. With his unparalleled bibliographic skills in several languages, including French and German, Legman probably also scouted erotica for Hacker and others; he may have conducted a small book-buying and -selling business of his own. His first wife, Beverley Keith, a skilled translator, helped out. Here he walked in the footsteps of the pornographer and poet Pierre

Louÿs and made friends with Maurice Girodias, founder of the Olympia Press and specialist in the most adventurous literary and trashy erotica. (Girodias was the son of Jack Kahane, original publisher of Anaïs Nin and Henry Miller.) Legman hung out with many other artists and intellectuals, European and expatriate Americans, making particular friends with Richard Wright.

But, eventually, the lure of Paris faded. Using a train ticket given in lieu of a paycheck, he and Beverley traveled south to Cagnes-sur-Mer and found they liked the Riviera. For several years they lived in the little towns of the Nice-Cannes back country, always shifting when the landlady needed her rooms for summer tourists. Finally, in 1960, they were able to use Beverley's small inheritance—she was the daughter of a wealthy Canadian family—to buy the remnants of a farm, a few acres of olive trees and an old goat barn. La Clé des Champs stands on the road between the sixteenth-century walled town of Valbonne and Opio, a tiny village perched above the highway to Grasse.

The place was remote and rustic; no running water, electricity, or indoor plumbing at first, not for years. They had no car and seemed to live on literally nothing except barter and the occasional stingy royalty check. When Beverley was diagnosed with lung cancer, Legman sold parts of his rare-book collection to pay for radiation treatments. After she died in 1965, he married a young Californian, Judith Evans, a librarian who would share his work for three decades, and with whom he would have three children. The goat barn expanded to accommodate them, spreading slowly into two structures, a studio and a modest but elegant house designed by Legman and built of native stone by local craftsmen.

This house in the woods offered Gershon a near-perfect life of quiet and isolation, a marked contrast to his years of scuffling in war-time Manhattan. He customarily rose at 4:30 AM and worked with ferocious and disciplined energy until 1:00 PM, a full eight-hour day. "Always give the hind part of the day to the boss, and keep the best for yourself," was his maxim or, less

Legman's collections of unprintable songs would form the core of two still-unpublished volumes, The Ballad.

politely, "Sweets to the sweet, and piss on the boss's shit." After lunch, Judith recalls, Legman would declaim to her what he'd written, answer correspondence, read, or work on pet projects. Nothing except illness or the occasional journey interrupted his schedule. Even honored visitors had to wait until after noon. He never took a vacation or a weekend off, laboring for nearly 30 years, almost 11,000 eight-hour days.

It was all more or less one work, a series of examinations of sexual folklore, based on his enormous collections of erotica, oral traditions, and popular culture. When he left New York in 1953, he somehow stored and later transported an astonishing volume of self-generated paper, and this archive would continue to grow as people around the world sent manuscripts and queries.

By a circuitous route his crates followed him to Valbonne.

Eventually he brought over, in addition to his extensive library, a collection of thousands of American dirty jokes gathered between roughly 1927 and 1950. He stored up bawdy drinking songs, parodies, and ballads expurgated from scores of more polite collections. From his research on censorship and sexual attitudes—outlined in *Love & Death: A Study in Censorship*, the book that got him in trouble with the United States Post Office in 1950—he kept file folders of magazine illustrations, book covers, and greeting cards. An unending drift of materials we now call popular culture—advertising, comic books, pinups, graffiti, pornography, and amateur or homemade erotic art—he studied as expressions of overt or covert sexual attitudes. Framed portraits of his mother and Sigmund Freud guarded his desk.

He had boxes of notes on children's folklore, games, songs, and rhymes. Naughty postcards—French, American, and English—augmented albums of his private erotica. He collected thousands of obscene limericks. Bales of correspondence from his earliest years as a writer tell the story of his life until leaving the United States, and to these he added over the years literally tens of thousands of letters to and from hundreds of international correspondents. Most of this material is still archived at La Clé des Champs. Even today, Judith Legman says she is unpacking boxes that were never opened after his 1960 move.

With the exception of a volume of 1,700 limericks published in Paris in 1953, all of Legman's big books were written or edited at Valbonne. His joke collection was worked into the classic *Rationale of the Dirty Joke: Series I* and *Rationale of the Dirty Joke: Series II, No Laughing Matter*. His detective works on the history of nineteenth-century pornography and his brief for the uncensored study of folklore appear in *The Horn Book*. There is a second volume of limericks called, naturally, *The New Limerick*.

He would bring to press Ozark folklorist Vance Randolph's volume of bawdy folk songs, *Roll Me in Your Arms*, and *Blow the Candle Out*, a collection of formerly unprintable Ozark speech, riddles, folk beliefs, and games. He would annotate Randolph's celebrated joke collection, *Pissing in the Snow*. There would be many other books, important introductions to volumes on folklore, and resurrections and rediscoveries of manuscripts by Robert Burns and Mark Twain.

Legman's collections of unprintable songs would form the core of two still-unpublished volumes, *The Ballad*. In the late 1980s, he pounded out thousands of pages of *Peregrine Penis: An Autobiography of Innocence*. Very little of this fascinating memoir has been published, and the bits in print appear in obscure journals, erotica magazines, critical essays, and introductions to other people's works. *Peregrine Penis* gathers memories of his early sexual adventures and experimentation, paints old lovers in vivid tones, and casts a perspicacious eye on the early giants of sex research and New York's literary fringes.

Even before his big books came out (and almost all were big), his knowledge and his archive established Legman as the go-to guy for American scholars stumbling across the folklore of sex or sex in folklore. He regularly got letters from the States that asked, in effect, "What do you make of this?" But he also struck up correspondences, writing to Roger Abrahams, a young folk-song collector working in a black neighborhood in South Philadelphia, to ask, "What can we do for each other?" Abrahams sent a remarkable manuscript and Legman replied, encouraging and advising him:

> **Spread out as far as you can.... [O]f course you're not making the mistake of collecting only the bawdy stuff in spite of its apparent uniqueness: all the material available should be latched on to.... Remeber [sic] that there are TURNS OF PHRASE ("went through Pittsburgh like shit through a goose"), similes, spoonerisms ("they're off! as the monkey said when he backed into the lawnmower"), proverbs ("that woman is cunt all over") and purely vocabulary elements ("boy in the boat": for clitoris) etc.—there is also a song about this: do you ever run into it?... There are riddles: there are chalk items that go on the walls repetitively, on both fences and toilets; also "catches" (for fools). YOU HAVE GOT TO GET IT ALL AT ONCE AND NEVER MISS A CHANCE... THERE IS NEVER ANY GOING BACK.... [July 7, 1959]**

Indeed, Abrahams spread out and wrote *Deep Down in the Jungle*, a breakthrough book on African-American folk poetry, "toasts," and "the dozens," antecedents of rap. He was only one of scores of scholars to consult by mail with Legman about obscene or sexual folklore. Whether or not they went back, Legman never did.

It's possible that somewhere in his unpublished writings Legman lets us in on the origins of his interest in this unstoppable flood of material. How, for example, did he come to realize that he could combine his absorption in sex—a subject few scholars would approach openly in the 1930s—with his interest in folklore—a topic condescended to by most scientists and writers? Most folklorists were prudish or intimidated by their publishers; most sex researchers feared federal intimidation. How did Legman free himself for a lifetime of intense study of the forbidden?

The answers are in his family, in the immigrant Jewish community in Scranton, Pennsylvania, where he grew up, and on the streets of Manhattan. He writes that his father was a re-

His knowledge and his archive established Legman as the go-to guy for American scholars stumbling across the folklore of sex.

markable storyteller, fluent in biblical and traditional Jewish lore and vivid in relating the Legman family histories, which were usually disastrous to the point of tragedy. Emil Legman was a butcher and a railroad clerk who would've liked to have been a rabbi. He pushed his aspirations onto his son, and rabbinical study occupied Gershon's early years. At thirteen, "tempted by doubt," Gershon rejected his father's goals for him in favor of free thought, and Emil rejected Gershon. But by then he'd learned the techniques of close reading and deep research, and he was able to transmute the dream of being "a perfect rabbi" into the goal of being a total expert on sex.

Following a short-circuited year at the University of Michigan, in the mid-1930s he scrounged a living as a ghost writer in New York. As he writes in *Peregrine Penis*, he was deep into a huge project, the *Encyclopedic Dictionary of Sexual Speech and Slang*. On his own time he was haunting bookshops and hanging out in "all the grimier public shit-houses around midtown, in burlesque theatres and hotels and subway stations," any sort of urban place where he could collect the anonymous folklore of sex. He spent years going through rare volumes in the New York Public Library, recording slang usage from every conceivable literary source across four centuries. The following notes from an unnamed eighteenth-century book are typical:

yarn, wind up her little ball of	**copulate**
yelper	**the penis**
yoked	**married**
wrinkle	**vagina**
wrong door	**anus**
wearing yellow stockings	**cuckolded**
what's her name	**vagina**
whirligigs	**testicles**

He scrutinized proverbs across languages: "a woman kissed is a woman half-fucked. (Italian)." And from more recent sources, joking euphemisms for cunnilingus: "'Eating at the Y,' 'Box lunches'—Texas."

He made notes on the way contemporaries spoke: "I bet she'd bounce like a rubber ball..."; "he sure was a <u>piss-cutter</u>, an old word according to Jake Brussel." Although the dictionary was never published, he worked on it for decades, with the dedication of one draft reading:

To William Dunbar (1467? — 1530?)
who first said <u>fuck</u>

By busily contacting anyone and everyone who might be able to help him, he met major intellectuals. He corresponded with men who had written outrageous books—Robert Briffault, author of *Europa* was one; Henry Miller was another—often asking them the meanings of terms or how they came by their knowledge of erotica. He met Columbia University professor Allen Walker Read, a lexicographer who had attempted to catalogue all the words purged from the *Oxford English Dictionary*, but found him "repressed."

He was able to transmute the dream of being "a perfect rabbi" into the goal of being a total expert on sex.

There was Zora Neale Hurston, trained in anthropology at Columbia University under the great Franz Boas. Her brilliant folklore collection *Mules and Men* was published in 1935, a few years before they bumped into each other in Greenwich Village. Legman described his childhood joke-collecting habits and his longtime interest in slang and graffiti—"obscoena," as he called it—to her. As Hurston knew from her research in Florida turpentine camps and juke joints, Legman was wading in a very big river. She assured him there was a whole world of such wild stuff out there. It might be beneath the consideration of the literary world and too impolite to be considered by most scholars of culture, but it was there nevertheless, waiting for someone who could bring it to light. Now he had a name for his dreamlike project: erotic folklore.

Another part of this great work was a prospective *Encyclopedia of Sexual Technique*. In New York in 1936–1937, Legman was researching this proposed book for Dr. Robert Latou Dickinson, dean of American gynecologists, and was being aided by a number of enthusiastic girlfriends. In theory, the *Encyclopedia* was to be an illustrated catalog of every sexual possibility—mostly heterosexual, although Legman also collected the lore of gay and lesbian sex. As it turned out, only the first part of the projected whole was published in 1940. Appearing under an anagrammatic French pseudonym, *Oragenitalism: Oral Techniques in Genital Excitation: Part I: Cunnilinctus* presented the fiction that it was a fragment of a disorganized manuscript left behind by the deceased author.

For this work, Legman drew on every source of information available to him, from art history and medical textbooks to French postcards and accounts of friends' sex lives. His research files from the 1930s and 1940s are full of tracings, diagrams, and jottings. But mainly the work was an exploration of his own sexual preferences, and his insistent nineteen-year-old libido was his best source of information. The energetic researcher rushed from bed to desk, pencil in hand, to write down his fresh impressions. Documenting his own sexual experiences on 3x5-inch notecards and scraps of paper was his habit, as much a habit as all his book and folklore collecting. In a sense, Legman collected himself, or at least his own experiences, for future reference and display. In the process he identified and outlined the themes that would preoccupy him for the next five decades.

This first work, rare and ill-remembered, is a key to Legman. At 67 pages, it is a thorough and analytical treatment of oral sex, sometimes heavy with anatomical description and scientific language. But under this remote style is a living, breathing author. This was his favorite sexual practice, he told friends, and he presents himself as a jocular virtuoso in an important art. *Cunnilinctus* is an older variant of the Latin term *cunnilingus*. Wordsmith that Legman was, he knew that *cunnilinctus* means not only the act of licking female genitals but also refers to the person who licks. It is hard not to think that the book's subtitle is eponymous: At least during his twenties, Cunnilinctus was Legman.

Oragenitalism is a bold and peculiar book, certainly from the perspective of the 1930s, even today. In many ways it is typical Legman. He had chosen, as he acknowledges, a taboo topic, "the most misunderstood and the most maligned" practice, one many women and men refuse to acknowledge. It was illegal in some places and often treated as grounds for divorce. Taboo-smashing was all Legman: If he sensed a cultural barrier, he looked around for a rhetorical bulldozer and opened throttle.

The book had just been printed and bound in red cloth when its New York publisher, Jacob Brussel, was arrested for sending obscene materials through the mail. His entire stock and all his records were seized; Brussel pled guilty and was eventually imprisoned. Legman got wind of the pending raid and caught a train to Washington, DC.

It's rumored that the whole first print run of *Oragenitalism* was burned, although the story may be circulated by book dealers as a way of keeping first-edition prices high. But somewhere Legman had squirreled away a cache of the books, so, although rare, they exist. At the death of Alfred Kinsey in 1956, Legman sent one from France to the Kinsey Institute, inscribed, "In Memoriam."

In the 1960s, he took up the book again, reworking it by ransacking the notes he had taken in the 1930s and the drawings he and friends had made. He expanded his assaults on received prejudices, reports of folk attitudes, jokes, and sexual customs, and peppered the slightly grave book with snappy bons mots and goofy humor. He folded in things he'd learned from the years, two marriages, and the births of several children. Now there was a chapter on fellation, collated from the writings of someone else since his interest in the doer, the person performing the act, meant he "didn't have the courage" to research it himself. He added his own thoughts on "irrumation," or mouth-fucking, a variety of oral sex left out of more polite books. A chapter on the "soixante-neuf" capped the new edition, which was appropriately published in English in 1969 and immediately pirated.

Most important, he greatly expanded an original, brief consideration of the psychological aspects of oral sex, explaining why it is so misunderstood. Legman takes us on a wild theoretical ride, posing a Freudian-inflected thesis: To understand oral sex we must look at why the active party—the cunnilinguist, as he puns him—performs the act at all. In the literature of sex, when cunnilinctus can be mentioned at all, it is treated as a technique by which men generously give pleasure to women. Actually, Legman notes in an acerbic aside, husbands (not men) are said to use it to gallantly excite their wives (not women) on the way to intercourse, since Americans do not admit that sex takes place outside marriage. But this is a neurotic displacement and a cultural lie. Heterosexual men very much enjoy performing oral sex on women, but while they joke about it and use jocular terms for it ("Hatsville, U.S.A!"), they can't talk about it openly. Why not?

The answer: Cunnilinctus is not a technique; it's the expression of a drive, the desire to return to the mother's breast and womb, or even to relive the infant's first oral caress, its passage down the birth canal. All this is "an encapturing for neurotic purposes of the perfectly normal mammalian preliminary." He points to evolution, noting that genital-licking and -sniffing preparatory to sex is common in quadruped mammals. Our prehistoric ancestors may have navigated the terrain of sex and reproduction by smell and taste as much as by vision. So the drive to lick and taste is a movement toward pleasure, and in some sense natural, even while the act is slurred as "animalistic," too natural.

Widening to human behavior again, Legman mentions homosexual fellation as further evidence of a basic drive to oral pleasure. He discusses the universal bathroom graffito demanding oral sex ("I want to suck you!") as expressing this profound need. So, too, acrobatic auto-fellation. So-called healthy customs and the behaviors that society describes as sick or bizarre are not so far apart because, in fact, the same undercurrents motivate them.

But conflicting with the oral impulse is the psychic potency of the head and the mouth in all human cultures. People—male and female, heterosexual and homosexual—practice oral sex upon each other and find pleasure in being both active and receptive of oral attention, but they have trouble dealing with the psychological discomfort caused by the apparent subjugation of the head to the genitals. Confusing thoughts arise: Cunnilinctus is seen as domination by the genital partner; a man may appear to dominate by his oral activity, but at the same time he seems dominated because of his desire and willingness. He is pussy-whipped, in a literal sense. This paradox is at the center of all kinds of oral sex. (Legman soft-pedals the question of whether all cultures experience the same psychic tensions, but he suggests that they do.)

Legman was no conventional feminist, but he acknowledges that women have discomfort about the submission of the mouth to the penis. Giving a blowjob, he knew, can create a subtly coerced sensation even in an enthusiastic relationship (but you would never catch him writing "in the context of unequal gender relations"). For Legman, women who hold back on this sexual favor are poorly adjusted to their femininity and possibly just plain mean. Women who refuse to swallow semen are deeply hostile toward men.

It's rumored that the whole first print run of *Oragenitalism* was burned.

There it is: hostility, another key to Legman. Hostility would surface persistently as a theme in his later analyses of humor, graffiti, and slang, and it was at the center of his analyses of popular culture. In *Oragenitalism* Legman suggests that all sex, even so-called normal sex, expresses a certain amount of anger and can tend toward violence, although we may not always allow ourselves to recognize it. Intercourse can be rough, and people often thrash, scream, scratch, or bite at orgasm. More important, and a major Legman point, there are vicious and unpleasant people out there "who wish to wallow in whatever eroticism seems to them nasty or lubricious." The practice—oral, vaginal, anal, or other—is less important than the deep, underlying attitude. The more important evidence of hostility, for Legman, is the refusal to participate generously. This is why oral sex of any variety can be so tricky: It demands the lovers navigate what is at once "the most submissive and most possessive sexual contact possible."

Not to put too fine a point on it, particular sexual acts have a range of subtle, semiconscious, and unconscious meanings that go far beyond individual relationships to connect to power. In this, Legman was following Freud, but, in his account, it is prudery and censorship as much as childhood traumas that create "vicious and unpleasant people," and there are a lot of them.

Legman (again following Freud, but in so much more detail)

He cross-tabulates the possibilities, going so far in his notes as to draw up sex-position multiplication tables.

was interested in how jokes, sayings, slang, and customs reveal these senses of the power currents of sex, scattering occasional light into the dim corners of everyday awareness. When we say, "He's pussy-whipped," we're revealing a lot about the relationships between men and women, fear and genitals. The folklore of sex is a kind of collective Freudian slip, culturally shared if rarely taken up for analysis.

When Legman turns to technique, the second edition of *Oragenitalism* becomes a strange mix of instruction manual, conduct guide, and household advice book, still underpinned with interest in psychological mysteries. As a how-to book, it is delightfully personal, the youthful vigor of the original still there. Legman is chatty and helpful, urging lovers to be suave and graceful, and offering solutions to common problems, such as the best way to slide a pillow under a woman's hips. He makes suggestions about ways to be comfortable out-of-doors. Following his original text, he is encyclopedic: He catalogs positions prone, seated, and standing, clothed and unclothed, lights on, lights off, man superior, woman superior. He lists all the ways the mouth, tongue, lips, chin, and cheeks can be put to use, then moves on to the thumb and fingers. He cross-tabulates the possibilities, going so far in his notes as to draw up sex-position multiplication tables.

Advocating practical elegance, Legman is interested in manners: It's rude, for example, to gag or make a face, even if you really are choking on a pubic hair. The man should find discreet ways of wiping his face, lest he give the impression that he finds the taste of his lover unpleasant. Whatever you do, don't rush to the sink! Fresh orange juice comes in delightfully handy, but squeeze cut oranges over your beloved—don't be a hopeless duffer and try to open a can of juice in bed. And so on.

As in all conduct books, precise descriptions blur into gentle but firm recommendations for things one really ought to try and things one must learn to do correctly. Despite his insis-

tence that oral sex represents the satisfaction of an "ego drive," Legman is clear that it is almost always a prelude, however elaborate, to intercourse. "The scissors" is a favorite position because it (somehow) allows lovers to move gracefully from oral sex to coitus, a desirable but not mandatory end to the proceedings. It is so comfortable that the couple can fall asleep or do almost anything else, like reading or eating or chatting, without withdrawing the penis from the vagina. Intercourse again? No problem. The continuous connection of "the scissors" is Legman's utopia.

Overall, Legman emphasizes that intercourse will take place, noting that none of the world's religious teachings forbids oral sex *as a preliminary*. And overall, it is intercourse that women want because their femininity is most satisfied when there's the possibility of having a child with their lover. Here's another key to Legman: Despite his own research with gay men and sexual experiences with lesbians documented in his notes and memoir, he was a heterosexual man of his time and firmly believed that men and women had essential and distinct natures. Maladjustments to these were the cause of tremendous suffering. Like many writers on sex, Legman could shift from radical to conventional in seconds when the topic was women.

Despite its jostling detail, for a contemporary reader *Oragenitalism* suffers from a lack of illustration. Legman himself is often annoyed by the difficulty of describing sexual positions and motions using language alone. He gets frustrated trying to describe the favored "scissors" and suggests drawing stick figures. Or perhaps, he proposes, falling back on his love of typeface, the reader can imagine two capital *V*'s lying side by side, or a capital *W*. Unfortunately, in 1969 as well as in 1939, photographs or drawings required backing and capital. Although his research files are full of sketches and diagrams, Legman couldn't pay to have them made into plates. And then there were the barriers to publishing erotica, which were crumbling but not fast enough. In 1971 a French edition of *Oragenitalism* became impossible to sell because of its explicit jacket.

By the early 1970s the fall of American censorship and, more important, the big money to be made meant that illustrated sex manuals like Alex Comfort's *The Joy of Sex* were becoming mass-market, over-the-counter products. Too late for *Oragenitalism*. Legman's first book—censored before it could be celebrated, and reviled, widely plagiarized, censored again—was published by small houses and more or less passed by.

Placing *Oragenitalism* next to *The Joy of Sex* gives a sense of how far out on a limb Legman was, even by comparison with the "New Freedom" washing over the English-speaking world. Although explicit, lavishly illustrated, and readably written, *Joy* is comfortably bourgeois, modeled on a cookbook. In consumerist style, it offers choices of sexual staples, main courses, and condiments. Legman found the book "cold," according to Judith. He certainly would have seen fakery in its slightly exotic eroticism, in the motif of a menu of boots and G-strings and fake French-bordello names for positions. Comfort's emphasis on freeing oneself of "hang-ups" in the context of tender, playful monogamy probably annoyed him no end. Legman thought sex was serious if hot business, and the young Legman, any rate, disdained monogamy.

"Hang-ups" (he would've called them fears, distortions, and repressions) were the whole point: You lived with them and suffered with them. Legman made a career of confronting them, and when they were confronted, they revealed not individual problems but the sickness of the entire culture.

As for oral sex, *Joy* calls it "the genital kiss," a term imported directly from what Legman saw as the hopelessly prudish marriage manuals of the early twentieth century. For Comfort, cunnilingus isn't a delicate psychic tightrope walk or a most passionate submissive possession; it's an item on the menu. What used to be cause for divorce had found a place in the kitchen cupboard. By the 1960s, Legman did not believe "more" was the same as liberation.

Although the finer points of oral sex have been graphically described many times over the years since its publication, *Oragenitalism* remains an unusual book. What had not been done before, and may not have been done since in mass-market literature, was this sort of deep thinking—based in introspection and broad observation—on the psychic undercurrents of a particular sex act. Only much later would feminists and gay-rights activists again take up questions of psychic power, submission, and mutuality in the meaning of sex, and this time from a perspective Legman might well have abhorred. Mean-

He certainly would have seen fakery in its slightly exotic eroticism, in the motif of a menu of boots and G-strings and fake French-bordello names for positions.

while, a revolution in depicting sex took place, not through the work of bold writers so much as through the energies of commercial publishers and porn video-makers. The worlds of erotica and cultural criticism moved past him.

Gershon Legman spent his whole life pursuing freedom and, having found his key to the fields, he paid the price. The costs were isolation, monetary but not intellectual poverty, and separation by distance from other American folklorists and a broader popular audience. His ideas were always "out there," but as he advised Roger Abrahams, once you were out there, there was "never any going back." Then there was age, and time and culture passing. By the time he died in 1999, all his big books were out of print, his name at least partially forgotten. But having wrested his freedom, Legman's prize was to work long and intensely on one huge project, unearthing activities, words, and images that shed light on the problems of sexual being. The materials he dredged up prove over and over again how broad and deep the river is.

Betty Dodson's Revolutionary Open Relationship

Rachel Kramer Bussel

A Sex-Date Surprise

I rarely read about a person's private life before I go to bed with him or her, but with Eric Wilkinson, I was briefed on his sexual M.O. before we even met. I know he's the twenty-something boyfriend of the "Mother of Masturbation," septuagenarian Betty Dodson.

When I meet them at a party in October 2004, their May-December relationship (he's 28, my age, and she's 75) is still going strong after five years. Eric is bold, and when he learns I've read Dodson's book *Orgasms for Two*, peppers me with questions about my opinions on the G-spot, clitoral stimulation, vibrators, and sexual attraction. With his slow Southern drawl, keen interest, and easygoing manner, he puts me at ease, and before I know it I'm telling him exactly how I do and don't like to come and which kinds of girls and guys turn my head.

He replies that he was checking out my cleavage and fishnets and asks if I want to "play" with him.

He reveals little of his own fantasy life but does make a point of telling me that he and Dodson have an open relationship. I'm not sure if he's flirting with me, but when I realize he's the only person I've spoken to for the past hour and a half, I jolt in surprise. I leave the party and send him a "nice to meet you" email. He replies that he was checking out my cleavage and fishnets and asks if I want to "play" with him.

We make plans for a sex date. Believe it or not, for all the flings I've had, I've never rented a hotel room with someone just for sex. I've had sex in hotel rooms, but on vacation. Renting a room with someone already in a committed relationship feels like the ultimate in sexual decadence. My friends are aghast when I tell them we're splitting the cost. "He should pay for it!" several of them insist. I'm shocked that they're shocked. The idea that the guy should pay is ludicrous, not to mention sexist, as if by granting him access to my pussy I'm bestowing upon him some huge favor, like I don't crave pure, carnal sex just as much as he does. If anyone's doing anyone a favor here, he's doing me one, helping revitalize my body after six celibate months. Even more than that, his overwhelming lust for me—our date happens within a week of meeting each other, at his insistence—does wonders for my self-esteem.

Before the big day, we trade a few dirty emails. I send him a story I wrote about a girl giving a guy a blowjob in a bathroom; he tells me to bring my favorite vibrator and that he can't wait to give me my first orgasm. Already, that's a huge switch from almost every guy I've been with. I believe guys want to please their women, but they assume that in the usual course of events, their dick will do the job more than amply.

I plan to reread Dodson's book but run out of time, perhaps because subconsciously I want to be swept away by the novelty of a new lover. There comes a point where I don't want to know what will happen; I want to be surprised, to see how my body will react in the moment. There's a great line that rings true for me in Karen Finley's play *George and Martha* about Jews being "too busy thinking while they're fucking." I spend enough time thinking about sex; when I'm finally doing it, I don't want to let my brain rule the show.

When we get to the hotel, he's as charming and gallant as if this were a normal date. He's brought everything I could have wanted and more—condoms, lube, and vibrators, along with bananas, Power Bars, vanilla-scented shampoo, and candles. There are a few moments of slight awkwardness, but they quickly fade. It's a relief to focus solely on our bodily pleasure without any dating drama. It's amazing how easily I'm able to adjust to his transition from relative stranger to new sex partner. Even though I know he wouldn't be a suitable boyfriend, once I accept that this is casual sex, nothing more and nothing less, I can focus solely on my physical pleasure.

I'm fixated on his long, soft fingers, and suckle them one by one until he makes me stop so he can undress me. I'm already wet and don't protest. "Welcome home," he says, referring to my six sex-free months, as his hands stroke my pussy until it feels like a continuous round of palms caressing me.

He's brought a Hitachi Magic Wand, as befits Betty Dodson's boy toy, and shows me various positions I've never heard of—one leg straight and one leg raised up on a pillow, one with me on my hands and knees while he stands behind me—all interesting but also distracting. I'm used to using my Magic Wand at home, alone, in a very precise way. We try these out and go back to more familiar positions.

I've had to pee since I arrived but forget about it in the midst of my arousal. When we're done with round one, I can't wait anymore and get up to use the bathroom. As I'm sitting naked on the toilet, poised with my legs spread, he comes in without asking. I'm all set to tell him to go away, but he shushes me and I let him stay. Then his hand reaches between my legs. I'm not prepared for the immense shock waves of arousal his touch brings me. I've only been in this situation once before, and I couldn't pee at all. But Eric stares at me as he strokes my oversensitive clit, and the more he does, the more I tremble. I still have to pee, but now that desire battles with my need to come. My toes are pointed and my legs shake so hard I have to hold onto the bathtub's edge. I shudder for several very long moments as I pee over his fingers. It's hotter than anything I could've planned, perhaps because I'm part horrified, part turned on.

After we're done fucking, I tell him he's adorable. "Dashing," he corrects me. As he rubs baby powder onto my back and massages my legs, I sink into the bed in blissful exhaustion. He tells me about the other women—about three a month—he shares similar trysts with. "Girls often call me their Oasis Cock. It's like you've been in the desert for so long and then here I am, waiting for you." It's such a sweet image, slightly at odds with his pee fetish, yet it fits. He's thought of things many guys never would have and is willing to try almost anything. Full of lust and pheromones, I walk him back to his apartment, not sure if I'll see him again.

A Revolutionary Relationship

I'm a little nervous when I pick up the phone to call Betty Dodson. After all, I had sex with her live-in partner, Eric, only a few weeks ago. While I know they have a long-term open relationship, that doesn't mean she'll exactly welcome me with open arms, even though she's agreed to the interview.

But from the start she's warm and friendly, punctuating her words with laughter and the occasional "ew" of annoyance, mostly when she's talking about concepts like monogamy and jealousy, which are anathema to her. I listen with rapt attention, because at 75 Dodson has truly seen and done it all. Before she became the Mother of Masturbation—displaying her erotic art at feminist conferences, leading workshops where women examined and played with their pussies, and writing her classic tome, *Sex for One* (originally entitled *Liberating Masturbation*)—she was married to a man she describes as not very sexual: "Sex was always a challenge for him." She cheated on him, and while he never found out, the experience haunted her. After her divorce, she delved into various scenes, participating fully in the sexual revolution with orgies, multiple partners, and later, the lesbian BDSM community.

Her attitude toward nonmonogamy (she hates the word *polyamory*) is that it's freeing. Instead of hiding and cheating, people can partake of their desires for others while still returning to their primary partner. And while her relationship with Eric is "open," not every detail of their extracurricular affairs gets discussed. "He doesn't need to report in," she says. The rules she and Eric have customized, including see-

As I'm sitting naked on the toilet, poised with my legs spread, he comes in without asking.

ing other partners only outside their home and him having sex with a given woman no more than once per month, were ones he brought to her. They've worked so far, but nothing is set in stone, and both are open to reconfiguring those arrangements.

Much of her current understanding and practice of nonmonogamy stems from the intergenerational aspect of their relationship. Because he's younger and has yet to fully explore his sexuality, she doesn't want to hold him back from experiencing life's erotic thrills. Then she says something that blows me away: "The day that Eric comes home and says, 'I met the woman of my dreams; I'm gonna move out,' I will find the strength to wish him well, because I love him. His happiness comes first, not my happiness, and believe me, I'll find some adorable lesbian to take his place."

It's this kind of statement, expressed with grace, honesty,

and purity of heart, that makes Dodson a person any woman (or man) can learn from. How many of us, even the most liberated and free-spirited, could have such an open attitude yet one imbued by love at every turn? It's easy enough not to be jealous when the flings are casual and feelings are fleeting, but when you're in love, the stakes are higher—I'd imagine especially so for someone like Dodson, who had sworn off what she calls "partnersex" more than a decade ago in favor of masturbation, only to find herself falling for Eric in a major way in 1999.

Does the author of the book *Orgasms for Two* partake in the open aspect of their relationship? Occasionally, but it's not a high priority. She may have a night of hot sex with a female friend, and they've enjoyed the occasional threesome, but when Dodson's not with Eric, more often she's working, finishing various art and writing projects, and fielding sex advice questions on her website. She tells me that her role model is

"When I die, baby, I'm gonna have so few regrets."

Granny D., a/k/a Doris Haddock, a 94-year-old woman who walked across the country in 1999 and ran for US Senate. How does this relate to nonmonogamy? It's clear that Dodson is a woman on a mission, and while she's excised jealousy from her heart, she also simply doesn't have time to brood. She's too busy trying to improve other people's sex lives.

Dodson realizes that open relationships aren't for everyone, though she feels strongly that the cultural imperative concerning monogamy is dangerous and damaging. "I'm just talking about myself," she says. "There are all these different ways to go. America practices serial monogamy with cheating on the side. It's never acknowledged, and it's lied about. Yes, there are people who are happy being monogamous, and if you're married and own a lot of things together and

have children, there's more at stake"—but that's not a reason to succumb to monogamy if it's not right for you.

Dodson can make it sound so easy (if only!) but admits that she was plagued by jealousy in the first year of their relationship. She was worried Eric would fall for someone younger and she'd be left in the dust, but over time she's been reassured by his constancy and love and has gotten over her jealousy. About the dreaded emotion, she says, "I hate it. I've never liked it in myself. I don't like it in other women and men; I don't like the way society accepts it as normal. I think it's a learned proposition. We're all a bunch of insecure wimps; we ought to have enough self-love and self-fullness that we don't have to be totally reliant on getting our self-worth from another person. It's my firm belief that jealousy turns into a cancerous growth."

I'd thought that I too might feel awkward—I'm talking to the female partner of the last guy I slept with. But I feel only amazement at Dodson's attitude, which turns our culture's totalistic devotion to monogamy on its head. We generally assume that actions speak louder than words, which in the case of sex means that physical monogamy is the only true way of showing our love. And yet, even for those who manage to keep their pants on (surely fewer than we'd like to believe), what about their dirty thoughts and fantasies? Growing up, we're taught that one person should be enough to satisfy all our carnal needs, leaving many with false expectations and crushed hopes. Dodson's lived through those and doesn't want to again. "When I die, baby, I'm gonna have so few regrets. Isn't that what it's all about, to live life fully?"

Our conversation is done, yet the feisty Dodson still has more to say, and she surprises me yet again. "The next time you're with Eric, know that I'm blessing you at every moment." I smile as I hang up, sure that on my date with him, I'll still be feeling Dodson's warmth, energy, and compassion.

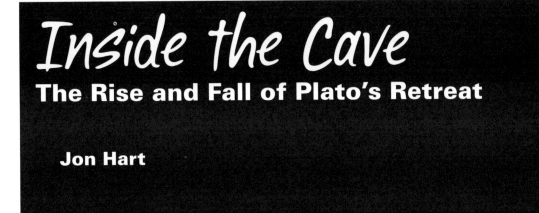

Inside the Cave
The Rise and Fall of Plato's Retreat

Jon Hart

In the late evening of September 23, 1977, a new era was in full swing. Captain John, a muscular motorcycle entrepreneur, took his date, Debbie, a perky, brunette Rutgers chemistry major, to opening night at Plato's Retreat, an X-rated Disneyland in New York City, where heterosexual couples came to fulfill their most fantastic fantasies. As they descended the steep, mirrored stairwell, disco blared from DJ Bacho's turntable. A scene reminiscent of a Roman orgy was already underway. Under pulsating lights, semi-clad couples ground against one another. By the pool and the mammoth Jacuzzi, couples fondled or had sex in plain view. Meanwhile, a Hells Angel–type sat attentively in front of the orgy room, guarding a sea of flesh.

"It was very natural there," recalls Captain John, who says that Debbie hooked up with a New York Mets pitcher that evening. "We ended up swinging with several different couples. From that point, we were hooked."

Following Woodstock, before "safe sex," there was a club called Plato's Retreat, the most famous swingers' club ever to exist. After opening in the majestic Ansonia building's basement on Broadway and 74th Street, dozens of imitators spawned across the country, and thousands of customers, from Hollywood stars to regular folk like Captain John and Debbie, headed to its cavernous confines.

"Everyone wanted to see Plato's," recalls Howard Smith, who covered the sex, drugs, and rock n' roll beat for the *Village Voice*. But after nine years of business, jealousy, greed, and, finally, disease conquered "the cave." It was an enigmatic palace of excess. Here is its story.

Perhaps it was fitting that a caveman of sorts, Bronx native Larry Levenson, created Plato's. "He was shallow intellectually," recalls pornographer Al Goldstein (founder and, until 2003, publisher of *Screw*), who was once so close with Levenson that some mistook them for relatives. "He never read a book, never went to a movie." Outside of their overfed pastrami physiques and sexual pedigrees, Levenson and Goldstein were quite different. While Goldstein, something of a Hebrew Hefner, perused Kafka, Levenson, a junior-college graduate, barely cracked a comic book.

Twice-divorced, at least twice hauled into court for failure to pay child support for his three sons, Levenson, a former McDonald's manager, was hawking soda and ice cream on the beach at Coney Island before Plato's. "He didn't have a pot to piss in," barked his future Plato's partner, Frank Pernice.

One night, though, Levenson got lucky. At the Golden Gate Motel's cocktail lounge, a seedy locale in Sheepshead Bay, Brooklyn, Levenson met Ellie, a voluptuous, married housewife who introduced him to a different life: subterranean swing clubs like the Underground and the Botany Talk House, where Madonna used to gig. After the initial, first-name-only introductions, Levenson, Ellie, and several couples retired to a Spartan, New Jersey high-rise apartment, where they tossed their clothes in the corner, rolled with one another, and snorted amyl nitrate.

"We'd swing the entire weekend," recalled Levenson. In that environment, Levenson thought, everyone is honest with one another. There's no cheating. Unfortunately, this new lifestyle was also extremely inconvenient. "It was tough to find parking," groused Levenson. "By the time we got to swinging, it was two in the morning."

Eventually, Levenson expedited matters by using just one venue for the entire evening. Hosting floating parties, Leven-

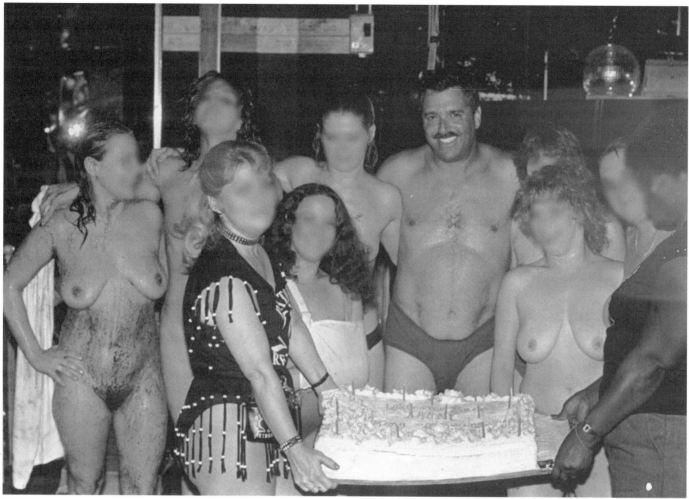

Levenson and friends celebrate at Plato's.

son quickly became known as "The King of Swing," attracting a loyal tribe of patrons, mostly unsophisticated, blue-collar types, who lived in the outer boroughs. Levenson also caught the attention of an organized-crime figure, who ordered him to promptly shut down—or else. Fortunately for Levenson, Al Goldstein came to his defense, delivering a scathing editorial in *Screw* magazine on the Mafia's attempt to monopolize the nascent public-sex industry.

However, there were other troubles for Levenson. When block associations learned of his antics, they promptly padlocked his establishments and told him to get lost. Every few weeks, Levenson was back on the road in his beat-up Valiant, which was stuffed to the hilt with mattresses. Eventually, Levenson found a home in the basement of Kenmore Hotel, a tawdry venue on East 23rd Street. It was here that Levenson became smitten. Mary, a thirty-something, statuesque beauty was an unemployed restaurant muralist with at least two daughters. Levenson felt that she needed him. He needed her, as well. Well-spoken, Mary became quite apt at articulating the allure of Plato's for women. Levenson and

Mary swung. Then they moved in together.

At about this time, Howard Smith got a tip about the unusual goings-on at the Kenmore. Smith was well aware of public-sex establishments for gay men, but he had never heard of this kind of locale for heterosexual couples. Skeptical, Smith, with a date, went down to investigate. At the Kenmore, he witnessed about a dozen-and-a-half out-of-shape, bridge-and-tunnel types in various states of undress, including two conspicuous men who wore nothing more than black shoes with black socks. After scoping the scene, Smith introduced himself to Levenson. "He was an innocent," recalls Smith. "He was a simple, nice guy in an insane, insane place."

After Smith featured Levenson's soirées in his *Voice* column, the Kenmore immediately became a hotspot for hordes of hip, Max's Kansas City-types, as well as other types from toney suburbs like Great Neck. Some of his small band of swingers felt uncomfortable around the newcomers. Levenson, however, embraced the novices. Swinging had given him a new lease on life, and now he wanted everyone to experience it. Levenson had become a missionary of the missionary, a crusader for couples in dire need of sexual experimentation. Simply, Levenson, who had experienced the embarrassment of being refused entry to Studio 54, refused to turn anyone away, as long as they were well-behaved. At Levenson's locale, patrons left their pedigrees at the door, wallets in their lockers. Cardiologists got down next to cab drivers, and so on. Levenson thought he had created a level playing field, where everything was equal, aboveboard, and honest.

One night, a well-dressed caterer from Brooklyn visited the Kenmore's basement. Frank Pernice stayed clothed, intent to remain on the sidelines and watch. At Levenson's, watching was perfectly acceptable. But Pernice was no typical voyeur. He was turned on—by the financial potential of Levenson's establishment. Eventually, he made Levenson an offer. "Right now you have a grocery store," Pernice declared in his Sicilian accent during one visit. "I can turn it into a supermarket." Pernice made it quite clear that he had the contacts to make good on his offer. Levenson, though, was not sold. At heart, he was a small-time deli owner who wanted no part of Pernice and his shady contacts. Although he liked having a few bucks in his pocket, Levenson didn't go into swinging as a business. It was a labor of love, his passion, his religion. So when Pernice left messages for him, Levenson did not get back to him.

Eventually, though, Levenson was forced out of the Kenmore. Reluctantly, he called the connected caterer. Pernice promptly made a phone call to Hy Gordon, a restaurateur who knew the Ansonia Hotel's landlord. Built in 1904, the Ansonia, a heavily-ornamented, 17-story urban castle, had already attracted its fair share of well-known tenants, including athletes Babe Ruth and Jack Dempsey and composers Igor Stravinsky and Gustav Mahler. A hundred of Paul Costellano's laborers swiftly went into action in the majestic Ansonia's basement, the former home of the Continental Baths, a gay bathhouse where Bette Midler and a young pianist by the name of Barry Manilow used to perform. In mere months, gloryholes were plugged, and it was transformed into the prototypical palace for the public-sex phenomenon.

✕✕

From the start, Plato's Retreat was a smash success, especially after *New York Magazine* featured the club in a cover story. It succeeded mostly because of the relaxed atmosphere. "I always used to say there's more pressure at a singles' bar than at Plato's Retreat," recalls Smith. "There was so much, so available, so why pressure anyone?"

As Plato's *maître d'*, Levenson welcomed his guests with the playfulness of a kid in a sandbox, providing tours of the un-air-conditioned premises: the ample hot-and-cold buffet, the clothing-optional dancefloor, the sixty-person Jacuzzi, the labyrinth of thinly-walled, no-ceiling private rooms, and the cushioned orgy room. Levenson was having the time of his life and wanted everyone else to, as well.

"He added a friendly touch to the place," says Smith, a non-swinger. "He always used to tell couples: If your marriage is in trouble, this won't solve it. This is fun. This is extra. He told me, 'I don't want to fuck up anyone's life.'"

Meanwhile, Mary played host, too. In addition to putting together the Plato's newsletter, she often ensured that special guests experienced the full Plato's sensual experience. According to Smith, Levenson offered Mary to him on several occasions. Smith declined. While she was a devoted swinger, Mary saved her heart for Levenson. "I intend to spend the rest of my life with Larry, whether he likes it or not," she told one television interviewer.

Of course, not everyone was thrilled with Plato's. Smith often escorted eager friends to the club, but some of them would leave, disgusted, shortly thereafter. After receiving a standing ovation from the Jacuzzi crowd, DJ Wolfman Jack blanched and didn't speak for the rest of the night. City officials were not amused either, hampering the high jinks by banning Plato's from distributing alcohol. If patrons wanted to drink, they would have to bring it themselves.

There was also the issue of the single men who were desperate to enter this new sexual frontier. To gain entry, they would garner a female, either a friend or a working girl. Invariably, their "date" would leave almost immediately, leaving an inordinate number of men and an uncomfortable, tense, testosterone-fueled vibe. In response, Levenson mandated that all exiting women must depart with their male counterparts. This seemed to do the trick—for the time being.

Plato's became the perfect alternative to the starfuckin' scene at Studio 54, which had opened five months earlier. Plato's embraced outer-borough punch-the-clockers like Rick "The Prick," a Queens desk slave who was armed with canteens of rum and Coke; Wally "The Cop," who supplied the scotch; and Vance "The Lance," who sold just about anything. Then there were the gals, ladies like the statuesque Sparkles, who gallivanted in only glitter; Candy, who dressed up as a nurse; and some spaced-out chick known only as "Wipe Out." Committed couples like Fred and Mary, Don and Jo Jo, and Mike and Anita were Plato's heart and soul. Ultimately, all were welcome.

"Plato's was welcome to anybody as long as you were a couple and you behaved yourself. We had 80-year-old people coming to Plato's as couples," said Levenson. "I had people weighing 600 pounds. If you could waddle through that door, if you're a nice person, come into Plato's."

While there was no velvet rope or VIP list, celebrities visited the cave, as well. More than a few times, writer-actor Buck Henry paid a visit. "We used to wander over there in the *Saturday Night Live* days to take a look," recalls Henry. "And, of course, we went there for the fine food." (If the hot-and-cold buffet wasn't enough, pipin'-hot pizzas were delivered every fifteen minutes. For a herd of "fat, Jewish rejects," this was the highlight of the evening, cracked Goldstein.)

Besides the cuisine, did you engage, Mr. Henry?

"Maybe," Henry replies coyly.

Regardless, just watching was thoroughly engaging, especially the orgy room—a huge mattress, sectioned off by a line of faux plants, right next to the dancefloor. "It was a huge group orgy, a couple of hundred people at a time. It looked incredible," Smith recalls. "The people who went in there wanted anonymous sex. They didn't care who they were or what they looked like. It was not unusual to see a woman being made love to by five men. You had to be in a zone. They were in a different place. They were high on sex." Many were probably also high on Quaaludes, Plato's drug of choice, which patrons stuffed into pouches emblazoned with the club's logo, the same ones featured in *Vogue* and sold at Plato's boutique for two bucks.

Of course, there were other things to see, notably Jill Monroe, the first transsexual centerfold, who would stand up amidst bodies in the orgy room and ask: "Isn't there a man here that can satisfy me?"

Mat Room Rules

No one admitted fully dressed

Couples and single women only

No drinks, food or smoking on mats

When female leaves, the male must also leave

Respect Thy Neighbor

While sex stars like Annie Sprinkle tackled just about anything ("I was fucked by a machine," she deadpans. "It had a motor and was pumping."), most of the time the big names took it all in, dressed. Sammy Davis, Jr. danced with the ladies as his wife, Altovese, danced in a risqué manner. One evening, John Wayne gave a nickel-plated .38 to Davis. Then-pro wrestler and later Minnesota governor Jesse "The Body" Ventura threw his physique around the cave and wore a Plato's shirt in the ring.

Ansonia resident Richard Dreyfuss strolled downstairs to check out the action and talk to his favorite pornstar, Jamie Gillis. "He was more impressed with Jamie than the other way around," laughed Levenson. Dreyfuss mentioned the club in a 1978 *Esquire* article. "I went to watch people screw and here they all were," he remarked. The Academy Award-winning actor went on to recall a naked man badgering him for entertainment-lawyer contacts at the club.

Meanwhile, Levenson became something of a celebrity himself. He wore a shirt that declared, "It's not easy being a legend in your own time," gave away thousands of dollars to patrons, and even lectured high-school and college students that swinging was a viable alternative lifestyle. More important, with Mary often at his side, Levenson sucked up the interview circuit, including at least two *Donahue* appearances. Smith had coached Levenson just to be himself: a poor, affable, horny schmuck from Brooklyn. "I debated a rabbi," Levenson quipped. "It was tough."

Mary argued that Plato's was the next step for the women's movement. "Many women, too, are brought up to be so careful and so monogamous and to live a certain way," she said on the *David Suskind Show*. "There's a certain line of behavior we're supposed to follow. When we grow up, we can make our own choices now. Very often, women have fantasies about doing certain things, such as being with another woman, just to experience it. I think this is a beautiful way to live. There's so much freedom, especially for women."

Soon, Levenson was telling anyone who would listen that plans were underway for Plato's franchises to open across the country. At least a dozen Plato's knockoffs, like Midnight Interlude and Noah's Ark, already had swung open their doors in Manhattan. None could match Plato's, which was so popular it inspired a hit disco song by Joe Thomas:

Getting' hot and bothered

Loosen up your collar

Let's all do the freak at Plato's Retreat

Levenson took the song to heart, having sex with bunches of women a night. "If fucking were an Olympic sport, he would have won a gold medal," says Goldstein. Once, to win a $5,000 bet with Goldstein, Levenson ejaculated fifteen times over the course of fourteen hours. "We had a doctor there to make sure it was an actual ejaculation. Hefner got in on the bet," remembers Goldstein. During a break in the action, Levenson confessed to *Screw*'s Josh Alan Friedman the secrets of his success: "The club runs itself. I'm in the back fuckin' all night. Anyone with half a brain can run a club. I wish they said I was a genius for thinking up Plato's Retreat, but it just happened. No great idea, nothin' brilliant. I just happened to be the first one to go public with swinging. Swinging shot through the roof. Now I'm riding the crest. I'm a fat, middle-aged guy. These chicks only want me 'cause I'm the owner of Plato's. Ya think I don't know that?"

But while Levenson screwed around, his relationship with Mary suffered. With so much sex at his disposal, he all but ignored her as a sexual partner. Eventually, Mary fell for Levenson's married chauffeur. One night Levenson became chagrinned when he saw them holding hands at the club. "You want to fuck him, that's all right," Levenson told Mary at the time. "But you can't show people that my woman is walking around holding hands with another guy. Doesn't look good. That's all I'm concerned about." Levenson laid down the law to the chauffeur: No-strings-attached sex was the rule at Plato's, nothing more. But the chauffeur couldn't accept it, claiming he was in love. Levenson promptly fired him. One morning, just as Levenson was exiting the club, the chauffeur and two accomplices jumped him and beat the crap out him, breaking his arms and legs. They dumped him on a deserted street near JFK Airport and ordered him to leave town.

Levenson survived. Ultimately, his relationship with Mary did not. Not long after, she disappeared from the Plato's scene. But something much more serious was transpiring. Something was killing gay men. In 1981, a *New York Times* headline stated: "Rare Cancer Seen in 41 Homosexuals." Back at Plato's, the party raged on, oblivious to the mysterious disease. Or perhaps they were just having too much fun to stop. "It was just something people didn't even want to discuss," recalls Candy.

However, Upper West Side community members were very ready to discuss their displeasure with the brigades of single men who loitered outside Plato's soliciting for "dates." Finally, Ansonia's owner, who wanted to transform the building into a condominium complex, paid Plato's owners a million dollars, much in deferred payments, to move downtown to a larger space on 34th Street, which would feature a Japanese tea room, a jungle habitat, and a "tent fit for an Arabian sheik."

The new home garnered mixed reviews. "It didn't work downtown at all," remembers Henry, who paid just one visit to the new locale. "The times had changed. It didn't have the same kind of friendliness. It was big and very empty. It was very creepy. I remember Jerzy Kosinski skulking out of a back room, wearing only a towel."

Others found fault with Levenson's bloated ego and aloof attitude. "He thought he was God's gift to the sexual revolution. He really felt he was important," recalls Goldstein. "In the end, he was in his private room doing coke. It was no democracy. The King didn't fuck with the rest of us."

Levenson had other things to consider. While Internal Revenue Service officers were probing his den of decadence, Plato's former manager, Anne Grippo, whom Levenson had recently fired, handed over a second set of the club's accounting books. "This was a chronic case of a company that had two sets of books," explains then-organized-crime prosecutor Peter Sudler, who also went after Studio 54's Rubell and Schrager. "One was phony." Unfortunately for Levenson and his partners, Grippo had handed over the true set of books.

On trial for skimming $2.3 million in receipts, Levenson was the lone Plato's owner to take the stand. The King should have kept his mouth shut. In response to the question of whether he had skimmed money, Levenson responded: "I never took anything that didn't belong to me, that wasn't owed to me." Levenson also stated that he believed Plato's was a tax-exempt, not-for-profit organization. "The jury was laughing at him. He was pathetic," recalls Sudler. "He was like a kid with his hand caught in a cookie jar."

Goldstein was flabbergasted by Levenson's lack of business savvy. "He was a retard, a disgrace to Jews," rails Goldstein. "If you're gonna do cash, you don't do it in front of people you're gonna fire the following week."

Sudler claims that there was no shortage of witnesses willing to spill the beans on the Plato's operation. "All the employees hated these guys," recalls Sudler. "They were having fist-fights to take the stand against them."

In July 1981, Levenson and his partners got eight years in Allenwood federal prison. Even locked up, Levenson ensured that he was not forgotten. His son Michael, known to many club members as the Prince, emceed at Plato's on Saturday nights, and Levenson tape-recorded announcements that the Prince played over the loudspeakers. But it wasn't the same. "The club definitely suffered," remembers Rick "The Prick." No doubt the club missed Levenson's enthusiasm for the lifestyle and his unique showmanship. With Goldstein as his tag-team partner, Levenson had mud-wrestled women. When the club closed for the evening, Levenson would transform himself into a Semitic Elvis, lip-synching "The Wonder of You."

Most notably, Plato's suffered regarding the admission of single men and working girls. According to Plato's former head of security, single men, including a number of Hasidic Jews, were allowed entry for a hefty payoff. In return for a house fee, working girls were allowed to ply their trade.

Captain John, the Jersey stud, whom women once lined up to be with, was staying clear of Plato's. He had heard about the mysterious virus referred to as acquired immune deficiency disease in a May 1982 *New York Times* article. The paper

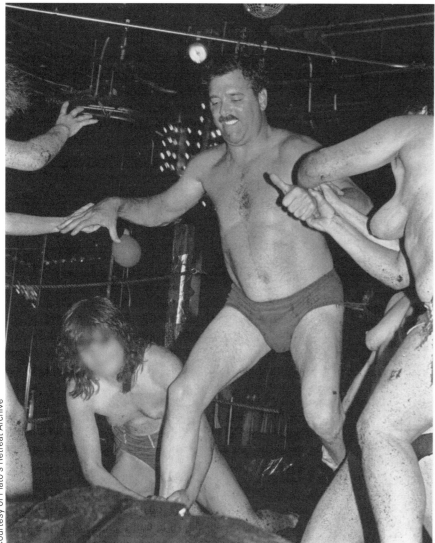

Courtesy of Plato's Retreat Archive

Levenson shows off his moves in the ring.

But now with AIDS on everyone's radar, a declining number listened to the King's pitch. The city was taking action to fight the plague, mandating literal writing on the wall: Health Department signs forbidding anal and oral sex were posted throughout the club. "There was an effort by the city to ensure safe sex, make sure people wear condoms," confirmed then-Mayor Ed Koch, who sent undercover inspectors into city sex clubs to investigate. "What the inspectors saw was so shocking, we had to provide them with psychiatric counseling."

Amid the hysteria, Levenson desperately tried to keep his club alive. Struggling to stay afloat, Levenson resorted to breaking the cardinal rule of swinging: the admission of single men at least one night a week. At one time, Levenson had preached that Plato's was about a couples' movement; now it had become about getting your rocks off in a glorified, touristy, post-*Cats* peep show. During these desperate days, a well-known singer showed up with a pair of dubious-looking pretty women. "Not even a class call girl," groused Levenson. At this point, working girls were a familiar, accepted part of the Plato's scene. "I started talking to a girl there," recalls an unescorted male. "She made it clear that she was paid to be there by the club."

reported that the disease had killed 136 people, including thirteen heterosexual women. "We didn't know if it was an airborne disease," says Captain John. Scared into marriage, he says he threw himself into the safer S/M world. "I would tie a girl to the floor, blindfold her, and have a bunch of naked guys stand around her naked. I would splash water on her to simulate an orgasm."

For one night, though, everyone's fears were put on the backburner. After about 32 months of incarceration, Levenson was treated like a rock star at his homecoming. "The place was packed with 900 people. They were grabbing at him, trying to touch him," remembers the Prince. Once again on center stage, with his mother René in the house, Levenson asked for eternal unity from his extended "family." "The friendships we have made here are lifetime friendships," the King preached.

Not only patrons were staying away from the club. Once the darling of the media, Plato's was passé and virtually ignored by television and newspapers. With the cameras gone, Levenson took the cameras to himself, hosting his own public-access show, *Inside Plato's Retreat*. For one show, Levenson, donning a knock-off blue Adidas sweatsuit, interviewed two call girls. It did not go smoothly. For most of the broadcast, audio wasn't available to audience members. Levenson smelled conspiracy. "I'll tell you one thing," Levenson declared defiantly. "If it is done intentionally, I'll fight this right down like I fought everything else. What can you do? The worst you can do is put a bullet in me like you did to Larry Flynt. I can handle that as well as anything else. If that's what has to be, that's what has to be. I'm getting sick and tired of this nonsense."

Later, Levenson turned his thoughts to AIDS, telling his audience that "very influential" medical professionals informed him that the transmission of the virus was unlikely at Plato's

EVERYTHING YOU KNOW ABOUT SEX IS WRONG

because of the large amount of chlorine at the establishment. "That happens to be a fact," said Levenson. He went on to state that his contacts had notified him that an Israeli bacteriologist was three to six months away from developing an AIDS vaccine.

During another broadcast, Levenson set his sights on Mayor Koch, calling him an epithet, referring to his sexuality. By now, it probably didn't matter at all what Levenson was saying. The city was already on a rampage, shutting down gay clubs like the Mine Shaft and others. Plato's was bolted, too, after inspectors observed prostitution on the premises. After some shifty legal tussling, Plato's reopened but was shut down for the last time on the afternoon of December 31, 1985. "New Year's Eve made $40,000 for the club. He needed that money to stay open," says pornstar Ron Jeremy, who consoled Levenson that evening. "I did not let him out of my sight."

In the following months, Levenson stayed at his mother's. He claimed that he was on the run from some organized-crime types. More likely, he was just lonely. But he was not beaten, at least not completely. Levenson launched a comeback, attempting to open a 1950s-style club in the Village. But it flopped. "People wanted to fuck more than rock," Levenson lamented.

Later, he moved in with his son in New Jersey, staying on his couch. Levenson escaped through television and sweets, gorging himself on gallons of ice cream smothered with chocolate fudge. "He said, 'I need the sugar. I'm sick,'" recalls the Prince, who assumed a somewhat parental role with his father, encouraging him to hold on to his dwindling savings. "At one point I just gave up. He just never wanted to grow up!"

After failing to show up at a pizza job, Levenson was imprisoned for a year for breaking his parole. When he got out, he took an array of jobs, ranging from renting apartments to selling carpets. "Who's gonna hire the ex-owner of Plato's Retreat?" Levenson asked. Eventually, he wound up driving a cab, once again playing the host.

He didn't give up on love either. At a Parents Without Partners social, he met Marilyn. They dated and eventually married and moved to New Jersey. Their relationship wasn't about sex; it was about long-term companionship. Now Levenson was just an average, suburban working stiff. And he was content with all of it. Ultimately, though, Marilyn was not, and they split. Levenson returned to Brooklyn, heartbroken.

One night, a bloated Levenson reflected on the fleeting nature of fame:

Nobody wants to know you. When you're not up there anymore, nobody. The phone don't ring, nothing. Believe me. What could I do for anybody then? Who was I? The ex-owner of Plato's Retreat. And that's the way the world is.

Everybody that called me to, this one, that one, they all forgot me. Everybody. Believe me. Movie stars. You don't see Sammy Davis, Jr. calling me no more. Isn't that funny. Hugh Hefner? He didn't know, know who Larry Levenson was anymore. You asked him today. He wouldn't even remember. Funny, but I used to go to Plato's bashes and sit down and bullshit with him. When I had the club.

That's how people are. People don't care. Once you're—it's over. The minute they came in and closed those doors—Larry who?

One late night, his eyes welled up as he drove near Columbus Circle. "My mother always told me it was going to turn out this way."

Meanwhile, swinging never stopped completely, continuing on a much smaller scale at Manhattan's Le Trapeze, or Plato's Repeat, which Pernice opened in Fort Lauderdale. Levenson swung into an even deeper depression, blowing his Plato's cash on high-priced call girls and crack, indulging in the latter while a disturbed Ron Jeremy looked on. "He was sweating profusely."

In his final few years, the erstwhile King of Swing slept on a box spring behind a wall of medicine bottles, his caller I.D. shut off. A videocassette of the movie *Big* lay conspicuously atop his VCR.

Before he gave in to a heart condition at the age of 62, Levenson made his final public appearance at *Screw*'s thirtieth anniversary, where he once again feuded with Goldstein, who called him "a has-been." As the adoring throng of Channel J jerkers parted for him, the fallen King kept his head up, his mouth shut.

Larry Levenson's last exit was more adult than regal.

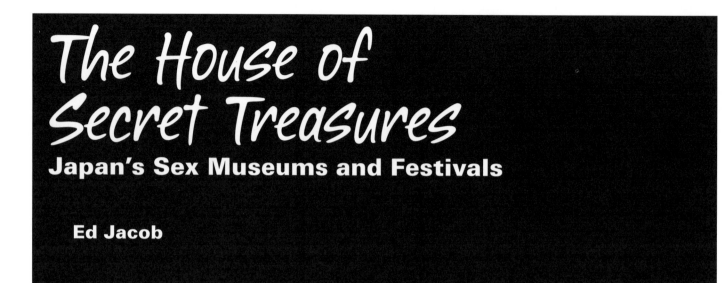

The House of Secret Treasures
Japan's Sex Museums and Festivals

Ed Jacob

Japan has museums for everything. From parasites to kites, from laundry to rubber baseballs, there's no aspect of human existence that's too mundane, unappealing, or strange to deserve a museum. It's hardly surprising, then, that there also should be a number of museums devoted to that most popular of human activities, sex.

Visitors to a typical Japanese sex museum wander through a surreal wonderland of erotic art, horror sex, adult toys from around the world, copulating animals, X-rated carnival games, and life-size dioramas of sex in various cultures. The gigantic whale vulvas, Viking rape scenes, and woodblock prints of lustful samurai with dramatically enlarged sex organs all merge to form a bizarre, erotic dreamscape as the gawking visitor giggles and smirks his or her way through the exhibits.

Japan's sex museums are called *hihoukan*, a word that means "house of secret treasures." *Hihoukan* is a typically euphemistic Japanese term that could be used as a name for anything from a candy store to a used record shop but has more and more come to be associated with sex museums, because it is almost always used in their names.

The Secret Treasurehouse of the Hermaphrodite God

Japan's first sex museum opened in 1969 in the town of Awacho, in Tokushima prefecture on the island of Shikoku. Located in the hinterlands of the least populated of Japan's four main islands, the Ome Kamisama Hihoukan (The Secret Treasurehouse of the Hermaphrodite God) certainly doesn't get many visitors.

It's so small and has such irregular opening hours, in fact, that there are occasional reports that the museum has gone out of business. If you're lucky enough to arrive on one of the random days when the museum is open, you'll be met by a friendly old man who will escort you. There's not really much to see, though, and you can be in and out in fifteen minutes. Most of the museum's collection consists of old *shunga* (erotic woodblock prints), which originated in the seventeenth century and served as both pornography and sex education material for newlyweds. Painted by some of Japan's greatest *ukiyo-e* (woodblock print) masters, these erotic images of women with tangled hair and unwound kimono sashes helped to shape Japan's artistic and cultural development. Then there are a few tabloid magazines with articles about sex museums in a glass case, and you're off to see the hermaphroditic deity.

Although it's technically a shrine, with an official permit to prove it, the place of worship is just a grungy old building. The Ome Kamisama is male on the right side and female on the left, and is believed to grant long life and happy marriages to people who pray to it. Apparently, it has both male and female genitalia, but they're always covered, so visitors have to take the owner's word for it.

The Ome Kamisama Hihoukan is tiny and not terribly exciting, but it was popular in its day, and it was a pioneer. It's important not for what it is but for what it inspired.

The First International House of Hidden Treasures

What the Ome Kamisama Hihoukan inspired is perhaps the most twisted, deviant, freakish facility ever to be called a museum. Located in the town of Toba, not far from Japan's holiest shrine, the Ganso Kokusai Hihoukan: Ise Branch is a long bus ride from a small tourist town about two hours by train from Osaka. From the outside, it resembles a comic-book version of a Russian palace, with blue and white onion domes rising over a sprawling, brown, strip-mall-looking building, and inside, well, it doesn't really resemble anything else on the face of the Earth.

Visitors are greeted by a giant, preserved whale vagina at the entrance, then things really get odd. After paying the 2600 yen (about US$25) admission fee, the visitor is taken on a whirlwind tour of sex throughout history and around the world. The bizarre voyage through space, time, and mythology starts with a woman having standing-up sex with a swan, then the bewildered museumgoer is confronted with a centaur raping a screaming woman. There are mannequins of a half-naked Salome triumphantly holding the bloody, decapitated head of John the Baptist; Caesar and Cleopatra making love; and violent Viking sex. One of the museum's most famous dioramas shows a technique, apparently from the *Kama Sutra*, in which a woman sits in a rattan basket astride her male lover, who enters her through a hole in the bottom of the basket. The ropes supporting the basket are twisted around, then released, allowing the woman to spin round and round on the man's penis.

Next, it's on to the animal paradise, which has all the scenes they couldn't show on *Wild Kingdom*, as well as a woman having sex with a monkey. The next room is all about horror sex and sadomasochism, with men eviscerating their partners as they climax, and naked women in iron maidens. To leave the horror sex area, the visitor walks through a Dalí-inspired hallway, where women's breasts and genitals, rather than clocks, are melting. The adjoining area focuses on Japanese sex, and the samurai, geisha, and yakuza here look especially run-down. A single mannequin is said to cost tens of thousands of dollars, and nothing in the museum looks to have been replaced in the last decade or so.

The exhibits take something of a scientific and historical turn in the next section, where there are numerous displays on the history of birth control and condoms, the stages of pregnancy, and sexual diseases. The subsequent room is the last of the mannequin areas, where dozens of characters from Japanese mythology and popular culture are mixed and matched in improbable sexual pairings that bring chuckles from Japanese visitors and confused looks from foreigners. After a final area with sex-related carnival games, it's time for the highlight of the tour.

What could top whale vaginas, basket sex, and evisceration? At 2:00 PM every day, an old, white horse with a mangy coat and a stiff-legged gait is brought into the museum's last room and called on to stand and deliver with his mare for ten min-

utes while an old trainer gives a play by play of the action.

As they leave, many visitors must find themselves asking, "How in the world did something like this ever come to exist?" Well, sex is considered neither dirty nor sinful in Japan, and although there are numerous societal mechanisms and constraints which curb actual intercourse, Japan has far fewer taboos regarding nudity, talking about bodily functions, and looking at pornography than other countries. Most of Japan's sex museums started in the 1980s during Japan's so-called *baburu keizai*, the infamous economic bubble, during which the country seemed close to overtaking the US as the world's foremost economic powerhouse. Money was so plentiful that sales at Louis Vuitton Japan rivaled Louis Vuitton sales for all of Europe, golf club memberships were being traded like stocks, and a membership at a top golf course in Tokyo could cost more than $1 million. A huge travel boom sprang up, and there was no such thing as too cheesy or too over-the-top when it came to tourist attractions. An entrepreneur named Masato Matsuno got the idea for a large-scale sex museum.

The Ganso Kokusai Hihoukan: Ise Branch was opened in 1971, and Matsuno blossomed into a minor celebrity known

Visitors are greeted by a giant, preserved whale vagina at the entrance, then things really get odd.

as "Professor Sex," appearing on numerous television and radio programs. His *hihoukan* became a well-known tourist attraction, starting a minor sex-museum boom that saw the creation of nearly a score of *hihoukan* across the nation.

The Science Fiction Hall of the Future
After the success of the Ganso Kokusai Hihoukan, Masato Matsuno decided to create a second, even more over-the-top sex museum. It was called the SF Mirai Kan, and it certainly surpassed his previous creation in terms of strangeness. The inspiration for the Science Fiction Hall of the Future was tabloid news reports about alien abductions involving anal probes and half-human, half-extraterrestrial love children.

At the entrance, visitors were informed: "In accordance with the prophecies of Nostradamus, the downfall of the human race came in 1999." After wiping out most humans, aliens from another planet began to hunt down the survivors in order to breed a new race with which to populate Earth. Exhibits began with the hunting of humans by sexy spacemen and spacewomen, then proceeded to sperm extraction, forced dildo sex, painful artificial insemination procedures performed without anesthetic, and finally disposal of the tortured victims' bodies. The museum played on xenophobic tendencies in Japan, and all the innocent victims were Japanese, while the sexually sadistic aliens had Western features.

For years, hordes of middle-aged and elderly package tourists dutifully paraded through the museum's rooms, quizzically examining the silver-suited spacemen dragging off naked humans to their spaceships, giant-breasted women with vacuum cleaner tubes up their vaginas, and Sadean space vixens flaying their captives alive.

The star of the show at the Beppu Hihoukan is Snow White, who is featured in a diorama being eaten out by one of the Seven Dwarfs while his fellow little people look on.

Although the main attraction was definitely the sexually dystopian future, the upper floors featured an erotic re-creation of the famous *ukiyo-e* artist Hiroshige's *53 Stations of the Old Tokaido Road*, with bathhouse orgies, samurai sex, and voluptuous pearl divers.

Despite the outrageous exhibits, the reactions of visitors at the sex museum differed very little from those of people at the nearby Mikimoto Pearl Museum or the Ise Aquarium, clearly demonstrating the openness and tolerance that exists towards nudity and sex in Japan.

The museum's popularity declined as Japan's economic bubble ended in the early 1990s; domestic tourism fell off, and the museum's exhibits aged. The Science Fiction Hall of the Future closed in 2001, and the First International House of Hidden Treasures has fallen on hard times, but together these two facilities inspired nearly a score of imitators, many of which sprang up in Japan's famous hot springs resort areas.

The Beppu Hihoukan
Sex and bathing are closely connected in the minds of many Japanese people. Japan's famous "soaplands" are basically brothels thinly disguised as bathhouses in which customers are washed down by "soapgirls," and for hundreds of years, male visitors to hot springs would engage *onsen geisha*, poor cousins of the entertainers who were the life of high-class parties in Kyoto and Tokyo. The typical *onsen geisha* had few of the qualms about sleeping with her customer that *geisha* from the city might, and Japan's biggest hot springs resort areas were home to thousands of prostitutes. Before overseas travel became common, these resorts were the top honeymoon destinations in Japan, so the large number of people with sex on their minds who came to Japan's *onsen* were an

invitation to open up sex-related tourist attractions.

The town of Beppu on the southern island of Kyushu is one of Japan's most famous hot springs resorts, so it isn't surprising that it would also be home to the country's most famous sex museum. The star of the show at the Beppu Hihoukan is Snow White, who is featured in a diorama being eaten out by one of the Seven Dwarfs while his fellow little people look on. Another scene depicts a smoking woman sitting with legs parted and a dog in front of her, and if guests push a button on the control panel, her dog moves forward and begins trying to tug off her panties.

You can't make a sex museum in Japan without a comparison of animal penises, and the Beppu Hihoukan offers the usual selection of horse, human, and whale organs. Far more interesting, however, are the displays of phallic objects used at places of worship, such as three-meter, wooden phalluses, an assortment of carvings, and a woodblock print of Japan's famous Seven Gods of Good Fortune having an orgy.

The Iron Phallus Shrine: Kanayama Jinja
If hot springs are the best places to learn about sex *à la Japonais*, a close second is the shrines, many of which have collections of erotic artifacts, statues, and phalluses.

Take, for example, the Kanayama-jinja in the city of Kawasaki near Tokyo. This shrine is small and out of the way but receives an inordinate number of visitors because it's one of the few places in Japan where you can still go to worship a sacred penis. There are several on the shrine's grounds, as well as some shockingly lewd artwork.

The Kanayama-jinja enshrines two deities called Kanayama Hikonokami and Kanayama Himenokami. These two gods appear in Japan's most ancient creation myth and are the children of the brother and sister gods whose procreation gave form to the world. As the story goes, Izanami had sex with her brother, and gave birth to the main islands of Japan. After the islands were created, the happy couple continued to have sex, giving birth to the gods that looked after the world. Everything was going well until Izanami gave birth to the god of fire, Kagutsuchi, whose birth was, understandably, more than a little painful. She was terribly burned, and two of her children, Kanayama Hikonokami and Kanayama Himenokami tried their best to save her. Because they were taking care of her womb, they have become associated with birth and cures for sexually transmitted diseases.

The shrine is visited by thousands of worshippers who rub

the iron penises to petition the shrine's gods for babies or cures to venereal disease. All shrines in Japan have festivals, and Kanayama-jinja is no different, but its Jibeta festival certainly is. In fact, it's about as wild and pagan as they get. People of all ages participate in a parade in which most of the participants sport a gigantic penis, and a massive lingam is carried through the streets. Females ride a penis-shaped see-saw, and men, women, and children get their pictures taken embracing a phallic statue. You can also buy penis-shaped candies or dress up as your favorite cartoon character with one part of his anatomy dramatically enlarged. The whole thing is presided over by a priest, and arcane Shinto rituals are carried out, as well.

The festival is said to celebrate the vanquishing of a demon that lived in a woman's vagina and would bite off the penises of her lovers. According to legend, a local craftsman fashioned a steel phallus which broke the demon's teeth. In the Edo period, courtesans would come to pray for good business and protection from sexually transmitted diseases, and today it is used to promote AIDS awareness and safe sex.

Tagata Shrine

The Tagata shrine, in a small town called Komaki in central Japan, is ancient Japan's answer to Viagra. There are so many hard penises here that anyone needing a little inspiration in the erectile department would be well-advised to visit this odd place of worship. Everything from the shrine's bell to the candy in the souvenir shop is shaped like a penis, particularly in the main building, which houses dozens of long, wooden phalluses as objects of worship. The Tagata shrine is dedicated to Mitoshi-no-kami, the god of the rice harvest, and Tamahine-no-Mikoto, a fertility goddess. The shrine also has a large collection of stones that look like sex organs, with two famous round rocks that represent testicles.

Every year on March 15, the Tagata Jinja is home to the Hounen Matsuri, or Bountiful Year Festival, an old, local spring festival that has grown to attract tens of thousands of visitors. Like the Kanamara Matsuri, this festival is all about penises, and the main object of worship is a giant, two-and-a-half-meter long, 620-pound phallus that is carried through the streets by a team of 42-year-old men (42 is considered an unlucky age for men in Japan). There's also free beer and sake for everyone who attends the festival, and although the bilingual pamphlet given out by organizers describes the Hounen Matsuri as a "solemn occasion," it never is. The highlight of the festival is supposed to be the giant penis, but for many people, it's the sight of their 40-year-old housewife neighbor dressed in a kimono, cradling a meter-long penis in her arms like a loaf of French bread.

Festivals like this one used to take place all over Japan, but unfortunately the Kanamara and Hounen festivals are the last of their kind.

Last Chance to See?

Japan's sex museums are becoming less and less common, and fertility shrines and festivals are increasingly being toned down. After Japan's economic bubble burst in the early 1990s, attendance rates at most museums fell off, partly because people had less money to spend and partly because the novelty had worn off. Japan is famously faddish, and sex museums have become passé. A *hihoukan* closes every few years, and what was once a score is now a dozen. The ones that survive receive few tourists, and the exhibits get more dilapidated every year.

Fertility festivals, while still popular, are being changed gradually, with penises being converted into spears or obelisks, and nudity being covered up. It's been happening since Japan modernized in the late nineteenth century and changed Shinto's focus from ancestors and fertility to emperor worship. Even worse were the terrible air raids of the Second World War; a great number of these shrines were destroyed and not rebuilt. After WWII, many local governments took steps

Everything from the shrine's bell to the candy in the souvenir shop is shaped like a penis.

to ban surviving festivals because they felt that they hurt their town's image or made their community look backwards. Even in places where festivals have survived, local tourist associations try to keep word from getting out and are taking them out of their brochures. In short, the more Westernized Japan becomes, the more difficult it is to find sex museums and fertility festivals out in the open, so if you want to see one, book your tickets soon. Here are a few addresses of the more famous museums and festivals:

- Ome Kamisama Hihoukan – Tokushima prefecture, Awa-gun, Awa-cho, Jio-nooka 143-8, Tel. 0883-35-2634
- Atami Hihoukan - Shizuoka prefecture, Atami city, Wadahama Minami-cho 10-1. Tel. 0557-83-5572
- Hokkaido Hihoukan – Hokkaido, Sapporo city, Minami-ku, Jozankei Onsen Higashi 2-103-1, Tel. 011-598-4141
- Ganso Kokusai Hihoukan – Mie prefecture, Watarai-gun, Tamashiro-cho, Seko 345, Tel. 0596-25-1251
- Beppu Hihoukan – Oita prefecture, Beppu city, Shibuyu Kannawa 338-3, Tel. 0977-66-8790
- Kanayama-jinja – Kanagawa prefecture, Kawasaki city, Kawasaki ward, Daishi Eki-mae 2-13-16
- Tagata Jinja – Tagata-cho 152, Komaki City, Aichi-ken. Tel. 0568 76 2906

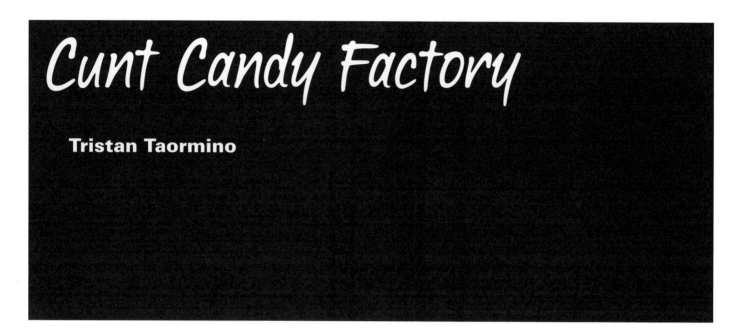

Cunt Candy Factory

Tristan Taormino

I owned Juli Ashton's ass and pussy—I spanked her cheeks, teased and probed her two orifices—before I ever met her. Let me clarify: I had Juli Ashton's Ultra-Realistic Pussy & Ass, a rubber replica of the famed pornstar's private parts, before I saw said star in the flesh. After her career on film, she went on to cohost *Night Calls* on Playboy TV and Radio, which she's done for ten years. When I first met Juli, I already felt I had a connection to her. After all, her rubber-genital self accompanied me around the country to dozens of workshops and lectures. When I couldn't have a real, live model, I always had Juli on (in?) which to demonstrate techniques. She brought my sex education to life.

In March 2005, the real Juli took me to the headquarters of Doc Johnson, one of the world's leading sex-toy manufacturers. I was expecting one huge factory, but it was more of a

Rarely do people ask themselves, "Where do dildos come from?"

compound, with multiple buildings all buzzing with activity in North Hollywood. I got a tour from the president himself, Ron Braverman, who proudly proclaimed, "We were the first company to manufacture and market butt plugs." My hero!

Doc Johnson makes over 5,000 different products, including vibrators, penis pumps, lube, blindfolds, and anti-porn crusader Catherine MacKinnon's worst nightmare: disembodied replicas of pornstars' famous bits (like Jeff Stryker's cock and Jenna Jameson's cooch). It hit me when I saw the recognizable crotch creations: I was visiting the place that created, and still churns out, Juli Ashton's Ultra-Realistic Pussy & Ass, and I was there with Juli. Life had come full circle.

We visited that very department, where designers had recently taken plaster casts of the pusses of four starlets: Lexie, Monique Alexander, and newcomer twins Lacey and Lyndsey Love. From the plaster cast a mold is created, explained Braverman. "We really try to make it as close to the real thing as possible." The four plaster cunts sat in a circle, but they weren't labeled, so I wasn't sure who was whom.

I noticed that a small, stray piece of plaster sat next to one. One of the workers said, "She had one very large labia. I had to fold it over her opening to make the cast, and it broke." To demonstrate, he carefully—dare I say lovingly?—placed the piece of plaster where it should be. "I'm going to reattach it before I make the mold," he said, and his statement was strangely sweet. Braverman informed Juli that they've improved the technology and the process, which only takes thirty minutes from start to finish. Juli considered doing a special tenth-anniversary pussy and ass as we walked over to the next building.

From there it was a whirlwind of sex-toy production. I can't adequately describe the sight of copper cock molds moving swiftly along a conveyor belt, of toys being pulled from those molds and tossed into a cold-water bath to cool, of sparkling pink jelly dongs laid out in a row, of fat, baby-blue butt plugs waiting patiently to be put into their custom-designed packages. Or the area where certain toys (known as "the realistics") get a personal touch: hand painting. Here, women gingerly brush pink dye onto cockheads and pussy lips and clits (to mimic the engorgement process during arousal) or draw bluish veins on peach-colored shafts. The color looked garish, but Braverman assured me that as it gets absorbed into the material, it fades and looks more natural.

Rarely do people ask themselves, "Where do dildos come from?" before they pick one out in the store, bring it home, tear into the packaging, and take it for a test drive. They are such personal items that bring us great pleasure. And there I was, at their place of creation. I watched with great reverence as double-dongs made their way down an assembly line, suction cups were methodically attached right under the balls of realistic dildos, and bottles were filled from huge vats of strawberry-scented lube.

At quality control, each product was carefully inspected for imperfections. I half expected to find a testing area in a typical focus-group room with one-way mirrors, this one filled with naked people trying out toys and rating them on a questionnaire. If that exists at Doc Johnson, I didn't get to see it.

I did, however, get a peek inside the new-product development department, which was the highlight of my visit. There, designers were brainstorming ideas, experimenting with new toy materials, and testing different design elements. I smelled the prototype of a scented toy they're working on (it was either peach or some kind of melon—I'm not sure). I spotted a uniquely shaped butt plug and asked when it would be on the market (about six months). I found inspired creations that I look forward to seeing on the shelf at my favorite toy shop. I felt like Donald Trump getting a look at new luxury jets before anyone else.

At first glance, Doc Johnson seems like any other factory, with the hum of machines creating the soundtrack of the workday, signs about worker safety prominently displayed, and staffers chatting on their lunch break. It seemed like a good place to work, judging by how upbeat everyone was. People smiled at me as I eyed chocolate-brown dicks standing upright on a shelf, and no one seemed stressed or frenetic. There was

The four plaster cunts sat in a circle, but they weren't labeled, so I wasn't sure who was whom.

good energy in the place, and I want my dildos coming from a place with good energy.

I wonder, though, how the over 600 employees who work there don't get distracted by the things they create, handle, inspect, and package every day. They are surrounded by sex life spicer-uppers, masturbation tools, and battery-powered orgasm generators. How can they keep from running to the bathroom to jerk off, as I wanted to do halfway through my guided tour?

Shockingly, I managed to score zero free shit from my visit (and I could really use a new Juli, since I've, um, worn her out). But that's okay, because Doc Johnson's bestselling toy, the Pocket Rocket, was already in my purse. I never leave home without it.

The Archive

Jack Boulware

"The clip we're about to see is from a film called *Make Mine Milk*," says a film archivist named Paul Potocky. "The gal who stars in it is lactating. It's one of my favorites, filmed right here in San Francisco." He pushes "play" on a video recorder, and the audience is treated to a grainy, five-foot image of greasy hippies having sex.

For the next two hours, similar clips roll past, from *Maxine's Dating Service* to *Miss Kinsey's Report*, *Starship Eros*, *Hitler's Harlot*, and *Reckless Claudia*. All examples from the dawn of America's adult-film industry, featuring the genre's requisite dirty feet, hairy bellies, pink faces, stoned expressions, and wretched acting. But we're not sitting in a sticky-floor theater with peeling wallpaper. We're actually in a meeting room of San Francisco's Cathedral Hill convention hotel. This is the twenty-fifth anniversary gala weekend of a state-accredited institution of higher learning. And we've just had lunch.

More than just retro raunch, these skin flicks represent a tiny nugget of pornography's mother lode, the world's largest repository of porn and erotica.

More than just retro raunch, these skin flicks represent a tiny nugget of pornography's mother lode, the world's largest repository of porn and erotica—three million items, including hundreds of thousands of films, which fill 22 warehouses throughout Northern California. The sex and porn industries know about the Archive. It belongs to the Institute for the Advanced Study of Human Sexuality. This specialized school has been squirreling away such materials for nearly three decades, valiantly cataloging what it refers to as America's "erotic heritage." Everyone knows of it, but few have ever seen it.

The Archive's contents arrive at the Institute primarily in the form of tax-deductible donations, from retired film producers, erotica collectors, even other museums and libraries. Policy is never to throw away anything, so warehouses fill with a never-ending stream of porn films, books, magazines, sex toys, virtually anything related to sex and pornography. I'm sitting in this hotel, crashing the Institute's anniversary weekend celebration, to catch a glimpse of this fabled historical repository. Which means, at the moment, a snip from the classic title *Hungry Hypnotist*.

This afternoon is not without its educational side. We learn that in the industry's infancy, low-budget directors would flash the lights on and off to simulate a strobe effect. To avoid prosecution, producers often added scenes of "redeeming quality" to their efforts, such as travel or documentary footage, or in the case of *Black Is Beautiful*, an actor in a suit at a desk, painstakingly explaining the marriage rituals of an African family. So-called "loop carrier" films began with a ten-minute loop of porn footage, then plot and characters were added around it. Soundtracks ranged from stolen rock and funk tunes to original music recorded by Blues Project guitarist Mike Bloomfield, who did the gigs to finance his heroin habit.

Our host introduces another film, also one of his favorites, he says, entitled *The Rites of Uranus*. We watch the footage of guys in satanic robes, chanting, "Hail to your anus!" while masturbating to a gyrating woman, who sports a lit candle sticking out of her rear. After an hour or so, it all sort of blends together in a sweaty collage of slapdash hippie lust. As I walk out, the noisy satanic chants still echoing behind me, I notice an elderly woman, one of the Institute's faculty, sitting in a wheelchair in the middle of the room, fast asleep.

Headquarters of the Archive is a nondescript building painted blue, with only the words "Exodus Foundation" printed on the door, and the copies of *Newsweek* and *National Geographic* in the lobby do nothing to tell visitors that this is the Institute for the Advanced Study of Human Sexuality. I'm met by Howard Ruppel, Chancellor and Academic Dean, a chatty fellow of about 60 who sports a graying ponytail, tie, and training shoes. Howard has taught human sexuality at university level and also worked as a sex therapist and counselor, which means he's very friendly and is the type of person that if you ever happen to interrupt him, he immediately stops talking and insists that you continue the point you wish to make. Although he's been on the Institute's board of directors for years, he had recently relocated to San Francisco to assume his duties as the boss. Howard's presence gives the school a jolt of new energy, because its founder and figurehead, former Methodist minister Rev. Ted McIlvenna, is considering retirement.

Applicants accepted to the Institute pay $13,500 for three terms, studying under 30 full- and part-time faculty. Most students participate through the mail from outside California and are working towards doctorate degrees in social sciences and helping professions. Among their requirements is the viewing of 100 hours of videos, selected from the Archive. Recent dissertation topics have included the external penis pump device, sex counseling for the mentally retarded, the interaction in gay baths, and the contributions to "sexology" of soul singer James Brown.

I hear the word *sexology* constantly. It's all over the school's brochures and mission statements. According to Howard, the study of sexuality is composed of various sex fiefdoms—the psychologists don't deal with the psychiatrists, who ignore the biologists, who dismiss the historians. Sexology, on the other hand, is the multidisciplinary philosophy that looks at all the disciplines and combines them. He compares it to the ecology movement in the 1970s, when biologists, psychologists, and geographers all came together to study the impact of "green" issues like pollution and zero population growth. The Institute's goal is to promote sexology through education, so as to have an impact on social issues. Howard says they definitely have achieved these goals, particularly in certain areas, including HIV, sexual counseling, and gender.

Erotology is another word peculiar to the Institute's philosophy. Howard explains it as "the scholarly study of erotic materials." They don't use the word *scientific*, he says, because it sounds too male-oriented, too patriarchal. Using *scholarly*

allows the feminists to become part of the discussion. So in other words, students specializing in erotology look at an awful lot of porn and analyze what it means—not an impulse that enters the mind of your average pants-to-the-ankles viewer.

Outside of a sexology program at the University of Montreal at Quebec, the Institute is the only school of its kind in the world. And it's also unique, of course, because of the Archive.

Now I really want to see the mountain of porn known as the Exodus Trust Erotology Library, or at least speak to someone who has. I track down a graduate of the school, Carol Queen, an extremely bright and strong-willed bisexual woman who has made a name for herself as a sex author and educator.

Recent dissertation topics have included the external penis pump device, sex counseling for the mentally retarded, the interaction in gay baths, and the contributions to "sexology" of soul singer James Brown.

She works days at the sex-toy retailer Good Vibrations, and after our meeting she will lead a masturbation workshop. Sociology graduate Carol first enrolled at the Institute in the 1980s, a time when it was nicknamed "Hot Tub U."

Unfortunately, Carol has not seen the Archive firsthand. But she's well aware of it. "Most people don't know that this exists," she says. "It doesn't matter what it is. It doesn't matter if you took that same scene from *Debbie Does Dallas* that you jerked off to for your entire adult life and looped it, and you got an hour of that one scene. They'll take anything. And it's all erotologically significant."

Carol has visited the renowned Kinsey Institute in Indiana and found that when she poked around their erotica collection, it was nothing at all like the Archive: "They're not proud of the smut like the Institute is. Which is a very different way of understanding things. Kinsey is like, 'Well, we shouldn't throw this away because someday it'll be important.' But the Institute is like, 'Look what we got! We've got porno!'

"The Institute respects this material as the cultural output of a society that's whacked-out about sex," she continues. "And that's worth studying. And what it produces is worth studying. And how people use it is worth studying. All of it is valuable. But good fucking luck if you're an erotica researcher and you want to go in and look around at that stuff!"

I've heard this from several people. I've even attempted to

use the Institute's resources myself while researching a book about the sexual revolution. Anybody engaging in serious research about the topic of sex in general, or the commercial porn industry in particular, would benefit hugely from the Archive. It's an incredible storehouse of knowledge and history. But it is not open to the public. I've asked various individuals from the fields of academic scholarship, museums, and journalism, and the verdict is the same: The Institute is very proprietary, and if you see any of it at all, you're extremely lucky.

According to one person who has been inside the warehouses, materials are still not catalogued or archived. Boxes and film containers are piled high, moldering with neglect, patrolled by platoons of spiders. There is potentially millions of dollars' worth of material here, which could be sold, published, put on exhibit in an art show or film festival. But outside of very occasional specific projects, there are no immediate plans for any of it. It's a dubious end to the career output of sexual pioneers like John Holmes, Seka, Traci Lords, and countless others.

꩜

The room looks straight from 1973: brown shag carpeting, orange walls, and dozens of large, embroidered pillows. My quest to glimpse the Archive has led me to the Institute's SAR Room (Sexual Attitude Restructuring), where for seven days students watch visuals and listen to lectures. On the final day, students are subjected to the Institute's most controversial educational tool, a 45-minute multimedia barrage called the Fuck-A-Rama. Culled from the Archive, the audio-

Boxes and film containers are piled high, moldering with neglect, patrolled by platoons of spiders.

visual assault covers every conceivable sexual behavior, from masturbation to gay, bisexual, transgender, bondage, bestial delights, whatever. The purpose is for students to discover their own "buttons," or personal limits.

"I advise everyone to have this experience every two years," Howard Ruppel says calmly, as I stare at the arsenal of video and slide projectors. "We cover everything—animals, elephants. I've been in this business for 30 years, but when I see a fist in another man's ass up to the elbow..." He chuckles and shakes his head, revealing his buttons may well have something to do with fists. Or elephants. I'm here today because Howard has asked me to deliver a three-hour lecture.

Lounging on the pillows are about fifteen students, aged from twenties to fifties, looking back at me. This is the same lecture series that Allen Ginsberg, Alex *The Joy of Sex* Comfort,

Gore Vidal, and a host of distinguished scholars have participated in. I've written a pop-culture book about the sexual revolution. Either the Institute considers my work significant, or they've reached the bottom of the list. I ask the students what the Fuck-A-Rama is like.

"Scorched earth," chuckles one guy.

"I had to change my underwear," says a woman from Minnesota.

"You dream about it for three or four months," says another woman. "It's headspinning."

"I've seen three or four," declares a young guy named Michael, whose career ambition is to become a porn director. "They change it a bit each time."

I plow through material from my book and, to eat up time, encourage the students to interrupt with questions at any time. They perk up at my experience as an extra (clothed) in the film *Dog Walker*, by veteran porn director John Leslie. At one point, as the crew readjusted lights, Leslie had announced to everyone on the set: "Over in Germany, they can shit on people, but they can't pull the hair!" After this is read aloud, a roar of laughter erupts from an adjoining room, where the Institute's faculty is watching the lecture from a monitor.

We talk about censorship, Monica Lewinsky, a dubious erectile device called the Accu-Jack. And then the question comes: Have you ever covered bestiality? I admit that yes, in my checkered past in underground publishing, I have been exposed to a certain film from Argentina, wherein a group of young couples go to visit a zoo and fool around with the animals. "It's actually from Brazil," corrects a voice from the back of the room. Another student in the front row adds that it's not uncommon for young Brazilian actors to get their start in bestiality films. I thank them and realize it's exactly as every teacher says: Education truly does work both ways.

We wrap it up, and a young man presents me with a ballpoint pen, commemorating the Institute's twenty-fifth anniversary. A girl from South Africa dives into the pillows, laughing, as other students toss pillows on top of her and jump onto the pile like a litter of puppies. I linger on my way out to poke a finger into one of the embroidered cushions.

"There's all kinds of jokes about dry-cleaning these," chuckles Howard. "We try to keep the orgies to a minimum."

⌣

Several times I ask if I can be given a tour of one of the Archive's warehouses, and each time I'm greeted with a polite brush-off. It's clear that this is the heart of the Institute and a sensitive issue. Either they're wary about divulging warehouse locations, or they're embarrassed about the unorganized conditions. Or perhaps I haven't sufficiently groveled enough to worm my way into the inner circle. As an alternative, Howard Ruppel does agree to give me a tour of the Institute's libraries, which contain thousands of Archive items considered important and useful enough to be made readily available for students.

"Get your galoshes on," he jokes, and we walk down a hallway garnished with colored drawings of wild sexual scenarios: a cartoon of a doctor sneaking pills to his beautiful, naked female patient, a Commedia Del Arté clown engaging in cunnilingus, a group of nude Rubenesque women in a pile, a woman tied up and getting spanked, an old man examining a young girl in his lap, a soldier surprising his friend in a bed of hay with a woman. According to a provenance, these items come from a four-volume work titled *Bilder Lexicon*, published in Germany from 1928 to 1930, which was banned by the Nazis. Howard explains that historians have turned up copies of these books with burnt bindings, suggesting that they were removed from fires in the nick of time. He points at one drawing: "Look at this one. That looks like an enema." He taps the drawing with a finger. "I never noticed that before. Huh. An enema bag."

The next room, with a circular table and chairs, is where students relax between classes. It's called the Mac Room, so named after the late Dr. Don McAllister, an early Institute member who also contributed designs for the Doc Johnson sex-toy company. Beautifully carved dildos fill a glass case. On another wall is a plaster cast made of a woman's bare torso, supposedly a prominent Hollywood actress "known primarily for her legs." Howard refuses to tell me who it is. I examine it more closely. She appeared to be wearing Levi's jeans. One of the original Charlie's Angels, perhaps?

He shows me the hot-tub room, an area with floors and walls covered with redwood. A few fake plants decorate a corner. The tubs were used a lot more in the past, he says. Students and faculty would hop in for a dip after classes. These days, students are more inclined to go home and do their work after hours by themselves.

We then enter a room of the library, lined with books, scholarly papers, and bankers boxes stacked to the ceiling. Howard then ushers me into the video room, walls and walls of Beta and VHS tapes. And what might the students be studying? *Bunbusters. Edward Penishands. Women Loving Women. The Dirty Debutantes* series. *Evolutionary Masturbation.* Bizet's *Carmen*?

What are the new trends in porn? I ask.

"The anal is very popular." Howard gestures to a wall of tapes. I follow him around a corner. "B and D [bondage and discipline] stuff in here. Over in this corner, all the extreme stuff, from Germany. The urination stuff."

Howard says that more sensitive materials, involving celebrities and semi-illegal activities, are safely stored under lock and key, available only upon serious request. Much of this library comes from people whom you and I might call "pornhounds." But to the Institute, these salivating pervs constitute a valuable resource.

"Some people think they're going to live forever." Howard shakes his head. Collectors often promise their archives to the Institute, then refuse, not wanting to give up the goods just yet. Sometimes these people will pass away without

On the final day, students are subjected to the Institute's most controversial educational tool, a 45-minute multimedia barrage called the Fuck-A-Rama.

leaving their collection to the school. The Institute will "discreetly" approach the deceased's heirs, hoping to snag the porn. But the executors often are disgusted upon discovering Dad's smut library, and they throw it away. Howard grows somber when he speaks of this. Clearly, it's been an ongoing problem.

He introduces me to librarian Jerry Zentara, who is reviewing a pile of postcards depicting muscled, nude men. Jerry also wears a graying ponytail and possesses the ultimate openness of someone who's seen just about every conceivable type of erotica man has ever produced. Whatever donations come through the door—films, books, videos, periodicals, pop-culture ephemera—Jerry opens the boxes, appraises their value, then files and catalogs everything and sends the least-usable items off to a warehouse.

I ask Jerry if he's completely jaded or if he can still be shocked.

"Disgusted, but never shocked," he replies. "Mostly, it's the same old stuff."

What are the most commonly donated items?

He sighs. "We're not interested in any more copies of *The Hite Report*." (A 1970s collection of women's questionnaire answers about their sex lives.)

"We want more fetish collections," he continues. "We have a pretty good collection of sex toys. It could always stand fluffing up. People just didn't save their dildos back in the 1920s and 1930s."

The library also contains private papers, films and videos produced in-house, recordings of guest lecturers, and all the dissertations. Perhaps a student will one day cue up a video of my little talk and learn more about Brazil.

Howard quickly ushers me through an empty room strewn with rubbish and beat-up furniture, into yet another room, where film archivist Paul Potocky is absorbed in viewing a video monitor, showing a piece of smut that—going by

It seems strange that the world's largest repository of sexuality—so often a source of joy in people's lives—is in the hands of such a curmudgeon.

hairstyles alone—looks like it's from the 1980s. Each day, Paul threads up 16mm porn films, views each roll of celluloid, and takes notes on its condition and deterioration. He is surrounded by stacks of film reels and containers, labeled with titles: *All About Gloria Leonard. Domination Blue. Loving Friends. Here Comes Johnny Wadd.* The most commonly donated films, Paul says, are the 1970s classics *Deep Throat* and *Behind the Green Door*, but the quality is often very poor because these are the two vanguards of adult smut, the temples of hardcore, and the copies have been screened too many times.

Howard and Paul walk me to meet Rand McIlvenna, the school's media director who is in charge of transferring the Archive's best-quality films onto video for archival purposes. Paul and Rand have spent two years digitizing the films, an enormous full-time undertaking they estimate will take eight more years—unless the Archive accumulates more, which is inevitable. Rand says that adult movies shot in the 1970s, rather than the 1980s, are surprisingly the best preserved, because they've either never been watched at all or haven't been screened in years. The films often sit in garages or storage facilities, until someone decides to donate them to the Institute.

They are well-steeped in American porn history and how the genre broke down geographically. New York's porn filmmakers in the late 1960s and early 1970s were convinced that porn was art, and they hired Off Broadway actors and used sophisticated camera and editing techniques. San Francisco's porn reflected the realism of hairy armpits and dirty feet, and invariably included several unnecessary minutes of cable cars and the Golden Gate Bridge. Los Angeles' porn was singularly poor because any jackass in Hollywood had easy access

to film equipment. Paul relays a joke common to the early LA porn industry, where politicians were most severe in monitoring its activities: "In Los Angeles, going on location meant going from the bedroom to the living room." Everyone chuckles.

⋈

I follow Howard down a flight of stairs. Sitting in an office is the Institute's founder and president, Ted McIlvenna. A former Methodist minister from Nashville, McIlvenna began offering sex classes in the late 1960s in San Francisco, which evolved into the National Sex Forum, then the present school. He's written several books, testified in dozens of court cases, and even claims to have invented a lubricating cure-all for STDs called Erogel. The man knows sex. And when it comes to the Archive, Ted is the Man. All acquisitions come directly through him.

The gravelly-voiced McIlvenna is introduced to me, and he sizes me up for a moment. He's at least 70, his hefty frame wedged into his chair. There is nothing on his desk but a phone and computer. If you get to know him, he's a cordial sort, but to strangers he radiates intimidation and a hint of contempt. His moods are legendary in that his own staff roll their eyes at his grumpiness. It seems strange that the world's largest repository of sexuality—so often a source of joy in people's lives—is in the hands of such a curmudgeon.

He launches into a familiar story about how they went to inspect one of the Archive's warehouses, which hadn't been opened in 20 years. Apparently the keys to the lock had been lost, so they had to use bolt-cutters to break open the door. Neighbors witnessed the act, called police, and a squad car arrived on the scene. He leans back and laughs, his joviality catching me off guard.

McIlvenna says he will retire at the end of 2003, but don't hold your breath.[1] In many ways the Institute remains a mom-and-pop sex shop, a store with a hanging shingle from a frontier town in the Old West. His wife is comptroller, his son the media director. In 25 years, they've had just 280 graduates. A common phrase around the school is: "We are what we are. We can't be what you want us to be." For years, outsiders have speculated about the future of the Institute, but in the end, it always revolves around McIlvenna.

He says he's never really been a collector, other than a few pieces of fine art. But what he does understand very well is that people respond to large numbers. Each time he speaks of the Archive, he says things such as, "We have 287,000 films alone," then pauses, knowing the listener is bound to be impressed.

But as we talk further, he appears to soften. He knows that everybody wants to see the stuff and that managing it is a massive chore.

"It hasn't been used well," he admits. "There's so much there. We're just discovering 16mm films we didn't even know we had. We definitely need help. I would hope people start coming along to help us. It's so much better than what you see on the Internet."

I press if there are plans to display any of it, and surprisingly, he agrees. "It really ought to be available to people. We have enough to open a museum now. We're talking about it. We can do it anytime. We have the financing. The problem is finding the place."

Over the years, the Institute has dribbled out tiny portions of the Archive. Several items were displayed in a late-1960s erotic art museum in San Francisco. Videos have been produced using excerpts from the bank of porn films. More recently, 100 vintage posters were shipped off to the Smithsonian for an exhibit.

He firmly believes that the Archive is important, even sacred history, whether it's old posters, brochures from 1920s swinger groups, or 8mm loops of gay porn. One reason why he chooses to spend a lifetime surrounded by smut may come from the fact that his church originally assigned him to stamp out this very material. Turning one's back on strict religious devotion often manifests in sexual ways—count the numbers of failed Catholics in strip clubs and porn films, for example. Perhaps collecting and preserving smut has in some deeper way become McIlvenna's way of releasing the binds of the church. And then there's the pride of possession, of simply having more than anyone else.

His weariness for most everybody else in the field is obvious. Researchers and filmmakers have borrowed countless items, he says, and never returned them. Or never paid for them. Or returned them damaged, as was the case with props used in

He firmly believes that the Archive is important, even sacred history, whether it's old posters, brochures from 1920s swinger groups, or 8mm loops of gay porn.

the film *Boogie Nights*. The current crop of porn-film producers and stars, in his eyes, doesn't compare to yesteryear's. It's changed for the worse. The older people who gave the industry some depth aren't around any more.

We continue chatting. The conversation turns to the topic of celebrity actors and actresses appearing in porn films—Barbra Streisand, Sly Stallone, Marilyn Monroe being the most well-known. Who is in possession of such artifacts? Ted McIlvenna is. He knew the Los Angeles man whose life goal was to collect all such footage, and he has since come into possession of these films and more. The Institute supposedly has all of them—every one of them—locked away in the Archive. It's hard to imagine a safer place.

Endnote
1. In fact, as of May 2005, he's still there.

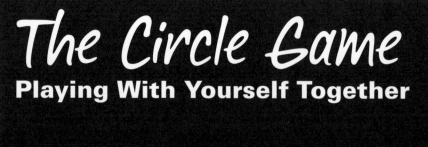

The Circle Game
Playing With Yourself Together

Martha Cornog

"We have termed onanism a solitary vice, and nothing is more just. It has also been termed a contagious vice, and nothing is more true."

—Walling, *Sexology*, 1904

Writing a book about masturbation wasn't a solo effort. In the process, I met all sorts of co-conspirators who fed me articles, factoids, tips, and encouragement. And I found out along the way that solo sex isn't always solo.

Naturally, I knew about circle jerks. I had been reading about them in a curious little magazine called *Celebrate the Self*, pub-

The other thing that I found out pretty quickly was that group masturbation had been virtually unstudied, in kids or adults.

lished for men who are masturbation aficionados. Personal vignettes dominated its pages, and more than a few described collective masturbatory camaraderie among childhood buddies. But a surprising (to me) number recounted pud-pulling circles of adult men—"close encounters," as one writer put it. I side-filed this intriguing information while continuing to order books, visit libraries, dig out more sex magazines, write to wildly assorted experts, and make copious notes for my manuscript of *The Big Book of Masturbation*.

Then one of my research trips took me to the library of a sexology organization in California. I found a fair amount on my topic, only some of it new and interesting to me. Then I chatted up the librarian, whom I shall call "Dr. Woof." (He knows who he is.) Would I, he commented diffidently after a while, be interested in hearing about the San Francisco Jacks? And what might they be? I inquired. A men's masturbation club.

Yow. I went on red alert, yanked out my pad, and sat down. For the next two hours, I scribbled frantically and murmured occasional questions. Eventually I staggered out with a large bag of documents to the drugstore across the street, which had a photocopier. The machine faced a floor-to-ceiling window on the street, so it was rather skittishly that I copied my way through copious and explicitly illustrated articles about the Jacks, back issues of their yearbook, flyers and handbills about sex parties, and the kind of sex "ephemera" that both Alfred Kinsey and Edwin Meese might have killed for—for different reasons.

Hot damn, the adult phenom was sure bigger than I thought, and that put the boys' camaraderie in a much more interesting light. What else could I find out? I went digging in all kinds of sex books, I surfed the Web, and I went back to *Celebrate the Self*. One lead eventually led to another, sometimes in surprising directions. For example, for a while Rodale Press put out a magazine called *Men's Confidential*, which had actually surveyed readers in 1996 about "group masturbation." Hmmm. Dr. Woof had preferred the term "social masturbation." Hell, either way, the whole concept was an oxymoron. Since Dr. Woof's expression evoked for me a nice game of bridge or perhaps charades, I decided to think of my topic as group masturbation.

What struck me pretty quickly was that the earliest known book on autoeroticism—the eighteenth-century anti-masturbation tract *Onania*—mentioned both boys' and girls' groups. In utter horror and disgust, of course:

Would all Masters of Schools have but a strict Eye over their Scholars; (amongst whom nothing is more common, than the Commission of this vile

Sin, the Elder Boys Teaching it to the Younger....) (1724)

~

My sad Case is, that when I was a young Girl of between 15 and 16 Years of Age, at the Boarding-School, being entic'd and shew'd the way by 3 of my School-Fellows, older than my Self, which lay in the Chamber with me, two Beds being in the Room, I did as they did...and I thought it was pleasing enough. (1724)

The later medical classic *Onanism*, by respected Swiss doctor Samuel Tissot, is considered the source of all of those terrifying myths about masturbation—that it would make you go blind and crazy. Tissot also referred to groups:

[A] whole school sometimes strove by this practice, to...keep themselves awake during the lectures upon scholastic metaphysics, delivered by a sleepy professor.... Some years since, it was discovered in the city, that a company of libertines, fourteen or fifteen years old, used to assemble to practice this vice, and that a whole school is still polluted by it. (*c.* 1760)

The other thing that I found out pretty quickly was that group masturbation had been virtually unstudied, in kids or adults. While the phenomenon theoretically had been under everybody's nose since the early 1700s, I couldn't find much about it, and I found far more in popular writing and on the Web than in scholarly work. Could this be a new intellectual find? An unexplored Island of Interesting Stuff? Lemme at it! I detoured from my masturbation book for a while to intensely focus on this almost unacknowledged variation.

Boys Have Circle Jerks—Do Girls?

I started with a little study of my own about circle jerks—because, paraphrasing Willie Sutton, that's where the data were, or at least *more* data. Circle jerks have been considered a guy thing, but *Onania* mentioned girls. Would I find girls' stories? From every printed source I could lay my hands on, I collected over 100 anecdotes about youthful shared masturbation. (I avoided the Net since I wanted old as well as new stories, and because on the Net fantasy mixes unpredictably with fact.) Most of the stories came from published books and from issues of that *Celebrate the Self* magazine (*CTS*). The editor—by now, one of my co-conspirators—included a flyer about my research with one issue, so I received more stories in letters and emails.

In addition, I added questions about group masturbation to a longer sex survey conducted by an academic friend of mine. He had recruited several classes of Midwestern college students to fill out his questionnaire, and I managed to piggyback onto the project. Among the students, four supplied stories about youthful groups.

Of course, these 100-plus anecdotes would never impress the statistically savvy. But I could not be accused of wasting taxpayers' money! And the stories did give an idea of the types and range of experiences among both boys and—as I found—girls. Here are a few of the men's stories about childhood and adolescence:

The circle jerk—that's one of my first memories. We all stood around in a circle, told stories about girls, or rubbed our penises until we got hard-ons. Then we ejaculated. The purpose was to see who could ejaculate the farthest. (#41 – Farrell, *The Liberated Man,* 1974)

~

Circle jerks have been considered a guy thing, but *Onania* mentioned girls.

Did you guys ever have a Boners Club? It was just about the time a lot of us were getting our puberty hairs [*sic*]. In the evening, around bedtime, we would all sit around and try to get a boner. We'd sit and think and think as hard as we could about some girl we couldn't quite get all the way with, and hope we could get it hard. (#42 – Farrell, 1974)

~

In a certain [high school],...boys had holes in the pockets of their trousers *ad stuprum mutuum faciendum* [to faciliate mutual defilement] during the lessons, in the presence of their professors. (#100 – Talmey, *Love,* 1919)

~

Friends had been telling me about "this neat feeling" and I had also been checking things out on my own. Eventually a friend and I tried masturbating together and we both found out what it was like. (#6 – Haas, *Teenage Sexuality,* 1979)

~

When I was in about the 7th grade...[t]wo of the other kids in the car pool and I were tight j/o [jack off] buddies.... I would sit in the middle and lean forward against the back of the front seat and talk to the guys in front.... [T]his made it impossible for anyone to see that my buddies each had one of their hands in my crotch, rubbing my hard cock

through my jeans. Just before we got to school (they would time it perfectly), they would make me shoot my load into my underwear. (*CTS,* 1995)

Boys' not-so-solo experiences could take different forms. Sometimes it was only two boys; sometimes many. Boys could self-masturbate together, give each other a hand, demonstrate favorite strokes to an audience, or simply watch. A circle jerk could start spontaneously and never happen again, or it could be a planned or semi-planned activity over months or years, older boys leaving and younger ones joining. Some kind of game or contest might be added to lend interesting complexities.

Much shared masturbation seemed to begin whenever cul-

"Did you guys ever have a Boners Club?"

tural traction brought boys together—on a sports team, in a fraternity, in a dormitory, at school, or at camp. Boy Scouts founder Robert Baden-Powell was a strict believer in conservation of the manly "sex fluid." Were he to find out about the sexual horseplay enjoyed by decades of his scouts, he'd kill himself if he weren't already dead.

Now, some stories about girls:

My best friend introduced masturbation to me [at age ten] when we were younger. We used stuffed animals and baby bottles (over our clothes).... [We also] pretended to play "boyfriend/girlfriend." One of us would pretend to be the boy. (#107 – college student, 1999)

~

Being about seven and having orgy-type sessions with one or two other little girls. We'd touch ourselves and rub on the side of the bed until orgasm.... We were also having oral sex at this age (with each other). (#55 – Winks & Semans, *The New Good Vibrations Guide to Sex,* 1997)

~

Sometimes there were just one or two people, but other times there were up to five or more guys and girls [in] a gang of 10 or more members. We would all get together and sort of play a game where first we would masturbate ourselves and we would masturbate each other and the one who lasted the longest (the one to come last) would be the winner and that person would get to receive oral sex from all the others who lost! [How old were you?] Sixteen. [How long did you participate?] About 3 yrs. (#106 – college student, 1999)

I collected 90 stories about boys but only 18 about girls. The girls' experiences seemed similar to those of the boys. But why fewer? Girls just might not masturbate together as much as boys, of course. (Over a century of sex surveys have all reported that, statistically, males are more likely to play pocket pool than females and to do it more often, too.) Or they just might be less willing to talk about it. Girls' stories described jilling off in pairs more often than groups. Games were more often "playing doctor" or "playing house" or pretending to be boyfriend and girlfriend than a contest. Also, while most people told about masturbating with the same gender, a larger percentage of girls' stories were about mixed-gender groups.

So here I was with an admittedly small collection of fascinating data about circle jerks. How much of this has been going on? The only survey I found was that one in *Men's Confidential*: 27% reported group masturbation as a boy—hardly a trustworthy statistic since this magazine's readership was in no way typical. But the sex experts had very little to say. Indeed, about all we know from the scholarly surveys relates to how people found out about do-it-yourself orgasms. In the Kinsey data from the 1940s, about 40% of the male sample had learned masturbation from observation. For women, it was around 10%.

Anthropologists have very occasionally described group masturbation among children, especially boys, in various cultures. The tantalizingly brief summaries in *The Continuum Complete International Encyclopedia of Sexuality* reported in 2004, for example, that in India, "boys at the younger ages may masturbate together without shame," and in Japan, "there is an indication that being 'taught by some friend' is the more common inspiration" for first masturbation experiences. But whatever, it sure looked to me like kids' circles were neither rare nor new.

The Boners Club Grows Up

So much for circle jerks. Boys did it and, occasionally at least, so did girls. Kids seemed to get into it partly as a learning experience (we learn hopscotch and ball-playing from friends—why not masturbation?) and partly as a kids-only social affair. But I had started with those pesky Jacks, and it was time to get back to them. What was going on with adult groups? And what about women?

Judging from what I knew about group sex in general, I guessed that adult coed group masturbation probably had been happening since time immemorial as merely one activity among others at orgies and fuckparties, from the Stone Age to modern suburbia. For centuries, amateur sex of all kinds in public or semi-public has appealed to lots of folks by offering casual, no-strings sex, orgasms to the max, plus opportunities to show off and also to watch—whether at ritualistic or recreational affairs. Alas, we can't go back and ask our ancestors about it! But a bawdy song about a famous and supposedly real-life 1880s orgy, "The Ball of Kirriemuir," has at least three verses referring to observers masturbating together or separately while watching the other guys and gals merrily banging away. For example:

The elders of the church
They were too old to firk [fuck],
So they sat around the table
And had a circle jerk.

We can't prove that this sex party really occurred and, if so, if any of the verses were more or less true. But we do know that the person who created the verses took it for granted that playing with yourself together was appropriate behavior under the circumstances.

Similarly, I thought that all-men groups—and perhaps all-women groups—probably had shared masturbation together with other kinds of sex in bathhouses and elsewhere, back to the Greeks and Romans and before. Certainly today, masturbation has been a part of the public sex scene for men in the backrooms of gay bars.

Now with the Jacks, masturbation became the centerpiece of an adult sexual occasion. And, as I had discovered, not just the Jacks—I remembered those "close encounters." In *Celebrate the Self* and a few other places, I found stories about solo sex together among grown men unrelated to the formally organized clubs:

> I and six other guys ages 54 to 72 get together for a mutual J/O time…. Three guys are married and four are single. (*CTS*, 1994)

> ~

> I'm 67, bi, married and…visited a gentleman in the Midwest. For 36 hours, there were four of us having all kinds of celebrations. I count to 10 the salutes. (*CTS*, 1998)

> ~

> I was at the West Side YMCA in New York City one night…about 1:30 in the morning, and I turned a lamp on right next to a window, threw open the window and stood naked in the light. In just a few seconds, across the courtyard of the U-shaped building, another light went on, and another. Two men stood at their windows nude, masturbating while watching me [masturbate]. (*CTS*, 1998)

~

> When I was in my 40s, I joined a group of men who would get together two times a month. For a few hours, we would trade stories about our sexual experiences with our wives. Then we would put in a sex movie and get out the magazines and just start masturbating ourselves. (*Men's Confidential*, 1996)

Like boys' circle jerks, these experiences sometimes happened spontaneously and never again, and some continued regularly among an informal peer group. As reported by Paul McCartney biographer Barry Miles, McCartney and co-Beatle John Lennon were part of such a group in their teens. Lennon later recast the experience into a playlet about a men's group. His "Four in Hand," part of the 1960s Off Broadway review *Oh! Calcutta*, drops in on a long-term trio joined by a new member—who is unexpectedly and hilariously turned on *not* by standard porn images but by the Lone Ranger!

Jacking Things Up
With larger groups of men and more infrastructure, the organized "jacks" or "JO" clubs have taken the adult concept to an, ahem, more elevated level. I went to the Web and found that at least 40 jacks clubs meet worldwide: San Francisco, New York, Philadelphia, Orlando, Cleveland, Paris, Melbourne, Mexico, even Finland…. Who knew? This was really under the radar!

Girls' stories described jilling off in pairs more often than groups.

The New York Jacks is reputed to be the first modern club of this kind, starting as an informal group and morphing officially into a club in 1980, before the AIDS epidemic. Dr. Woof's San Francisco Jacks, another early club, has described itself as "a service organization whose purpose is pleasure," and a 1996 article in the *Bay Area Reporter* compared it to the Elks Club. JO clubs have typically stressed joy, fellowship, and acceptance of diversity in backgrounds and bodies—but not hearts and flowers. As the New York Jacks stated, "We're looking for recreation, not romance." Another club has announced, "We are not here as a 'hook-up' for guys to meet other guys."

The Elks Club is a good comparison. JO clubs may have membership cards, newsletters, songs, rituals, yearbooks, theme parties, weekend retreats, even charity fund-raisers. Bonhomie, enthusiasm—and engagingly bad puns!—are everywhere. The clubs have their own quirky individualism: One quotes the Talmud in its newsletter. Another uses grape-seed oil as the club lubricant. A third offers masks to members who want to stroke anonymously. (Is that my boss coming on me, or does this dude just wear the same power Rolex?)

Generally, firm rules bar oral and anal sex, variously worded as, "No lips below the hips," "On me, not in me," or, "We discourage insertion of anyone's anything into anywhere." Most clubs forbid drugs, alcohol (BYOB may be okay), and sometimes cologne. The New York Jacks holds weekly "meatings," whereas others may get together less frequently. Theme parties—a No Pants Disco Dance or a "We Have a (Wet) Dream" night for Martin Luther King's birthday—may add to the fun.

Members keep in touch through telephone messages, mailings, or websites. Larger clubs rent a hall or spacious area, while smaller groups may meet in basements or garages. Protocol stresses on-time arrival, since latecomers disturb the

As reported by Paul McCartney biographer Barry Miles, McCartney and co-Beatle John Lennon were part of such a group in their teens.

momentum. Clothing other than footgear must be checked at the door, although underwear and costumes may be encouraged. Juice, soda, lubricants, and sometimes snacks are provided. The men gather in open areas, usually with music or videos, comfortable furniture—and protected surfaces. With cum flying in all directions, wet, sticky, and slippery win out over Martha Stewart as *décor du jour*.

Men may do themselves and each other, plus kiss, massage, caress, fondle, grope, titillate, rub, hug, body surf, whatever… so long as rules are observed. Performers and watchers are all welcome. Some men show off solo, while others go at it together in pairs and clusters. Early ejaculations start a chain reaction of more ejaculations followed by breaks for snacks, laughter, and conversation. Then round two…or three…. After a couple of hours, the party winds down and everyone leaves. Men have described these evenings as joyous, ecstatic, even spiritual, "a religious communion flying on sex to come towards joy and glory":

> **The [San Francisco] Jacks offer not only a solace of safety from the nightmare storm of AIDS, but better still, an effective new way to meet socially, intimately, physically and spiritually men who are defined by behavior as lusty, visually forward, and generous with their smiles, cocks, hugs, and conversation. (San Francisco Jacks website, 2005)**

> ~

> **Yes, Virginia, sex can be sleazy, safe and satisfac-**

> tory. We men were made for orgies and brotherhood sex which can be both fun and loving—yes, loving! Men kissed, hugged, smiled. Warmth was omnipresent. I left exhausted but also reassured that the gay male mystique will survive this deadly crisis. And yes,…it was theatre. (San Francisco Jacks website, 2005)

> ~

> **As I am a male in his mid-thirties I find an extra sparkle in my loins to see the Senior men stroking and shooting from some of the hardest penises I have ever seen! I guess things in life do get better with age. (San Francisco Jacks website, 2005)**

> ~

> **Hey, what a great club. [I'm a m]arried daddy who is a ch[r]onic 'bator. I loved watching everyone shoot their hot sperm the first time I went. (San Francisco Jacks website, 2005)**

> ~

> **It is a very HOT, SPIRITUAL, and FREEING experience…. I've met several men who identified as being straight, bi, and no preference—but they simply enjoyed being nude, hard, or soft in the company of men—in other words some guys just like to hang out among other men…with their dicks out and stroke (maybe cum/maybe not)… (San Francisco Jacks website, 2005)**

> ~

> **And I remember walking into this amazing environment with a hundred men bathed in this red, glowing light, all just jacking off, and I just thought, "Wow! This is heaven! This is hell! I don't care! I'm here! I love it!" And there was the same kind of group energy…where like, people would be having orgasms—you could almost feel this chain reaction rippling through the room. Someone would get off in a really incredible scene, and he'd have maybe seven guys around, kind of supporting it. And then someone across the room would catch the wave of that, and they would start coming, and there would be five people shooting off in the space of a minute, and everyone else was getting off on their energy…. It was very synergistic. (*Black Sheets* #12, 1997)**

Women's masturbation clubs? Although I found descriptions of lesbian sex clubs, ladies-only backrooms, and women's sex groups, self-pleasuring did not seem to be the focus of these affairs. And the lesbian clubs listed in the alternative sex directories *Gayellow Pages* and *The Black Book* all looked S/M-oriented. Indeed, I found *no* accounts of jilling off soirées other than workshops given by masturbation guru Betty Dodson and occasional reunions of Dodson alumnae. Again, we don't know if fewer women than men have gotten together just for masturbation, or if they simply have not written much about it—perhaps both.

But I did read about some mixed-gender sex parties that focused on sharing self-help:

Mother Goose (Delores) spearheads these monthly gatherings...and tells me, "The folks that come to our events range from 18 to 80.... Men and women all together in the same space at the same time—some gay, some lesbian, crossdressers. Some bring leather, some only want to watch, some are show-offs. We are all dedicated to Jacking and Jilling. Some do massage, some whip the daylights out of each other, some do dirty dancing, etc." There are some simple rules: no fucking, no unprotected sex, no rude behavior. (*CTS*, 1995)

~

Club Relate is a club for people that enjoy and include masturbation in their sex play and desire meeting other people in a party setting for group masturbation.... Currently, the Club's parties are held three Saturdays per month in Orlando and Tampa.... Swinging and/ or penetration is an option among consenting participants...[but] the primary reason for Club Relate's existence is masturbation. (Club Relate website, 2005)

~

[T]he Center for Sex and Culture will hold its fourth annual fund-raising Masturbate-a-Thon on May 28.... [T]he CSC's Masturbate-a-Thon is a live group event at which participants will raise funds by getting others to sponsor them for each minute they masturbate.... Separate areas...will be set aside for men who would prefer to masturbate together and women who want a single-sex space, with the rest of the room a mixed-gender venue.... (Masturbate-a-Thon.com, 2005)

The San Francisco Mother Goose parties began in 1987 as an enlargement of the "jacks" concept. These parties appear to have ceased, but their function has been subsumed by the more general sex parties, such as the Queen of Heaven parties, which have stressed safer sex, eclectic attendance, and a variety of activities, from masturbation to fisting. On the East Coast, the all-male New York Jacks held a mixed-gender Jack and Jill Party for at least several years in the 1990s. By contrast, Club Relate grew out of the swingers' movement, from the large responses to one couple's advertisements for others

interested in sharing masturbation. Club Relate is a member of NASCA—North American Swing Clubs Association.

The San Francisco sex-toy company Good Vibrations started the Masturbate-a-Thons in 1998 to raise funds for safer-sex causes and to educate the public about using self-pleasuring as a safe-sex strategy. The first live, group version was organized by Carol Queen, founder of the Center for Sex and Culture, in 2000. Over the years, 1,700 participants have "come for a cause" and raised over $25,000.

Since by no means all swinging takes place in formal, organized groups, there might well be small, informal, mixed-gender masturbation circles besides Club Relate. Judging from ads on the Internet, a good many heterosexual men are interested in sharing masturbation with women. But only a few women seem to advertise on the Net for either male or female masturbation companions.

෨෨

So I've concluded that sharing masturbation has long been an enjoyed activity for at least some men, perhaps not a few. But only recently have groups organized and gone public—male-only and coed. The sexual revolution, the gay rights

Some men show off solo, while others go at it together in pairs and clusters.

movement, the AIDS epidemic, and the Xerox machine have surely all contributed to a more open milieu for an historically undercover activity. And now the Internet allows wannabes to find out about JO and JJO clubs, as well as contact each other for private gatherings and even to start new clubs.

One needs to experience this activity (first hand) to understand just how satisfying it can be. At least part of the satisfaction has to be the knowing that transmission of disease has not been risked. Also, I assume that some of the participants are in relationships to which their significant others are unaware and unapproving of their partners' actions. This is the efficient solution for the man who wants dalliance. Having his cake but not coming home with crumbs in his stash. ("Ask Isadora" website, 2002)

Although the sex scholars hadn't picked up on adult group masturbation, a few anthropological writers have mentioned it in different cultures. In the US today, adult group masturbation has mostly earned notice only by gay and lesbian writers of sex manuals, advice books, and journalistic accounts.

Although heterosexuals are certainly in there stroking, they aren't writing about it in the mainstream press.

Some Conjectures About What's Going on Here

Is group masturbation a distinct sexual behavior? Certainly, I might think so. But the people involved might not. Among youthful groups, masturbation can co-occur with oral sex, anal sex, and other sex play, and the kids may not think of masturbation as "different." Some boys' groups do seem to have stuck with either self-masturbation or a mix of self- and mutual masturbation.

Lesbians don't seem to select out shared jilling off from other forms of group sex. Gay men, however, do consider shared JO a distinct behavior. At least a few coed sex groups also consider shared masturbation a unique activity, probably led to this distinction partly by preference and partly by the need for safe sex. For straight couples involved in nonmonogamy, group masturbation may seem less threatening to the main relationship than other forms of sex. After all, fewer than 20% of respondents to both US and UK surveys in 2001 considered even mutual masturbation—playing with a partner's genitals or vice versa—as "having sex."

Why does group masturbation seem more common among males? Solo masturbation has been reported as more of a guy thing than a gal thing in numerous surveys over more than 100 years. And why is *that*? Some writers have linked

"And there was the same kind of group energy...where like, people would be having orgasms—you could almost feel this chain reaction rippling through the room."

male interest in monkey-spanking to visibility of the penis itself and erections, tangible evidence left by wet dreams, greater social acceptance of male sexuality, and higher levels of testosterone.

Additional factors make it more likely for males to masturbate together. Western bathroom customs require males to expose their penises in each other's presence from an early age. Group nudity on, say, swimming teams and in showering is part of male culture beginning in boyhood. For females, casual, shared nudity is far more socially unusual at all ages, even given the requirement for group showers in high-school gym class. And even when females do share nudity, their genitals are less obvious and any sexual arousal can't easily be observed.

Certainly as a matter of pure performance, male masturbation has a showy and contagious quality that can attract admirers—and imitators.

I remember my older friend's penis was beautifully built, about six and a half inches long erect, and would erupt in a white pearly spray that shot at least twelve inches in the air. It was a beautiful sight, like watching the geyser Old Faithful erupt. (#13 – *The Hite Report on Male Sexuality,* 1981)

In female orgasm, however, the experience is mostly internal. I conjecture that some gay men divert polyamorous inclinations to JO groups because of fear of HIV. The virus has appeared less virulently among US lesbians and heterosexuals, so they might not have as much motivation to focus on sex that is do-it-yourself—but shared. And then, we do not know how accurately people remember and report their experiences. Perhaps many more women masturbate than report it—or share masturbation than report it—but have not thought of it as masturbation or have not wanted to admit it.

How many people participate? We hardly have any idea at all. When group masturbation has made its way into surveys, it has likely been lumped into youthful sex play, generalized masturbation, homosexual sex, or group sex. More probably, it has simply not been collected. Certainly more shared jacking (and maybe jilling) is going on than is generally suspected because researchers have not asked and certainly the public has not volunteered! Masturbation, homosexual sex, and group sex are big-time no-nos for many people. While these activities may be accepted and discussed privately, they still may not be reported to outsiders.

It has been especially difficult in surveys to get people to report solo sex. A US research team conducted a comprehensive sex survey by in-person interview in the 1990s. But both interviewers and interviewees shied away from the masturbation questions, which were eventually delivered by a confidential form to be filled out. At about the same time, a large British sex survey completely excluded questions on masturbation because of "disgust and embarrassment" all around.

A complicating factor is that surveys typically ask, for example, about homosexual sex acts or for experiences "thought of as being sexual." Yet many people don't label their shared masturbation as homosexual or even sexual. My files are full of such disclaimers, even from married men with "JO buddies" who do not think of their current and clandestine activities as "homosexual." Quite a few Internet ads seek "str8" (straight) partners or "married pals" for shared JO. The *Men's Confidential* survey drew "hundreds" of responses from men, the vast majority self-described as heterosexual and married, and 44% reported shared jack-offs as adults. In one informal adult group, "We all agreed that the experience enhanced sex with our wives."

It would be absolutely fascinating—and quite a challenge!—to investigate how many "heterosexual" married men regularly share masturbation with other men, and how many gay men do so. Or, of the membership of the 40+ masturbation clubs, how many identify as straight versus gay versus bi? As Kinsey said, you do not know what your neighbors do, and I might add, you do not know how your neighbors think. A man once told me that he was a "heterosexual who likes cocks," and perhaps others would agree with that description. There's a word that might apply here: *heteroflexible*. (Hey, guys, are your wives reading this?)

Is group masturbation becoming more or less common? Many of the boyhood circle-jerk stories come from older men, and it may be that boys' circles were more common in the past. Although still taboo among many people, masturbation has become more "normal" in the last 30 years, so fewer boys might need peer permission to indulge. Today, many young people learn about masturbation and ejaculation/orgasms via parents, public schools, and the media, so perhaps fewer are taught by friends. Further, with greater public awareness about gays and lesbians, more young people may shy away from activities that might be construed as "homosexual." Perhaps fewer children have as much unstructured and unsupervised time to play together. And it may be that earlier eras of same-gender boarding schools fostered a collective intimacy that is less common now.

On the other hand, group masturbation among adults may be increasing because of the desire for safe sex and the opportunity to find companions through gay newspapers, small-circulation periodicals like *Celebrate the Self* and *Jox*, and especially through the Internet. Also, participation in group masturbation may increase because it's much more acceptable today—especially in youth culture—for both women and men to be single, sexually active, and interested in doing sexual stuff besides intercourse.

Group masturbation has unique appeal as a sexual opportunity for people without partners. This can include people over 50, a demographic that is increasing. It may be no accident that the coed Club Relate has thrived in Florida for nearly a decade—Florida is a known locale for retirees. The club's website tells of a widow in her sixties who hadn't had sex in years and decided to put her late husband's memory firmly to rest by attending one of the parties. "It was like someone had turned a light switch on." After a wild stroke-off with several of the men and an encounter with the hostess, the widow "went home, built a privacy fence around her backyard, installed a hot tub, and is dating a younger man."

Do people who have participated in group masturbation differ from those who have not? One survey (Bell, Weinberg & Hammersmith, *Sexual Preference*, 1981) found that people who self-identified as gay or lesbian more commonly reported childhood sex play with the same gender—such as boys masturbating with other boys—than those identifying as heterosexual. Yet because many people have not consid-

"Club Relate is a club for people that enjoy and include masturbation in their sex play and desire meeting other people in a party setting for group masturbation."

ered their early experiences "homosexual" or even "sexual," surveys may not have picked up much same-gender shared masturbation. And it may be that people who self-identify as homosexual or bisexual remember such experiences more often and more clearly than those who don't.

Among adults, it does appear that group masturbation is more popular among gay men than among lesbians or heterosexuals of either gender. One reason: Gay male partner-sex carries risk of HIV. But more obviously, gay men find male sexuality attractive, and what could show off male sexuality more emphatically than a group of men ejaculating? People who enjoy long periods of sexual activity and frequent orgasms could also find group masturbation appealing—no risk of tiring out a partner!

But what do adults get out of group masturbation, anyway? We can see how kids can end up in circle jerks by comparing genitalia and teaching each other about sex. But why might people of all ages be spontaneously interested? Of course, we know that masturbation is safe sex; you don't need a partner to satisfy you—or to satisfy, and it's a sure route to orgasms. But simple exhibitionism is probably a major reason. Victoria's Secret stays in business because women like to dress—and undress—sexy. Taking it further: Topless bars and stripper joints stay in business not just because they attract men as customers but also because women will show off their bodies—for money and also for the delicious feeling of power and sexual turn-on that can come from a whole room of horny admirers.

For men, the turn-on seems to come partly from watching the other guys ejaculate and identifying with them *all*. Males have a natural refractory period and can't have (potentially) unlimited orgasms the way women can. Some younger men can come repeatedly, but as a man gets older, he can't come as often. Yet in a group, a man of any age can come vicariously over and over and over.... His ejaculations multiply, cascade—one ejaculation mirrored into a gusher, a fountain, a torrent, a joyous, rushing tide of semen. Both gay and straight sex videos feature external "cum shots," partly to prove the sex is real but also as a source of vicarious jollies. Hence, the popularity of "cum shot" compilations and bukkake porn, in which many men come on camera, masturbating onto the face or body of a woman or another man. Porn performer Jerry Butler wrote about how cum shots have become more elaborate in recent decades, with special effects used to

For men, the turn-on seems to come partly from watching the other guys ejaculate and identifying with them all.

make ejaculations seem more copious and longer-lasting. Ejaculation equals sexual pleasure, a male symbol reaching across years and sexual orientations.

One sexologist told me that men want to have a sense of closure and finality about sex. Watching ejaculations provides this. (She also told me that many men like videos showing "squirters"—women ejaculating—for the same reason.) So, many men who consider themselves heterosexual might (heteroflexibly?) enjoy watching other men's ejaculations and even participating in shared JO because they feel their own sexual pleasure magnified vicariously in the other men and because they get that sense of closure.

Conclusion

> I celebrate myself, and sing myself,
> And what I assume you shall assume,
> For every atom belonging to me as good as
> belongs to you.
> —Whitman, "Song of Myself," 1856

Oxymoron or not, group masturbation, or "social masturbation," is apparently becoming an emerging cultural phenomenon. Participants and reporters describe same-gender and mixed-gender adult masturbation groups as wonderful opportunities for sexual exhibitionism, voyeurism, experimentation, and variety in congenial settings, all without risk of disease, pregnancy, expectations for commitment, or need to cater to a partner. One gay man wrote: "I've had a lover for almost ten years. He's 30, still as sexy as when he was 20, and we're compatible and monogamous except for participation in our

J/O club" (Califia, *The Sexpert*, 1991). It seems likely that organized JO and possibly JJO groups will grow in number and visibility in coming years, and that small, private circles will proliferate even more widely.

I did finish writing *The Big Book of Masturbation*. It became a big book partly because I came across group masturbation—and many other fascinating facts and phenomena. Like the Catholic theologian who gave married women explicit permission in 1748 to masturbate after sex with their husbands if they hadn't come yet. A quotation from the Dalai Lama giving the green light to solo sex for anyone not under religious vow. A vigorous debate across several Islamic websites as to whether and under what circumstances masturbation might be *wajib* (obligatory), *halal* (permitted), *makruh* (discouraged), or *haram* (absolutely forbidden). The shooting script for "The Contest" episode of *Seinfeld* from 1992. Thousands of creative and delightful slang terms in a dozen languages. A poem about dildos from 1700. State laws about sex toys.

People interested in evolutionary conundrums have asked, Why do people masturbate? It doesn't seem to increase survival, fitness, or number of offspring. In one evolution listserv discussion, the general consensus was that people masturbate—like that joke about dogs licking their balls—because they can. And if masturbation doesn't contribute much to fitness or survival or progeny, it doesn't detract much, either. Nearly everybody who masturbates, alone or not, also has some kind of sex with a partner and enjoys both. Recent research suggests that people who masturbate more may tend to have more partner sex, and more different kinds of sex. Interest in masturbation apparently relates on the average to *greater* personal sexiness, not *less*.

Is group masturbation really so weird? After all, millions of people share masturbation by phone sex or cybersex. The phone-sex industry took in up to $1 billion per year by the late 1990s. As for cybersex, it's been reported that 17 million users surfed adult entertainment sites in *one month* of 2000—and I think we can assume that many of these people were typing one-handed while cybering with playpals. It may become less of a step from virtual playpals to in-the-flesh playpals when the sex is (just) masturbation—completely safe, with no romantic obligations.

So why do people masturbate in groups? Because people somewhere, sometime, do just about anything in groups, including just about any kind of sex—partly just to do it, partly to show off, and partly to watch.

And because they can.

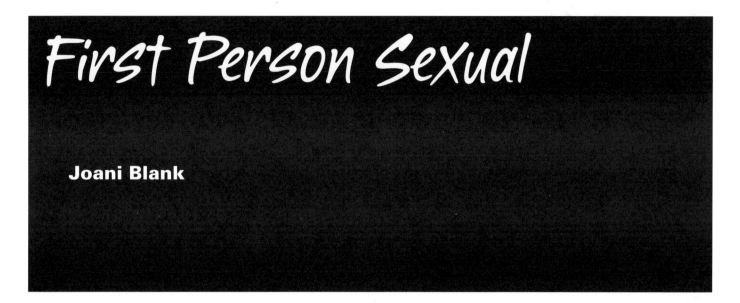

First Person Sexual

Joani Blank

In 1996 I edited a book, *First Person Sexual: Women and Men Write about Self-Pleasuring*, which presents 45 intimate, personal accounts of masturbation. It was a groundbreaking publication about an important and, for many people, uncomfortable subject, but one I felt had broad implications for human health and happiness. Happily, a decade later, the book is still in print. This article is an adaptation of my original introduction. We're still fighting the good fight over masturbation, and these words are still relevant.

Back in the 1970s, I had the privilege of working as a counselor in the Sex Counseling Program at the University of California at San Francisco. The program's participants were women who previously had never experienced orgasm but learned how by gradually approaching masturbation as their homework. They verbally shared their experiences in the group.

My contact with these women and with the program's therapists gave me a new appreciation for masturbation—my own and that of others. Whether or not our clients ever learned to have orgasms during partner-sex (indeed, whether or not they even had sexual partners), virtually all of them learned to masturbate to orgasm reliably and joyfully, and they finished the program far more relaxed, self-confident, and optimistic than they had been previously. Sue-Marie Larsen, in her *First Person Sexual* story "Taking Myself in Hand," explained it perfectly: "I don't know one woman who I consider the mistress of her own sexuality who has not spent considerable amounts of time masturbating…. Hands down, masturbation has been the single most important tool I've used to create an outstanding sex life for myself."

One of the few texts for these pre-orgasmic women's groups was an early version of Betty Dodson's soon-to-be-self-published *Liberating Masturbation: A Meditation on Selflove*, a feminist classic for the next twelve years. Since then, Dodson's book has been expanded and is now in its second edition as *Sex for One: The Joy of Selfloving*. In the late 1970s, this book and the later, male-focused *Joy of Solo Sex* and *More Joy...* by Harold Litten stood virtually alone in their focus on this subject. Remarkable, is it not, that with all the popular and scholarly books about sex, there were then so few about the planet's most common human sexual practice? More books have arrived recently, but given self-pleasuring's ubiquity, only a very small number.

One rarely sees an erotic short story, novel, or sexually explicit movie or video with the central theme of masturbation. Is it possible that increasing openness about variety in partner-sex has driven masturbation even further into the closet? With all these "new" things to do with a partner and with the willingness of more and more women to initiate sex and specific sexual activities, who has the time, energy, or inclination

One rarely sees an erotic short story, novel, or sexually explicit movie or video with the central theme of masturbation.

to masturbate? Well, I do—and so, apparently, did the 43 contributors to *First Person Sexual*. They even had the additional time, energy, and inclination to write about it, sometimes hilariously: "The panic was rising. The emergency room is going to love me—an eight-and-a-half months pregnant woman with two Superballs stuck up her ass. They wouldn't even be able to roll me over onto my belly to get these things out."

(Shannon René in "Big Mama and the Superballs.")

♡

Masturbation has never been highly regarded. "Why are people so uncomfortable about masturbation?" asked Leonore Tiefer, author of *Sex Is Not a Natural Act*, in a radio interview. "Many religious teachings say it is bad or wrong. And much sexual discussion is tinged by embarrassment, discomfort, shame, and awkwardness. Saying or believing that masturbation is wrong or bad with the authority of scripture behind you somehow justifies the negativity about it."

People go to great lengths to disassociate masturbation from other sexual expression. Only rarely do we refer to masturbation as sex or as a sexual activity. There is "having sex," and then, separate but hardly equal, is jacking (or jilling) off. Even the enlightened few who don't limit the phrase "having sex" to intercourse virtually never include masturbation when they think or speak of "having sex."

Do we denigrate and conceal masturbation because we fear the judgments others might aim at us if they knew we did it? Are we fearful that a partner's masturbation says something

"Those who report on, go on tirades about, and legislate against pornography never talk about masturbation."

about our own inadequacies or about defects in our shared sexual experience? Do we judge ourselves negatively because we enjoy masturbating? For most of us, at one time or another, the answer to any or all of these questions is a self-conscious "yes."

Society's concerns reflect a profound suspicion of any sexual activity that has no conceivable rationale other than pleasure. We appreciate pleasure in partner-sex, but in rationalizing that pleasure we frequently fall back on love, the sacramental quality of sex in marriage, bonding, or just plain friendship—not to mention fulfilling an obligation or meeting the expectations of our partner. Moralists eschew the credo, "If it feels good, do it," particularly if "it" has no apparent, redeeming social benefit.

First Person Sexual contains this from Robert Morgan about his early discoveries: "What a concept: 1) put vibrator against penis; 2) orgasm; 3) repeat until exhausted. (One day I came thirty-five times just to see how many were possible.)" Masturbation does feel good, *very* good in fact, and it does no conceivable harm. This is indeed sufficient reason to do it—with enthusiasm, in any manner, and with any frequency one chooses.

Leonore Tiefer draws our attention to the connection between the crusades against pornography and the fear of masturbation. "The main use of pornography," she says, "is for masturbation. Everybody knows that. Those who report on, go on tirades about, and legislate against pornography never talk about masturbation. They say that pornography harms people's minds, warps them, and causes them to go out and do bad things. They never acknowledge that most people use pornography to enhance their masturbation fantasies. A lot of the fuel for anti-pornography crusades comes from anxiety and awkwardness about admitting that people masturbate."

✕✕

A decade ago, as I collected the stories for *First Person Sexual*, I was struck with the differences between stories written by men and those written by women. Two differences are especially noteworthy. Although I asked contributors not to fill their stories with masturbation fantasies that left little or no room for describing the masturbation itself, quite a few of the men did exactly that. I also asked that contributors not describe a lot of sexual interaction with a partner. However, a significant number of women (and a few men) did that. This led me to questions about the places masturbation holds in the sex lives of men and women.

Do men who masturbate—virtually all men do—tend to distance themselves from the purely physical sensations while they focus on fantasy? Do fewer women than men masturbate in part because those who feel too guilty or too fearful simply don't do it? Apparently, men masturbate most frequently during periods when they aren't having enough partner-sex, or none at all, while the more partner-sex a woman is having, the more likely she is to masturbate. Why?

Although some women masturbate before a sexual encounter to get "warmed up," men apparently rarely do so unless they are trying to avoid ejaculating prematurely when later engaged in sexual activity with a partner. Women who masturbate are often willing and eager to try new positions, locations, and techniques for their masturbation, while adult men commonly masturbate pretty much the same way they did as adolescents. Why?

In the course of my years of work at the progressive sex shop Good Vibrations, I was frequently asked if, given the danger associated with unprotected partner-sex in these times, people are masturbating more—and presumably using more sex toys and fantasy materials.

Are they? Masturbation is, after all, the safest of all sexual activities. Certainly more sex toys, books, and videos are sold today than ever before, especially to women. And some of these toys and materials may be used by people who are enhancing their masturbation practice as an alternative to partner-sex, with its attendant real or imagined dangers. One of the high points of *First Person Sexual* is Anne Semans' description of discovering a vibrator for the first time, personifying it in this way: "I caught my first glimpse of her lying heated and spent on the bed. I approached curious and mystified: she was so small! I'd heard rumors about her incredible amorous powers, but she didn't look anything like I'd imagined."

It is also possible, however, that many of those who fear and therefore avoid partner-sex may masturbate significantly *less* than they did previously. Some of the men and women contributing to *First Person Sexual* didn't want sex with a partner and might have felt that masturbating would turn them on and leave them frustrated. Others found that masturbation brought up feelings of loneliness. Still others simply felt so "shut down" sexually that they rarely experienced any desire for arousal or orgasm.

To the extent that people are having less partner-sex, men may be masturbating more and women less. Fortunately, most people seem to be masturbating as much as they always have, and increasingly, couples are making touching themselves in each other's presence a regular part of their lovemaking.

Only three or four of the stories in *First Person Sexual* are fiction. I didn't identify which they were because it doesn't matter. Well over half the authors were not professional writers; a few virtually tore pages out of their journals. My experience suggests that people who are willing to share writings about their own sexuality often express themselves very well. Those who wrote for *First Person Sexual* didn't disappoint me in that regard.

A half-dozen of the stories in my book were originally written in the third person; in each case, I asked the author to rewrite his or her piece in the first person. Although a few expressed fear of doing so, all obliged, and I was pleased with how much more immediate and personal their stories became. Several contributors agreed that readers would be

Women who masturbate are often willing and eager to try new positions, locations, and techniques for their masturbation, while adult men commonly masturbate pretty much the same way they did as adolescents.

able to identify with them more easily now that their stories were in the first person.

For some reason, it didn't occur to me that the stories in my book would be sexually arousing to readers. So I was pleasantly surprised to find how many of them were.

Thea Hillman, in the first piece in the book, "Home Alone," offers us this surprising intimacy: "I love the sounds I've been hearing lately, that no one taught me to make—funny, awkward, deep sounds that come from my belly and from my clit. Sounds…that sound exactly like me."

At its best—and even at its worst—masturbation is "having sex with someone you love" (a thought attributed to Woody Allen). So, from time to time, we might all apply Good Vibrations' slogan: "If you want something done right, do it yourself."

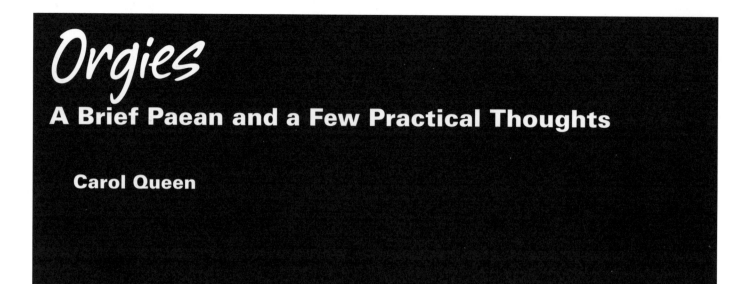

Orgies
A Brief Paean and a Few Practical Thoughts

Carol Queen

No experience compares to your first orgy. Only fantasy and porn might begin to prepare you for the experience of stepping into a room full of rutting, sucking, or masturbating people, and even then you won't be ready for the sensurround-sound, the body heat, the smells.

Group sex of any type defies the cultural norm adopted by all but orgy and public-sex enthusiasts: the belief that sex ought

If you somehow still carry an inculcated belief that sex is only for the young and beautiful, attending an orgy might well disabuse you of it.

to be private. As such, it's one tool in the kit of those who wish to shake off handed-down or enforced norms, and a powerful tool it is. The orgy places its participants in context: Sexual pleasure is one thing when it comes in the arms of a partner or by your own hand, but sex at an orgy happens in a kind of community.

Orgy sex appeals to people who desire that sense of group participation, who long to lose and find themselves in a throng, who are curious about what other people do and what they look like in the throes of whatever-that-is, who want by extension to imagine themselves fully erotic, the way they can see the others who surround them. Having sex in a community can heal the isolation so many feel about their erotic desire. It's also not a bad way to meet people.

Orgy sex is for exhibitionists, too, of course. If the presence of others excites you, if the opportunity to show off and be seen—be watched—is a turn-on, the group-sex environment is perhaps the most perfect and safe venue in which to be consensually observed.

And certainly orgies are for voyeurs. They're voyeur heaven: better than the fantasy, better than porn. They're better because what you see is unexpected; it's real. Think how many people will never get to see other people fuck. Think how much delicious sex goes on in private, sex you'll never get to see. Watching the erotic experience of another person is a privilege; when you can watch more than one, it's a downright epiphany.

It's real in another way, too. Though most situations of public assembly are controlled in some fashion (you're supposed to sit at an unoccupied table in a restaurant; you generally don't go in the out door)—and orgies are no exception—unlike most porn, they are not scripted. Nor will you find a porn's-eye view of humanity at most orgies: only the buff, the lithe, the endowed. If you somehow still carry an inculcated belief that sex is only for the young and beautiful, attending an orgy might well disabuse you of it, because you will see (unless the organizers have excluded them) a more diverse stream of humanity than you'd expect. Shapes, sizes, and ages less commonly eroticized in our youth-fetish culture will be there...getting it on, whatever their "it" of choice may be.

The common image of orgies is probably mostly heterosexual, a group fuck party. Of course, there are orgies that fit this image; many swing clubs host them every weekend. But I'm using the term more expansively here, to include jack-off (and jack-and-jill-off) parties and Masturbate-a-Thons, queer group play and S/M gatherings, pansexual orgies where everyone and (virtually) everything is welcome. Thinking about orgies more inclusively is, well, more inclusive; plus, these parties' differences are as instructive and interesting as their similarities. One reason to attend an orgy is to receive the visceral message, "Everybody does it"; a reason to attend a pansexual or other type of gathering is to be reminded that everyone does "it" a little differently.

While I'm touching on reasons to go to an orgy, let me tell you a good reason not to attend: to get laid. Sure, you might. But people leave orgies all the time having not gotten what they wanted, and the reason is usually simple: If you have a hard time getting laid outside a roomful of people (because you are painfully shy, have bad social skills, smell funny, etc.), the people inside the room probably won't want to screw you, either. Certainly your odds get better when you're in the company of a dozen (or a hundred) potential partners instead of one, but the variables are many. I've seen men bring their actual wives to sex parties and not get laid. No, the best reason to go to an orgy is simply to be there. Everything else is gravy.

Look, before I go on, let me say this explicitly, because one factor in Americans' reaction to our neighbors' sexual kinks is to feel that their very existence somehow challenges our own sexual choices. This is—may I be frank?—bullshit, but it's common. So here goes, and this is especially for those of you who may be reading in quiet yet fascinated horror, the people who would run screaming from a room full of naked people and who somehow feel my very discussion of it is meant to invalidate your own life-history and choices: There's nothing wrong with having sex alone (well, or with one other person). It's time-honored; it can be intimate; it can be passionate. It's the basic unit, and rightly so. I am not suggesting you do anything but...unless you are so inclined.

Me and Orgies

I was always, it seems, so inclined. I fantasized about threesomes and moresomes from the time I figured out there were such things. Threesomes were relatively easy to find my way into, but I didn't grow up in a community that hosted orgies—at least, none I was ever invited to. I was 30 years old by the time I had an opportunity to go to an orgy, and it changed my life. It was the first-ever Jack-and-Jill-Off, a pansexual safer-sex party with a no-intercourse rule.

In San Francisco in 1987, all sorts of people were open to attending such an event, so there were gay men and swingers, lesbian sadomasochists and frisky sexologists, with plenty of latex to go around. Besides the upfront prohibition on fucking, the only other rule was, "Ask before you touch."

I wound up masturbating on a couch with several people around me. A fag wearing boxer shorts with kissy-lips printed all over them talked dirty to me, and a bunch of men stood in a semicircle watching, dicks in hands. I came about eight times. I walked out on a cloud. By the next time a party was held, I had joined the organizing committee.

I met my next partner at an orgy. I met my partner, Robert, at a Jack-and-Jill-Off a year later. And when the JJOs ran their course, we started our own sex-party community, Queen of Heaven. I still miss the venue we used to rent for our parties because it had a sound and light platform, like you'd put a loft bed on in a high-ceilinged apartment. I could climb up there and look down at a roomful of people fucking, sucking, spanking, and dancing naked...all at the same time.

So I found my exhibitionism and my voyeurism at orgies. I had easy access to partners and sexual adventures in the context of a friendly community. I found love in the room; I rarely enter a group-sex space where I do not feel it, though I realize people who haven't experienced this themselves might not believe it. This is a culture that wants to package love into monogamy, and that is emphatically not the only place love resides.

I was 30 years old by the time I had an opportunity to go to an orgy, and it changed my life.

I also found the nerve to say no at orgies, which is a good skill to have when it comes to sex—just about exactly as important as saying yes. I found that my orgy-mates were total literalists: If I said, "Not right now," to an invitation to fuck when what I really meant was, "Probably not ever," the person would invariably be back 20 minutes later, hoping that enough time had ticked by that my answer would change. I don't know that Miss Manners has ever weighed in on orgy etiquette, but I like to think she would recognize that a simple, pleasant "no, thank you" will fit the bill in any situation like this.

Likewise, the person asking has to be willing to be told no. Orgies are a bad place for the sexually desperate, but, then, there is no truly good place for them, as anyone who has ever fended one off at closing time can attest.

Speaking of drunken people: The number-one social-skill problem may well be too much alcohol, and I do not allow it at my orgies, nor am I happy to attend sex parties where it is present. If this seems shocking to you—like, "How could anyone do that sort of thing without a couple of stiff drinks?"—you're not ready for your first orgy. Good sex doesn't result from drink and drugs. Learn to let your vices stand on their own before commingling them, that's my motto. Don't obscure such an amazing experience; be in it.

I once had a guest at Queen of Heaven who complained that he wasn't getting any action. He wasn't likely to get any, either: He was a sullen guy with an entitled attitude, the kind of guy who gives guys a bad name. We didn't invite him back, of course (even orgies, as I implied above, are subject to social control, and the first level of control is the guest list). Before he left, though, I asked him to do a little math problem with me.

"How many people are in this room?" I asked him.

"Uh, about a hundred."

"And if you were going to hire sex workers to put on a sex show for you, how much would that add up to?"

If you go to an orgy and see a guy in the corner, wide-eyed and stroking his cock, he's just marveling at how much money he's saved by not having to spend 200 bucks an hour times 100 to see the vision of erotic play ranged out before him.

How Do You Find an Orgy?

If you aren't already on the right guest lists, you have three choices: Try to get on them, start your own party, or travel somewhere to visit a publicly accessible party. There are not many of the latter, unless you're a gay man. Gay men can usually find group sex opportunities through the socio-sexual grapevine of any city with a visible gay community—and this grapevine now also exists online. In some places you can even find group-sex options in the gay newspapers.

Swingers' parties are nearly as accessible; they're held all over the nation. The trick is, they're almost all couples-only, although many will welcome single women, and a very few will allow single men to attend. But if it's your goal to be the only stag at a swing party, you'd better have better social

That, my friends, is why there's not an orgy hall in every town, like there was in Pompeii.

skills than you do now. Find swingers via contact magazines in adult bookstores, online, and through their national group, the Lifestyles Organization.

How can a guy persuade his wife or girlfriend to go to a swing party? Assure her she'll probably have a better time than you, then don't be surprised (or a jerk) when you find it's actually true. Bottom line: If she doesn't want to go, don't nag her or drag her. It's not erotic (or especially consensual), and it won't work. Look for a place you can go alone, or look for a friskier woman who'd like to check out the scene.

If you're in a city with a sex-positive community, affiliate with it. Go to its events and get to know people. That's the best

entree into more private parties. If there's a publicly accessible club in your area (like San Francisco's Power Exchange), by all means check it out, but don't be surprised to find many, many curious men and fewer play opportunities than you expected (unless you're one of those guys who can get happy with another guy when there aren't lots of women around; in that case, you're probably ready for anything).

The orgy's biggest challenge (for heterosexuals, anyway) is this: more men who want to rush down and give it a try, which results in a gender-skewed room of people in which all but the most wild-at-heart women begin to feel overwhelmed, even unsafe. That, my friends, is why there's not an orgy hall in every town, like there was in Pompeii.

If BDSM is your cup of tea, go to events held by your local National Leather Association affiliate; you can find these online, too. These are not fuck parties, so don't go unless you really want to do BDSM. Expect, if you're new to the scene, to be required to go through a screening process, probably including an intro workshop. Some sex parties are beginning to include these, too.

How Do You Behave?

How would you like to be hit on by someone whom you're not sure you want to fuck? That's how to approach others: Don't come on too strong; don't be pushy; don't assume the whole room wants to fuck you. Almost nobody comes to an orgy to fuck everybody. If you find one who does and you're in line for the ride, well, yee-ha! And use a rubber.

If someone approaches you, but you don't want to play? Remember what Miss Manners would want you to say.

Don't touch without asking and getting consent, and if you spill anything (your soda, your lube, your seed), clean it up.

Orgies are like no other social space...and yet they're just like any other social space. Rules of interaction and good conduct apply, and they're not all that hard to understand. Once you grasp that orgies facilitate sex but don't guarantee it, you can see them for what they are: relationships, multi-person and ever-shifting but subject to the same sorts of success and failure as two-person relationships.

Go to an orgy, if you go, to see and explore, to experience the power of sex all around you (whether you're having sex or not). To cross the social boundary, you must go there in the first place, but respect the boundaries of the people inside. It's just like real life, only probably a little sweatier and maybe more atmospherically lit.

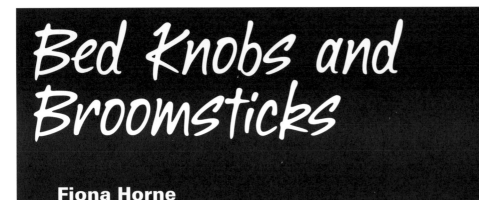

Bed Knobs and Broomsticks

Fiona Horne

Everyone wants a magickal love and sex life, and you don't have to be a full-time Witch to be able to enjoy the influence of magick in your life. You do, however, have to have things in common with a full-time Witch—the ability to see nature as sacred; thus, so is the human body, human desire, and our sexuality.

Below are questions I've received from various people pertaining to their love and sex lives, followed by my magickal and practical advice to them. Most readers will relate to one, if not more, of the questions featured here and feel compelled to try out my advice—so go right ahead!

Included are ways to work with the power of various herbs, crystals, colors, phases of the Moon, and Goddesses and Gods of different cultures to improve and enhance your love and sex life. The most powerful tool you have to work with, though, is your will—magick will work as well as you want it to, so really concentrate and believe in your own infinite abilities.

To work magick you need to suspend any disbelief and fear and be prepared to accept that extraordinary things can and do happen—the world is a magickal place!

All the different herbs, crystals, colors, and objects that are used in the spells are aligned for their magickal abilities—these work like magnets to help ensure that you "attract" your goal. Be aware of this, and they will work for you.

Finally, the most important thing is to enjoy what you're doing. Witchcraft is just that—a craft—and the key to success is to get creative and have fun!

On the Prowl

I am single, and I love meeting women and having one-night stands—not very politically correct, I know. My problem is that as much as I love doing this, I don't get much action! I'm not bad looking, but is there a spell that would improve my chances?

Well, at least you're honest. I do have a spell for you, and it has an added advantage—it promotes safe sex—something you need to be very conscious of if you're running around and hopping into bed with all and sundry. This spell will help you to magickally charge your condoms and guarantee their usage!

Before you head out for the evening, light a purple candle for success and burn musk or coconut incense for lust. Get dressed with intent, consciously focusing on your goals for the evening as you adorn yourself.

Now pick out your favorite condoms—as many as you think you can use—in your power color—maybe red for passion,

> ## This spell will help you to magickally charge your condoms and guarantee their usage!

black for mystery, blue for happiness, green for fun, natural for pride—whatever resonates most strongly for you.

Hold the condoms in your hand and focus on your goal. In your mind's eye, see yourself meeting interesting, sexy people and having your pick of the bunch. See yourself in bed with the woman you want, taking out your power condom and making good use of it! When the vision is very clear—open your eyes, gaze at the candle flame, and say:

Power of fire, heed my desire
My vision is clear—fueled by desire
On this night, without delay
Passionate sex will come my way

Snuff the candle flame and say, "So mote it be."

Pocket your condoms, head out, and I expect you to use every single one of them! Also, seeing as you are using magick to increase your chances of achieving your desires, you owe the Universe something back. Why not offer it "honest intent"—that is, be very clear with your conquests and partners about your intentions. Don't mislead a girl into thinking your objective is more than a bit of overnight fun. Be honest with your intent, and your magick will work better and no one will get hurt.

Looking for Mr. Right

Every guy I seem to pick up is a dud—not only in behavior but in bed! I guess I'm drawn to guys who are tough and masculine, but they end up being rough and insensitive. Is there some spell to help attract the right partner?

Well, you probably need to do some work on yourself, examining your values and self-worth and working out why you keep falling for the same kind of guy. All brawn and no brain makes Jack a dull boy, so why do you go for him?

Sit naked in front of a mirror, surrounded by a circle of seven white candles for purity and spiritual enlightenment.

So the first part of this magick is a self-awareness ritual, and the second a "come to me, man of my dreams" spell.

Sit naked in front of a mirror, surrounded by a circle of seven white candles for purity and spiritual enlightenment. Burn sticks of frankincense and sandalwood incense for wisdom and clarity. In each hand hold a rose—a symbol of love and female sexuality. Close your eyes, take a few deep breaths, and take your awareness inward to a sense of inner peace. Concentrate on what qualities you really desire in a man. When you have a very clear vision and feel calm and ready, open your eyes and gaze at yourself in the mirror. Say:

I am worthy of love, I am worthy of grace
Passion and fulfilment take their place
In my heart and in my mind
The perfect man is now mine to find

It's important that you have a really clear image of the man you want in your life and also a strong sense of self-worth—

you deserve the best, and you'll settle for nothing less!

The next step of the spell is to conjure the man of your dreams.

By the light of red candles, on a piece of red paper in black pen write a description of the man you desire. Don't specify a particular person—that would be interfering with his free will, and the spell would backfire. Visualize the things you desire, perhaps:

~ **Gentle caresses**
~ **Long, sensuous kisses**
~ **Firm lovemaking**
~ **Laughs and good conversation**
~ **Friendship and fun**

When your list is finished, pluck three petals from each of your roses and place them on your list. Taking one of the candles, drip wax on the petals to seal them and your desire to the paper, as you say:

Come to me
Man of my dreams
As is my will
So mote it be

Fold the paper over, so that the wax seals. Place this under your pillow. As you sleep, you'll have visions of your man—be on the lookout for him after this, because he will appear to you within fourteen days.

Remember, magick works with the intent you fuel it with and with your desire—so suspend any disbelief and fear. The universe is full of unimaginable potential, and you can tap into this to realize your goals. Just believe in your own infinite potential, and know that all the magick you need is inside you—you just have to unleash it.

Leave the Lights on!

I love having sex and have been told I'm good in bed, but I get really insecure if the lights are turned on. I can only really loosen up in the dark—is there a spell to give me more confidence?

To Witches, being naked is an utterly divine and pure state—not just when you're a newborn baby but all through your life. Our bodies are miraculous and one of nature's most profound expressions of the life force. One of our greatest challenges in this modern age is to rise above society's notions of what looks good and express our own individual, unique, and perfect beauty.

So the first thing I'm going to tell you to do is…get naked!

In the privacy of your home, start going starkers. Eat your breakfast in the nude, do the vacuuming, make the bed—whilst doing simple daily tasks, get used to being naked. Spend as much time as you can outside sans clothing, too. Swim, sunbathe, even do some gardening. Commune with nature as much as possible in your natural state, and you will start to feel at ease and proud. This might sound a bit silly, but it's actually very empowering.

You can also mix up a magickal body-love elixir to drink and a self-love potion to massage into your skin to affirm your unique beauty.

To make the body-love elixir pour a pint of almost-boiled spring water into a bowl and float two handfuls of fresh, scented rose petals in it. Cover with a cloth and allow to steep overnight. In the morning strain and mix in one tablespoon of brandy, two tablespoons of rosewater, and four teaspoons of sugar (or two teaspoons of sugar syrup).

Keep in the fridge and drink half a cup morning and night. The rose is a sacred flower of love and beauty—as you sip your elixir, ask for the blessings of Aphrodite the Goddess of Love:

Bless me, lovely Aphrodite
As today I honor my special beauty

To make a self-love potion: Take a handful of scented rose petals and a handful of marigold petals. Place these in a pan and pour over a cup of almost-boiling water, cover with a cloth for a few hours, then strain. To each four ounces of unscented moisturizer cream (not lotion—sorbolene is good), mix in one quarter-cup of the flower infusion, whisking so that it doesn't go too runny. You can also add one or two teaspoons of very finely ground orris root powder (a powerful love and romance attractor) to thicken if necessary. Now add five drops of rose geranium essential oil and mix through.

Store the potion in the fridge, and after giving it a good shake, massage the cool, divinely scented cream into your body morning and night, and as you do so, concentrate on feeling proud of your body and blessed by your unique beauty. The potion will be good for your skin, the massage good for your spirits, and the flower essences good for your heart.

Also, next time you're making love with the light on, try easing into it with the wonders of candlelight! Lots of red and pink candles will encourage passion. Burn some ylang ylang essential oil for sensuality and confidence, and you will be free and willing!

Desire Me

There is a guy at work I really like—in fact, I would love to seduce him! Is there a spell I can do to make him fall for me?

You're heading into dangerous waters here. To cast a spell over someone else for selfish purposes is to break one of the three main Witches' Laws—"Do what you will, but don't interfere with another's free will." If you attempt to make this guy fall for you, be prepared for nasty repercussions. He may well fall for you, but you might find you're better off without his interest. Someone I know did a "come to me" spell, and it worked very well—unfortunately, the guy turned out to be a bit of a psycho, and she ended up very unhappy.

> **To cast a spell over someone else for selfish purposes is to break one of the three main Witches' Laws.**

It is far better to do a general "come to me" spell: Instead of specifying a person, you ask for a person with your chosen qualities and attributes—and let the Universe decide who is best for you. Having warned you, and you're thinking, "Blow it! I like trouble; give me the spell," here it is—for the girls and boys.

You need to get hold of something that has his/her energy. Some soil scooped from a footprint he/she has made, or perhaps some body bits—hair, fingernails (the girl I knew who did this spell offered her guy a manicure at work. Creepy!), or even spit (a glass from which he/she has taken a sip).

Prepare for the spell by taking a bath to which you have added half a cup of Epsom salts and five drops of lemon oil (or a half-cup of the juice). Lemon and salt work to purify you and protect you from negativity. As you lie in the bath, focus on your intent, picture the guy/girl in your head, and say the mantra, "Come to me; come to me," over and over.

Do this spell in an enclosed, private place—it is a work in progress and must not be disturbed.

Sprinkle a circle of salt within which to work, and assemble a large red candle, white cord, and "come to me" potent paste. Make this by mixing half a cup of water with cornstarch until it thickens. Add a teaspoon of damiana (for passion), a teaspoon of cinnamon (for potency), and six black peppercorns (for speedy results). Mix this through, then add some of your own saliva—or for really potent results, masturbate and add some of your vaginal fluid or semen.

Carve his/her name into the candle, place it in the center of a large plate, and sprinkle the body bits or soil around it. Take some of the paste and smear it over the carving of his/her name, and have a clear vision of his/her face in your mind as you say:

**Come to me, my will is great
Now you can't escape your fate**

Take the white cord and trail it across your body, visualizing it absorbing your energy, your lust, your desire. Then wrap it around the base of the candle as you say:

**Bound to me you now be
As is my will, so mote it be**

Light the candle and gaze at the flame as you intone: "Come to me; come to me," repeatedly. When you have a clear vision of the two of you together, snuff the flame and say: "It is done."

Cover the candle and plate with black cloth and leave. Every night for the next seven days, smear more paste on the candle, relight, and again chant: "Come to me." He/she will be yours within the week.

This is quite a sinister spell—I am assuming your motives are harmless fun—but as I said earlier, interfering with another's free will is breaking the laws of Witchcraft, and you will have to accept repercussions. So think hard before you use magick to seduce another—and perhaps do a self-love spell to enhance your natural charms. Then when she/he falls for you, you'll know that it is really you that she/he desires and not trickery and enchantment.

Supplies for the Spells and Rituals

There is an extensive list of international suppliers at my website <www.fionahorne.com>. Otherwise, everything I have suggested should be available at a well-stocked health food store and/or New Age/alternative-living gift store.

Remember:

**ALL ACTS OF LOVE AND PLEASURE ARE
SACRED TO THE GODDESS.**

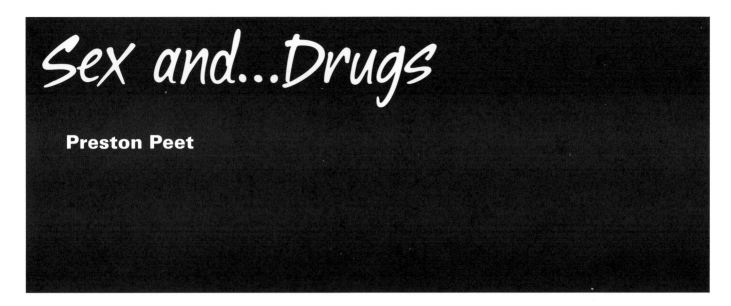

Sex and...Drugs

Preston Peet

"It is obvious that sex and drugs together can lead to more extraordinary and paranormal trans-ego experiences than either sex or drugs alone," the incomparable Robert Anton Wilson once wrote.[1] As aphrodisiacs, as lubricants in social settings, as a tool to assist in seducing a potential partner, to help make the sexual act a more magical and mystical experience, there is no set reply—everyone this writer discussed sex and drugs with while researching this article reports a different view of both the purpose(s) of taking drugs with their sex (or sex with their drugs, as the case may be) and of the results.

Despite the rampant sex phobias and drug phobias that many in roles of authority labor under, which in large part are used to manipulate the populace into supporting our current worldwide drug prohibitions, millions of people across the globe still use drugs, both legal and illegal, and many if not most do, at least sometimes, combine their drugs with sex. Is Wilson correct, that the reason many people take drugs in combination with sex is to enhance their sexual experience? Or is the sex often a result of the drug use itself, an inadvertent accident where one wakes in the morning, looks across the bed, and says through a throbbing headache and pasty mouth, "Oh shit, what have I done?"

Both sex and drugs are often targets of puritans, politicians, and law enforcers who need a scapegoat to blame for this or that problem or social ill and to insure a continued source of revenue for their coffers. But both are so much fun, with the possible yet at times very real negative consequences so far out of the mind and down the road for most, that few heed the calls for stricter controls and for less of both. Whether they're aphrodisiacs for arousal, illegal drugs for thrills or enlightenment, or pharmaceuticals for staying power, drugs and sex go hand in hand, nearly inseparable.

Alcohol

"Alcohol is the big one. I already have my lessons for my daughter worked out. 'Look, some guy plying you with drinks isn't doing it out of charity. He's spending his good money on booze for you for one reason.' My guess is we all have a few ancestors and, therefore, ourselves here because of drunken sex."—Steven Anker, television and commercial/video director (*Outer Limits, Dinosaurs, Jimmy Kimmel Live,* more)

~

"Chemicals such as opiates, methamphetamines, and downs of any kind, including alcohol, can make me limp as a wet lettuce leaf. Women can sometimes hide these effects, but no man I've met can. In youth, of course, we think we are immortal and God-like strong, but in sexual success it is only

> **"My guess is we all have a few ancestors and, therefore, ourselves here because of drunken sex."**

a matter of your youth, not the chemical. Let's face it, inhibited desire is the point to beat, not a limp 'junior'!

"I know with sex I want to give or receive something special, and most folks I talked to agree: A little bit of your favorite sugar can make you feel like a Tyrannosaurus (I mean like maybe two drinks, one joint, etc.), but go over whatever is *your* dose to do the job, and you fail. Drunk girls can be very uninhibited, but they smell and pass out easily. If I still drank, it would be no different!"—TR, subscriber to DrugWar.com email list

By the nineteenth century, the tide of moralistic prohibitionism was firmly rising in the US, with a variety of failed attempts by some US states to discourage and/or control alcohol use through high taxation and outright banning only strengthening the temperance movement's resolve. The Reverend Howard Hyde Russell's Anti-Saloon League, founded in 1895, launched one of the very early anti-drug campaigns in the US, aimed at hard liquors and spirits and the saloons that sold them, with advertisements and handbills printed up proclaiming such scientific messages as, "Alcohol inflames the passions, thus making the temptation to sex-sin unusually strong."[2]

This perception, that alcohol use often leads to rampant immoral sexual practices, continues right to this day, based in part on reality, and in part on moralist fearmongering. The BBC reported in March 2005 that by the upcoming October, British "TV advertisers are to be banned from portraying alcohol as an 'aid to seduction' or showing it alongside themes

"I was extremely high at that point, so any curve of her skin, the smell of her hair, it was all a wonder, as if I had never done or seen this before."

strongly appealing to under 18s." The aim is to discourage positive linking by youth of drinking and sex. "They should also refrain from making links to sexual motive or include sexual contact, and ads should not imply that sexual activity has taken place or is about to take place."[3]

Alcohol is the first drug of choice today for most people, mostly due to its being the only completely legal drug that might be ingested in a social setting without fear of arrest. Legal, and one of the most potent, most easily overdone drugs, alcohol is also inhibition-releasing yet potentially damaging to the sexual act.

Who hasn't gone to a bar to try to get drunk and laid at the same time? It's such a socially accepted practice, so common and unremarkable, that most people don't even consider that they're taking a drug when slugging down their cocktails, watching and hearing members of the opposite (or same) sex grow ever more attractive as they themselves grow ever more confident, often simultaneously growing ever more sloppy and drunk. There's no denying that alcohol has been at the root of many a date rape, abusive domestic situation, and simply bad sex—there's a fine line with alcohol where "too much" is only a fraction more, often just one drink, than "just enough."

"One time I had a regular at my bar ask me to make him a drink that would make him horny, so I made

him a Peach Vellini, as that usually makes me horny, too."—anonymous female NYC bartender

~

"I suppose if fumbling, energetic, and overall goofy sex is your thing, I would say alcohol is the ticket. Hard thing about that is just enough and you should have some fun. Too much and, well, your man rising to the occasion could be a challenge."—Johann, subscriber to DrugWar.com email list

~

"Alcohol? Sometimes a struggle, and not ideal conditions, but I have been known to make the odd Command Performance."—Tim M., subscriber to DrugWar.com email list

Marijuana

"I have had sex while under the influence of marijuana, and it did seem to make the experience more warm and soft. I was extremely high at that point, so any curve of her skin, the smell of her hair, it was all a wonder, as if I had never done or seen this before. It made things new again."—Johann

~

"You always hear that marijuana is supposed to be a libido inhibitor, but for me, marijuana has always been a true aphrodisiac. Not in the 'I smoke, then I get horny' kind of way, but in a general, overall sense, and I have smoked daily for 24 years. Cannabis is known to be a dopamine agonist and without dopamine you don't feel horny, so it stands to reason that a dopamine agonist is gonna help in that department, not hinder things.

"And certainly during periods of time when I am not smoking daily (those rare, rare times), I feel, well, less horny. Then I light one up and bingo, horny again. All day every day, that's my motto. Not saying if I am referring to smoking or fucking. I will let *you* figure that one out."—Richard Metzger, cofounder and creative director of The Disinformation Company Ltd.

~

"Pot? Love it. IMHO [In my humble opinion] it connects you with your partner and makes it more pleasurable, more 'into' things and more attention is paid to other aspects other than the piston action. Staying power is very high. Too high, sometimes."—Tim M.

"Probably the most natural sensual stimulant would be marijuana but—take heed—this is an illegal natural substance."[4] The Internet is full of websites put together by or in cooperation with the Partnership for a Drug-Free America and other anti-drug groups, along with the help and funding of the US White House Office of National Drug Control Policy (ONDCP), that decry the use of drugs and engaging in sex by teens, warning of the dangers of sex and marijuana (and other drugs, too, of course) in combination. These websites are chock full of dire predictions of pregnancies, disease, and death—and the warnings, if quite a bit over the top, are often worthwhile when it comes to young people mixing substance use with sexual activity, though the threats posed by marijuana are usually overinflated in the extreme, even laughable. This can lead to young people totally disregarding any of the beneficial and serious warnings of possible danger ahead.

Marijuana is by far the most widely used illegal drug in the world, enjoyed regularly by anywhere between 20 to 50 million Americans each year, and it has been used in conjunction with sex for millennia. It wasn't until the early twentieth century that the outcry against marijuana and those "degenerates" who used it—often Mexicans, blacks, and jazz musicians, and the white women they were reported to be leading astray—really began to rise in volume, accompanied by strenuous calls for its outright banning, with William Randolph Hearst's newspapers leading the charge.

Robert A. Nelson describes a reefer-madness styled, sex-fearing article published during the original attack on pot. "An unqualified article linking marihuana, crime and insanity, written by M.A. Hayes and L.E. Bowery (a policeman from Wichita, Kansas) was published in *The Journal of Criminal Law and Criminology* (1932), and thereafter it was often cited as a definitive study. Hayes and Bowery asserted that the marihuana user is capable of 'great feats of strength and endurance, during which no fatigue is felt... [S]exual desires are stimulated and may lead to unnatural acts, such as indecent exposure and rape.'"[5]

Despite these early horror stories blaming all sorts of sexual criminality and depravity on the use of the demon weed, millions of people from all walks of life, with all sorts of sexual preferences and practices, merrily smoke it to this day, using it to help ease their inhibitions, increase sensitivity, and generally help make their sex that much more enjoyable. The ONDCP has taken note of this tendency and claims at various times that smoking pot will decrease libido and cause other unspecified sexual debilitations, yet simultaneously runs taxpayer-funded anti-drug commercials that link pot-smoking to teen pregnancy. This is just one more indication of the insanely schizophrenic nature of the War on Some Drugs and Users.

"In the end, the right variety of cannabis—a good sativa/indica hybrid—is the best enhancer. One with a 'high head' but that also delivers an underlying physical rush without wonking you out like a Quaalude on a stick. Throw in the little mentioned narcotic, music—for me, some haunting jazz with a soprano sax.... Hmmm. Anyway, in reviewing my most memorable sexual experiences (and I've had quite a few), the best ones could be described as beginning in that manner."—Libby, subscriber to DrugWar.com email list

~

"I smoke my slave out when we begin a session together. It seems to give things, or at least put him into a more spiritual place when we're playing. It leaves him less inhibited or reserved, and helps him into a more special place. We never actually have sex per se, only role-play, but he's my full-time slave, living with me, and it's definitely a sexual situation."—Velocity Chyaldd, front woman of the NYC band Vulgaras

~

"I like pot brownies a lot. They are definitely an aphrodisiac for me, particularly the combination of chocolate and marijuana. The same goes for mushrooms and chocolate."—DJ Ness, female NYC DJ

Psychedelics

"I'm always fond of tripping and sex. 'It's so cool when your face melts when I come, honey. And your pussy looks cosmic.'"—Steven Anker

~

"Well, for me, sex on X (ecstasy) is the shit, the best, indescribably delicious. That would be old school X—MDAA, MDMA, powder form, not the

I experienced perceptions and feelings I never imagined possible, a meeting between her and myself on the very deepest levels, a melding together as one person.

bullshit they call X today. A blend of X and LSD is also a delight, and straight up fresh and clean LSD is also beautiful, while mushrooms, they're mystic and tantric."—Sharon Secor, freelance journalist

~

"For myself, I never liked doing it under the influence of psychedelics. For me, acid and mescaline and mushrooms were always more about the cerebral than the physical planes. It was too much work to stay present in the body that was performing the act when my mind was out chasing phantom scraps of other realities. Besides, the room was always melting on me. I much preferred to be outdoors walking in that state."—Libby

Infamous LSD proponent Timothy Leary labeled acid "the most powerful aphrodisiac ever discovered."[6] But this isn't the universal view concerning psychedelics and sex by any means. The Blue Honey website says: "To determine whether psychedelic plants are, indeed, aphrodisiacs, we must first determine what we mean by an aphrodisiac. If we mean that the drugs specifically excite the sexual organs, then psychedelics are not aphrodisiacs. If we mean that they produce or encourage sexual desire, again they are not aphrodisiacs. But if we mean that the drugs can profoundly enhance the quality of sexual acts that occur between people who would, in any case, have had intercourse, then the drugs are aphrodisiacs, and my only objection to the term in this context is that it will continue to be misused by psychedelic or sexual extremists."[7]

So what we're seeing is the police asserting both that LSD destroys the sex drive yet simultaneously turns users into sex-mad maniacs.

For this writer, there once was a time when I felt like Libby, quoted above. I clearly remember saying to someone during a conversation—just nineteen and living in Paris, where I sold and ate a lot of LSD—that I did not enjoy sex while I was tripping on LSD, that I was usually too distracted and involved in the visions and deep thoughts to spend much time concentrating on my sexual partner. I went so far as to insist that I'd "never" enjoy sex during an LSD trip.

But then came that one special night a few years later in Tampa, Florida, when my partner (at the time) and I melted into one another during a particularly heavy yet easygoing trip. I experienced perceptions and feelings I never imagined possible, a meeting between her and myself on the very deepest levels, a melding together as one person, with moments of telepathic communication and multiple, simultaneous orgasms during hour upon hour of incredible, literally magical sex. Ever since that night I have always found sex while high on certain psychedelics to be extremely enjoyable; substances such as LSD and mushrooms add a special level to lovemaking, leading me to some of the most profound mental revelations I've ever experienced, as well as some of the most intense physical sensations I've ever felt during sex or otherwise.

P.G. Stafford and B.H. Golightly—discussing the linking by fearmongering politicians and police of LSD use and violence, helped along by a new generation of yellow journalists and the rags that published their outrageous anti-drug screeds—note that fears of violent trippers weren't the only worries manipulated to frighten middle America into supporting the latest drug prohibitions and subsequent war upon users of LSD and other psychedelics. "Others were quick to link LSD to sex. Thus *The Confidential Flash* asserted in a full-page headline, 'LSD Kills Sex Drive Forever' although the story itself in no way bore out this claim. And, interestingly enough, the *Police Gazette,* in its August, 1966 issue, reprinted an article from *The Journal of the American Medical Association* which they retitled 'LSD and Sex Madness.'"[8] So what we're seeing is the police, and others who depend upon the War for their livelihood, asserting both that LSD destroys the sex drive yet simultaneously turns users into sex-mad maniacs—yet another example of prohibitionist schizophrenia.

Oddly enough, these anti-drug zealots may have a valid point tying psychedelic drug use to sexual escapades, even if they can't keep their scare stories straight and their facts are often, if not usually, skewed or just flat-out wrong. In this case, they've gotten things entirely backwards, if their own religion's roots are any indication. There is strong evidence that even the most important Christian holy day, or at least its pagan predecessor, was once marked with the use of strong psychedelic plants during sexual festivities.

"The celebration we know as Easter dates back long before the time of Christ, and has its origins in traditions that involved ritualized sex and consumption of a wide variety of potent psychedelics and aphrodisiacs, including marijuana," writes Reverend Damuzi.[9] For any fundamentalist Christian who sides with the prohibitionistic moralists in calling for stricter controls of both sex and drugs, the idea that Easter stems from an ancient pagan event celebrated with debauched orgies involving the taking of heavily hallucinogenic substances while having sex with all sorts of unmarried people must be particularly galling. But it just goes to show that people have been mixing sex and psychedelics for far longer than Christianity itself has been on the planet, which leads some to suspect there may be something to the idea that we are meant to be mixing the two, or at least that there's nothing sinful or unnatural about doing so.

"It was MDA (the love drug) back in the 1970s and later MDMA. (Both precursors of today's XTC, which I haven't tried *yet* because I haven't found anyone who could promise me what they could get was real XTC.) If my date agreed to party with me on

MDA, I knew I was getting laid. All I had to do was mention sex once and touch them *anywhere*, even their arm and they wanted more."—Anonymous 48-year-old resident of Indiana and subscriber to the DrugWar.com email list

~

"Personally, for my own sexual activities, I'm more of a mushroom person. I've never tried heroin or cocaine or even LSD, preferring mushrooms or perhaps a good tab of ecstasy."—Velocity Chyaldd

Heroin, Cocaine, and Methamphetamines: The Powders

"'Dope Dick, an Ethnographic Examination' or 'Faking the Big O: A Male's Perspective.' When I had girlfriends who I was hiding my dope hobby from, I got good at faking the O. 'Honey, how come you always come so quick first thing in the morning?' they'd ask. 'I guess I'm just a morning person.'"—Steven Anker

~

"Cocaine, sniffing, is odd. It feels real nice, but can frustrate as full orgasm seems elusive. Smoking cocaine, the vibes are all wrong for sex, kinda creepy, really. Heroin, I've no desire for much more than noddin' and chillin', maybe a snuggle while I drift, with a place to rest my head."—Sharon Secor

~

"Crack or freebase.... Sex is the only thing that gets my mind off of being paranoid when I do either. Makes me horny as a dog, but then I have trouble 'getting it up' so combine that with a prescription which helps me get it up (not Viagra, there are others I enjoy better), and voila! Whew! Take a hit at the same time I am coming and *bam*! The biggest best fucking physical *and* mental orgasms I've ever had in my life!"—Anonymous 48-year-old Indiana resident

For this writer, heroin and cocaine both started out being extremely sexy drugs. I would shoot heroin with a lover, then make love all night, unable to come yet able to stay hard for hours. It was an awesomely beautiful experience each and every time—until I caught a habit. Then my use of heroin got in the way of sex and rapidly became much more important than sex ever was.

Cocaine was very similar for me—when simply snorting the powder form, I felt like a god in bed and would find myself feeling especially kinky. But once I began smoking, then eventually shooting, cocaine, forget about it—sex was suddenly nothing more than a way for me to make more money to cop more cocaine and heroin. Forget about love and forget about pleasure.

But this isn't how it works for everyone. Some people thoroughly enjoy taking cocaine while having sex. Some folks have no problem with taking heroin and maintaining an erection all night and never catching a habit—or if they do, not letting it get in the way of their sex. Some folks love taking speed and screwing all night. It's a case where "to each his/her own" rings true.

Cocaine (and speed) has been alleged by some researchers, not to mention anecdotally by many users, to release such a flood of dopamine in the brain that it blows away any release naturally occurring from orgasms, making sex seem somehow insignificant to the habitual user. "As a result of cocaine's actions in the nucleus accumbens, there are increased impulses leaving the nucleus accumbens to activate the reward system, and with continued use of cocaine, the body relies on this drug to maintain rewarding feelings. The person is no longer able to feel the positive reinforcement or pleasurable feelings of natural rewards (food, water, sex)."[10]

While it is questionable as to whether this becomes an issue or problem with most recreational, part-time sniffers, from my own personal experiences and taking into account the numerous tales told by hardcore cocaine, heroin, and speed addicts I've known and loved, this lack of interest in sex amongst addicts is more often than not the rule rather than the exception. "As with cocaine, continued use of opiates [e.g., heroin] makes the body rely on the presence of the drug to maintain

"If my date agreed to party with me on MDA, I knew I was getting laid."

rewarding feelings and other normal behaviors. The person is no longer able to feel the benefits of natural rewards (food, water, sex) and can't function normally without the drug present."[11]

But as our anonymous Indiana resident above makes clear, there are exceptions to every rule, and cocaine and heroin have always been, and will continue to be, sex enhancers for many users.

"I used to want to do coke and go out, but now when I do cocaine I just want to go home and spank the monkey."—Anonymous male NYC burlesque performer

~

"I don't recommend this to anyone trying to stay away from opiates, but, just the right amount of heroin or maybe an 80 mg oxy [OxyContin], would make me think I was Howard Huge. Staying power? Hell, you would have to really concentrate to ever get to where you want to go, so to speak. Too much opiate? That's where you snort coke off of her body. You pick the spot. Smoke a joint, ring a bell, round two."—Randy, subscriber to DrugWar.com email list

~

"As far as white stuff, it didn't do it for me either. I never really did heroin, but coke and meth didn't make me want to go lie around in bed. I was too busy talking to get into the mood for physical intimacy. The only time I found coke useful in fact was once when we didn't snort any, but my partner dipped his erect penis in a bag of it. He had some issues with staying power. It wasn't an issue that time. In fact, it was probably the mightiest and longest lasting erection he ever achieved."—Libby

Pharmaceuticals

"Cialis is a wonderful drug. It is also easily available from online pharmacies or your best friend's dad. Being in my early 20's, I admit I don't really need Cialis, but then again who in their right mind would turn down a three-day erection? This drug doesn't exactly give me a high besides the fact that I feel like Superman and can perform for days. Not to mention the woman has no idea I popped one of those little gifts from god, so in turn she thinks I am a god as well. Ah, good times. Well, besides the hellish heartburn as a side effect but honestly, in light of the pros, I can deal with it."—Johann

"Viagra's effect is to inhibit an enzyme known as *phosphodiesterase type-5* (PDE5), which naturally occurs in erectile tissue. PDE5 can break down cyclic GMP, the substance that is produced during sexual arousal and causes vascular and muscular changes that eventual [*sic*] lead to an erection."[12] The current slew of advertisements on TV, in print media, and

"Too much opiate? That's where you snort coke off of her body."

online (for instance, rampant email spamming) for such pharmaceuticals as Cialis and Viagra, aimed towards men with erectile dysfunction, make clear that both sex and drugs continue to be moneymakers. Beyond the obvious physical pleasure derived from being able to engage in sexual activity—if one has checked with their doctor first to be sure they're healthy enough to still do the physical deed—these drugs do not get their users high at all. This sort of drug works directly on the penis, enabling a man to get an erection. The user might get that elusive hard-on, but as one friend described it to me while researching this article, "There's no arousal whatsoever, no lust. It's like walking about with a baseball bat between my legs but no turn-on at all."

Then there are drugs like Uprima, otherwise known as apomorphine (unrelated to morphine despite having the word in its name), which work a bit differently. "Uprima doesn't act directly upon the penis like Viagra or Befar, but instead exerts its influence in the brain for arousal, pleasure, and orgasm. Uprima acts upon receptors in the hypothalamus and can enhance erection by increasing the signals from the brain to begin the process."[13] Use of Uprima can result in nausea the first few times, not something one normally associates with sexual arousal, but as any new user of heroin can tell you, the same thing results from dope, too, and few stop using solely because they got a little queasy the first few times.

"My boyfriend began having problems with erections (he's older), and I suggested he look into Viagra. Boy, am I glad he did! The first time he tried it, one 50 mg pill did nothing, so he took another and that was a mistake. Three hours later he was still rock hard and had come multiple times (so had I)! Since then a single 50 mg dose does it very well—he's now good for almost two hours of good hard sex that leaves both of us worn out."—Bobbie, USA[14]

Conclusion

As evidenced by the $400-$600 billion a year in illegal drug trade profits, according to the US government's own figures (not even getting into the legal pharmaceutical profits, where Viagra alone made a $411 million profit for its maker, Pfizer, in the first three months of its release, and $1.8 billion in 2003), as well as $4 billion from the sale and rental of porn videos in 2002, it's obvious that sex and drugs both sell, and there is a reason for that: Sex and drugs simply fit together as naturally as the sexual organs. Sex and drugs are two of humanity's greatest passions, its most profitable businesses, and its greatest sources of pain and pleasure. It's obvious that for most of recorded history, humankind has been fascinated with both pursuits and will continue to be so enthralled for the foreseeable future.

The desires for sex and drugs are natural drives, inherent in our very essence, in who we are as human beings. No matter how many sermons are preached against them, no matter how many laws are passed governing them, no matter what the risks and dangers and negative repercussions that can and do sometimes arise from both, people will continue to get drunk and stoned and boff like bunnies until the end of time. And they'll be willing to pay a lot of money, dodge a lot of laws, and leap through a lot of hoops to do so.

Endnotes

1. Wilson, Robert Anton. *Sex and Drugs: A Journey Beyond Limits.* New Falcon, 1987. Originally published by Playboy Press, 1973. **2.** "History of Alcohol Prohibition," in "Marihuana: A Signal of Misunderstanding," the final report of the National Commission on Marijuana and Drug Abuse (1972). Commissioned by President Richard Nixon, who utterly ignored the findings. [www.druglibrary.org/schaffer/Library/] **3.** "Alcohol and Sex Link Ban for Ads." BBC News, 15 Mar 2005. **4.** "Aphrodisiacs: A Short History of Sex and Drugs." [www.aboutaphrodisiacs.org] **5.** Nelson, Robert A. *Hemp and History.* Chapter 3: "Marijuana and Madness." [www.rexresearch.com]. Citing *International Medical Digest* 7 (1937):183-7. **6.** Leary, Timothy. "Millbrook '66: On Sex, Consciousness, and LSD." In *The Delicious Grace of Moving One's Hand: The Collected Sex Writings,* by Timothy Leary. New York: Thunder's Mouth Press, 1998. **7.** "Sex and Psychedelics." [www.bluehoney.org]. **8.** Stafford, P.G., and B.H. Golightly. *LSD: The Problem-Solving Psychedelic.* Chapter 1: "The LSD Crisis." Award Books, 1967. **9.** Reverend Damuzi. "Easter: Sex and Drugs Celebration!" 10 May 2004, CannabisCulture.com. **10.** Office of Science Policy and Communications, National Institute on Drug Abuse. "The Brain and the Actions of Cocaine, Opiates, and Marijuana." National Institutes of Health, 1997. **11.** Ibid. **12.** Micans, Phil, PharmB. "Beyond Viagra: The Latest Treatments For Erectile Dysfunction." International Antiaging Systems, no date. [www.antiaging-systems.com]. Citing: Micromedex Martindale, International Drug Information, June 2002. **13.** Ibid. Citing: Altwein JE, Keuler FU, "Oral treatment of erectile dysfunction with apomorphine SL." *Urol. Int.* 2001; 67(4):257-63. **14.** "Viagra Stories: First Hand Tales of Viagra, Personal Experiences and Testimonials." [www.viagrastories.com]

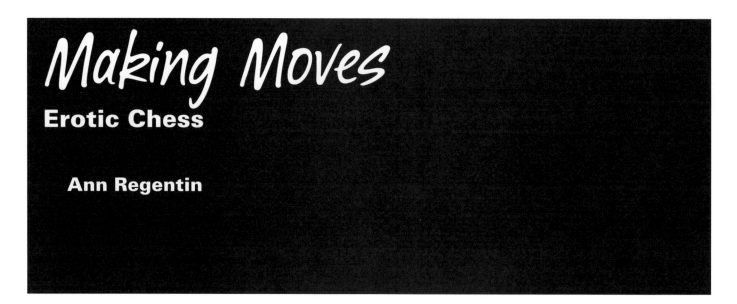

Making Moves
Erotic Chess

Ann Regentin

Faye Dunaway and Steve McQueen sit opposite each other, assessing, wondering where their game of cat and mouse will end. She rises suddenly, walks over to a chess set and looks down at it speculatively.

> "Do you play?" he asks.
> "Try me," she says.

And so they play. A finger caresses the curve of a bishop, plays with a lip, runs up and down a bare arm, fidgets with a tie, brushes a knee under the table. They smile, exchange glances as the fire crackles in the background.

Check.

He stands, his back to the board, to her, then turns and looks over the game. He did not expect this. It's his move now. He pulls her to her feet. "Let's play something else!"

What are you supposed to think when somebody declares that they're going to mate you in five moves, so you might as well surrender now?

This chess game in the 1968 version of *The Thomas Crown Affair*, along with the kiss that follows, is one of the great seduction scenes on film. The movie itself is about the collision between a rich, spoiled bank robber and a beautiful, intelligent insurance investigator, and is only otherwise memorable for some tricky production techniques. But the chess game does its double duty splendidly, providing both a metaphor for the battle of wits between the two protagonists and a perfect arena for a long, slow dance of mutual temptation.

I love chess. I was introduced to it by my father and uncles, who played constantly at every family gathering. I learned pinochle the same way, but I've never eroticized that. Pinochle is associated in my mind with peanuts and kidding, but chess is another story entirely. I've never been particularly attracted to my uncles, but I am very attracted to chess.

The language of chess is very sexual. What are you supposed to think when somebody declares that they're going to mate you in five moves, so you might as well surrender now? Things get taken in chess. They can also be pinned and skewered. If you're going to nab the queen, you have to move in carefully, obliquely, much like a tricky seduction. It's a traditionally masculine game, but in spite of that, or perhaps because of it, she is the most powerful piece on the board and calls many of the shots. A knight, if he's careful, can take her without putting himself in harm's way. He just has to make the right moves.

I'm not a particularly gifted player. I can think ten moves ahead, but I usually forget the first three, and I can get so invested in a plan that I fail to see clearly what my opponent is doing. Sometimes I get impatient and careless. But I play ruthless, material chess, and I win at least as often as I lose.

I love the challenge of the game. I like pitting my wits against someone else's. I like the tension of the endgame, when every move counts and there is no room for error. My heart pounds and I fidget, waiting on tenterhooks for my opponent to make his move, then sitting there staring at the board for ages, trying to anticipate him. That's part of what makes chess so erotic. In order to play well, you have to read your opponent's mind, get into his head the way you do when you're in bed and trying to figure out what will please this particular lover best. In both chess and sex, you use that intuition to break down the other, bring them to their knees in one way or another, whether it's defeat or ecstasy.

Chess is a sort of acid test for me. I once beat a man who was foolish enough to think that he could sacrifice his queen and still win. He was wrong, and I never slept with him. When my now-ex-husband and I played, the tension was so high that a house full of out-of-town guests bailed like rats off a sinking ship. I won, but it wasn't worth it. I still married him, but that wasn't worth it, either. I played with a woman who was trying to seduce me out from under him, and I won both games. I played with a good friend, a close game that I lost due to the aforementioned carelessness, and wished that things were different, and going to bed with him was a reasonable proposition.

I once dated a man who beat me consistently at chess. The games drove me insane. I'm extremely competitive, and although I'm usually a good loser, I'm not happy about losing all the time. I started to get reckless on the board, just like he was reckless in bed. Actually, "in bed" is a bit of a misnomer here. He liked a lot of different places, like playgrounds, stalls in communal showers, deserted buildings, and wooded areas. He did things to me that no one has done before or since, things that I have missed like hell even though he never took them quite far enough. But on the chessboard, he pushed me harder, backed me into corners, mated me, and I grew addicted to that.

This, I think, is where the heart of my attraction to chess lies. I like the chase. I like to take and be taken. It's not a physical thing, although I'm not averse to a good wrestling match, nor is it quite BDSM, although I'm not averse to the judicious use of restraint. What I like is to play with power. I like to win. I like to mate someone or, failing that, tell him that if he moves I'll stop and then make it impossible for him not to move. But I also like to lose, especially when the game is very close. I like to surrender, but only after a good fight.

It's the men's game that is taken seriously, but there have been some excellent women chess players. Russian-born Vera Menchik was the women's world champion from 1927 until her death in 1944 during a bombing raid in Kent. Hungarian Judit Polgar, the reigning women's chess champion, became a Grandmaster at the age of fifteen years and four

months, beating the record previously set by Bobby Fischer, and is currently ranked the twenty-third best player in the world, male or female. In 1998, she beat Anatoly Karpov, then the FIDE World Champion, in a rapid-play match. But perhaps the most memorable game played by a man and a woman—at least from an erotic point of view—was between Jacqueline Armand and Robespierre.

During the summer of 1793 in France, mere nobility was a capital offense, and that was to be the fate of Jacqueline's fiancé, a duke. In desperation, she cut off her hair so she could enter the men-only café where Robespierre liked to play chess. When the seat in front of him became vacant, she took it, asking a special favor if she won, offering money if she lost.

Legend has it that he knew the real stakes from the very beginning, but one wonders when Robespierre realized that his opponent was a woman. Was it a slim, manicured finger hesitating over a piece? The beardless chin resting on a clenched fist? The hint of curve under her shirt or a mouth that was too soft and too round? As the story goes, he said nothing until the end of the game, which he lost in spite of a material advantage. What did he think when she requested as her prize

I like the chase. I like to take and be taken.

the life of a fiancé instead of a father or a brother? Would he have taken her money if she had lost, or would he have asked a special favor of her, perhaps offering the life she wanted in return? In any case, he honored his word. Her lover went free.

⋈

I have never played tournament chess, but I imagine the stakes would be too high to be thinking about anything but the game. In the casual matches I've played, however, if there's the slightest attraction between my opponent and me, the temperature starts to rise whether or not there is an active seduction. If there is, the game becomes much more than a game and the closer it is, the hotter it gets.

About halfway through the game with the woman I mentioned earlier, I knew that if she won, I would go to bed with her if she asked, even though it was the eve of my wedding, and when she lost, she knew that it would never happen. But we never said a word. We just played chess.

Pervert

Jill Nagle

He's on his stomach, breathing slow. I'm moving my hands over and over his back, kneading the knots out of tight muscles, smoothing the surface of his skin, feeling the occasional sprout of hair or random mole—and then it happens.

The feeling overtakes me; in that instant, I know there's no turning back. From that moment on, I contrive to orchestrate all my movements to reach my goal, without tipping him off to the truth.

I pinch and press the skin all over his back, holding and twisting in many places, as if I meant to execute a special neuro-muscular technique—so that when I press and wriggle my thumbs around that special pore, he won't wonder why.

I've found that long strokes of my fingers alongside the target area help to loosen the skin in preparation for removal. In these circumstances, it's always a multiphase process, with each step needing to be worked in around the, well, more expected activities. Irving writhes whenever I stroke his ass,

Am I tampering nonconsensually with a part of him I have no business touching?

and tilts his large, white, hairy buns skyward. I spank him lightly, and he groans. I yawn.

I don't know why I've never just come right out and asked someone, Dude, can I pop the zit on your back? Maybe it's because I'm afraid they'll say no; maybe it's because I love the challenge and the satisfaction I get of using my stealth extraction skills undercover.

My breathing becomes labored as I pass the designated co-ordinates again and again, searching for signs of readiness for

the kill. Suddenly, Irving turns his head up toward me.

"I have to ask you something," he says. My hands freeze. Fuck. BUS-ted, I think.

"Sure, Irving, what's up?"

"I've never had a woman, you know," he pauses. I know what's coming.

"Fuck you up the butt?" I offer, brightly. His face reddens.

"Uh, yeah."

As we ready ourselves for this deed, I'm pondering how to proceed with the important task at hand. It's not as if I have no practice.

During my tenure as a San Francisco call girl, I have successfully extracted approximately 26 columns of compacted sebum, otherwise known as blackheads, which are now probably forever lodged in the camouflage of my beige carpet. Despite my best efforts, I've never managed to retrieve one later for closer inspection of my triumph.

Yet I know from looking before tossing that some are long and hard, and, I suspect, have been hiding in their host's back for many, many months, if not years. This sort of incubation period yields a product that is quite firm and deeply rooted. I have no use, of course, for the young ones that have had no time to ripen and solidify. Besides, they are usually too messy, and I tend to be squeamish. I've become quite a connoisseur over the years and often pass over prospects others would jump at. Let them, I say. I know my vintages and will harvest no fruit before its time.

While my dildo is plugging away at Irving's butt, I take advantage of the angle to further my cause. If I scratch the surface of his skin in just the right way, I can often catch the head of my target and dislodge it just a bit. It's tricky to keep it intact, which is 90% of the satisfaction of a job well done.

Pressing and heaving and scratching in rhythm with Irving's bucking and grunting, I gradually move things along. I've made some serious headway when Irving decides it's time to turn the tables. And no, I don't mean me on my stomach; my smooth back is no fun, anyway, and I wouldn't let him tamper with it even if it were. That's only for sacred intimates. Irving, not surprisingly, is in the mood for...the Big Missionary Finish.

While Irving is screwing me, I wonder about the ethics of what I've done. Am I tampering nonconsensually with a part of him I have no business touching? Is there a Mrs. Irving? Has she monitored The Big One over the course of Its life? Has Irving expressly forbidden her to disturb It? What if she's like me and has been mourning the opportunity to have at It? Upon witnessing the gaping hole soon to be in Its place, will she pack up her things and leave him, now certain by this evidence that he's been with someone else? I'm nervous now.

Still, I can't let It be.

Irving has had a completely silent, unremarkable (at least in its palpable manifestations) orgasm, and is resting on his side, probably thinking about the next round of semiconductors he must peddle to Silicon Valley. I offer to finish up with... a back rub!

With Irving on his stomach again, I notice that the prior course of events has rendered my hidden prize ever-so-ready to be liberated from its tight, fleshy prison. My groin is pulsing—only from having been plumbed, I'm sure.

It's in the Death Zone, which means that merely a few well-placed strokes and prods will free the particle permanently. I pray silently that he doesn't miss it. I have to time this carefully, because once the thing is gone, I will want to simply roll over and go to sleep, no matter whether there's still more time on the clock. Okay, four more minutes. Here goes: Thumbs up the vertebrae, concentrate there, almost. Fake him out with a double press along the right, so he thinks nothing of pressing hard on the l-l-l-left, come on, you little fucker, I haven't got all night, once more, oh who gives a shit if he

It's unusually large, solid steel-gray at the top, fading down to a roasted golden color, and finishing off with a delicate ivory.

knows what I'm doing, WHAM! There it is. Almost! I run my fingers over it; it doesn't move. Okay, scratch. Scratch down below, work my way up, run my fingernails RIGHT OVER that baby, and yes! *Yes!! YES!!!*

I perch the bibelot on my thumbnail and stare. It's unusually large, solid steel-gray at the top, fading down to a roasted golden color, and finishing off with a delicate ivory. I can't dwell here too long, or he'll wonder. Still—it's a rare beauty. I wish for a moment that I had a magnifying, three-dimensional Polaroid. Reluctantly, I flick my treasure away. Ephemeral and unsung, like Irving's orgasm, my peak moment has come and gone.

I breathe, enjoying the resolution period, and pass my hands absentmindedly across the impressive hole I've left in Irving's back. Goodbye, little work of art, I think. Irving's DNA, and the weeks of history you contain, are now forever immortalized in my carpet, along with the other 26 unsuspecting tricks' epidermal artifacts. A few more strokes, and I get up to wash my hands.

As Irving sheepishly dons his creased slacks, white button-down shirt, and tie with sailboats cruising a sea of navy, he says, "Tell me something, Isabella."

Terrified, I say, "Sure, Irving, what is it?"

"Do you think I'm a pervert?"

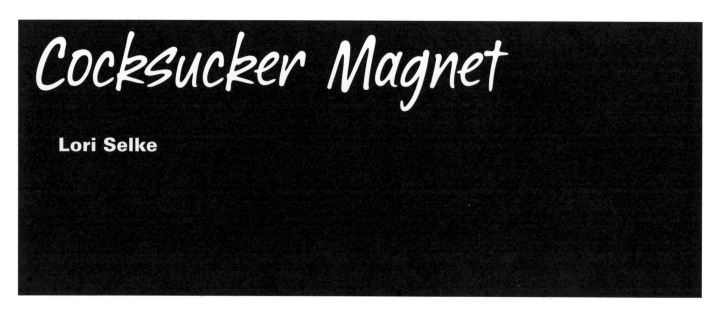

Cocksucker Magnet

Lori Selke

"I know what boys like."

—The Waitresses

This is a true story.

I have a cocksucker magnet.

I don't mean this the way that some women do—"All the cute ones are gay," or even, "Yep, after he broke up with me, well, you know. Just like my last two boyfriends, too."

No, I'm serious. I can sniff out a cocksucker at twenty paces.

Better than that, they actually seek me out.

There's a myth in our culture about men's sexuality. It's a persistent myth; lots of people believe it, and it's dead, flat wrong.

If anyone ever tells you that girls' sexuality is fluid—they're comfortable moving from boys to girls and back again, whatever works—while men are more, well, rigid about their preferences, don't believe them. It's a crock. The canonical Big Lie.

I know better.

Here's how I learned the truth.

I'm currently employed as a phone-sex girl. Yes, I have joined the ranks of the educated, middle-class sex workers that San Francisco is so famous for. My chosen profession is legal, therefore less lucrative, but I figured it showcased my best asset—no, not my tits and not my tattoo—my mouth. I'm good at talking dirty; that's why I write smut, too.

Plus, it's kind of like acting. I enjoy the make-believe.

On the phone, I'm twenty-four. I'm shorter. My tits are smal-ler, because everyone thinks I'm lying if I tell the truth. My waist is slimmer. And of course, I am femme and like to lounge around the house in black silk slips, a baby-T, and a thong, or a lace bra, short skirt, and no underwear. I also traffic in silky panties and little red dresses and high-heeled, marabou-trimmed mules.

I have brown hair, except when I'm blonde. I'm curvy and plush, except when I'm petite and slim, and I always have brown eyes.

And I have a cocksucker magnet.

I'm not sure if I've gotten a reputation in, I don't know, the underground phone-sex-fiend network or something, but more than half of my customers end up telling me, by the end of our ten, twenty, thirty minutes together, how much they want to suck cock. That's right—they want to give another guy a big, sloppy blowjob. They want to open their throat, get facefucked, and swallow a load of cum.

Some of them are honest about it, more or less. "I'm going to go visit a gay bar for the first time ever this weekend," one guy said to me. "I've always fantasized about it, but this time I'm going to do it."

I don't know if I really believe him or not. He could just be feeding me a line. But that's okay, because what he really wants to hear about is how, when he goes to that bar on Saturday, he's going to meet a guy who's going to drag him into a bathroom stall and force his cock down his throat, then take him home and fuck him up the ass. You didn't know this always happens in gay bars?

Or the guy who asked me to tell him what it was like to suck cock, because, "I tried it once in college, and I think about it now and then, and that's not so weird, is it?" I always assure them that no, of course it's not weird. I think they might be a bit put off, though, if I admitted that I get calls like theirs every single day. "Sure, there are thousands of guys out there just like you!" doesn't seem to be what they want to hear, either.

But you would be surprised by how many times these guys sneak their desire for cock into a scenario. I once was asked to spin a fantasy about slipping a Mickey into a guy's drink at a party and then "having my way" with him. So I did—I dragged him into a spare bedroom and made him lick my pussy, suck my toes, and so on and so forth. But clearly, he wanted more. Someone to watch, perhaps. So I told him the bedroom door was ajar and that anyone could see inside.

"Like your boyfriend? Maybe he wants to join in?" he suggested. A-ha. Soon enough, boyfriend was fucking me, too, then suddenly the guy was licking my boyfriend's cock as it slid in and out of me. And soon after, just like in a porn movie, imaginary boyfriend had to pull out and come—all over this guy's face.

Or here's another one. I got a call from a guy who told me that his fantasy was about watching his girlfriend fuck another guy. She had met this guy at a party (aren't parties fun?), and he could tell that she was really hot for him, and ever since then he'd had a fantasy about surprising them in the bathroom at the party. So I narrate a little of that for him, and he's peering in through the crack in the bathroom door.

I say, "I bet they know you're there. Would you like to go inside? Do you want to join in?" He sighs with relief and tells me yes. So he's inside, watching the guy fuck his girlfriend.

"He's going to fuck her up the ass for the first time," he tells me.

"Oh, you must be so hot watching her beg for that cock up her ass for the first time," I say. "She's never let you do this, but she's going to let him, and you get to see it."

"Yeah," he says. "I wonder how it feels."

"I bet you're wondering how it would feel to have that cock up your ass," I suggest. Sure enough, he just about blows his wad right then.

"You're good," he says admiringly, afterwards.

Sometimes I tell them I like to watch two guys get it on together, which is true. They're always amazed. "Really?" Like I just made it up to get them off. Like it's too good to be true. But it is true. "Sure, just like some guys like watching two girls together," I say, trying to normalize the situation a little bit. Usually, that's all the permission they need, and next I get an earful of exactly what they'd like to do with a guy if I was watching.

If it's not cocksuckers, it's crossdressers. And do you remember when we were told that just because a guy likes dressing up as a woman, it doesn't mean he actually wants to have sex with a man? That may be true, but not of my clients. Every single one of these guys wants to be made up like a slut, taken out to a bar or a club, and get picked up and taken home by a guy who'll fuck them up the ass.

I find these fantasies hard to narrate sometimes, because they mess with my ideas about continuity. Because, follow along with me here, they want me, their new best friend, to get them dressed up and tell them how pretty they look and then accompany them to the bar or wherever, where they get picked up by a guy and taken home. Presumably I'm still sitting at the bar, right? So how can I tell what's going on in this guy's hotel room or apartment or wherever he's taken my crossdressing friend? Oh, well. This is where being a writer gets you in trouble, because nobody cares about those details except me.

Now keep in mind, these are all heterosexual men. They found my number in the back of a magazine like *Gallery* or *Hustler*, so presumably in most cases they were looking at pictures of naked women shortly before they called me. They want to talk to a girl about sucking a guy's cock or dressing up like a slut and taking it up the ass. They could've called a gay chat line, but they didn't; they called me. They want a warm,

More than half of my customers end up telling me, by the end of our 10, 20, 30 minutes together, how much they want to suck cock.

friendly, female voice to walk them through the scary corners of their own sex fantasy life—i.e., the ones that are filled with men, with waiting cock.

Because I'm a girl, I must know about cock, right? So I'm the perfect, safe guide. And I really am! I always think, boy, they lucked out—if they only knew how okay I am with guys who are into guys. If only I could tell them about my cocksucker magnet. But I'm afraid that would frighten them off. For some reason, each one of them wants to think that he's the only one with this frightening, slightly shameful, but oh-so-compelling fantasy. It makes him unique. But he's not. They're steady business.

Sometimes I wonder: What if they knew? If they had any notion about how common their fantasy is, how would that change them? How would it change the world? For one thing, it would dispel this myth about men's rigid, predefined sexuality.

I know that my sampling is not scientific or even statistically significant, but it does say something. There are more closet cocksuckers than you think. And for some reason, they all want to confess to me.

Cat-fighting, Eye-licking, Head-sitting, and Statue-screwing

Brenda Love

Acrophilia

Acrophilia (*Acro*: highest point; *philia*: attachment to) refers to a person who is sexually aroused by heights. Skydiving and bungee-cord-jumping are high-altitude activities that elevate one's adrenalin. This excitement can then be transferred to passion and sex. Both of these activities include a form of bondage, vertigo, and suspension.

S/M partners who suffer from acrophobia are sometimes blindfolded and made to climb ladders. If this is done often, the phobia seems to dissipate and, along with it, the sexual charge it first produced. ("Terror," QSM lecture by J.C. Collins, Nov 28, 1990.)

Another popular form of acrophilia is having sex at a high altitude. This is humorously referred to as becoming a member

Aerobatics can be sexually arousing for a few people.

of the "Mile High Club" and is done in airplanes or other aircraft. (Conversely, one wonders if there is a "Mile Low Club" for submarines.) There was a group of pilots in New York that had its own version of a Mile High Club. The requirements were that the pilot and passenger go up in an open-cockpit bi-plane, and when they reached an altitude of 6,500 feet, the passenger would disrobe, climb out onto the wing and into the back seat, returning to the front seat after having sex with the pilot. All without falling off! (Personal communication, 1980.)

Aerobatics can be sexually arousing for a few people. Stunts in a small plane offer 4-5 negative G-forces and 3-4 positive G's. These affect the body by pushing the blood into either the head or the lower body, resulting in feelings of lightheaded-ness, floating, or sinking, depending on the maneuver. There is a tremendous adrenalin rush and a simultaneous sense of power over the airplane and submission to it. The feeling of being bound is greater in stunt flying than with other sports because the belts have to hold both body weight and the chute through every maneuver. There are very few sensations that compare with hanging upside down while one's weight pulls one toward the glass bubble that separates the pilot from the rapidly approaching ground. This feat provides enough sexual stimulation to cause at least one female pilot to experience spontaneous orgasm. (Personal communication.)

Finally, there are people who claim to have been captured by creatures from outer space and impregnated while aboard flying saucers. Their stories have provided many with a sexual fantasy, one that is acted out with the aid of readily available space costumes.

Agalmatophilia

(Galateism, Pygmalionism, Statuophilia.) Pygmalion was a mythical Greek sculptor who fell in love with Galatea (one of his female statues). At his request, the goddess Aphrodite brought her to life. Today this term refers to people with a statue or mannequin fetish.

Several historical cases of agalmatophilia have been documented. Clisyphus evidently "violated the statue of a goddess in the Temple of Samos, after having placed a piece of meat on a certain part." In 1877 "a gardener fell in love with a statue of the Venus of Milo and was discovered attempting coitus with it." (*Psychopathia Sexualis* by Richard von Krafft-Ebing, p 351.)

The practice of having sex with a statue was common among worshippers of the god Priapus, where virgins were first to be penetrated by him. This practice was later relegated to a priest or magistrate. However, even in the twentieth century, young Indian virgins were known to use sacred phalluses to break their hymens before marriage.

A few ancient statues had removable penises to facilitate their use as dildos. Several statues of Catholic fertility saints—including, among others, St. Foutin, St. Guerlichon, St. Gilles, and St. Rene—were equipped with a large phallus. The Protestants demolished a church at Orange in 1562 to find a large wooden phallus that had been covered with leather, and 23 years later found people at Embrun still worshipping the statue of St. Foutin by pouring wine onto its penis. (*Sex in History* by G. Rattray Taylor, pp 269-70.)

Today some men still prefer the multidimensional aspect of these forms to two-dimensional printed erotica. One case was reported of a man who as a twelve-year-old boy became enamored of a life-size statue at a museum when his mother called it obscene. Later, he spotted two small statues in a store window and purchased them. He began using them while masturbating and at the age of 34 had not broken the habit, even though he was married. Another case was that of a window dresser who felt compelled to masturbate whenever he saw a nude mannequin. His first sexual experience was at the age of fourteen when he was forced to perform fellatio on his supervisor as they sat on mannequins. He developed the desire to not only rub against a mannequin to masturbate but to have another man watch. (*The Sexual Fetish* by Robert Tralins, pp 27, 46.)

A few people in today's S/M community use a psychological form of restraint where the person, like a statue, is not to move or respond to the fondling actions of his or her partner. And people everywhere seem fascinated with the royal guards at Buckingham Palace for their statue-like imperviousness.

Bee Stings

(Melissophilia; Entomocism—use of insects; Entomophilia—arousal from insects; Formicophilia—arousal from ants.) Bee stings are used to extend the duration of orgasm, enhance sensations of the penis, and increase its circumference.

Bee stings were once used as a folk remedy by arthritis sufferers. The insects were captured and held on the affected joint until they stung. The poison and the swelling it caused alleviated much of the pain in their joints.

One male, having observed his grandparents using bees for

this purpose and later having a female friend throw a bee on his genitals as a joke, discovered that the sting on his penis extended the duration and intensity of his orgasm. Realizing that the bee sting was almost painless, he developed his own procedure, which consisted of catching two bees in a jar and shaking it to make the bees dizzy to prevent their flying away. They were then grabbed by both wings so that they were unable to twist around and sting. Each bee was placed just below each side of the glans and pushed to encourage it to sting. (Stings to the glans do not produce desired swelling, and the venom sac tends to penetrate the skin too deeply, causing difficulty in removing them.)

Bees leave their stingers in the penis and are not able to sting other parts of the body. Stingers have a small venom sac that pumps the remaining poison into the flesh before removal. Stings on the penis, unlike other areas, resemble the bite of a mosquito. The primary discomfort is produced by subsequent itching, although the penis will also become tender and swell. A thick twine or leather strip tied around the base, allowing enough space to insert two fingers between the penis

In 1877 "a gardener fell in love with a statue of the Venus of Milo and was discovered attempting coitus with it."

and string, restricts the swelling in the penis from dissipating into the body but will not cut off circulation. In this case the circumference of the man's penis increased from 6.5 inches to 9.5 inches. Swelling is greatest on the second day. There are two unexpected effects, however. The swollen outer skin may restrict blood flow into the penis, and the swelling can become lopsided or uneven if pressure is applied on only one side.

Caution: Poisonous venom can have serious effects on about 5% of the populace. Any of the following symptoms of anaphylactic shock following a bee sting require emergency medical care: difficulty breathing, chest pain, dizziness, nausea or vomiting, edema or general swelling, blue coloration of lips, weak pulse.

Cat-fighting

Cat-fighting is a fight without rules between two women. They scratch, bite, gouge, pull hair, and rip clothing. Cat fights appeal to men who hope to catch a glimpse of forbidden flesh as fighters tear clothing. Fighting also provides vicarious thrills similar to when one watches professional male boxers and wrestlers. However, the difference between them is that men do not want to see serious injury or nose bleeds on the women. They want the abuse to be verbal, preferably squabbling over a man or undergarments, and the physical violence restricted to ripping clothes or pulling hair. A description of a cat fight was given by a female participant in an adult newspaper, *Fetish Times* (No. 191):

> **Some people say I'm a bossy dom but the way I see it is I just don't like to be pushed around. When my roomie took my best black bra without asking for it I blew my stack. Ripping it off her tits I gave her a hard slap across the face. She grabbed my hair and yanked and the fight was on. Tripping her with my foot I dived on top of her and got her in a tight wrestling hold. Just as I thought she was beaten the little bitch slipped free and smacked my ass. Rolling over to protect myself I left myself open for a shiner. Seeing stars I grabbed out blindly and grabbed her by the pussy hairs. She screamed and I pulled. Then I caught...**

Cat fights between saloon girls and even the leading lady seemed to be more common in western movies before the 1980s. Today, mail-order videotapes are available showing cat fights, female boxers, and males and females engaged in hand-to-hand combat. Live performances are also staged for gamblers in the United States. The women and their sponsors travel to different locations, setting up events that are evidently similar to that of a cockfight. (Personal communication.)

Mud wrestling is a similar sport that became popular in the 1970s.

Today, mail-order videotapes are available showing cat fights, female boxers, and males and females engaged in hand-to-hand

Coitus à Unda

(Albutophilia, Undinism; Coitobalnism—in bath tub.) *Coitus à unda* refers to sex in water, as opposed to water sports, which generally involve urine or enemas. People are often fond of masturbating or having sex in the shower, rain, ocean, swimming pool, and Jacuzzi. Fellatio, during which the partner holds hot water in his or her mouth, is another form of water sex that is sometimes mentioned.

Tiberius Caesar was inventive with aquatic sex sports. He had young boys trained to swim after him and come up from below to suck and nibble on his genitals. He called these boys his "minnows." (*Perverse Crimes in History.*)

Some women use the water flow from their bidet (a basin that sprays water upward for a woman to clean her vagina) for masturbation. This is called bidetonism.

Bars sponsor entertainment such as naked women swimming in a large aquarium and wet T-shirt or jockstrap contests. In bathtubs soap is often used as a lubricant to insert fingers, toes, and toys into openings. Gloves, brushes, or chemical scrubs are used for body massage, and some people bind their partner's wrists with rope or blindfold them. Those involved in infantilism may run a bubble bath for their partner and add their favorite rubber duck or toy boat for the "baby's" entertainment.

Caution: Electrical or battery-operated devices are dangerous near water, as is sex in a swimming pool or outdoor body of water during a storm. Nudity in the ocean has led to some men having their uncovered genitals stung by jellyfish.

Dogging

(Amomaxia—sex in a parked car.) *Dogging* is the English term for a sport where people watch couples having sex in parked cars. The couples in the cars perform for those who gather around outside their car. There are specific parking areas that have become known for this activity, and the couples identify themselves as willing to be watched by turning on a colored interior light. Much of the same social etiquette applies here as does at group sex clubs. Touching of the performing couple is not appreciated without their invitation, as is unnecessary noise. Those asked to leave are expected to politely obey.

Other couples engage in oral sex or nudity on the highway for the purpose of attracting attention from truck drivers.

Homilophilia

(Autagonistophilia—arousal by being on stage or on camera.) Homilophilia (*homilo*: sermons; *philia*: attachment) refers to feeling sexual arousal while listening to or giving sermons and speeches. Public speakers are often dynamic, and this, combined with adrenalin, can produce sexual arousal for both the speaker and the audience.

Religious services were once designed to arouse devotees sexually in preparation for the ensuing orgies. Today, tent revivals still appeal to the emotions of those gathered by promising that God will forgive their sins and love them. Occasionally, people will fall to the ground in mild convulsions that are indistinguishable from some Tantra practitioners whose bodies go limp during exercises due to sudden orgasmic vibrations that last ten to twenty minutes.

Spiritual arousal at revivals, however, was not always limited to God and the individual worshiper. In 1873 D.J. Davis recorded his experience of old-time American camp meetings: "Those who think that a camp-meeting is no place for love-making are very much mistaken. When passions were aroused and moral restraints gave way for miles around the camp hundreds of couples could be seen prowling around in search of some cozy spot." (*History of the City of Memphis*, p 173, as quoted in *Sex and Race* by J.A. Rogers.) Rogers continued with this explanation: "Since the camp-meeting was a primitive affair, those human beings who were nearest to original Nature, were the leaders, thus the chief stirrers of the sexio-religious emotions of the whites were Negroes, most of whom could neither read nor write. Surcharged with primordial feeling, these totally illiterate blacks would whip their white audiences to the heights of frenzy" (p 331). In small towns, lacking more sophisticated meeting places, the back rows of tent revivals were popular cruising spots for both gay men and heterosexual prostitutes during the 1950s and 1960s.

Trial attorneys are another group of speakers who seem to project sexual chemistry. These people have to deliver intense emotional pleas in defense of clients. This responsibility and strong emotional display sometimes induces erection in male attorneys. They are often warned by their professors not to fixate on a female juror because she can pick up on the sexual energy and feel uncomfortable.

The ability to emotionally or sexually arouse an audience appears to be necessary; without it an audience will not respond to the desires of the speaker, whether this is to purchase an object, convert, volunteer, or change their position on an issue.

Speeches that are about sex do not have to condone it. Often the guilt associated with a minister's admonitions against this "vile" act can create greater arousal than a lecture discussing its merits.

Kabazzah

(Pompoir; Kegel exercises; Snapping pussy.) *Kabazzah* is translated as "holder" and refers to the Eastern technique where the male partner is passive and the female uses only abdominal and vaginal muscle contractions to "milk" the penis. Both partners simply relax and enjoy the sensations of the union while she moves her muscles. Women train for years before becoming proficient. It is a form of Tantra designed to increase and enhance time spent with a loved one. There are still some Eastern prostitutes who have this expertise.

Kokigami

Kokigami (*koki*: a cloth worn around the waist by Japanese actors and used as a prop; *gami*: paper) is the art of wrapping the penis in a paper costume. The eighth-century Japanese aristocrats practiced the art of *Tsutsumi*, or packaging. A man would wrap his organ with silk and ribbons in complex and intricate designs, and upon entering the bed chamber, offer it as a gift to his lover. He then enjoyed the physical sensations as she carefully unwrapped her prize.

Today, the authors Busch and Silver have invented a similar

Coitus à unda refers to sex in water.

form of art. However, instead of ribbons, paper is used as a disguise or costume. The lovers then act out their roles based on the type of figure selected. There are geese, fish, squid, and dragons. Busch and Silver, in their book of *Kokigami* cutouts, suggest the following dialogue and play for the latter: "The crafty Dragon likes to breathe his fire into the dark jeweled cave. Ravaging, vengeful, sly.... 'Where are my precious jewels? My treasures? My trophies? Are they hidden there in your dark cave?' The Reply: 'Come on, hot stuff! Careful the iron gates don't snap shut and sever your burning tongue!'... With arms outstretched and fingers curled like claws, move forward warily with the knees bent. The hips may be flicked about spasmodically accompanied by the low seductive roar of a raging furnace." (*Kokigami: The Intimate Art of the Little Paper Costume* by Heather Busch and Burton Silver, p 18.)

The Japanese also used samurai face masks over the groin region with a dildo protruding as the nose. Those not interested in artificial phalli cut out the nose and put their own penis through it.

Nasophilia

Nasophilia (*naso*: nose; *philia*: attachment to) refers to arousal from the sight, touch, or act of licking or sucking a partner's nose. The reasons people are enamored with this activity varies. Eskimos rub noses when greeting others, and Sioux Indians traditionally rub noses to express affection; they do this just as other cultures kiss on the lips.

Magnus Hirschfeld related the case of a young writer who made wax noses and put them over his own, admired himself in the mirror, and with a "slight manual manipulation he brought about an ejaculation." Another would hire a gay prostitute, take him home, and, having placed a wooden clip on his nose, have the prostitute pull on an attached string while saying, "I hope this nose is going to be so big that everybody will be surprised at it." This was necessary to induce orgasm.

Another man became fixated on the size of female nostrils, thinking that if large enough, they could be penetrated. He drew and kept sketches of his large-nosed feminine ideal. One day, while on the bus, he spotted a young woman who had large nostrils. Infatuated, he followed her home and proposed marriage on the spot. She refused, and when he continued to come to her home, she had him arrested. *(Sexual Anomalies and Perversions* by Magnus Hirschfeld, pp 411, 551-2.)

People sometimes use nasolingus (licking or sucking nose) as a substitute penis during intercourse, occasionally asking the partner to blow his or her nose in simulation of an ejaculation.

Caution: This is an activity that exposes a partner to the bodily secretions of another and is therefore not considered a safe sex practice.

Another man became fixated on the size of female nostrils, thinking that if large enough, they could be penetrated.

Oculolinctus

Oculolinctus (*oculo*: eye; *linctus*: lick) refers to the act of licking a partner's eyeball for sexual arousal. This seems to be rare, but there are several cases, including one of a female who in order to orgasm would have to lick the eyeball of her obliging male lover.

Caution: Oral herpes (cold sores) can be transferred to the eye.

Pie-throwing

Pie-throwing is one of the most amusing forms of defilement. There are several scenarios found in pie-throwing. People at parties have thrown pies at each other, couples engage in the activity in private, and there is even a gay pie-throwing club.

One individual nicknamed "Pieface Brown" asks attractive women at social functions or theaters to pie him. Nine out of ten agree to smear the pie over his face and body. He professes to have been pied by over 200 women within a span of three months. Pieface Brown began having pies rubbed in his face at the age of eight, and suddenly at the age of eighteen, it began to be sexually stimulating. He often records the event and, once alone, replays the giggling and comments made by the women as he masturbates. Women sometimes add to the sexual aspect of this practice by saying things such as, "I would like to do this to your crotch."

Elements of arousal associated with pie-throwing are an-

ticipation, fear of rejection, thrill of acceptance, humiliation, desire that the partner will say or do something sexual and unexpected, sharing intimacy with an attractive person who might not otherwise notice them, and deceitfully engaging in a sexual and socially unaccepted act in public.

Psychrocism

(Psychrotentiginosity.) Psychrocism (*psychro*: cold or freezing; *cism*: act) refers to those who are aroused either by being cold themselves or by watching someone else who is cold.

Hirschfeld relayed the personal confession of a male patient who had a cold fetish:

The thought and sight of chilly dress or pictorial representations of it, induce in me considerable erotic pleasure. My wife naturally has no idea of my abnormal sensations in this respect, and when I make a drawing of the type with which you are familiar, say, a drawing representing a girl with bare arms and shoulders, and dressed only in the flimsiest of undies, on the ice in the skating rink, she always regards it as a joke, for she naturally does not take seriously the exaggerations in which my imagination revels. Such fantasies, accompanied by masturbation, have frequently come to me at times when sexual intercourse with my wife has been impossible for physiological reasons. These fantasies were confined to a single subject—immature girls wearing the lightest clothes in winter. (*Sexual Anomalies and Perversions** by Magnus Hirschfeld, p 569.)*

Some people have masturbated by putting a towel in the freezer, then laying it on their genitals; others have used icicles. One California man has reported that on several occasions after swimming in the ocean for 30 minutes during the winter, he would obtain an erection that lasted two to three hours. (Personal communication.)

Exposure to intense cold creates a sharp sensation that is similar to other physical stimuli that produce tension. The mind changes its focus from intellectual pursuits to physical awareness. Many S/M players use cold contact to heighten awareness of skin sensations. They often alternate cold with heat, such as ice cubes and candle wax.

Queening

The term *queening* refers to the European practice of a dominant female using a man's head as her throne. The woman sits in one of several positions, either on the side of the man's head or so that his nose is near her anus with his eyes covered by her genitals. The object of queening is bondage or breath control, not cunnilingus. The man may wear supplemental restraints on the wrists and ankles.

A slightly comparable American sex scene is where a stripper completely disrobes and stands over a sitting male with his head titled back so that her genitals are only a couple of inches above his face. She stays in this position, moving her pelvis to the music for about five minutes. The male is not permitted to touch her in any manner during this exhibition.

Scrotal Infusion

(Ballooning; Scrotal inflation.) Scrotal infusion is the process by which a solution is injected into the scrotal sac. It is also referred to as *ballooning* or *scrotal inflation*, although these terms might be taken to mean expansion by air or gas, and for safety reasons that impression is best avoided by using the word *infusion*, which denotes expansion by fluid.

The visual effect of the scrotal infusion resembles a water balloon. Men do not report any pain from this procedure and claim that one advantage is found the next morning when the solution filters into the penis, causing it to swell to the size of a beer can. Men claim exclusive license to this type of sex play. There is no sealed part of the female anatomy that has a hollow sac that lends itself to expansion.

Paraphernalia used for this procedure were scissors, first-aid tape, a 20-gauge angiocath or hypodermic needle, a one-liter plastic bag of saline solution, an IV pole or hook on the ceiling, plastic tubing, latex gloves, and packaged alcohol prep pads. The saline solution was warmed to body temperature ahead of time. The bag was then held against the inside wrist to determine a comfortable temperature. Incidentally, the temperature is not for the comfort of the patient but rather to prevent the scrotal sac from shrinking, as it normally does when exposed to cold water or ice. This shrinking would hamper the expansion process that is essential for infusion.

The bag was hung from a hook and spiked with the tubing, which was then pinched closed, not contaminating either of the ends. The scrotal area was swabbed with the alcohol prep pad, and the needle was inserted about one inch directly below the base of the penis in the middle of the scrotum. The partner waited for a moment to make certain that he had not pierced a vein (evident by blood backing up into the needle); the needle or angiocath was then taped flat and upright against the top of the scrotum. The tubing was opened and adjusted so that it drained at a rate of about 60-90 cc's per minute.

The male stood because gravity helps to facilitate the expansion. However, fainting is a natural response, and the person was monitored closely and had a bed or table behind him on which to lie if necessary.

Scrotal infusion is an activity that is difficult for most observers to understand. The men who experiment with this form of body modification have explained their various motives or desire to experience different feelings, to be unique, for the shock value, to prove that these are their genitals and they will do with them as they please, and to visually set their genitals apart from all others.

The saline in the scrotal sac absorbs into the body within about three days. Some people inject more saline than the scrotal sac can accommodate, and this will immediately overflow through a small opening into the abdomen.

Caution: This is a blood sport that requires proper sterilization procedures and is therefore not considered a safe sex practice. Improper placement of the needle may also damage local nerves. ("Scrotal Inflation and Other Genital Modifications," by J.B., QSM lecture, Dec 1, 1990.)

Oculolinctus refers to the act of licking a partner's eyeball for sexual arousal.

Sitophilia

(Botulinonia—sex with sausage.) Sitophilia (*sito*: food; *philia*: attachment to) refers to those who use food for sexual purposes. Masturbation aids are found in the form of corn cobs, squash, cucumbers, bananas, sausages, warm melons, liver in a milk carton, or a jar of honey.

One gastronomic game is used in bondage scenes. The male partner is first immobilized, and a paper plate is cut so that a two-inch hole is made off-center. The plate is held over the male genitals, which are pulled through so that the genitals now look as though they are being served on a platter. Lukewarm spaghetti and meatballs are served on the plate and, with fork in hand, a helpless male is told he is about to be fed his own balls. It doesn't matter who eats the meatballs, but each strand of spaghetti is sensuously wrapped around the penis and sucked through the lips before being eaten.

Another use of food is that of taking a slightly slit, pitted plum and pushing it onto an erect penis. Once secure, this can be inserted into a partner's vagina, adding volume and pressure for both partners. Banana-carving contests are used as erotic teases at adult parties. A row of contestants is lined up, given a banana, then told to compete with each other for who can carve the most realistic penis with only their teeth. Some strippers use a cucumber in a pseudo-castration scene where they have a man hold a cucumber between his upper thighs and proceed to fellate the green erection. As the audience becomes enthralled, the stripper bites off the tip of the cucumber. People sometimes suck on a lime before cunnilingus to make their taste buds swell, creating more texture when rubbed against sensitive genital tissue. There are special caterers that design cakes and pastries with a sexual theme. People also stuff objects like grapes, small tomatoes, peeled and cooled hardboiled eggs, and small pieces of ice into the rectum for erotic pleasure.

A row of contestants is lined up, given a banana, then told to compete with each other for who can carve the most realistic penis with only their teeth.

Another use of food consists of combining it with bodily secretions. One couple developed a game where the wife, after dismissing herself during a formal dinner to go to the restroom, upon returning would dip her finger in some food and put her finger to her husband's lips, asking him to try it.

People at the table, if they noticed at all, thought he was only tasting food, while in fact she had first dipped her finger in urine. The same is done with vaginal secretions.

People aroused by lactating breasts sometimes drop cream onto a partner's nipples and lick it off. Sex surrogates use food to get some clients back in touch with their bodies. The surrogate gets clients excited and salivating by slowly rubbing their favorite food on their bodies. This reconditions their bodies to respond to touch. Food orgy parties are organized by individuals where friends bring either an erotic arrangement of food to share, or food that feels sensuous when rubbed onto a partner and licked off; afterward, everyone soaks in a hot tub.

There are all-male games such as "Shoot the Cookie," where men stand in a circle around a cookie and masturbate. The rule dictates that the last one who ejaculates on the cookie has to eat it.

Food can be used for a form of flagellation. A regular client of an Oregon bordello during the 1940s would pay to have two prostitutes watch him strip naked, put on high heels, get into a tub of water, and walk back and forth. His only request was that they throw oranges at his buttocks as he paced. He would then get out, pick up the oranges, replace them in his paper bag, dress, and leave. (Personal communication.)

Rules

Dirty Found

Found Magazine has become a sensation by presenting bits of other people's lives that had been discarded or lost in public places. The spin-off magazine, *Dirty Found*, does the same thing with people's sex lives.

Contributors send in discovered explicit photos, dirty drawings, handwritten stories, invitations to sex, and material that's hard to describe.

Case in point: From the first issue comes this list of rules, apparently written by a man in a submissive relationship with a woman.

It was discovered by Grant Lawrence, who explains: "Found in the grass in idyllic English Bay, in Vancouver, BC. One constant news story here has been squatting in parks, though the pencil-written rules here go a little beyond the usual 'no dogs, no fires, no overnight camping...'"

ADD-ONS:
G - NOT ALLOWED TO ASK PERMISSON MORE TWO TIMES
ON THE SAME QUESTON. (ON THE SAME NIGHT)
- MUST CHOISE OWN PUNISHMENT & CANNOT USE THE SAME
ONE TWICE UNTILL ALL HAVE BEEN DONE ONCE
- AFTER ALL THE PUNISHMENTS HAVE BEEN USED
3 TIMES THE PUNISHMENT MUST BE CHANGED

ALL RULES MUST BE FOLLOWED WITH NO CHANCES
OR EXCEPTIONS OR ELSE MUST FACE IMEDIATE PUNISH MENT.
I AM ALLOWED TO BARGAN MY WAY OUT. ALL RULES
ARE ALLOWED TO BE CHANGER AT ANY TIME BUY HER.

ONCE SIGNED ALL COMPLY

MANSON X

- No cuming 3 time a
days → each time
- You mess up 3 days
will be addaton
- No Mastecb
Just teasing 5 X a
day for an hour each
time

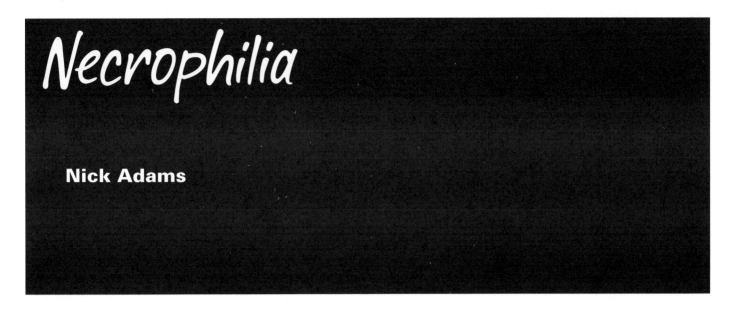

Necrophilia

Nick Adams

It's a damn shame what we've done to necrophilia. Not the concept. The concept has, I think, been properly demonized and swept under the rug in our society. I mean the word *necrophilia* itself. Taken purely at face value, it is one of the more poetic and beautiful words in the English language. In fact, it's too good to be English. It's worthy of one of the Romance tongues. Example (imagine this in Italian):

"And then we went on a romantic gondola ride through the canals of Venice. We marveled at the amazing architecture of the buildings and the sweeping necrophilia that adorned the sides of the bridges."

Unfortunately, *necrophilia* is a term that is used to describe one of—if not *the*—most distasteful acts that a human being can carry out. As you may or may not know, necrophilia means having an erotic attraction to or sexual contact with corpses. That's how repulsive and depraved human beings are. We had to come up with a word to describe that. If it was just the one crazy guy living in Florida, we could laugh it off with, "Oh, that Earl. He sure is an odd bird!" But, no. Apparently, there have been more than a handful of people throughout time who have been fascinated with this concept; at least enough to warrant a dictionary entry.

As crazy as it sounds, there is a segment of our species who would eschew all of the various and sundry ways there are to pleasure oneself—with a person of the opposite sex, a person of the same sex, yourself, or an inanimate object—and instead choose to seek the dry, dusty pleasures of the dead. Remember that the next time you climb up on your *Homo sapiens* high horse. Your dog might drink out of the toilet bowl and hump your leg, but would he fuck the rotting corpse of the Shih Tzu across the street? I think not.

I can't help but wonder what the process was like choosing the word. I can't imagine the intellectual elite of long ago ever thought they'd come across something as perverse as this. Fuck a young boy? Sure. Sell your enemies into slavery? Why not? March human beings into ovens? If need be. But getting it on with a dead body? I can only imagine what that first conversation was like.

"Looks like another guy whipped it out in the mausoleum last night. What are we going to tell the reporters when they show up?"

"Beats me. We don't even have a name for this yet."

"How about *dead fuckery*?"

"It's catchy but a little too literal."

"*Corpsilingus*!"

"I think you're on to something, but it's too close to *cunnilingus*. We don't want to discourage people from tasting a bit of the bearded clam from time to time, now do we, Cyrus?"

"Well said, Winthrop."

"I've got it. We shall call it *necrophilia*!"

"Brilliant. Now let's pull this cadaver's pants up and go get some lunch."

How does one become a necrophiliac? Obviously, these people didn't just start out that way. You can't take a dead body to your junior prom without raising some suspicions. If you're a teenage necro-virgin, you probably just started out by dating really thin girls. Then you progressed to dating really, really thin, hideous girls. Finally, you start exclusively dating really, really thin women who are also hideous and have tremendous body odor. After that, it's just a hop, skip, and a jump to dating a dead body. (Imagine having sex with a stinky Lara Flynn Boyle. No, wait. Imagine having sex with a stinky Lara Flynn Boyle after she's gained about fifteen pounds.)

For every other sexual orientation, there are also specific types that some people are interested in. Does this hold true for our confused, corpse-fucking friends? Are there picky necrophiliacs? I would imagine so. I'm sure that somewhere out there is a man who has sex with dead blondes only. No dead brunettes or redheads.

"Hey, I'll fuck a dead chick, but no fatties! I bang thin corpses only."

What about those who are necro-curious? The people who think they might like it. Can you imagine spending months or years working up the nerve to commit the deed, only to discover that you didn't even like it? And God forbid you were caught. You'd be forced to wear the scarlet "N" on your chest without any of the satisfaction of having scratched your itch. I'm sure the reception for necrophiliacs in jail is not especially warm and fuzzy. When the necrophiliacs show up at the big house, all the child molesters breathe a huge sigh of relief.

At some point the person has to actually make the switch from live women to dead women. (I suppose there are female necrophiliacs, but I don't see how it would be possible for a woman to consummate with a dead man. The term "stiff" isn't that literal, is it?) What if you find out that your ex is now humping dead people? Can you imagine what something like that could do to a woman's image? What happens to your self-esteem when you find out your man rejected your warm, moist, living vagina for a dry, rotting, corpse vagina? How do you cheer up a friend whose boyfriend has just left her for a dead body?

In Lieu of Necrophilia

Once I started working on this essay, I asked myself if there was any way I could ever see myself in a sexual situation with a non-living person. Obviously, the answer is a resounding "hell no!" Besides the fact that the very notion of having intimate relations with a corpse is revolting, there are simply far too many other objects that I find more arousing. To find out just how far removed I am from fondling the deceased, I sat down and wrote out all of the options that I would have to exhaust before I resorted to a midnight mausoleum raid. The

following is a random sampling of some of the 715 things into which I would rather insert my penis than a dead body:

17. Wet laundry
28. Warm mashed potatoes
312. Cat food (the wet kind)
517. Don King's hair
601. Bubble wrap
682. The tailpipe of a 1982 Toyota Corolla Station Wagon
713. Old Faithful
714. Kelly Osbourne

During my freshman year at college, one of my suitemates was an incredibly intelligent, slightly eccentric guy named Tommy. He was a farm boy through and through. He would head back home almost every weekend and invariably return on Sunday evenings with some sort of confection from his mother's kitchen. She was an excellent and prodigious cook, and he always had more than enough to share. I don't know how, when, or why this happened, but at some point it became our inside joke to refer to the various cookies, brownies, cakes, and pies that his mom would bake as *necrophilia*.

Your dog might drink out of the toilet bowl and hump your leg, but would he fuck the rotting corpse of the Shih Tzu across the street?

At that time, it was just one of those words that I thought sounded impressive, but I had no idea what it actually meant—like *lugubrious* or *verisimilitude*. (Go ahead. Take a dictionary break. Those are two words worth knowing.) If I wasn't around when Leon returned to campus, he would just leave a note on the dry erase board on our door. "Nick, I've got some good necrophilia in my room. Leon." There was more than one occasion that found me attempting to explain to a pretty young coed that she wasn't about to enter the lair of the black Jeffrey Dahmer.

That brings me to my final point on this sordid issue. *Necrophilia* is too good a word to be reserved for describing the toxic human actions of the species. I say we reclaim this and other rarely used words and appropriate them for more enjoyable usage. The possibilities are endless.

"Did you see the necrophiliacs on that redhead?"

"I sure did. As a matter of fact, I almost hydroplaned in my pants!"

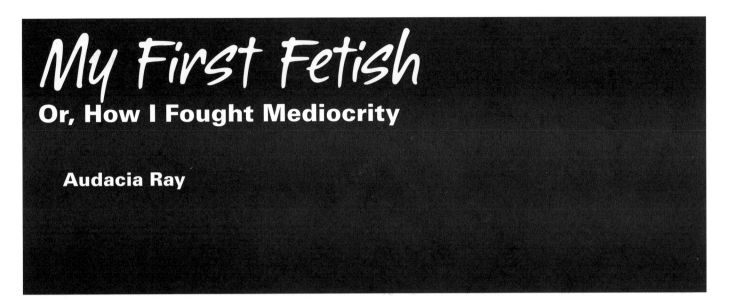

My First Fetish
Or, How I Fought Mediocrity

Audacia Ray

I've spent the last few years as a professional appreciator of sexual perversion: first as a researcher and curator at the then-nascent Museum of Sex, then as a marketing researcher for a smut company. It's been an interesting journey because research on sex is something that I'm capable of being overly intense and academically serious about, but it is also a topic that—ahem—arouses my prurient interest. I pride myself on being able to talk nerdy about dirty things.

In both of these jobs, I met people of all sexual stripes. I interviewed many of them about their perversions and lifestyles, and I borrowed heaps of well-loved pornography from all kinds of people, for research purposes, of course. In the course of these adventures, I often was asked questions that would qualify as sexual harassment in any other work environment, or at the very least an invasion of privacy. "Do you prefer girls or boys?" "How big are your tits, anyway?" "Have you ever been gangbanged?" However, of all the personal questions thrown my way, the most challenging has always been: "What's your fetish?"

I've never had an answer to this question that satisfies the inquirer. Quite simply, the reason is that I don't have one special item or act that I fixate on and get pleasure from. In the world of radical sex, this seems to indicate to people that there is something lacking in me, that I'm somehow unenlightened and unfulfilled because of this shortcoming. Either that or I've landed in a world of sexual deviants where sexual one-up-manship is the name of the game. People with fetishes have Unique Perspective and have a Community and are Heroically Marginalized. I am none of these things; I'm just a girl who saw the opportunity to combine my love for research and museums with my love for sex. But after many withering looks upon the admission of my un-deviance, I decided that it was high time for me to look into getting myself a fetish.

So I did what I always do before I actually act on anything: I researched. I wanted to find an edgy fetish, something daring and provocative that I could still be rather blasé about, because I'm so jaded and worldly.

I discovered a few things in the R&D phase, which mostly consisted of looking at porn and reading the blogs and Live-Journals of various perverts. To be convincing, a fetish needs to fall into at least one of three categories:

1. Many fetishes are largely irrelevant to one's daily life (well, you know, except as a jerk-off fantasy). Balloon fetishism is a perfect example of irrelevance. There is a community of people (usually men) who like to see girls with balloons. Not nekkid girls getting wild with each other while balloons float by, but usually clothed girls dancing with balloons, sitting on them, and popping them.

> **After many withering looks upon the admission of my un-deviance, I decided that it was high time for me to look into getting myself a fetish.**

2. Traditionally, a fetish is thought of as being somehow taboo, though there are varying degrees of this. There is no better or more extreme example of a taboo fixation than the fetish for shit play—watching people shit, eating shit, and masturbating with shit. This is so taboo that it kindles the kind of revulsion that you, dear reader, are probably feeling right now.

3. Since fetishists are often closeted and secretive about their fixations, they sometimes incorporate fetishes into their

lives in bizarre/creative/creepy ways. For instance, I met a guy in my travels who has a major foot fetish. He regularly visits the local Foot Worship Palace, where he pays women to let him massage, kiss, and suck on their feet. In his day job, he's a shoe salesman in a chichi shoe store, where he gets to slip a variety of expensive shoes onto the feet of unsuspecting rich ladies, while also fulfilling his desire to touch and serve women's feet.

Another important thing that I learned about fetishes through my research and chats with sexual deviants is that doing a scene or performing a ritual with their object of affection is basically an alternative to a sexual act involving genitalia. I knew that this would be the most difficult thing for me, because I have difficulty understanding the purpose of a sexual act that doesn't result in orgasm or involve my girl parts.

After much research and soul-searching, I narrowed my fetish options to three final contenders: sneezing, amputees, and guns.

After much research and soul-searching, I narrowed my fetish options to three final contenders: sneezing, amputees, and guns.

Getting my jollies from watching people sneeze would be a low-budget alternative to other fetishes that require elaborate outfits made of expensive fabrics. Also, it could be fulfilled in simple yet strange ways—for instance, by spending lots of time on New York City public transit, where I could vocally urge on a sneezer and hope that he or she is perhaps a serial sneezer, with each sneeze bringing me closer to ecstasy.

Amputees, though less accessible and less common than sneezers, are also somewhat publicly available, especially as pictures of young, strapping, crippled troops returning from Iraq are increasingly published in news outlets. Wartime is an amputee fetishist's dream come true. The creepiness of this is obvious, because especially with vets, I'd be fetishizing the sacrifices people have made for the good ole US of A.

I think I've been able to approximate the fetish mindset best

with the potential that guns offer. The fact that I've been trained to fear and despise guns and all they stand for (via hippie parents) makes them taboo—and sexy. And because they are often seen as phallic symbols, they are objects that I could work with (though I guess amputee limbs could work similarly)—guns could be good for sucking and fucking. But this brings me back to the original problem I have with fetishes—in adopting a gun fetish, I would be thinking up ways to get off, but really I should be thinking solely of the illustrious beauty and danger of the object itself.

I tried really hard to think sexy thoughts about sneezes, amputees, and guns. I was definitely able to get closest to sexy while thinking about guns, but then it rapidly became ridiculous when I realized that I was trying too hard to think sexy thoughts, when I could be looking at pictures of naked people and get there much more easily.

Sum conclusion: I'm much better at objectifying people than objects.

The problem, as I suspected, is that my fetish is orgasm, only that isn't really a legit fetish. I tried hard to fit into the deviant pattern, because I knew that if I only had a fetish, I'd be embraced by deviants everywhere, and they'd be able to identify with me and trust me as one of their own. But I guess I have to accept that I've got a mediocre sexuality and a deviant lust for knowledge.

So my answer to, "What's your fetish?" I don't respond. I do the shifty-eyes thing, or if I'm feeling particularly witty, I declare, "I like fucking!" But it's the next assumption that still raises my hackles and inspires the urge for one-upmanship—the dismissive reaction, "Oh, you're vanilla." Being called vanilla, a norm, a member of the ignorant masses, makes me angry, and my ornery nature is what started all this fetish nonsense to begin with. Maybe I just need to do some more soul-searching until I find my one and only true fetish. I mean, seriously, how do people discover that they get off by sitting on a cake while wearing a diaper? It must be through research.

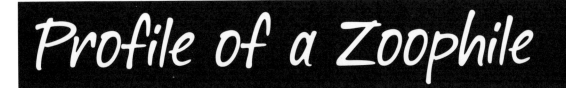

Profile of a Zoophile

Bill Brent Interviews Clive Grace

Bill Brent: What's the most common misconception that people have about zoophilia or bestiality?

Clive Grace: The biggest misconception, I think, is that we do it because we can't get girls or boys. I think most of the time, people assume we're a bunch of sad bastards who can't get it up.

Bill: How easy, or how difficult, has it been for you to be open about this aspect of your sexuality? Are you pretty out about it?

Clive: I'm very out about it; hence, I'm here. I guess it's because I've lived with it and done it for so long, I feel like it's just so ordinary. Like, I guess, people who do anything—S/M, or you see queer stickers everywhere. There isn't a "zoo" sticker per se. I wish I had a few, but, y'know, there's not a big "we fuck animals!" sticker. So, if people ask, I generally try to present a very thoughtful, sensible side to it.

Bill: What would you consider the formative experience for you around discovering that you were into "non-human life forms"? [*Both laugh.*] How did that happen for you?

Clive: Oh, that happened—it happened on two occasions. The youngest was when I was eight—I wasn't really sexually active by that point—and there was a female black dog that lived down the alleyway where I was—one of the neighbors'. I don't know, just something in me really wanted to be that dog's puppy. I really wanted just to be completely nursed and looked after by her.

And then—oh, gee—I used to travel into London a lot, and I used to travel back home by train. And where we lived, there was a field with horses in it. And one day, I just looked out the window and saw these horses. My god, they were fantastic, magnificent-looking creatures. And something in me just said, "Just go and see them." And that night, I snuck out of the house, and it was a four- or five-minute walk to the field. And I guess I spent many evenings creeping out of the house, going out to the field and seeing these horses. It didn't initially start off as something sexual, but it pretty much segued into it.

Bill: How did that happen?

Clive: Well, I guess what happened was that—I was getting pretty confused at the time. I was feeling very strong attractions and very strong urges toward animals. I really

What would you consider the formative experience for you around discovering that you were into "non-human life forms"?

didn't know how to deal with it. Even then, it was like, "This isn't normal—help!"

Bill: Sort of like same-sex stuff.

Clive: Yeah. There were no positive role models; there was nothing—I didn't even know where to look. I didn't even know what to find out, information-wise. So I just went out to the fields and just stood there and petted them and, y'know, talked to them. They're very, very, very attentive, by the way. If you ever go out to a field and talk to horses, they'll come around and look at you and interact with you and sniff around and look for carrots or things. In the end, I did actually bring things like apples to feed them.

Bill: How sweet.

Clive: Yeah, y'know, I was, like, fourteen, shivering for fear of being caught, and also because it was so cold in England at night. And one night, I just—it was a very weird time; I felt really, kind of, bad and sick, and twisted, and "this is wrong," but still, I wanted to do it. I thought that these creatures were so beautiful, and that I was so really ugly, really somehow kind of stumped and ugly. Something in me just sort of—I took all my clothes off in the middle of the field. It was almost a full moon, and it was really well lit, and I could see almost every hair on the backs of these horses, and there was a herd of about five or six of them. And they were kind of interested in what I was doing—like, "What's going on?" They stood around me—

I just put my arms around her neck, and I started kissing her, and I started moving my hands over her body.

Bill: Wow!

Clive: Yeah. I mean, it's one of those formative spiritual moments for me. And I just held onto a particularly beautiful horse—a black-and-white, dappled horse, a mare—and I just put my arms around her neck, and I started kissing her, and I started moving my hands over her body. She moved her rear towards me, and I started eating her out. All the other horses were going, "Wow! What's going on here?"

Bill: "They don't usually do that to us!" [*Laughter.*]

Clive: Yeah, yeah! [*Pauses.*] Well, maybe they do! Who knows? I was almost shivering with cold, and also with fear, but they kind of stood around me, and when you're inside a circle of horses, you're really warm. So that was really the first event. Very, very special.

Bill: Did you, like, kiss her on the mouth, with your mouth open? You said you kissed.

Clive: Yeah. She would, like, sniff me over. In fact, in terms of equine socializing, one of the things I learned pretty early on is that horses snort down the noses of each other, and if you're going to start really wanting to communicate with animals in that respect, you have to learn to talk on their level. So I saw that they were pretty much interested in getting involved with me—well, I needed to learn their language. So I sort of learned to [*snorts*] down their noses.

Bill: Wow. And they liked that?

Clive: Oh, yeah, they love it. I've seen some people do it, and they get freaked out, so perhaps they can sense something else—I've been very successful.

Bill: Sounds like you were a natural! [*Laughter.*]

Clive: Well, I think maybe. I mean, there are people—I've talked about this with other people. "Is it a kink, or is it a sexual identity?" And it's really difficult to work out which it is. For me, I believe it's an identity. I do identify first and foremost as someone who loves animals. Everything else is secondary. People come a close second, though! I mean, they really do.

Bill: There's something that I've always thought was really attractive about animals having sex—just the pureness of it, stripped of the human interaction of, "Oooh, baby, baby," and all those kinds of trappings, which I think is refreshing.

Clive: But there's nothing quite as hot and raunchy as seeing a stallion with this enormous cock mounting a mare—I mean, oh, my God, I've sometimes come just looking at two horses fucking, and it really is just so—I don't think I've seen people that raunchy. Not yet, anyway.

Bill: Wow.

Clive: I had an experience one summer when I was in the same field, actually, and it was actually in the daytime, during the summer holidays. And you know what it's like—you're fifteen, you're bored—

Bill: You stick your dick in a vacuum cleaner! [*Both laugh.*]

Clive: I mean, it was like, "Get out of the house." And I just got the pleasures of being out in the open. But there was an added component, because in the day, it was summer, and it was sweaty, and there were all kinds of—you know, there was mud getting in your feet and stuff, and there's a very different quality to having sex with a horse in the daytime. They're actually a lot muskier-smelling, and they're much stronger-tasting or -smelling, or whatever. It's probably the heat and the sweat and everything. That's kind of a turn-on.

♀

Bill: So are you mainly interested in horses, or do you play with other animals?

Clive: Oh, no. I play with horses and dogs. There was a period of time, when I hadn't been with animals for, like, oh, four years, and I'd started looking at cows and going, "Hmm! Maybe cows—." [*Laughter.*] But I had a really aborted attempt at that, and they would come look at me, bug-eyed, going, "What's he doing here?" They'd quickly take a very watery dump in front of you and run off. So no, I don't find any grace or beauty in that!

So it's been mainly horses and dogs, although between the two, it's been mainly horses. Although I would say that my dog experience has been equally as pleasurable. There's something quite sweet, actually, about someone's dog crawling onto the bed with you, and you just get the urge to, and you touch him or her, and if they're not interested, fine. They'll let you know. And if they are, well, if it's a small dog, then there are certain things you can and can't do, and if it's a large dog, there are certain things you can and can't do.

Bill: What was your reaction initially after you first played with these horses? You must have gone through a tremendous amount of—

Clive: Absolute terror! And kind of a weird sense of, "Hey, that was really special." Even then, I think I had a sense that this was a turning point in my life. Not only had I gotten a sense that there was something—this sexual feeling that felt good, and okay, I wasn't caught this time, so maybe I'll get lucky and have another go. But also the fact that there was something deeply meaningful to me. That it somehow put it all into some kind of sense, as far as my life, and as far as how I was growing up. At that age, I don't think I really had much of a clue about anything, to be quite honest.

Bill: Who does?

Clive: Yeah! I mean, in retrospect. And at that time, it was such a very important experience for me. What happened was that I would go out there, sometimes two or three times a week. And sometimes something would happen, sometimes not. It wasn't easy going to begin with, either. I mean, yes, I had that first wonderful experience, but afterwards I had to start learning their language and communicating with them. The number of times I had bites or had been kicked because I had not been aware of boundaries, let alone acknowledge them—that process of learning happened immediately afterward.

Bill: Do you think there's such a thing as nonconsensual sex with animals?

Clive: Oh, yeah! There are definitely cases of puppies that have been bred and physically trained to respond favorably to sexual advances. My personal feeling is that—and this is different for everyone who practices bestiality—you really make yourself open to the animal in question, and you offer them something, and if they're interested,

then they'll let you know. But if they're not interested, then you should stop.

I'm sure there are cases of people who have raped animals. They can't speak—well, at least, they can't physically speak. I've seen many different kinds of abuses. When you see a cringing dog walking down the street, that's a form of abuse. I think that's a much greater sin than offering yourself to a dog, and if he's interested, letting him take you, or a female dog, and if she's interested, she'll raise her tail, and you can start making love.

So yeah, it is possible. And that's the most important thing when you're starting, is to learn their language, to find out whether or not they're okay with that.

Bill: Which sounds like being attentive.

Clive: No more so than as one would be with any sexual partner. I guess it's just that there are a lot of clueless people out there who aren't attentive, of whatever orientation, whatever gender they are.

Bill: In your experience, how do animals communicate about sex in relation to how well people communicate about sex?

Clive: It depends. If, for example, it's a bitch in heat, then she's very communicative! She's really, really communicative! In terms of horses—mares in heat again are very responsive. Animals who aren't necessarily in heat are still interested in sex, and they'll still try to mount you, or they'll still go through the motions, if after a while you've

I'm completely open to the advances of both male and female, dog and horse.

been playing with them—you know, stroking them and playing ball or whatever—or with horses, giving them the "skritch" along the mane, which they absolutely adore—and you can go through various courtship rituals and things like that. Again, it all goes back to learning their language. And it really isn't that difficult if you go into it with an open mind and an open heart.

⌢

Bill: Are you heterosexual or bisexual with animals?

Clive: I'm—definitely—bisexual. I'm completely open to the advances of both male and female, dog and horse.

Bill: Do you think that's true of most people who are into this, or do you think that varies a lot?

Clive: Hmmm. Good question. I certainly know some women who really get hot off the idea of, say, for example, licking a female dog's cunt. And they're very interested also in being fucked by an animal. Either male or female. In terms of porn—what a lot of people get is the *Color Climax*-style Danish porn, which is very straight-oriented. It's basically, "A bunch of bored women can't get guys, so they turn to the pet." Yawn. But then again, it could be quite a hot thing. Most of the porn out there is really designed for what I feel is a straight male audience.

I can't really speak for other zoos, because, quite frankly, each zoo is different. We've each come to it in our own ways. That would be the case with gay people or with people into S/M. I think each person's case is individual. I know I'm bisexual in human terms, as well, so I think it's fairly natural to be bisexual with animals, as well. I really see it as life, as interacting with living creatures, with communicating in ways that don't necessarily require language. And that's really, really—kind of frighten-

He was really digging his claws in and getting quite insistent.

ing, and also amazing. You realize that there's this whole universe of communication in front of you that you've not been aware of.

Bill: It seems to verge on the spiritual component that you mentioned earlier.

Clive: It's very spiritual. I derive a tremendous spiritual sense from it. And over the years, it's developed into something that's really my own. But it does involve an almost shamanic level of shape-shifting, of spirit-shifting, of opening up to spirits of creatures, or offering yourself to the animal in question. It is very spiritual. It is definitely a way of communing with natural forces, without a doubt.

Bill: How would you define "shape-shifting"?

Clive: "Shape-shifting" is a technique whereby people who practice it can take on, if not necessarily the physical form, then the immediate spiritual mindset—the mindset of, for example, a fox, or of whatever.

Bill: It sounds like a really intense form of empathy, maybe.

Clive: Yeah, yeah. It's effectively dropping down what makes us civilized beings, what makes us human, and really trying to cast away with all that tosh, with all that rubbish. And really just being what we all are anyway, which is animals. The only thing that separates us from the animal kingdom is our sheen of civilization. You lose that, and you're no different.

When I say "shape-shifting," I also mean a form of drop-

ping your guard, of letting whatever comes along happen. But you have to be careful, because obviously, there's the boundary issue. In the early days, I may have let a particular dog that I was with—I may have let him go a little bit too far, but that for me was a learning process, anyway. What happened is that I was with a friend's dog, and he was—let's just say he was a little bit too big for me! [*Laughter.*]

Bill: So he was mounting you.

Clive: Well, yeah. And he was digging his claws into my sides, and I think this may have been my first-ever sadomasochistic experience. He was really digging his claws in and getting quite insistent, and though I was aware of how the dog's penis is, which is a sheath and then a bulbous piece. Now, the bulbous piece actually swells up, just as they're about to come for the final time. It's a device that locks the male into the female's vulva, and where they're connected, and then they stay there for a while. Then the swelling goes down, and he detaches. It's actually a device to ensure that no sperm is wasted.

He was a Weimaraner—a beautiful dog—but he was big. Back then, of course, I didn't have access to wonderful things like Astroglide or Probe or even K-Y—

Bill: All of that works with animals, huh?

Clive: Oh, yeah. In fact, it's essential with female dogs, because male dogs come all the time, and that's actually where you can spot the bad porn, by the way—people who've never had sex with a dog often write things like, "And then he came!" And it's like, no, no, he's been coming for at least ten minutes, if he was really there. And the process of the dog coming all the time provides lubricant for the bitch. So you really have to lube up if you're with a bitch.

This dog was just inside me, and then all of a sudden, I felt him expand [*laughs*], and we got kind of locked for a few minutes, and I think it was probably a mixture of my tightness, but he was digging in, and I couldn't really do much about it, other than to discover pain in a sexual context with animals for the first time! [*Laughter.*] It was a very intense experience. So that was a case of not knowing boundaries. But I look back on it fondly. Happy memories.

Bill: How do you deal with the moral issue of engaging in sex with other people's animals? They might not consent to it if they knew it was going on.

Clive: Well, it's between me and the animal. They may have paid money to a pet shop, or they may have paid for the vet's bills, and stuff like that, but the question of ownership—it's still the animal's body, it's the animal's right to decide for him or herself.

Bill: I'm picturing people reading this, going, "Well, how does he know the owner wanted the dog to do this? They must have thought it was weird."

Clive: It doesn't come into it. If the dog wants it, then they're really happy.

✕✕

Bill: I notice, as I'm getting more information about this, that some people differentiate between "bestialist" and "zoophile." Do you differentiate, and if so, what does that mean?

Clive: It's funny. I guess I started recognizing the definition, the more people I've come across. Basically, "bestialists"—they're the people who are described a lot—I've never heard any describe themselves as this, but they basically want to fuck animals and use them as sex toys. A dog is, basically, a big, portable dick. Or a bitch is a willing hole that you can stuff something into. And that is totally uncool. And a "zoophile" is somebody who really—I hope—does what I do, which is to open themselves up on many different levels. As if they were having sex with or making love with a person. I don't really know about the two different terms, personally. I guess it exists—I hope there aren't bestialists out there, though. The presence of "sex puppies," as I think they're called, kind of suggests that, but who knows?

Bill: How would someone physically train a dog to do that? I can't even imagine.

Clive: Well—the stuff I've heard is only hearsay, so I really shouldn't comment, But—it's stuff like, um, training them to have a sexual response at a very early age, and to give them sexual responses to certain stimuli, such as food. Things like that.

Bill: So you'd reward them for sexual acts.

Clive: Yeah. It's like training a dog. Certain types of training are important, because, for example, certain types of dogs are very jittery, highly strung. What you do is, you train a dog to give it a sense of, there is some kind of order in their world. And actually that does give them a lot of trust in their surroundings. But training them for sex is a trust kind of gone wrong, basically.

Bill: Right. It's using them as a sex toy. Which isn't very un-

derstanding of the animal's feelings or preferences. That sort of goes along with young people being trained to be prostitutes, and what goes on in Third World countries. But I'm sure here as well, occasionally, at least.

When I was about fourteen, I remember reading the "Happy Hooker" series of books [by Xaviera Hollander]. There was this one great story where she was sort of cooped up in South Africa with, I think, her sister and her brother-in-law. She was going kind of stir-crazy in this huge, fabulous mansion with nothing going on, and eventually she and this German Shepherd, I think—the pet—got together—

Clive: It's always German Shepherds. [*Bill laughs.*]

Bill: Are they easy? [*More laughter.*] Are they the right size?

Clive: Yeah, they're the right size; they're amenable; they're—

Bill: So they're easy!

Clive: —intelligent...yes. Although Great Danes are easier.

Bill: Oh, my!

Clive: I often wonder about the number of Great Danes on the Castro and think, "Hmmm." [*Laughter.*] Yes, you were saying—

Bill: I'm turning red now. Anyway. It was a really good story. She talked about having sex with this dog, this really amazing experience, and I got the impression that she didn't necessarily pursue that in her sex life, but it was this affair of conve-

Clive: It's always German Shepherds. *Bill:* Are they easy?

nience, and at the time it served her quite well. I don't know whether you would define someone like that as a bestialist or a zoophile! But it seems like she got what she wanted, the animal got what it wanted and seemed to be very turned on by her. I thought that was great! It was the first time I was really aware someone could have sex with an animal, and I thought, "Well, isn't that nice!" [*Laughter.*]

Clive: Oh, wow. Not having read any of those books, actually, I can't say whether she was a bestialist or a zoophile. I think labels are things that you pretty much discard once you feel comfortable with what you're doing. I think labels in this case are really more restrictive than defining, so I try not to use the term. I'm just somebody who loves animals. And I've been doing it for a long, long time.

This interview was conducted on November 2, 1996.

Margins to Mainstream

Pornography Refreshes American Culture

Joseph W. Slade

On April 22, 2002, Linda Lovelace was killed in Denver in an automobile accident, yet another of the car wrecks that scarred her body and marked her life. The obituaries in the New York Times and other newspapers were signs of the country's acceptance of her status as a trend-maker. Most noted that the star of Deep Throat (1972) had published several books decrying the pornography industry that made her famous. None of them revealed, however, that in the last years of her life Lovelace had once again begun giving interviews to men's magazines and had been attending Glamourcons, the conventions of aficionados of softcore and hardcore pornography, there to bask in the adulation of fans who never stopped worshipping her.

The curve of Lovelace's experience resembles the larger, just-as-tentative acceptance of sexual explicitness by a growing number of Americans. The opposition of anti-porn feminists, easily the most significant challenge to pornography for the last two decades, has been muted. The argument that pornography directly causes sexual aggression against women, a thesis central to the anti-porn feminist position, has been undercut by successive annual reports of the US Department of Justice, which indicate that rape and sexual assault have fallen dramatically over a period that coincides precisely with booming sales of sex videos and erotic websites. Indeed, feminists now write "Bad Girl" fiction, shoot explicit movies, and endorse sadomasochism.

In short, sexual materials enjoyed in secret, long characterized as insulting to religion, offensive to various genders, intellectually worthless, and socially and politically subversive, seem now to be operating as a source of cultural energy. As pornography has moved front and center, scholars have begun to study once-tabooed expression and imagery for what they reveal about bodies and sexual orientation. The number of academic texts on such subjects has swelled. Perhaps more significantly, so has a popular conviction that pornography is now important, as suggested by Pornified: How Pornography Is Transforming Our Lives, Our Relationships, and Our Families (Times Books), the title of a forthcoming book by Pamela Paul. Pornography seems to be refreshing a culture that continuously mines its own edges in search of novelty.

Some dismiss the trend as trivial, akin to the perennial surfacing of phenomena such as astrology, a mere triumph of kitsch. Others see it as a function of a society besotted with physical beauty and fame at any price; after all, said the late Katharine Hepburn, celebrity is just a sanctioned form of prostitution. Some believe that citizens of an increasingly inhuman post-industrial society simply need titillation. Still others think of increased tolerance for pornography as all of a piece with relaxed attitudes toward minorities, corporate theft, or capital punishment. Others think of the change as more profound. While suppressed voices and transgressive images have always driven American culture, they say, pornography's roles as stimulus and inspiration have never been so clear. Somewhere in between these two extremes, a sense that there has been a massive shift in the plate tectonics of culture or merely a conviction that pornography is an idea whose time has come, lies the margins-to-mainstream dynamic.

Talking about pornography is a lot like talking about religion: Nearly everyone brings to the subject assumptions that color the debate. One can avoid some of the confusion by using terms such as sexual materials or sexual representations, but even there we swiftly find that we have no common discourse for speaking about sex. For good or ill, pornography is itself a principal source of sexual language and images, and their very instability energizes the cultural dynamic. Three of my own assumptions follow.

1. Except for materials that involve minors or are sold to them, most pornography is legal in this country. Obscenity is not legal, but the difficulty of deciding what is obscene, a slippery concept (involving assessments laid out in *Miller v. California* [413 U.S. 15 (1973)] and subsequent iterations) that changes over time, and one that preoccupied the judicial system during the last century, makes the issue largely moot, at least where adults are concerned. In fact, criminalizing child pornography is part of the cultural dynamic I wish to discuss, since its effect has been to reinforce the legality of representations of, by, and for adults. It has also globalized markets. When the European Parliament passed guidelines for dealing with child pornography, including prison terms for those convicted of sexually exploiting children, it did so partly to protect minors, but just as obviously to permit European countries to compete against American pornography.

2. Pornography comes in many genres, and the cultural emphasis we give those genres—the hierarchies we rank them in—also varies over time. Constant shifts in such scales are also part of the margins-to-mainstream dynamic. For many Americans, *pornography* refers to hard-core videotapes or DVDs, which constitute one of the most visible and familiar sectors. Depending on the individual, *pornography* can also refer to peep shows, striptease, live sex acts, adult cable programming, sexual aids and devices, explicit telephone and computer messages, erotic websites, explicit comic books, adult magazines, nude photographs, and raunchy fiction. The less discriminating add late-night television broadcasts, soap operas, rap and rock music, romance novels, fashion magazines, and R-rated movies. In any case, pornography is not monolithic: The genres target audiences diverse in their age, gender, and ethnicity, and their content can vary sharply in degrees of textual and graphic detail.

3. What determines the market for any pornographic genre is demand, which in turn rests on the desire for pleasure, which in its turn derives from individual tastes, sexual orientations, and psychic histories. Most consumers of pornography are average and normal, merely looking for materials to gratify erotic tastes. At one extreme, taste is simply a programmed or learned preference for certain kinds of sexual fantasies. Sexual orientation tends to fix desire across a heterosexual, gay, lesbian, or transgendered spectrum whose fluid eroticism we are gradually learning to appreciate. Where pornography is concerned, we often fail to notice that moral standards frequently reduce to taste. As Al Goldstein, former publisher of *Screw* magazine, has observed: "Eroticism is what turns *me* on; pornography is what turns *you* on." *De gustibus non disputandem est*, the Romans used to say: There is no arguing with taste.

At the other extreme, taste rigidifies into fetish—a term nowadays loosely defined as an element that must be present for an individual to become aroused: women with large breasts, men with large penises, say, or blonde hair, high heels, leather costumes, or specific scenarios. But, as Pierre Bourdieu has observed, a taste is always also a distaste. Those who do not share specific fetishes often condemn them as immoral or deviant or simply dopey. Some tastes become notorious when celebrities embrace them. President Clinton mistook a cigar for a penis; Attorney General Ashcroft apparently thought the breasts on a Department of Justice statue were political statements. We despise or cherish political leaders

Pornography seems to be refreshing a culture that continuously mines its own edges in search of novelty.

for their odd sexual notions, for they add idiosyncrasy to personalities. They also keep our collective erotic expectations a little off-balance.

Few countries are more conflicted about pornography than the United States, and few countries so relentlessly package and recycle it. According to architects, pornography has eroticized and gendered our public and private spaces.[1] Where once sex configured the red-light districts of urban areas, now it shapes the experience of average citizens. The Playboy mansion still serves as the model for bachelor pads, but seductive lighting, hot tubs, and flexible furniture also appear in family homes. Suburban apartment complexes enclose "clothing-optional" swimming pools. Lesbians and gays rehab slums in Atlantic City and other towns to create gendered communities. Hooters restaurants are no longer remarkable features of the American landscape, and Victoria's Secret stores can be found in every upscale mall. Department stores stock fur-lined handcuffs and jeweled whips next to plastic party plates.

The girl next door has become a sexual icon, transformed by *Playboy* and its imitators, not to mention amateur videotapes and popular series such as "Girls Gone Wild." Young feminists have adopted the terms *slut* and *bitch* as markers of empowerment. The word *pimp* seems incredibly cool. Women throw stag parties for soon-to-be married friends; their mothers scream at Chippendales dancers. In imitation of porn performers, college girls are depilating their pubic regions, piercing their nipples, and getting their buttocks tattooed. Cosmetic firms are selling nipple blush. Going Calvin Klein one better, Abercrombie and Fitch fills its catalogs with nude models. The great pornographic photographer Araki shot a layout for the *New York Times Fashion Supplement*; the same issue ran an article on the influence on style of the erotic motion picture *Emmanuelle* (1974). Fashion designer Alexander McQueen modeled his recent clothing line on his reading of Leopold von Sacher-Masoch's *Venus in Furs*, a classic of pornography.[2]

Celebrity prostitutes appear on afternoon talk shows. The *Jerry Springer Show* generated a London play. The satellite radio service Sirius hired Howard Stern for $500 million. Cable

In imitation of porn performers, college girls are depilating their pubic regions, piercing their nipples, and getting their buttocks tattooed. Cosmetics firms are selling nipple blush.

networks offering sexy shows are stealing male audiences from broadcast television. When Janet Jackson's wardrobe "malfunctioned" during the telecast of the Super Bowl, the furor in an aroused Congress doomed the FCC's proposed relaxation of rules governing media ownership. Jackson single-breastedly forestalled a growing monopoly and became a Joan of Arc for consumer forces. Mainstream artists are rushing to photograph porn stars. Jenna Jameson's autobiography was a bestseller. Paris Hilton's "secret" videotape jumpstarted her career.

The *Atlantic Monthly* published "Conservative Men in Conservative Dresses," an extensive survey of mostly Republican heterosexual male crossdressers that concluded that the real problem, sexual fetishism aside, was that they looked pretty frumpy.[3] Upscale magazines such as *Talk* and the *New Yorker* have run articles on porn performers. The *Talk* piece, by novelist Martin Amis, was accurately entitled, "To Millions of American Men and Women, These Women Are Movie Stars."[4] Clive Barnes, the distinguished drama critic, wrote a similar article for the *New York Times*. Elegant erotic novels are commonplace; think of Susan Minot's *Rapture* (Knopf, 2000), whose narrative is a single act of oral sex, or of other bestsellers, such as Nicholson Baker's *Vox* (Random House, 1992) a few years back. The Book of the Month Club routinely offers erotic fiction.

Recently audiences could attend the stage version of *The Graduate*, in which the fifty-plus Kathleen Turner stripped completely naked. Other startling Broadway productions have included *Lysistrata*, *The Vagina Monologues*, *Puppetry of the Penis*, *Menopause: The Musical*, and *Urinetown*, and still raunchier fare frequently appears Off Broadway. Chloë Sevigny fellates her lover—the director—onscreen in the mainstream film *Brown Bunny* (2003). In Michael Winterbottom's film *Nine Songs* (2004), stars Kieran O'Brien and Margo Stilley engage frequently in actual intercourse.

Museums and art galleries in Manhattan are exposing sexual explicitness in modern painting, sculpture, photography, and fashion. "Surrealism: Desire Unbound" at the Metropolitan Museum of Art quite deliberately included unmistakably pornographic works by famous Surrealists.[5] The Whitney mounted a successful exhibit of G-strings and thongs.[6] "Erotica and the Like," a show at the CDS Gallery (79th Street), featured graphic works by artists such as Goya, Bellmer, Bonnard, Bourgeois, Balthus, Wesselman, Lucian Freud, De Kooning, and Picasso. The Deitch Projects gallery in Soho displayed the photographs of Vanessa Beecroft, who strips and depilates models, and photographs them in nude battalions in order to comment on modern eroticism.[7]

Because practice as well as ideas are involved, the dynamic that legitimizes pornography is far from precise, and definitive tipping points—clear-cut examples of acceptance of previously anathematized expression—are hard to establish. Explanations nonetheless abound.

Pornography as Political Expression

First, according to historians, pornography has been linked for over 300 years with politics and identity—even, if you like, with the politics *of* identity. The essays in *The Invention of Pornography: Obscenity and the Origins of Modernity, 1500-1800* (Zone Books, 1993), edited by Lynn Hunt, point out that from the sixteenth through the eighteenth centuries, pornography promoted democracy, urbanization, secularism, scientific method, equitable legal systems, technology, and modernity itself. Beginning with the nineteenth century, middle-class males striving for respectability and fearful of sexual license tried to prevent sexual information from reaching women and the lower classes, says Walter Kendrick's *The Secret Museum: Pornography in Modern Culture* (Viking, 1987). Forbidding sexual expression shored up a sense of privacy in a society increasingly convinced that democracy and literacy had led to open, public vulgarity. According to Lauren Berlant in *The Queen of America Goes to Washington City: Essays on Sex and Citizenship* (Duke University Press, 1997), pornography strengthened democracy by reminding Americans that a culture can become authoritarian by trivializing the sexuality of its members.

Another argument that pornography is essential to democracy is Joss Marsh's *Word Crimes: Blasphemy, Culture, and Literature in Nineteenth Century England* (University of Chicago Press, 1998), which maintains that "lower-class," blasphemous, and obscene speech challenged established institutions. Underclasses often embrace pornography as a political act, say critics who find racism and class bias behind attacks on erotic expression.

We still think of pornography as vulgar. In the past, we thought of pornography as the expression of Others: East European immigrants, African-Americans, communists, subversives, and deviants. And we have traditionally justified laws restricting expression by our desire to protect Others from those voices, by shielding children, of course, and women, and the weak-minded from the dangers of sexual knowledge. Pornography can't hurt me, the argument seems to go, but it will absolutely corrupt my twit of a neighbor.

During the 1980s, pressure groups defined pornography as a tool for oppressing women; during the 1990s, women, minorities, gays, and lesbians recast pornography as a method for discovering and enhancing sexual identities. Telling a sexual story helps to construct a sexual self,[8] create a sense of community among similar individuals, and—by giving weight to constructed identities—foster social acceptance. Since the larger culture for decades automatically classified gay and lesbian speech as pornographic, as John Preston has said, then an obvious strategy is to embrace the language and turn it to different purposes.[9] Gays and lesbians today are deliberately recovering a pornographic past by way of establishing their history and legitimizing their presence.

Why would they choose such forms? Perhaps because our society insists on transparency. Cellphones, surveillance cameras, credit card tracking programs, massive databases, voice- and face-recognition technologies, digital scanners, and reality-based television shows routinely reveal the intimate secrets of our neighbors. Hundreds of thousands of Americans now exchange erotic messages and photos of themselves over the telephone and the Internet.[10] We have become a nation of voyeurs and narcissists. Getting others to recognize an agenda means working within that voyeurism and self-absorption.

Part of the dynamic involves conscious agency. Moving alternative visions of eroticism into the arena of popular culture allows straight women, lesbians, gays, African-Americans, Asian-Americans, Hispanic-Americans, and so on to compete for attention and acceptance. Collections of ethnic erotica have poured into bookstores in the last five years, and Black, Hispanic, and Asian performers are in high demand as video performers. Given enough effort, say advocates, such groups can assert their own preferences and advance their own mythologies, their own ideas, their own standards of beauty and objects of desire. Recognizing that pornography replicates gender stereotypes and sexual myths but also undermines them, female performance artists, often former porn stars,

create explicit stagings that deconstruct gender and sexuality. They appropriate and invert older forms, which I take as a sign of cultural health. If pornography were not important, of course, it would not be worth hijacking.

Pornography as Folklore

Second, pornography is associated with folklore, in a double sense. In one sense, porn draws on vast reservoirs of myth, legend, belief, customs, and mores that work both for and against establishing norms of behavior. Pornographic representations often contain archetypal stories of women and men in heterosexual and homosexual acts, often-told narratives of smutty humor and sexual anxiety, and endlessly recurrent motifs of desire, frustration, and satisfaction. Traditional folklore embodies and stores obscenity, the (originally) oral sources of "low," vulgar, even scabrous forms of expression. Modern media transmit the *same* pornographic images: males with enormous penises, women with dangerous vaginas, tales of ingenious seduction and gender trespass. Today's pornographers suck filthy jokes, transparent stereotypes, hoary motifs, nasty themes, and quaint sexual notions directly from folklore. "All folklore is erotic," said Gershon Legman;[11] it "is the voice of those who have no other voice, and would not be listened to if they did."[12]

If pornography were not important, of course, it would not be worth hijacking.

Obscene folklore—the demotic rendering of human sexual imagination—serves as the fountainhead of pornography, a collective cultural id. Vulgar images and vulgar stories—the kind born in folklore—often conflict with more refined, upper-class revisions of sexuality—the nice kind called "erotic"—especially since the latter types deny the sweaty physicality of intercourse that dirty jokes and stories insist upon.

In another sense, pornography—and our reaction to it—continuously fabricates modern sexual folklore, some of which is surely mistaken. Call us puritan or not, Americans remain deeply suspicious of the sexuality that pornography represents so well and so badly for us, and thus attribute to pornography a force that it may not deserve. Our attitudes toward sexuality are tangled not only with social and political values but also aesthetic and moral standards. As a culture, we seem unable to acknowledge the biological origins of sex and are only just beginning to sort through its social construction. Some cultural critics refer to pornography as a "contested cultural site" where gender and sexuality are "negotiated." I would go further: Pornography is our principal source of information on gender and sexuality. Most of what we think we know about sexuality and gender is folklore. We may say that sexuality lies between the legs, and gender between the ears, but we don't know much more than that. Pornography is perhaps our best tool for demystifying sex and gender, but progress is slow.

Serious scholars agree that pornographic materials carry contradictory messages. Hardcore videos depict behavior that subordinates women, yet at the same time urge women to seize sexual autonomy.[13] Romance novels aimed principally at women prize "sensitivity" in men but also delight in depicting males as powerful, aggressive, and protective. Inspected closely, nearly all pornographic genres depict gender instabilities that wobble between gay and straight, between women with masculine characteristics and men with feminine traits, as if to project warring impulses that men and women do not themselves fully understand. Factoring in tastes complicates

Pornography is perhaps our best tool for demystifying sex and gender, but progress is slow.

matters further. Some men enjoy only softcore scenarios, while others insist upon gonzo hardcore sequences. And, as Susie Bright has noticed, "Some women...[want] the ordinary, some the punch of the kinky. And some want all of it. Our sexual minds travel everywhere, and embrace every emotion."[14]

That said, I still think that most pornography discriminates against women, though not for the hackneyed reasons we so often hear. For example, I do not think that pornography objectifies women any more than it objectifies men. All media, especially the visual, objectify their subjects. Moreover, objectification may be a necessary precondition for choosing one's roles in life. Depicting women as sexual beings, without reference to the males who in the past claimed to own their bodies, in a sense is liberating. Treating someone as an object, rather than merely depicting them as objects of desire, of course, is unethical, and pornography can to some degree be implicated in that injustice, though here again porn in skillful hands can remedy matters by endorsing different kinds of behavior. At base, however, except for porn made by women for women—and increasingly that is happening—pornography is male-oriented, which is to say that it ignores women's sexual pleasure. Worse, too often pornography functions as a training manual for women. Most pornography depicts women working hard to give men a good time—not the reverse. Again, change comes slowly.

The Technology Factor

One trendy explanation implicates technologies ranging from languages to electronic media. Pornographic representations have long functioned as engines of post-industrial capitalism because the need to create and to enjoy those representations quite literally drives the development of new media. In previous ages, cave painting led to pictures of vaginas and penises, clay tablets to sexy cuneiform messages, printing to steamy typographies and startling images. Such older technologies seem "harmless" now; few Americans appear to worry about erotic novels. By contrast, photography still seems dangerous, perhaps because, as Susan Sontag said, it cannibalizes all other art forms. Louis Daguerre invented the daguerreotype in 1839; by 1859, the poet Charles Baudelaire complained that people seemed to be buying cameras only to take pornographic photos. More recently, erotic applications fueled the evolution of VCRs. In 1975, Sony introduced the Beta home videocassette recorder/player, but refused to license the format to the adult film industry, the principal producer of videotapes at the time. One year later, in 1976, JVC introduced the VHS videocassette recorder/player, and gave the format to the adult industry for free, which doomed the Beta machine, despite its superior qualities.[15]

Pornographic entrepreneurs were crucial to development of the Internet.[16] In constructing websites, pornographers invented such novelties as Flash, the click-through banner ad, and pop-up windows.[17] Those irritants aside, three major innovations stand out. The first is the creation of "transaction technologies" on the Internet, or electronic protocols for making credit card purchases secure. The best of these methods was established by the Internet Entertainment Group (I.E.G.), producer of pornographic videos and websites, and immediately copied by legitimate industries from banks to retail merchandisers. If you order online, you use those transaction technologies. A second is the "streaming" of audio and video content on the Web, another technology advanced by I.E.G. and companies such as Vivid Video.[18] If you download audio files or video clips, you use those technologies. A third involves the creation of "virtual reality" scenarios that will make artificial sex seem "real" to electronic participants. Here again, Vivid seems to be outpacing universities and other commercial leaders.[19] Berth Milton, Jr., CEO of Private Media Group, a leading adult-entertainment company, has been advising the NASDAQ exchange on making its electronic stock reporting both friendly and secure.[20]

Capitalism at Work

Another contention is that porn is not subversive at all, that elites make use of sexual expression for their own purposes. Herbert Marcuse argued that a capitalist culture appropriates and sanitizes sexual ideas precisely in order to co-opt them, to defuse their explosive power, and thus to restore the power structures of the status quo. That argument has weight, if only because we recognize one of culture's imperatives, which is continuously to stabilize itself. A bleaker version of cultural survival suggests that the introduction of new ideas and information is imperative lest the institutions, customs, and values that make up the culture succumb to rigidity, and go entropic. Max Weber's process of rationalization and charisma, for example, is a sociological version of the Second Law of Thermodynamics. According to this formulation, new ideas tend to emerge on the margins or fringes of a culture, where they are anathematized until their growing strength coalesces into charismatic, irresistible energy. Thus, pariah entrepreneurs become captains of industry. That the voices of young, black ghetto males (an economic underclass) rapping urban porn could become a multibillion-dollar industry in the space of a few years lends credence to such views.

Nobody knows the exact revenues of the American market for pornography, let alone those of other countries. Back in 2001 *Forbes* magazine challenged the *New York Times*' estimate of a domestic market of between $10 and $14 billion, saying that the total was too high, and the argument continues. Dispute arises in part over what to include. Women's romance novels (Regency Romances, bodice-rippers, Gothics, and so on) sell a billion dollars' worth a year and account for half of all the paperbacks annually purchased in the United States.[21] Should those figures be part of the total? Some estimates compare apples and oranges, as in the claim that annual revenues from X-rated videos and DVDs exceed the annual box-office receipts of the mainstream Hollywood industry, and so they do, but pale when measured against the sales and rentals of Hollywood videos and DVDs. One irony is that producers of adult materials may inflate revenues to make their industry seem more important in an economy that excuses almost anything if it makes a profit. My own best guess is that the *Times* is closer to the mark, and that the domestic totals are higher in 2005, probably closer to $16 billion. Given US dominance of adult industries, the global total is probably roughly double that. Precision is less important than acknowledging that these are impressive numbers, although here are some more apples and oranges: Americans spend about $30 billion on gardening, more than $40 billion on hamburgers at McDonald's, Burger King, and other fast food chains,[22] and $130 billion a year on weddings.[23]

Much to the ire of fundamentalists, corporate America is assisting with the required capitalization. Time Warner, Marriott International, Hilton, and News Corporation market hardcore video directly to hotel rooms and homes, and General Motors and AT&T did the same until the early part of this decade.[24] The effect has been to stabilize the finances of porn production houses, which rely on cable, satellite, and foreign sales to remain profitable. Foreign demand for pornography, especially for videotapes and DVDs, is increasing steadily. Since European companies turn out fewer than 2,000 porn videos per year, French, German, Italian, and Spanish distributors program Europe's television channels with American product.

As they mature, some pornographic industries expand while others contract or consolidate, and thus replicate the patterns of conventional corporations. In the 1970s, more than 50 adult book publishers controlled three-quarters of the market for erotic paperbacks; now only seven firms control roughly the same percentage.[25] The adult video industry is consolidating as the sheer volume of annual production threatens to lower profits. Companies vertically integrating production, post-production, packaging, and distribution in Chatsworth, California (picture hillsides dotted with studios) turn out over 11,000 pornographic videos each year. But five or six companies (Metro, Vivid, VCA, Evil Angel, etc.) now dominate the distribution of pornographic videos in this country, much as the big six Hollywood studios dominate the distribution of legitimate movies; the porn majors claim most of the shelves in video rental outlets, just as the Hollywood majors sew up the screens at the cineplexes in middle America.

But not all genres have done so well. Once robust traffic in telephone sex—800/900-number calls—has been declining

Five or six companies now dominate the distribution of pornographic videos in this country, much as the big six Hollywood studios dominate the distribution of legitimate movies.

since 1992.[26] The Internet is swiftly putting older forms, especially magazines, out of business. *Penthouse*, one of the leading men's magazines, teeters on the verge of bankruptcy. At the same time, while the number of websites devoted to sexual expression has steadily increased, the growing number is reducing profits for all. The Internet is no place for porn amateurs while it is undergoing consolidation; most photos now flow through only a half-dozen distributors. In the near-future, however, assuming adequate bandwidth, streaming video will transform the video porn industry, which is why Vivid Video and other big companies are staking their claims now. The dotcom industry could learn a lot from Chatsworth.

Culture as Information Processor

Obviously, explaining the margins-to-mainstream dynamic

depends on the cultural metaphor of choice. In the most basic sense, a culture can be construed as a transmitter of customs, values, mores, and attitudes, all of which outline a domain of meaning. For a critic such as E.D. Hirsch, for example, culture is simply the background information that we need to make sense of the world. More formal information theorists think of culture as active, a gigantic information processor, its operations determined by constantly shifting hierarchies of channels. The more channels, the more they need content, and they must get it from somewhere, in the interstices of a post-industrial society or along its edges.

Theorists such as Niklas Luhmann introduce biological metaphors, making culture into a quasi-organic, self-organizing, intelligent communication system. In that kind of formulation, noise becomes paramount as a source of novelty, much as mutations arise in DNA when biological meta-editors accidentally reproduce new combinations from the string of meaningless codes imbedded in genetic plasm. The notion of noise as a generator of cultural information resonates, for example, in Tricia Rose's *Black Noise: Rap Music and Black Cultures in Contemporary America* (Wesleyan University Press, 1994). Here noise is cacophony, subversion, marginal messages deprecated by mainstream culture until such time as those messages can be understood by the mainstream.

Our culture still tries hard to marginalize sexual representation in order to endow it with outlaw status.

Because many Americans until quite recently condemned rap music as obscene, it resembles other forms of sexual representation. Other critics suggest that the recycling and transformation of noise or trash in a culture can best be described by "viral communication," "contagious media," or the kind of synchronicity popularized in games of six degrees of separation.

In any case, other questions arise, chief among them the question of how pornography retains its marginal status, its edginess, long enough to function as a source of powerful novelty. Our culture still tries hard to marginalize sexual representation in order to endow it with outlaw status (the Janet Jackson episode is a case in point), trying to reestablish pornography as reliably transgressive. This was easier a few decades ago, when organized crime was involved with the distribution of various porn genres, especially magazines, when such materials were still illegal. During the 1960s and 1970s, the Mob moved aggressively into peep parlors, arcades, and adult-movie houses, where visual materials could be exhibited and sold, and rival factions fought, cheated, and killed each other for turf. In New York, for example, organized

crime figures most often leased or purchased real estate in seedy neighborhoods, then subleased the premises to sex-businesses at exorbitant rents, or operated protection rackets, in effect taking profits from adult arcades and shops.[27] Organized crime thrives, of course, on providing goods and services that are forbidden but in high demand. Until gays revolted against police persecution at the Stonewall Bar (operated by the Mafia) in New York City in 1969, for example, organized crime owned or controlled virtually all homosexual meeting places in municipalities.[28] Once homosexuals began to enjoy the rights of other citizens, the Mafia saw its profits erode.

Similarly, as the distribution of sexual materials was decriminalized (*de facto* if not *de jure*), organized crime began to retreat from adult enterprises. Courts have continued to convict pornographers with ties to organized crime, most recently Ken Guardino, head of Metro Video (the first porn video company to go public on a stock exchange), in 1997.[29] Relentless prosecutions by the Justice Department, however, have seriously weakened crime families. Competition has cheapened all forms of pornography and reduced profit margins. Zoning regulations and home videotape players have put most porn arcades and theaters out of business. The Internet, a technology impossible for the Mob to control, now distributes pornography on a massive scale. Public tolerance for most forms of sexual expression undermines the hold of criminals. In fact, some experts believe that strip clubs and bars may be the only type of sexually-oriented venue in which organized crime still has a large financial interest, and the connection probably has more to do with opportunities for skimming profits and laundering currency than with erotic activities per se.[30] But some taint remains.

Likewise, Americans have linked pornography with violence as a way to marginalize the former. One of the most enduring legends associated with porn is the secretly circulated snuff film. Cherished urban myth to the contrary, American authorities have never discovered a snuff film (i.e., a film in which a person is actually killed in a sexual act). There was, to be sure, a softcore film in the 1970s with the title *Snuff*. To the delight of the distributor, feminists in what has been described as a moral panic picketed it for months, thus assuring the commercial success of a movie that is almost totally incoherent. Generally speaking, the violence in most genres of porn comes nowhere near levels of aggression in, say, Hollywood movies. Pornography can of course be unpleasant, nasty, and repugnant to many not-particularly-queasy Americans. Moreover, formal sadomasochistic and bondage scenarios do use ritualized aggression in genres of that fetish. Nevertheless, American pornographic genres preponderantly foreground sex, not violence. No reputable researcher has concluded that there is a causal relationship between exposure to garden-variety pornography and antisocial behavior. The jury is still out on whether pornography that does contain violence is harmful, but the issue, to say the least, is clouded. The conflation of sex and violence, however, endows some genres with semi-criminal status, poises them on margins from whence they can refresh cultural discourse, and enables them to retain subversive energies.

But caution seems advisable: If federal and state governments could suppress pornography in the past because a majority of citizens tacitly agreed, popular opinion could scapegoat sex again if opinions change, in the sort of cycle that might be assisted by the bin Ladens and Falwells of our time. Fewer than four decades ago pornographers were despised, artists went to jail, performers suffered mistreatment by producers and police, and consumers (the case of the literary critic Newton Arvin comes to mind[31]) lost reputations and careers to the zeal of censors. Worse to think, some degree of repression may ultimately be essential if pornography is to retain its power to enrich culture.

Perhaps the best strategy is to admit that sex and, as a consequence, its representations, resist research. Despite hundreds of quantitative and qualitative studies of many genres of pornography, we know for certain only that some sexual expressions and some images inflame the fantasies of some people, under some circumstances, some of the time.[32] Although we can outline the economics of pornography and guess at its cultural significance, we know very little else. To me it seems wise to remember that pornography is profoundly human: If sexual representation involves exploitation and degradation, it also enshrines love and longing. Human sexuality itself remains mysterious, try as pornographers might to plumb libidos, and pornography itself remains scarcely less so. The inability to explain pornography's attractions and effects, of course, ensures our continued fascination with it, and its power as a cultural force.

Endnotes

1. Preciado, Beatriz. "Pornotopia." In *Cold War Hothouses*, ed. Beatriz Colomina, Annmarie Brennan, and Jeannie Kim. Princeton Architectural Press, 2004: 216-53. **2.** Trebay, Guy. "Want to See a Hot Runway Show?" *New York Times*, 11 Mar 2002: A20. **3.** Bloom, Amy. "Conservative Men in Conservative Dresses." *The Atlantic Monthly*, 289.4 (Apr 2002): 94-102. **4.** Amis, Martin, with photos by Oliviero Toscani. "To Millions of American Men and Women, These Women Are Movie Stars." *Talk*, 2:5 (Feb 2001): 98-103, 133-5. **5.** "Museum Guide." *New York Times*, 8 Mar 2002: B38. **6.** Glueck, Grace. "E.V. Day: 'G-Force.'" *New York Times*, 7 Dec 2001: E31. **7.** Descriptions of these and other shows can be found in the *New York Times*, 12 Apr 2002: B34, 36. **8.** Plummer, Ken. *Telling Sexual Stories*. Routledge, 1995. **9.** Preston, John (ed.). *Flesh and the Word*, 2 vols. Plume, 1992, 1993: II, 2. **10.** For example, see [www.voyeurweb.com]. **11.** Legman quoted by Dudar, Helen. "Love and Death (and Schmutz): G. Legman's Second Thoughts." *Village Voice*, 1 May 1984: 42. **12.** Legman, Gershon. "Erotic Folksongs and Ballads: An International Bibliography." *Journal of American Folklore*, 103 (Oct/Dec 1990): 417. **13.** Hume, Alison. "Fear of Porn: What's Really Behind It? An Interview with Carol S. Vance." *Vogue*, 175 (Sep 1985): 679; see also Kipnis, Laura. *Bound and Gagged*. Grove Press, 1996. **14.** Bright,

Worse to think, some degree of repression may ultimately be essential if pornography is to retain its power to enrich culture.

Susie. "Introduction." *Herotica*, ed. Susie Bright. Burlingame CA: Down There Press, 1988: 3. **15.** Van Scoy, Kayte. "Sex Sells, So Learn a Thing or Two From It." *PC Computing*, 13:1 (Jan 2000): 64. **16.** See Tierney, John. "Porn, the Low-Slung Engine of Progress." *New York Times*, 9 Jan 1994: sec. 2, pp. 1, 18. **17.** Op cit., Van Scoy. **18.** Rose, Frank. "Sex Sells: Young Ambitious Seth Warshavsky is the Bob Guccione of the 1990s." *Wired*, 12 Dec 1997: 5. **19.** Dibbell, Julian. "The Body Electric." *Time Digital*, 12 Apr 1999: 24-7. **20.** AVN, Dec 2001. [www.avn.com]. **21.** "Words of Love." *New York Times Magazine*, 7 Feb 1999: 21. **22.** Lubow, Arthur. "Steal This Burger." *New York Times Magazine*, 19 Apr 1998: 38-43. **23.** Holson, Laura M. "For $38,000, Get the Cake, and Mickey, Too." *New York Times*, 24 May 2003: A1, B2. **24.** Egan, Timothy. "Technology Sent Wall Street Into Market for Pornography." *New York Times*, 23 Oct 2000: A1, A20; "American Porn" episode of *Frontline*, Public Broadcasting Service (PBS), 7 Feb 2002. **25.** "Ticker." *Brill's Content*, 2.1 (Feb 1999): 128. **26.** Fried, Joseph P. "AT&T's Decision to Withdraw From Billing for '900' Lines Leaves Call-in Industry in a Bind." *New York Times*, 25 Mar 2002: C4. **27.** "Neighborhood Porn Wars." *Newsweek*, 18 Apr 1993: 39. **28.** Cummings, John, and Ernest Volkman. *Goombata*. Boston: Little, Brown and Co., 1990: pp. 60-1. **29.** Ford, Luke. *The History of X*. Amherst NY: Prometheus Books, 1999: 141. **30.** Goldberg, Jeffrey. "The Don Is Done." *New York Times Magazine*, 31 Jan 1999: 71. **31.** See Werth, Barry. *The Scarlet Professor: Newton Arvin: A Literary Life Shattered by Scandal*. Nan Talese/Doubleday, 2001. **32.** See the chapter "Research on Pornography in the Medical and Social Sciences" in volume 3 of my *Pornography and Sexual Representation: A Reference Guide*, 3 vols. Westport, CT: Greenwood Press, 2001.

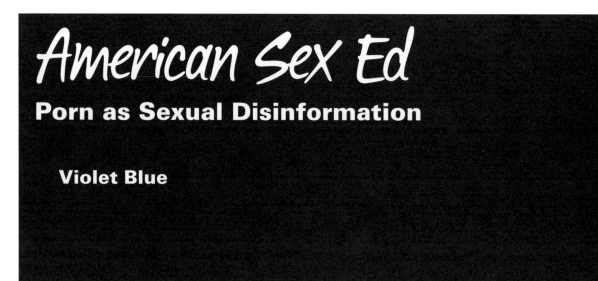

American Sex Ed

Porn as Sexual Disinformation

Violet Blue

I perched on the edge of a king-sized four-poster bed in a rented mansion on Mulholland Drive. The combination of bright, hot studio lights, the glare of cameras, crew, and director, and the windows shut tight to keep out external sound conspired to make the air thick, humid, and stifling. On my right, the male performer's exposed, sweaty, disappointingly flaccid crotch smelled like feet. Between us sat a naked, nineteen-year-old woman wearing nothing except clear, plastic, six-inch heels and LA-trendy, skunk-striped, frosted blonde hair.

After I described the oral sex technique I wanted them to perform for the camera, she leaned over and whispered to me in a soft, candy-baby voice. "Hey, I just started my period and I stuffed a buncha toilet paper up there, so will you tell me if it shows?"

To me, the greatest mystery of sex remained how something so hot and arousing in fantasy could have absolutely nothing in common with *actual* sex once put onscreen.

Like everything she'd said to me that afternoon, this request filled me with dismay and terror. I nodded yes.

Porn has always struck me as the kind of genre that in the right circumstances could produce a film so powerful and culturally relevant that it could change the way the world views sex and independent filmmaking. Free of the rules and taboos placed on mainstream media, and with no ratings system to worry its pretty little head, I always thought porn would be the birthplace of the next Bertolucci. As a professional porn reviewer, a female pro-porn pundit (and porn-lover), I started my porn-watching career by placing a great deal of faith in the human capacity to create, to make art, to break the rules of sex foisted upon us proles, who are just waiting for the chance to break free of the shackles of oppression that bind us in our boring little sexual cages.

Faced with an exciting question, porn proved to me over the course of eight years and over a thousand films that it could only respond in the dullest possible way. To me, the greatest mystery of sex remained how something so hot and arousing in fantasy could have absolutely nothing in common with *actual* sex once put onscreen. I certainly express physical enthusiasm every once in a while for a stocky cock and a greedy mouth, but while screening the latest copy of *Beverly Hills 9021-Ho* or *The Sopornos #6*, I'd often find myself thinking that I should rent some hot porn so I can jack off, completely forgetting that I'm watching porn at that moment.

Porn, known for Mafia ties (graft and menswear), check fraud, and fluorescent lighting, took my hopes and dreams of cinema verité fucking *alfresco* and turned it into my own personal freakish experiment of boredom. By my third professional review, each film looked more and more like it was made by someone desperate to create time capsules of 1981. Somehow, somewhere, someone made a rule that all porn videos must contain six or seven sex scenes, and that each sex scene must repeat the same sex positions, duration, and execution. It took me half an hour and two double-A batteries to figure out the Mad Libs-inspired formula, then gaze over to consider the date of my next pedicure. I had a sneaking suspicion that Rain Man was running the porn industry, counting reverse cowgirls and doggie/mish/oral sequences, in between rocking himself in the corner and telling the directors, "Uh-oh, fifteen minutes to Wopner...."

It was no wonder to me why porn performers always seemed to be thinking about anything except what they were doing. Granted, when I press "play," I know I'm not going to jack off to lovemaking, but sometimes I'd like to see at least *like-making*. Puffy lips polish knobs with the precision of bottle-topping machines in a factory. Close-ups on genitals go beyond the actual human capacity of seeing, creating panoplies of indistinguishable meat rubbing together in ways that would make Karen Finley cry, "Plagiarism!" Abattoir sounds of fake orgasm compete with screeching saxophones and synth beats to conspire against my sanity and irritate my neighbors' dogs. Ropes of semen shoot onto flinching or bizarrely grinning faces like a child's prank, the bottle rocket aimed at the teacher. And the positions seem like a cruel Cirque du Soleil masterpiece, though they often do serve as a reminder to attend my weekly yoga class.

So when my years of sex-ed training, porn reviewing, several books on sex and sexuality, and a willingness to talk about it on camera landed me in "porn valley," I was excited to have my first real, live on-set experience. I brought my digital camera and extra batteries, and had a list of questions for the performers and director. But it wasn't just any porn set: The highest profile "men's magazine" had flown me to Los Angeles to make a how-to sex-ed segment based on my two most popular books.

When I got off the plane, I discovered that the wealthy gentlemen's glossy outsourced all their film ventures, and were as cheap as the day is long. The first day of filming in their tiny, stuffy offices went fine, and I did a series of basic anatomy descriptions in a "talking head" introduction to the segment. They told me that the next day we'd be on location to film the sex scenes and that they had porn performers coming in for the shoot. In the scenario I was a sex counselor for a couple who wanted to learn more about oral sex. It was to be the most explicit segment the magazine's cable TV franchise had done yet; they'd had to get personal approval from the famous billionaire owner, and they were cleverly cloaking the pornographic demonstrations in an educational wrapper. I was nervous.

Perhaps the problems started before I'd even arrived, when the producer was too shy to interview performers for the shoot. The outsourcing company had never "done porn," but due to the sexually explicit nature of the segment, had to hire porn performers. We needed to show sex techniques,

not porn sex, so they wanted me to supervise and coach the performers. At the same time, the biggest HIV scare to hit the porn industry in many years was all over mainstream and adult news outlets, proclaiming an industry-wide shutdown until all tests were in. Unlike the gay porn industry that condemns and forbids unsafe sex practices, the straight porn industry insists that safer sex and condom use would doom their businesses to failure, claiming that condoms take away from the "realism" of their work.

After the first public HIV scare in 1997, a few renegade performers got together and founded a testing clinic and nonprofit, attempting to make HIV testing (at minimum) socially mandatory for performers. Even with such positive strides, an HIV breakout occurred. The leading adult industry magazine put out an issue with a sexy nurse on the cover, proclaiming "Killer Sex," and ran opinion pieces on both sides of the testing debate. As if it were debatable, like, "Drinking lye can kill you," versus, "Drinking lye is only something you need to worry about if you're gay."

The next morning started out sunny and warm, and as the production assistant and I entered the mansion, I realized that I'd seen the rooms of this house in some of the "high-class" porn films I'd screened. I noted the credit card on the glass coffee table in the otherwise spotless house (which was for

I had a sneaking suspicion that Rain Man was running the porn industry, counting reverse cowgirls and doggie/mish/oral sequences.

sale), and a ratty-haired blonde asleep on the couch in the game room. I quickly snapped a photo of her, and the flash made her bolt upright in an instant—not asleep, after all.

The performers arrived half an hour later looking like they'd just come from an all-night porn party. The female was a tattooed brunette who was a recognizable name in the porn world; he was a tall, blonde surfer-boy type, and they both told us they were a real-life couple who did porn together. I was elated, and though they seemed standoffish, I knew that once we had a chance to talk, they'd see that I was a knowledgeable, supportive porn fan. We'd chat and gossip about the porn business, laughing and making fun of long fingernails in "lesbian" porn. I looked forward to working with the sensitive, artistic temperament of performers who'd see the educational vision of the segment and would conspire with me to explicitly convey a slightly subversive yet sex-positive message. But until then, I couldn't help but notice that no matter what the male performer was doing, his hand always strayed to his crotch, grabbing his cock, his balls, or something. I wondered if porn people developed their own kind of nervous tics. For instance, before leaving a room he'd grab at his crotch; I wanted to suggest the doorknob, as that's what works best for the rest of us.

The crew's first task was to shoot the couple's opening scene: entering the house. Throughout all five takes, the cameraman had to carefully position the camera to avoid the formerly sleeping blonde as she obsessively scrubbed a spot on the carpet with a sponge and a saucepan filled with soap and water.

Next, it was time for me to explain sexual anatomy using the brunette as a live model, pointing out my descriptions to the camera. I sat on the bed and waited for the actress to take off her clothes, which took all of five seconds due to the fact that she wore no underwear, but then had to wait as she searched her belongings and asked everyone on the crew if they had any baby wipes. "I think I need 'em," she rasped.

I focused really, really hard on avoiding skin contact, visualizing at one point that her pussy was made of molten lava or skin-melting acid.

Finally, she flopped onto the bed and spread her legs, and motioned to a Braille pattern of sores and scabs on her shaved vulva and inner thighs. In a Suzanne Pleshette voice, she croaked, "Fucking razor burn!" I took stock of the bumpy terrain, like some planet best discovered only by some sort of remote-controlled machine, and carefully pointed out anatomy to the camera in my best teaching voice. I focused really, really hard on avoiding skin contact, visualizing at one point that her pussy was made of molten lava or skin-melting acid. After the director yelled, "Cut," I walked over to him and thoughtfully whispered, "You know, I'm a bit concerned about the sores."

"You can see those, too?! Shit."

He put a stop to the filming. Then he told the brunette why we stopped and why we couldn't use her for the shoot, sending her into a screeching, wig-throwing rage. Her boyfriend obsessively yanked on his dick and quietly told us he was going to stay and do it for the money, assuring us he could get another girl, no problem. He fished his cellphone out of his pocket with his free hand. "What about the HIV moratorium?" I asked him. "Oh, that's nothing. (Company name) is sending out 200 girls a day; their drivers can have one over here in an hour. You want (now famous, awarded starlet)? I think she's free this morning. Let me make a few calls."

So we did. Seven hundred miles from home, I talked about sex with the crew and took turns playing Crockett and Tubbs with the cameraman in the spacious, abhorrently tacky *Mi-*

ami Vice mansion. There were no wastebaskets or trashcans in the entire house. We found a condom wrapper under a dresser, creeping each other out with suggestions as to where the contents now lie.

Two hours later, a pretty, comparatively plain-looking blonde arrived. She was, in fact, beautiful, soft, and naturally lovely, not hard-edged and thin like the brunette. I was relieved that no one had arrived with some sort of "porn look," to which years of porn-watching had made me violently allergic. It had become impossible for me to enjoy porn starring living blow-up dolls, every breast a perfect chemical melon, pendulous miracles of science. If their boobs were filled with air, you could tie a string to an ankle and fly them. Their tanned and toughened skin always looked like the interior shots of a car commercial, and threesomes at a glance could trick me into seeing an epileptic man in a fit with a hard-on, bookended by a pair of overstuffed Naugahyde recliners.

The director whisked our blonde upstairs to the bedroom, had her take her clothes off, and asked me to come in. She was waiting for me on the bed, with her legs spread, looking at the ceiling. The director indicated her splayed crotch and asked me, "Is she okay?" I glanced at her and waited for a second, wondering how David Lynch had managed to become director of my life. I told them, "She's fine."

⋈

We started over from the beginning, and this time the blonde performers flirted like mad, dropping names about industry contacts and bantering about sex. She was a rising star; he was hoping to get a rise. Back on the bed, about to point out anatomy for the second time (but still careful not to touch), she whispered to me in a baby voice, "I thought you were going to say I was ugly." I told her no, the last girl had sores. She looked at her new paramour, his hand absently massaging his scrotum, and exhaled, "Ah."

I explained clitoral anatomy to the camera, my fingers careful not to graze her kryptonite pussy. She was perplexed. "How did you learn all this stuff?" I told her I'd done around seventy hours of sex-ed training courses and that I'd been pretty surprised about the clitoris, too. I wondered what else I should be telling her about sex in the seconds I had between takes, and whether she'd listen, or care, or see something shiny.

The next segment was male genital anatomy. The male performer took his clothes off, and I wondered if he was going to need baby wipes, too. The blonde kept flirting with him, and he played pocket pool, now minus the pocket. "Wait," he told us. "I gotta get a hard-on for this part." His genital gropes were getting rough, beating, and the crew and I exchanged nervous glances. I told the room, no we don't need a hard cock yet, it's okay. I proceeded with my anatomy lesson, continually telling him to stop touching, to move his hands away. Between takes he said to me in a wide-eyed whisper, "It won't get hard!" The blonde giggled and assured him, "I'll help you...."

We changed scene and moved onto the bed to film a series of techniques from my books. My role was to explain each technique to the camera, then off-camera I'd tell the performers what to do, and the couple would demonstrate. Between takes, I was marooned on the bed with the performers, where they'd chat with me while lights were adjusted and the crew assisted the director and cameraman.

The blonde's voice was high and whispery, like pink cotton filigree full of air. She told me, "He's leaving her for me!" her eyes shining. She also told me about the toilet paper stuffed in her vagina. Every once in a while, the performers asked if they needed to keep pretending they were a couple. I asked them how work was going during the moratorium. They both bragged about how they'd never had so much work in their lives and were making a lot of money.

"Everyone's really busy, and a lot of companies are filming more to fill in the gaps," they assured me.

I said, trying to be cool, "So, is everyone just using condoms or something?"

They looked at me with puzzled faces, as if I were a foreign exchange student, and told me, "No."

The male performer could not get an erection. The techniques were mostly foreplay-oriented, yet the afternoon dragged on. The female performer grew bored. "This soft-core shit is boring," she told us, her captive audience, with a smile. "I want to *really* fuck now!" Her impatience grew, and she was speaking to the whole crew, not just me anymore. "I did this awesome scene yesterday—it was so hot. The guy in the scene fucked this girl in the ass, then he held her over my face and dripped the cum into my mouth so I could drink it. I loved it!" She smiled at me, apparently my cue to say, "Wow, that's so awesome," as if she weren't making gruesome boasts about felching. She simply didn't know that her standards of awesome experiences, like her sexual practices, were devoid of anything one might consider polite conversation among strangers. Silence descended on the room, but the male performer picked up the conversational thread. "Who was shooting it?" he asked, smacking his dick.

Unlike the rest of the non-porn people in the room, I knew that for porn performers, sucking things out of a stranger's asshole was as everyday as slurping froth off a latte. Though

admittedly it might be latte seasoned with hepatitis, herpes, HPV, and a bacterial infection. No, no chocolate sprinkles for me. The list of unsafe (and for many people, distasteful) practices common in porn is lengthy and ever changing. Besides the incredibly trendy ass-to-mouth fetish, there's bottle-fucking, bile-drooling, throat-gagging to the point of vomiting, eye and nasal ejaculation, anal-to-vaginal penetration, anal penetration without lubricant, multiple male "cream pies" (internal ejaculation), and, of course, good ol' sex with multiple strangers without condoms.

The blonde was just like the rest of the world in that she'd never learned about any kind of sex except through reproductive information; those of us lucky enough to get sex ed in school don't ever see real, non-drawn genitals until we find our stepdad's *Playboys* or *Playgirls*. Our first glimpses of porn are filled with wonder, horror, curiosity, dread. Sometimes arousal. Like the blonde, everyone's real sexual education comes from a combination of our own scary and exciting experiences, and porn.

It wasn't difficult to imagine the blonde as a vessel for anatomy instruction for her thousands of wanking viewers, but it was chilling to think that people were getting sex ed from her movies. In fact, certain kinds of brutal sex—what I call "fear

I knew that for porn performers, sucking things out of a stranger's asshole was as everyday as slurping froth off a latte.

factor sex"—have become so trendy (hence, popular, widespread) among industry insiders that they have become standard sexual practices in porn, giving the porn community the misguided impression that specialized brutality is the norm in bedrooms across America. Porn, as our most vital vehicle of sex ed, has become the most viral form of sexual disinformation. If you used porn as a guide to real sex, you'd think that young women like having their anuses held open and spit into, that girls have earth-shattering sexual experiences when you choke them and slap their tits, and that large objects can easily be shoved in virgin assholes sans lube.

The director asked everyone to get back to work, opting to film a few more cunnilingus scenes. "Okay," I commanded the male performer, with no small amount of internal giggling: "Lick!" He took this as his cue to loudly spit on her vulva. The crew and I groaned, the director yelled, "Cut!"

I said, "Uh, no, don't do that, please."

"I thought you told me to spit."

"No. I told you to lick her."

My last shreds of irony ebbed. I didn't want to explain to him that genital-spitting was a common porn practice, but it wasn't common to the rest of the world—who were the ones who would be watching the show. Most people don't hawk loogies on each other's genitals unless their sex play is pretty evolved, and then usually for different reasons. "Just lick, okay?"

Eventually, we were way over the rental time on the mansion, and still no erection, despite the brutal beating surfer boy's cock and balls had sustained and the fervent cock-

Porn, as our most vital vehicle of sex ed, has become the most viral form of sexual disinformation.

sucking the blonde was administering in the adjacent bathroom. Finally the blonde had had enough fluffing, which, she reminded us several times, she was doing for free. She clop-clopped into the room naked, save for her Lucite stripper heels. Everyone tried to look busy with something, and I busied myself attempting to suction a dildo demo model onto the hardwood floor next to my chair. She announced, "We need a hard dick."

She surveyed the room; each of the men seemed to be visibly concentrating on what he was doing. But she had my full attention. She turned around to the cameraman busily changing tape on the gaudy *faux*-finish fireplace in the corner of the room. "What about you?" He focused on the task at hand while trying to shrink into the hearth. Naked, hands on hips, she cornered him. "I'll suck your cock. Then we'll have a hard dick." The cameraman declined without looking up from the task at hand. "What the fuck?" she asked the room, in which I was the only other female. But she didn't see me. I was invisible, while she was the elephant in the room.

The production assistant dragged a heavy light out of the room by himself, down the hall and out of sight. With one man left, she asked the director, "How about you? I'll suck your dick and make it nice and hard."

"Uh, no, that's okay."

"What the fuck!?" she yelled at all of us. "Am I not pretty enough?"

I escaped when they ordered the Viagra.

Black and Blue
New York's Roughie Grindhouses and the Films That Played at Them

Michelle Clifford

The Cameo

The theater with the reputation of being the oldest and most notorious grindhouse in Times Square was the Cameo Theater, located on West 44th Street and 8th Avenue. It was only two speedy blocks north from the Port Authority Bus Terminal. The Cameo was a huge, cavernous two-floor affair, with the second floor for employees only. The projection room had a storage space for prints both current and rotting. Two busy toilets flanked patrons as they walked past the theater's glass front doors. The Cameo began building its reputation back in 1964 when distributor Stan Borden presented *Olga's Girls* and its spin-offs, like *White Slaves of Chinatown* and *Olga's House of Shame*, with marathon runs.

Chelly Wilson paid lip service to community standards while making a quick buck off of the small cluster of Greek immigrants who lived in Hell's Kitchen. She'd show Greek-language films every Sunday at the Cameo so they wouldn't attack her smut-peddling the other six days of the week. It was one of Mrs. Wilson's tithes to the Greek business association, of which she was a proud and rowdy member. Of course, other Greeks were disgusted by her pursuits, but her money didn't stink. In fact, the Greek Mafia she worked for couldn't get enough of the smell. They had a taste for it.

In the mid-1970s, the Cameo became the superdome of the rough-sex action picture. It premiered *Femmes De Sade*, *Masters of Discipline*, *Love Slaves*—anything with a super-kinky reputation that preceded winning titles. The audience was busy, with massage parlor girls and streetwalkers pecking around for business in the aisles. Black transvestites offering "honey, you want anything for $5?" were a constant. Leftover disco-era clones in cowboy hats hovered near the well-traveled toilets.

A roughie classic that played the Cameo back in 1976 was *Love Slaves*. It's the only hardcore film directed by the late softcore roughie legend Bob Cresse under his pseudonym "Robert Husong." Cresse is renowned for classic S/M films like *Love Camp Seven*, *Hot Spur*, and many others. The plot revolves around a drug ring that kidnaps women. The girls are shot up with heroin, hypnotized, and turned into lethal, sexually driven assassins. John Leslie plays a federal agent sent to bust it down. The dirty airport-novel plot holds together an abstract fetish movie sprinkled with blatant, graphic sex scenes in the raunchy loop tradition. Like Cresse's other films, you enter a drone and exit it at disturbing, severe, and sexually driven moments. Rope bondage, catfights, close-ups of syringes piercing flesh, and as the *pièce de résistance*, the love slaves fucking impassive, dildoed mannequins. *Love Slaves* provides a spicy, rich, and varied menu of kinks able to engage the most jaded of palettes.

The Cameo premiered *The Abduction of Lorelei*, starring *Metasex*'s favorite masochist, wild and sexy Serena in a velour kidnap psychodrama. As Serena gets into her gold Lincoln Continental after a wearying day at the mall, she is dragged from the parking lot into a nondescript van by two biker scum. They bring her to their white trash hideout, where she meets the female part of this vile troika. They subject her to rope bondage and repeated rough violations, in one bitter instance with a Coke bottle. In between abuse sessions, they groove on Pink Floyd's *Dark Side of the Moon* and guffaw in methamphetamine glee about their upcoming ransom windfall. Serena, superstar that she is, plays on the male kidnappers' libidos to outwit them, leading to the surprise joy-buzzer ending.

The Abduction of Lorelei delivers its promise with exceptionally heavy B&D scenes alternating with graphic hardcore sex.

The three supporting players are effective unknowns, with no associations to other films. Serena, as always, more than lives up to her infamous S/M reputation. Remembering this film will lead you to ask, "Where is Serena today?" and, "Is she still *alive?*"

A most peculiar Cameo offering was *Red Heat*, written and directed by cult movie figure Ray Dennis Steckler and his wife using the collective pseudonym of Cindy Lou Sutter. *Red Heat* is equal parts off-kilter Vegas travelogue, bloody sex-killer flick, and raunchy loop package, all in one. The grizzled-sounding offscreen female narrator tells of her sleazy adventures directing skin flicks. Then she tells you about her star, Red Heat, who went on a wild murder spree. The sex scenes are raunchy early-1970s hotel-room balling populated by hardboiled, aged Vegas pros. Las Vegas is really the co-star, showing off a constant tapestry of nightclub marquees advertising the likes of Barry Manilow, Buddy Hackett, and Flip Wilson, filmed under a blinding white Sun. This is intercut with after-dark drive-by shots of degenerate massage parlors and adult bookstores. Watch for director Steckler's cameo as Red stabs him in the shower. It's far from a conventional hardcore film, but *Red Heat* still had enough oomph to satisfy horny Cameo denizens.

When the Cameo turned into a $1.99 triple-bill house in the 1980s, tourists, suckers, and guys from Jersey in groups made the pilgrimage.

The Venus

The Venus Theater was originally called the Eros E but changed its name in the mid-1970s so people would stop confusing it with the gay Eros next door. The Venus was Mrs. Wilson's second roughie showcase. The Venus showed *all* aspects of the violation theme, whether interracially in *The Big Man*, starring Jim Cassidy and John Holmes, or be it guys in gorilla

In the mid-1970s, the Cameo became the superdome of the rough-sex action picture.

costumes. Abductors, psychedelic pissing, or filmed volcanic eruptions of *all* bodily fluids (shit, piss, semen, menstruation), sometimes all at once, flew across the Venus' grubby, stained screen. The Venus audience was mostly black men agreeable to any kind of kinky, anonymous sex and white men seeking a dingy experience. All manner of 8th Avenue flotsam floated in after midnight like a tide breaking. Hustlers, drug casualties, homeless perverts. In the 1980s, the Venus was an incredible place for reruns, be it *Teenage Fantasies* or any number of Shaun Costello movies.

The Intrusion was a frequent Venus replay. Pseudonymously directed by "Art Nouveau" (most likely Shaun Costello), *The Intrusion* is a meditation on the molecular structure of a rape. Kim Pope plays a shy, bored housewife married to ineffectual businessman Levi Richards. Michael Dattore cruises suburban streets in his car looking for just the right house to invade. After posing as an insurance salesman, he suddenly pushes his way into the quiet home. Dattore's shrunken Skeletor coke head and loud plaid pants only makes him more rank and believable.

He hustles the frightened wife upstairs, where he beats her face with his cock, violates her with a knife handle, and face-fucks her. The Filipino maid surprises him, and she gets some of the same. She's stripped, revealing pubic hair shaved into a heart. He ties her hands behind her back. After acquiescing to Dattore, she is ordered onto the bed with Pope. It all builds to a crescendo of an oral orgy. A flip-book reprise of the whole film is presented, leading up to the final moment, with the maid drawing a fatal close to the rapist's whole insane outburst. Menace is the leitmotif of *The Intrusion*. Sharp character performances and professional direction contribute to its overwhelming sense of erotic threat, which is amplified by its malevolent avant-garde soundtrack. *The Intrusion* is a tight, compelling, minimalist psychodrama.

The Capri

The friendly neighbor of the Venus and Eros was the Capri Theater on 46th Street and 8th Avenue, owned by Tom, a nondescript little Greek guy. The Capri was a long, shoebox-styled grindhouse with a busy balcony. A staircase above the balcony led to the owner's office. Tom was a sometime XXX producer but looked like he should be running a coffee shop. The Capri had a reputation in the 1970s for showing so-called quality adult films tinged with a patina of kink. These features brought a dedicated crowd bearing five-dollar bills to the box office. The Capri was considered reasonably safe, despite the 8th Avenue hookers who'd mosey around during closing time.

The Capri was immortalized in Shaun Costello's *Afternoon Delight*. George Payne, Vanessa Del Rio, and Dave Ruby, all attired in leather, get it on with a shattered-looking Alan Marlow in the theater's balcony.

One of the Capri's popular 1977 offerings was the Jamie Gillis vehicle *Winter Heat*, shot in the middle of winter, with all the inherent isolation that cold weather imparts. Snow covers the remote cabins where Jamie, Helen, and their two aging, Stonewall-era traveling companions bust in on three passive girls. These creeps take over the cabin and have their raw way with the pitiful girls. *Winter Heat* is an ambient roughie that strikes a relaxed groove through its insulated setting and occasional disco music interludes.

Gillis is in top form. His seedy brutishness sets the film's tone. At one point, he humiliates and force-feeds oatmeal to a girl who, when provoked, explains her shaved pussy as the result of recent surgery. This only inspires Gillis. This is one of the few films to feature Helen Madigan in a dominant role. Creative verbal abuse, avaricious sex, and curious casting made *Winter Heat* a comfortable white noise for the Capri's roughie fans. It's a must-see for Gillis aficionados.

By the mid-1980s, the Capri turned into a $1.99 second-run house. It was so infested by crackheads that the theater's management was forced to team up with the NYPD to stop the place from being a full-tilt crack palace. Tom handed over the Capri's daily operations to a couple of patois-babbling Haitians, who suffered from terrible B.O., and Mary, an old, stone-faced Greek troll, who oversaw the cashbox.

After Mary quit, Tom hired Wayne. Wayne was an aged career chickenhawk with a Grecian Formula pompadour who worked every single adult theater in Times Square at one point or another. Wayne was known for tricking with troublemaking Latinos. One wily youth went so far as to rob a local black coke dealer named Muscles. When Wayne got rid of that kid, everyone at the Capri was glad. Wayne was quiet, but his friends were trouble.

The Rialto One

Forty-second Street's biggest, friendliest, and best-liked adult house was the Rialto One. It was situated right on 42nd Street and 7th Avenue. The heart of the Deuce. Surprisingly, patrons made the effort to stay out of each other's way and be unobtrusive to one another. The Rialto was a first-run house, so the audience held high expectations for each premiered film. You could bring a date. The Rialto attracted a more cerebral crowd. Opinions flew through the air. Everyone had a say.

In 1977 the Rialto unveiled *Waterpower*, the most bizarre film ever credited to Gerard Damiano but actually directed by Shaun Costello. It's a taboo-breaking film dealing with scat and enemas without ever displaying the brown. Since *Waterpower* was made around the time of *Taxi Driver*, you'll see the similarities.

It opens with an antisocial, troubled, and confused Jamie Gillis wandering through the fetid 9th Avenue Food Fair, stopping briefly to have his bewildered mug placed on a "Spirit of '76" badge. Gillis contemplates the button, then goes home to peek at a stewardess neighbor. Frustrated, he heads to an S/M massage parlor, where Eric Edwards and Marlene Wil-

loughby play a sadistic doctor and nurse. They give a bound and gagged girl a disciplinary high colonic. After seeing this scene unfold, Gillis' gaskets are blown. He goes bonkers, haunting 42nd Street adult bookstores, buying slick enema mags, muttering, "That's where it's at...water and power!" Now crazed and overheated, Gillis goes on a nozzle rampage, beginning with his stewardess neighbor. He progresses to two aged schoolgirls, and ends up with undercover cop C.J. Laing in handcuffs. Gillis gets away scot-free, and a postscript mentions the number of unsolved rapes in the United States.

Waterpower is held together by a straightforward B-picture narrative and goes for a documentary look with brown, muddy photography. The film helped cement Gillis' reputation as dean of the roughies. On its initial release, *Waterpower* flabbergasted 42nd Street's inner-city audience, a nearly impossible feat. People could not believe what they had just seen and sat through it numerous times. The film was a real rarity.

Red Heat is equal parts off-kilter Vegas travelogue, bloody sex-killer flick, and raunchy loop package, all in one.

Everyone kept their hands under control as they sat elbow to elbow, spellbound, watching the acting stylings of Gillis. The crowd laughed and speculated aloud about how crazy Gillis was.

It sounds funny, and it was, but it was a very special event. The right audience had shown up for a movie that not only met their expectations but challenged them, keeping everyone engrossed in what was about to happen next. *Waterpower* does its job in spades. It is a dirty movie that delivers heavy sex scenes with an A-level kinky cast. It also works as a grindhouse picture with a full-scale maniac portrayal by Gillis, an obsessive-compulsive loner who was real enough in terms of Times Square.

The Globe

The Globe was a big, rude theater squatting right next to Nathan's Famous Hot Dog emporium on 43rd Street and Broadway. In the early 1960s, it had been a revered nudist theater for aging World War II veterans. In the 1970s, the Globe peeled its fisheye towards freaky stuff, like 1974's *Climax of Blue Power*. Originally, the movie was reviled by critics for its intermingling of violence and twisted sex, but its eye-catching ad campaign, classic title, and high-voltage content made the picture enormously popular. The film is one of the boldest, at times funniest, and most unrelenting roughies ever made, entering taboo realms within role-playing and terminal kinks.

Jason Cams plays a security guard who gets off impersonating an LAPD officer. During his voyeuristic prowls, he rapes, debases, and bullies hookers. One night while peeping in windows, he accidentally spies a woman killing her husband during a heated argument. Cams stews in his own perversions, watching anal loops and terrorizing a massage parlor owner after having a two-girl session. His erotomanias draw him back to the murder over and over. He fantasizes about brutalizing the murderess, and he acts on his obsession, even assaulting her in drag. She rewards him with the appropriate, final remedy he is seeking—his death at her hands.

Climax of Blue Power is made in a TV movie/Crown International thriller vein, complete with car chases and L.A. location work. The film is an edge-of-the-seat ride. Shockingly hostile

All manner of 8th Avenue flotsam floated in after midnight like a tide breaking.

in intent and execution, sex scenes emerge as integral parts of the narrative. It's raw, yet the film adroitly walks a tightrope of prurient impact. Jason Cams, with his nondescript good looks, gives a transcendent performance as the perverted antagonist. He's so convincing that you shudder at the thought of this creep living next door to you, which sustains the believability that most hardcore films lack. The hardened Hollywood Boulevard female cast members are equally apropos. (Watch for the curious glimpse of Uschi Digart in the massage parlor.) *Climax of Blue Power* is a terrific movie and a must for anyone into rough sex.

By 1976 the Globe had deteriorated into just another shabby adult house with odd happenings, like Mark (Mr. 10-½) Stevens, high on a fistful of drugs, approaching bewildered and shocked nerds by the toilets. Stevens enjoyed getting off while his image played on the big screen.

In late 1976 the Globe renamed itself the Rialto East and went high-quality super-sleaze. The first feature to kick off the name change was *The Double Exposure of Holly*. It's the story of Jewish American Princess Holly Levin (Catherine Earnshaw), who is married to an old man for money but fucks around constantly behind his back. One of her throwaway lovers puts her under video surveillance in an attempt to destroy her marriage. This chaos triggers a ripple effect of betrayals and murder. *The Double Exposure of Holly* captures the glossy dissipation of sexual decadence in mid-1970s Manhattan. Jamie Gillis remembers that director Bob Gill was a drop-in director and only around for this one hardcore film.

The conflict-driven narrative structure resembles an existential soap opera. As the investigating team, Gillis and Terri Hall, always terrific together, are impressive as sex-driven depressives. Hardcore scenes appear fluidly. Terri Hall nods out and imagines a dark, disembodied orgy set to an aural tapestry of ambient jazz music. Annie Sprinkle appears as a pea-brained, giddy hooker who seduces Gillis in a prearranged three-way with Nancy Dare. Leading lady Catherine Earnshaw, who also used the names Cary Lacy and Catherine Burgess, was a hardcore anomaly. She appeared in a few big-budget porno films, performed simulated sex, but required a body double for hardcore inserts. She was hired, it seems, to lend a patina of glamour. It's also curious to see videotape, which is sadly now the almost necrophilic norm, used as a futuristic, kinky voyeuristic device. *The Double Exposure of Holly* is a moody, erotic film noir with its own unique aesthetic.

In the early 1980s the Rialto East turned into a Spanish-language theater. Then, Sweetheart Theaters, an arm of the Jewish Mafia with many fingers in Times Square pies, bought the theater. Sweetheart also owned high-profile first-run theaters like the Circus, Mini, and World Theaters. All of the Sweetheart Theaters were running steadily on the decline. They broke the Rialto East in half to make a twin theater and renamed it the Big Apple. After this change, the theater turned extremely rank. Black sleepers, unskilled pickpockets, failed beat drug salesmen, couples chasers, and one-armed bandits were all drawn by the Big Apple's large size. They had the luxury of changing films or "scenes" at any point by moseying over to the twin's other side. Films like *Big Abner* with John Holmes and Jim Cassidy played, but no one really watched the movie. Everyone watched each other. The theater was a big jerk-off palace. The Big Apple stunk, it had sticky floors, and after leaving, anyone sane would burn their clothes and douse themselves with Rid.

If you came in a couple, you were immediately the audience's sexual focus in a hostile, cum-shot way. The whole vibe of the joint was blank, not home, and more than disaffected, like a crowd of aggressive sexual autistics. Once during a showing of *Orgy Party*, a white couple came in and quietly sat down near the front. The woman looked around, nervously, not trusting her surroundings. She looked like an innocuous out-of-towner. Suddenly she hollered: "WHAT THE FUCK IS *THIS*?" The audience came to a stunned standstill. "Your head is ten feet tall!" She called the guy with her an asshole, and, getting out of her seat to leave, she scanned the audience watching her. "You're all assholes, too!" she barked, almost knocking the exit doors off their hinges. Just another quirky Times Square outburst.

The Big Apple's rotting neighbor, Nathan's Famous Hot Dogs,

held strong until about 1989, when it finally closed up shop because so few people would eat there. It was too out of control with crazy crack casualties acting as if it were their psych ward. Nathan's wide, cascading staircase led to a vision out of *Caligula*. The very public toilets in Nathan's were so terrible that all the doors were removed, giving an unappetizing piss show to unaware diners. The ladies' room fared no better, as it was utilized as a bidet station by the lowest of Deuce streetwalkers. Tourists seeking refuge and food would enter Nathan's and became confused. If they ordered a meal, they ate grimly, leaving most of their leaden food behind, grabbing their stomachs, running horrified from the place.

The Lincoln Art

The Lincoln Art Theater charged a little more to keep out the riffraff, with a $5 admission price for only one feature. It was a little north of Times Square on West 57th Street near Carnegie Hall and had come to prominence through *The Devil in Miss Jones*' year-long marathon run. The Lincoln Art showed freaky raunch and an occasional gay film like Fred Halsted's *Sextool*. Women—anything wearing lipstick—were admitted to *Sextool* for a cut-rate $3 admission. Even though it showed straight films, much of the Lincoln Art's audience was homosexual, with a lot of cruise activity. To its credit, however, you could enjoy heterosexual oral sex openly as long as you didn't mind providing a show for the rest of the house. The Lincoln Art had a mostly white crowd, as opposed to Times Square's inner city black stronghold.

Films like Roberta Findlay's *The Clamdigger's Daughter*, better known as *A Woman's Torment*, opened at the Lincoln Art. Frankly, the films made by Roberta solo, without husband Mike, are terrible. Yakking Manhattan shrinks, unsatisfied sex, and kvetching women. The plot revolves around a drunken psychiatrist (Jake Teague) and his sexually frustrated wife (Jennifer Jordan). Meanwhile, Tara Chung sits in a beach house like a zombie and murders men after she has sex with them. Director Findlay has a cameo as Chung's nosy neighbor. The swirling camera angles, disjointed close-ups of body parts, and terminal underpinnings recall Roberta's 1960s efforts but are updated for hardcore. They're also reminiscent of the sex-and-horror hybrids of Andy Milligan during his *Ghastly Ones* prime. Violent deaths, combative fucking, and ensemble acting by ubiquitous New York players Jennifer Jordan and the bewigged, aged Teague create a sexual disharmony on every level. The film is an unwatchable headwrecker, only bearable to neurotic, diehard Roberta Findlay fans.

The Lincoln Art had a huge run with *A Dirty Western*, the film that dragged the time-honored genre of the sex western into the hardcore age. It differs from bare-bones psychodramas like *Hot Spur* or teepee cheapies like *Ramrodder* by actually delivering on its promise. *A Dirty Western* boasts aerial shots of the Great Plains, twangy original music, a meticulously illustrated title sequence, horseback-riding outlaws and posses, and many outdoor sex scenes that are natural extensions of the storyline.

Barbara Bourbon, iconized by Radley Metzger/Henry Paris as *Pamela Mann* and familiar to exploitation film fans from *Girls for Rent* and *The Candy Tangerine Man*, plays Sarah, a rancher's wife. Three jailbirds, outfitted in convict black-and-white stripes, strip and rape Sarah, leaving her suspended by rope. The cons take off with Sarah's three sexy, skinny-dipping daughters, shoving and dragging the nude girls along. An orgy in a stream unfolds, with the girls performing incredible underwater sexual gymnastics. As Sarah and her husband follow in hot pursuit, the villains hole up with the daughters in a cave, where the girls go about their escape by exhausting their captors. Although there are amusing, hokey touches—Barbara's wig is a wobbly nylon prop-store cheapie and Levi Richards can't shake his New Yorkese—the production of *A Dirty Western* is sound, with the roughie template of victimized women turning the tables on their male aggressors fully realized.

They give a bound and gagged girl a disciplinary high colonic.

The Doll

Ten blocks south of the Lincoln Art, in the middle of Times Square's tourist promenade, was the Doll Theater on 47th Street and 7th Avenue. It was right across the street from the TKTS booth and the shat-upon statue of Father Duffy. In *Taxi Driver*, the Doll was featured as part of Travis' neon, schizophrenic sexual netherworld.

The Doll was part sex parlor, part revival house. It was a live sex-acts theater running double features of hour-long one-reelers, with the occasional two-reel Zebedy Colt feature thrown into the mix. The programming was exquisite, thanks to the cinematic selections of Stella and the Martinez brothers. It showed the finest vintage roughies and movies with dedicated followings. Drop into the Doll and you could see John Holmes, a Joe Davian film, or the pact-with-the-Devil movie *Mary Mary*, with Constance Money.

The Doll was a tiny shoebox seating perhaps 80 people, tops. It was basically a mellow, secure place. Less assault-prone than 8th Avenue's Venus, although Japanese tourists were frequent targets for toilet muggings. A live, on-stage sex performance interrupted the movies every hour and a half. For such a small, unassuming place, the Doll was popping. Porno stars who were starring in a picture playing, or ones who were recovering from just making one, hung out there. The theater appealed to a metasexually bent personage. The disaffected people who fall into all categories. A building full of offbeat heterosexuals. Homosexual admirers of these metasexuals would prowl around, like Burt Reynolds' pal, Dom DeLuise. Dom cruised and was gregarious enough to give autographs. It was shocking that he didn't care who recognized him.

You could find human makings for a good party at the Doll, whether to be enjoyed on-premise or purchased for later. Drugs were available: The projectionist sold Percodans; the live sex-show teams sold coke and pot. Latino knuckleheads were used in a sandwich-boy capacity to fetch dope in neighboring Hell's Kitchen. Patrons who wanted to be voyeurs were left alone. Their peripheral vision burned off anyone unappealing. People could meet partners by flashing or sitting with a ready-to-go erection in a little, recessed row, accepting or rejecting offers of sex. If someone wished to receive favors, they'd make a hand gesture resembling hailing a cab.

The live show on stage would spread an infectious party fever, with hookers hopping on guys' laps, getting their cash, and going for it right in the audience. The rest of the crowd would worship these moments of sexual abandon. It was an

She rewards him with the appropriate, final remedy he is seeking—his death at her hands.

authentic experience, and that's what anyone really wanted there. On slow days the Doll was like a metronomic heartbeat.

The week that Forced Entry played the Doll, it wrecked everybody's heads. Written and directed by "Helmut Richler" (Shaun Costello), Forced Entry was notorious. Its initial release in 1971 left audiences agape. The film continued to haunt Times Square adult theaters through the early 1980s. Forced Entry is a groundbreaking film in that its female lead (Laura Cannon) was the first hardcore star to pose for girl-next-door-loving Playboy, which was played up in the film's ad campaign and title credits. More important, the film is the first fully realized feature to cross the sex and horror genres.

Pre-Deep Throat fame, Harry Reems is sans his trademark Beefsteak Charlie mustache and is credited under his hokey loop moniker of "Tim Long." Harry does a 360-degree turn from the hambone he's known as, playing a shellshocked Army vet just back from Vietnam, pumping gas and following women home after they use his service station. He forces the girls into sex at knifepoint as he unleashes torrents of verbal abuse, climaxing in stabbings. Forced Entry features some of the most hate-driven talk ever documented on film. Harry threatens to cut the eyes out of a bewildered trampy girl as she gives him head. He screams about shit on his dick after he anally violates his next victim. Making the movie even more disturbing is the unrelenting newsreel Vietnam atrocity footage interspersed throughout. The sex scenes are imaginatively photographed in a post-psychedelic manner, graphic and blunt. The cast is fleshed out by freak-era, big-titted actresses.

After the reaction Reems received from Forced Entry, he refused to accept any more hardcore, psycho dominance roles. Curiously, the film was remade under the same title in an R-rated version starring Tanya Roberts. Not for the fainthearted, Forced Entry is a sexual anxiety attack. The live-show guys who had themselves been to Vietnam took great offense to the film and literally turned their backs on it.

The Hudson

The Avon Hudson, located on 44th Street between 6th Avenue and Broadway, was a veteran of the days when Warhol films were merchandised as sex movies. It drew elbow-to-elbow crowds. According to Avon maintenance man Benny Torres, "The Hudson had three balconies with everything goin' on in them."

Shaun Costello's Dominatrix Without Mercy played a marathon run at the Hudson. Marlene Willoughby answers a want ad in Screw magazine offering thousands of dollars. It turns out to be a busy Manhattan dominance apartment run by a frumpy madam. The film's overlapping vignettes depict different sadomasochistic situations played out by perverted sexual compulsives. Incidents appear with the fluidity of daydreams brought to life. The cast is a compilation of mid-1970s New York, S/M-bent porno superstars, all of whom let their hair down. Marlene has the looks and charisma of an Eric Stanton cartoon come to life, dramatic without being laughable. Masochist Terri Hall changes caps to become a dominant. Jamie Gillis is a sexual nihilist rope freak kept in a closet. He's later raped orally with a dildo by Marlene. Vanessa Del Rio gives the submissive performance of a lifetime; you are amazed she went through it. The button-downed, wee-mustachioed Grover Griffith provides the comic highpoint as an overamped slave. Dominatrix Without Mercy was produced by Jason Russell under the pseudonym "S.S. Plug."

Another big draw at the Hudson was Joe Davian's films, including the supernaturally bent Night of Submission and the deranged women's prison melodrama Domination Blue. Davian's dark masterpiece Revenge and Punishment opens in a cemetery with an Oriental dominatrix out to avenge the death of her sister. A porno photographer who beats his models receives her wrath with penis restraints, riding crops, and whips. The heroine receives a thorough gynecological examination by the perverted doctor who gave her sister the fatal abortion (a startlingly effective Al Levitsky). She gains the confidence of another peek-a-boo shutterbug, incarnated with sexual bluntness by Dave Ruby. Hair Club for Men member Jake Teague is believably sleazy as an evil senator. Although uneven, with slow passages between the shocks, *Revenge and Punishment* confirms that Davian is an adroit constructor of erotic menace.

House of De Sade and *Fetishes of Monique* put the Hudson crowd in a more jovial mood. *House of De Sade* is a wild haunted-house romp with Vanessa Del Rio and her sexually overactive cohorts conjuring the spirit of the Marquis de Sade during a nonstop orgy. Davian's staples of heavy B&D with appropriate equipment is in full force. Vanessa's resilience in slave scenes, from chastity belts to nipple clamps, boggles the mind.

The Hudson also had success premiering *Fetishes of Monique*. The film focuses on a mad scientist and his kinky, glitter-era assistant who develop an aphrodisiac made from the scientist's own sperm. The scientist keeps human experiments in prison cells, where they perform a plethora of sex acts that a photographer records. Enormous Ben Wa balls come in to play. Nurse Monique and the shutterbug make off with the lust-inducing liquid. After they fuck, Monique is kidnaped and dragged back to the lab. The scientist and his assistant give her a gynecological exam and a whipping. This movie is Davian's version of lighthearted.

The Bryant

The Bryant Theater was smack in the middle of 42nd Street, between Broadway and 6th Avenue. The Bryant also housed Avon Picture Company's headquarters, nestled on its top floor. The Bryant's cashbox was a tiny closet with half a wall of glass exposed to the sidewalk, as if the cashier were an exhibit, becoming the human face of the theater. The admission was a bargain-basement $1.99 at all times.

In the 1970s the Bryant took a lot of flack from *Screw* magazine for showing old softcore movies in the age of hardcore. Around 1976 the Bryant changed its policy to triple bills of second-run hardcore. One of their most memorable triples was *Lunch*, *Night After Night*, and *Sweet and Sour*. *Lunch* was a realistic look at a sexual pest bothering some San Francisco freaks who are sharing space at a creepy boarding house. *Night After Night* is a New Yorky piece in which Jamie

Gillis, Alan Marlow, and Eric Edwards find renewed marital bliss after cheating on their wives with Darby Lloyd Raines. *Sweet and Sour* is another good New York movie in which Jamie Gillis imagines a pick-up with a girl he sees in a coffee shop, bringing her home for an afternoon fling. The punch line comes when the girl is revealed to be an undercover cross-dressing cop.

The Bryant's front glass doors led down a long lobby that was literally a hall of mirrors. There was a payphone booth in the lobby, which afforded Avon's staff a smidgen of privacy while making and taking drug orders. An anonymous door by the payphone led to a long, rickety, wooden stairway, which led to the Avon Pictures office. One big, dusty room of worn-down wooden office furniture. That's where you'd find Stella, Murray, and Phil. Stella's desk had an intercom where she could place a chubby finger on a button and buzz the box offices of any of the other Avon theaters in Times Square. Some days at the Bryant, there would be Cheri Champagne picking up a paycheck and hustling some more film work, or Brad Sanders, the projectionist, inevitably cornered by Phil, hearing out another of his psychotic schemes and hysteria-driven film ideas. The Bryant was a madhouse and a beehive of criminal activity.

The theater itself was one giant floor. In the winter everyone froze. A space heater was shoved dangerously next to the live sex-show performance mattress on stage. The stage was high up over the audience. Having ample room behind its curtains, it was often used for casual, quickie sex encoun-

The Big Apple stunk, it had sticky floors, and after leaving, anyone sane would burn their clothes and douse themselves with Rid.

ters between Bryant employees. The audience was always crowded, especially Sundays when family-deprived Popeyes were all the more lonely. These old farts always demanded that penny change from the $1.99 admission.

The programming at the Bryant was tremendous. The screen was really big, although the sound could be difficult to make out in the projection booth due to the weird acoustics in the large auditorium. Phil Prince's better second-run features played, giving them an extra dimension of depth. Prince's films were backed by Zebedy Colt's almost hysterical features, like *The Affairs of Janice* and *The Devil Inside Her*.

Angel in Distress looked great on the Bryant screen. A conventional narrative is deconstructed and rebuilt into an intense S/M psychodrama. Blonde, big-titted Joey Karson is kidnaped and held in a tenement on 42nd Street and 8th Avenue, right in the crotch of Times Square. Mistress Candice oversees her verbal threats, torment, bondage, and other assaults at the hands of seen-it-all George Payne. Dave Ruby is a shocker. Bearded, muscled, issuing terroristic sexual threats—there's a little bit of Richard Speck in that Ruby.

The movie sweats off its storyline as Mistress Candice takes over, abusing, berating, and snarling at virtually the entire cast, creating a many-sided S/M orgy. One of its more brutal scenes features three bare-breasted women tied to a wooden frame. Largely filmed in one claustrophobic set, peppered with choice location shots, and driven by its cast members' overamped personalities, *Angel in Distress* achieves a Warho-

Forced Entry features some of the most hate-driven talk ever documented on film.

lian aesthetic. Excellent performances, breakneck pacing, unrelenting sado-sex, and dynamic camerawork using looming p.o.v. angles intermingle to accomplish its symphony of hate.

The Bryant played Phil's segmented loop package, *Tales From the Bizarre.* Four skanks in negligees sit discussing their freakiest sexual experiences in four stories which are equal verbal and physical abuse. Cheri Champagne phones a *Screw* ad, and George Payne appears bearing clothespins and an angry mouth. Phll Prince is featured in the film. He interviews Ambrosia Fox, who reveals her birthdate to be 1966, making her sixteen at the time of the filming. Prince Mickey Finns her and drags her into an orgy where he handcuffs her feet to her hands. Alan Adrian and another simpleton jerk off as Phil presides like a basehead gargoyle, laughing in big, ugly close-up. He treats Ambrosia to hot wax, bananas, and plenty of psychobabble. Blunt, basic, and graphic.

A Bryant staple was Shaun Costello movies. *Prisoner of Pleasure* concerns a hedonistic housewife who swings, gets kidnaped, and experiences a masochistic awakening. Excellent New York location work and good character turns, including an assault-prone performance by George Payne and a slovenly cameo by Carter Stevens. Long Jeanne Silver's stumpfucking scene tested the audience's limits. The internal voiceover narration by the heroine is both creepy and effective.

Mistress Electra is Shaun's demented hybrid between *Bachelor Party* and a Mickey Spillane novel. A mild-mannered computer programmer watches hardcore loops at the weekly stag parties given by his buddy Harry (Carter Stevens). He's stunned when his prudish wife (Mistress Electra) turns up in one. Detective Steve Tucker follows the wife to a sleazy photo studio on 42nd Street, where Electra leads her double life with the assistance of photographer Marlene Willoughby and

her musclemen assistants George Payne and Dave Ruby.

Shaun's talent for making his cast members into larger-than-life exaggerations, sometimes hideously comical, is amply displayed here. George Payne is a complete bottom, flexing his pecks for Marlene, while at the same time groveling at her high heels. She rewards him with cock torture. Blockheads Steve Tucker and Dave Ruby stick their cocks in the same pussy at the same time. Ruby's routine as a porno photographer is amazingly sleazy and accurate. Out-of-shape Carter Stevens looks like a leftover from the old Hellfire Club. Steve Tucker is filmed against "ALL MALE" theater marquees, coming across as a big closet queen. Film buffs got a kick out of the lifted soundtrack from *Taxi Driver* and the neon-soaked imagery of Times Square.

Like many second-string pornographers, Carter Stevens has a background in filming industrials. Unfortunately, this is evident in the movies he makes, all of which ran repeatedly at the Bryant. The sex-play in his films is frequently as appealing as an auto-parts demonstration. He has an annoying habit of using unattractive, C-list men who work cheap. Stevens' *House of Sin* is a dull supernatural tale with scant interesting moments, such as willowy blonde Tigr performing upside down blowjob acrobatics. Mistress Candice puts her slave (and then-manager) David Christopher through a lengthy 360-degree session showcasing verbal degradation, hair-whipping, tit-smacking, and a piss-soaked climax.

Bizarre Styles stars Vanessa Del Rio as a garment district fashionista with a cadre of perverted female sidekicks, including Annie Sprinkle. Skanky Honey Stevens parades herself in a red leather corset, armed with a red cat-o'-nine-tails. She humiliates her male slave with verbal sewage and whipping, leading to an explosive golden shower. Lovers of dirty sex and sleazy women (paired with off-putting, effete men) were the only individuals who found this film erotic. *Bizarre Styles* has so much balling in bathrooms that the entire movie seemed shot in one.

The most popular Carter Stevens picture to play the Bryant was *Wicked Schoolgirls*, Avon Films' only starring vehicle for their tiny, brunette sadomasochistic dynamo, Velvet Summers. Velvet plays out schoolgirl fetishes, dominates, masturbates, has toilet sex, and fucks practically everyone in the cast. The film's raunchy humor is well integrated with its prurient sex. The best comic scene has Velvet subjugating blockheaded Dave Ruby, who's dressed in garters and a leather bikini. He barks and acts like a dog as "How Much Is That Doggie in the Window?" wafts over the soundtrack. Carter Stevens put this film together with more style and skill than his typical work. *Wicked Schoolgirls* is among his cheapest yet most accomplished films.

Avon 7

Avon 7 was known for premiering the Phil Prince film efforts Avon produced. Heralded by ads in the *New York Post*, they were as explicit as you could get. The ads were created by the Samson advertising agency. Samson did a lot of ad work for pornographers. Those ads let you know just what you were getting. A clear photo of Sharon Mitchell or Annie Sprinkle packed into a whorish corset with ad copy calling her "the biggest pervert in the business," with little chain-links surrounding the borders of the ads.

The Avon 7 was located just across the street from the Doll, on the corner of 48th Street and 7th Avenue, next to Popeye's Fried Chicken, which provided the staff with many a warm meal. Off the sidewalk and down a flight of stairs, you'd enter a relaxed turnstile/counter which also offered Phil's videos for sale for around $100 apiece. The admission to the Avon 7 was steep: $7 for a first-run feature. The theater had been down at the heels in the mid-1970s, but Phil had it spruced up with comfy seats and straightened-up bathrooms, which provided many a happy base party for the live-show teams.

Unlike the other Avon Theaters, it was difficult to skim from the box office. Raymond, a retentive, older Hispanic queen with hair plugs, was the manager and a known fink. He also ran a bodega in Spanish Harlem after 5:00 PM. Leon, the projectionist, suffered from Parkinson's disease. Leon took every prescription and street drug he could get his hands on, and had hookers/porn actresses like Helen Madigan servicing him in the projection booth. Phil Prince liked showing up to peep at the Avon 7 audience watching his pictures. High out of his mind, he'd break into stoned, satisfied grins. Phil was a somebody, for a change.

The Taming of Rebecca was Phil's zenith as a filmmaker, made just after the murder of his wife. Sharon Mitchell runs away from her abusive, incestuous dad, David Christopher. She seeks help from malevolent schoolmarm Stella Stevens and is put in a kinky boarding school, where the students have hetero fisting orgies in the dorm. Everyone is prey for the sadistic Dean of Discipline (George Payne) and his sinister female assistant (Nico). The no-holds-barred climax features Velvet Summers pierced, pissing, and receiving a geyser of torment from Payne and Nico. Genuinely psychotic.

The murder was still playing on Phil's mind when he made *Kneel Before Me*. George Payne marries Annie Sprinkle, and he becomes delusional, believing that he's the Marquis de Sade. George has nightmares of leather masks, piercings, orchestrating the degradation and torture of slaves at S/M orgies. He calls Alan Adrian an asshole as Adrian pees into his own mouth. He puts Annie in bondage and strangles her to death. In desperation, George seeks counsel from a sadistic doctor (Nico). She hypnotizes him, and the nightmares become real and uncontrollable. *Kneel Before Me* is one of Phil's most personal films and had a very successful Avon 7 run.

Dr. Bizarro features Phil speaking directly to you, the viewer. Clad in a barber's coat and frayed bell-bottom jeans, Phil looks like he just got off the basepipe. He plays a psychiatrist who dispenses sexual healing to those in need. Phil presents four case studies of sexual obsessives. George Payne plays a silver-haired man with familial problems, which he solves by giving elfin submissives Ambrosia Fox and Velvet Summers sassy spankings. The female dominance angle is harnessed by leather-clad Cheri Champagne, who knocks around the long-suffering Alan "Spike" Adrian. Entertaining, and worth seeing for Phil's personal, criminally insane presence.

The Avon 7 was packed yet almost reverentially quiet for the opening of Phil's *Forgive Me I Have Sinned*. George Payne plays a perverted priest with a peculiar list of sinners he feels he must reform. Inviting his victims to his church, he hears their confessions, drugs their wine, and holds court over a sadistic orgy. Cheri Champagne humiliates wimpy Martin Patton and gets her comeuppance in a pillory. George gives Ambrosia Fox his special brand of religious instruction. The atmospheric photography, with a visual scheme of red, black, and white, makes this one of Phil's most distinctive films.

Phil Prince's *Story of Prunella* is a criminal's home movie. He captures the ugly look of New York on a gray, rainy November

> ### Vanessa Del Rio gives the submissive performance of a lifetime; you are amazed she went through it.

day. The film was shot in 1983, but it has the look of a decade before. Three prisoners (George Payne, David Christopher, Martin Patton) escape and wreak sexual mayhem. This trio of degenerates crashes Ambrosia Fox's wedding shower, where they explode on Ambrosia, her mother (Dixie Dew), and their two big-titted friends (Joey Carson and Nico). Another vitriolic Payne performance, as he swears, spits, and issues a barrage of terroristic threats that include Oedipal violation. Ambrosia gets put through heavy paces and blows her brains out at the end. Phil places himself in the film in a comic-relief cameo as a bungling cop. *Prunella* had a brief Avon 7 run and was an infrequent replay at other Avon Theaters.

A less depressing and more eccentric Prince premiere was *Oriental Techniques of Pain and Pleasure*. David Christopher drops a Chinese manuscript belonging to an Oriental torture society somewhere in Queens. Annie Sprinkle finds the manuscript and loses it in her apartment. David kidnaps Annie and her pal Debbie Cole, a busty white-trash submissive with a tattoo over one tit. They're taken to a basement with "COCKSUCKING SLUT" spray-painted on the wall. David and George Payne, sporting an odd goatee, abuse them as Nico and Ambrosia Fox masturbate. Annie and Debbie are put in a bondage show where they're tortured by Mistress Candice. Mistress Candice also debases human ashtray Alan Adrian with verbal abuse, clothespin cock torture, and a golden shower. Annie's assailants force her to fist a rotted leather queen playing her brother. Phil Prince turns up at the end to rescue the girls. True to its 42nd Street roots, there's nothing Oriental about the movie, except for the Times Square novelty shop kung-fu jackets and China bowl hats worn by the male leads. *Oriental Techniques* was a real Avon 7 crowd-pleaser.

Painmania is Avon Films' most self-referential movie, entirely shot inside their Paris Theater. Melissa, the late granddaughter of Avon's owner, Murray, has a non-sex role as host "Nora Nookie from WCUM." She interviews various performers in seedy Paris Theater dressing rooms. They describe their supposedly personal dominant or submissive natures and play out S/M skits on the theater's runway. Especially amusing is the interview with the low-paid, ubiquitous muscleman Dave Ruby. Clad in a leather bikini, flexing his pecks, Ruby professes that he "prefers to be dominant" and takes umbrage when Melissa asks him if S/M prevents him from liking normal sex.

There was a payphone booth in the lobby, which afforded Avon's staff a smidgen of privacy while making and taking drug orders.

"What kind of a question is that?!!" David Christopher nervously juggles his balls, declares that he enjoys all forms of sex and loves worshiping beautiful women. Padding out the movie are heavy scenes from other Avon films, like the fisting scene in *Oriental Techniques*. The location work and pseudo-documentary approach make this a must for aficionados of Phil Prince or the Avon Theaters scene.

Savage Sadists and *Den of Dominance*, less than an hour each, played the Avon 7 as a premiere double bill. The films were early, minor directorial efforts by Phil Prince. Authentically seedy, they again mirror Prince's actual life. In *Savage Sadists* Martin Patton sells porn videos as his wife (skank to end all skanks Nicole Bernard) gets assaulted by two thugs (Danny Stevens and David Christopher) at their low-rent split-level house. There is a long, Dadaesque scene of Patton

answering the phone over and over. After Patton fucks his secretary, who's attired in an absurd glitter hat and dress, the wife turns up at his office with the two thugs in hot pursuit. He hides under his desk as they abuse and attack the women.

Den of Dominance features the same cast as *Savage Sadists*. Martin Patton turns up at a saloon where David Christopher is bartender. No alcohol is served. The bar is actually a massage parlor, and the movie turns into a full-fledged, one-room orgy. Featuring petite, brunette, 42nd Street peep-booth women recruited out of Avon's live sex stage shows.

The Avon 7 played its share of clunkers, though, like the Ray Dennis Steckler not-quite-hardcore Nazi movie filled with fart noises, which was yanked after two days due to audience complaints.

In 1983 Avon Films acquired some early 1970s no-budget San Francisco curiosities produced by Mary Thomas and directed by Katrina Lee, and re-released them with new ad campaigns. *Young Girls in Bondage* revolves around the dog fetish. A placard announcing the film's redeeming psychological value appears as *The Good, the Bad and the Ugly* score plays on the soundtrack. A girl is in a cage. Her male partner treats her like a dog, as well as subjecting her to caning, verbal abuse, vibrator torment, and nipple torture. He strings her up in a bed and a doorframe. Turning the tables, she assumes the dominant role and puts him in the dog cage. Then it's the St. Bernard's turn. He's been silently surveying the proceedings. She attacks the hapless pooch, dry humping him all over. *Young Girls in Bondage* concludes with the couple responding to an off-camera interviewer, extolling the psychic benefits of pornographic films.

Young Girls in Bondage was played with another Katrina Lee/Mary Thomas movie, *Begging for It*. *Begging for It* contains some candid and fascinating documentary footage of early 1970s San Francisco peep parlors and dirty theaters. It's intercut with sleazoid loops of hotel-room balling. Two greasy boys have a mixed combo with two soul sisters to the tune of inexplicable classical music. The grand finale features a freewheelin' freak-era denizen in a cowboy hat and a hardboiled broad encased in a corset. This duo fucks atop a Shetland pony. They follow with B&D acts on the horse while they keep their balance. After watching this spectacle, you'll feel like you've spent a night in ol' Tijuana. The amount of overall freakiness in *Begging for It* and *Young Girls in Bondage* made it a thumbs-up double bill for the Avon 7 audience.

In late 1983 the Avon 7 was busted for having hookers work the audience. It then changed into an all-male house, renamed the Park Miller. Phil's last picture and one and only all-male movie premiered there. It was an idea that had been festering in Phil's mind for at least two years. He dictated the script to the Bryant projectionist, Brad, who recalls, "It seemed to be yet another reflection of Phil's life. The story was about a young boy who runs away to New York and winds up at the Port Authority Bus Terminal, giving Phil lots of excuses for location work. The kid gets abused working as an 8th Avenue hustler. He meets an old man who takes care of him. The old man is a member of NAMBLA. The police arrive at the end, breaking up the romance. It was obvious that the whole thing was a dramaturgy of Phil's life with, and affection for, Pat."

The movie was made as *Johnny Boy Blue* and bore scant resemblance to Brad's original script. Many disgusting scenes were thrown in, like fistings with wriggling fingers displayed through stomach lining.

Johnny Boy Blue premiered at the Park Miller and played only three days in November 1984. By the end of those three days, Phil was psychotic, strapped to a gurney, and in jail for a laundry list of crimes. Armed robbery, attempted murder, illegal possession of a firearm, possession of controlled substances, resisting arrest.... The list went on and on. Phil was the patsy that led upward to the Times Square hierarchy. At this point, his insanity made him of little use to anyone. He was cut loose from operations, although Stella kept tabs on him, and George Payne forlornly missed him.

The End

In the mid-1980s, Times Square was being dismantled. Mrs. Wilson had one of her Haitian handymen, Nelson, carry prints like *Confessions of a Psycho Cat* out of the Venus Theater attic and over to the Cameo. The prints were her property. She knew that the video scavengers were hunting for them, and she wanted them safeguarded before the Venus doors got padlocked. One of the last acts Mrs. Wilson performed before her death in the 1990s was to remake the Cameo into her all-male palace named the Adonis, which had been origi-

nally located on 50th Street and 8th Avenue. When the Board of Health belatedly shut the all-male theaters, the Cameo's space was converted into an Indo-Paki peep scumatorium called the Playpen.

The roughie theaters had become lethal due to AIDS. The audience attendance rapidly declined, leaving only the insane behind. The police turned up at the Venus, stated that the theater was being shut by the City of New York, and quietly and gently told the audience and staff to leave. No arrests were made, but Danny, the projectionist, and Wayne, who was the cashier, were out of the careers they had held around the Deuce since the 1960s. Mrs. Wilson died, and her daughter, Bondi Wilson, took over the reins of the operations. Bondi sold the Venus to developers who immediately razed it and turned it into an after-theater Italian tourist trap, the Daniella Restaurant.

Inviting his victims to his church, he hears their confessions, drugs their wine, and holds court over a sadistic orgy.

The Big Apple and the Capri bit the dust at the outset of the 1990s when the city authorities padlocked their doors. As did all the adult houses. Their spaces vacantly sat with neon-orange legal notices plastered to their front doors. It was like a postapocalyptic *Last Picture Show* of AIDS.

The World Theater eventually became another tourist trap bar/restaurant. The Lincoln Art went through various names and permutations, showing art films and Hollywood revivals. At one point it was a showcase for Hindustani musicals, showing how much New York had changed. The Rialto One turned into a Cineplex Odeon. It's now been transformed into a virtual-reality family entertainment center.

By 1996 all traces of the roughie grindhouses were wiped off the face of the earth. But the films, which were the life force of those houses and the blood that ran through their veins, remain. Hate springs eternal.

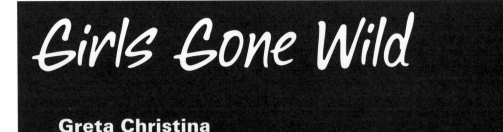

Girls Gone Wild

Greta Christina

The Tease

I'm sure I started seeing the ads around the same time everyone else did. Suddenly, the late-night TV shows were full of them: the pulsating graphics, the loud, leering voice-over, the drunken college girls pulling up their shirts to show their pixelated boobs. The first one I watched in appalled fascination; the next several dozen I flipped away from, disdainful and dismissive and rolling my eyes in amused disbelief.

And, I will now admit, somewhat turned on.

It was the first time in a long time that I'd felt embarrassed about being turned on. To be more precise, it was the first time in a long time that I'd felt embarrassed about *what* was turning me on. I am a happy consumer of very graphic porn, and I typically like my porn kinky and perverted and pretty fucking nasty. I will happily watch (or read about, or look at photos of) young ladies in school uniforms being spanked and fondled by teachers and nuns, or a woman being given an enema and forced to keep it in while she's beaten with a cane, or Rocco Siffredi shoving his cock down a porn actress' throat and holding it there while tears pour down her face. I will watch it, and I will jack off to it, and I will write about it in the national press if I can. But somehow I couldn't admit, even to myself, that I was getting turned on by the "Girls Gone Wild" videos. Or, to be more precise, by the TV ads for the "Girls Gone Wild" videos.

The problem wasn't that they looked exploitative, or that they looked pornographic (if anything, they didn't look pornographic enough). The problem was that they looked tacky. Adolescent. Dumb. The kind of thing yahoo Dartmouth frat boys would jerk off to. I didn't want to admit to even a remote possibility that I shared pornographic tastes with yahoo Dartmouth frat boys.

I have to say, the whole phenomenon puzzled me. I mean, why on earth were these videos so popular? Why were they selling at all? Hardcore video porn is readily available to anyone with a credit card. You can rent it at your local video store or have it discreetly mailed to your home, fast and cheap and no questions asked. You can easily see explicit, seriously graphic videos showing almost any kind of sex you can think of. Why would you pay money for videos where the main feature is drunken college girls showing their boobs?

But I started thinking about it a bit. (Always a dangerous move.) And it occurred to me that "Girls Gone Wild" did seem to offer some things that hardcore porn didn't. Some of it might be the verisimilitude, the easy suspension of disbelief. If you're an ordinary Joe, it's pretty hard to honestly imagine yourself having sex with pornstars. But it's not hard to imagine yourself in a huge, noisy street party, watching uninhibited-for-the-weekend girls pull up their shirts. And it's not much of a stretch to imagine one or more of those uninhibited girls going off with you and doing even wilder things in private.

There was more to it than that, though. For one thing, the "Girls Gone Wild" ads were all about the "reveal," the moment when the woman goes from being covered and decent to being naked and shameless. I love that moment. It just makes me swoon. They don't do it nearly enough in hardcore video porn—and they don't make nearly a big enough deal of it when they do. Hardcore porn is often like a crappy lover—it rushes through the foreplay to get to the "good stuff," so impatient to get off that it ignores the nasty, teasing buildup that makes the good stuff so good. The "Girls Gone Wild" ads held the promise of videos that didn't rush, videos that would give you that lovely, swoony "reveal" moment...over and over and over again.

But I knew that couldn't be the only thing "Girls Gone Wild" had going for it. As much as I personally love the sweet moment of sexual revelation, I found it hard to believe that this was the force driving millions of customers into this company's arms. There was something else "Girls Gone Wild" seemed to offer, something the video-porn industry just doesn't have a grip on: transgression.

I know that sounds weird. How could college girls pulling up their shirts be more transgressive than explicit triple penetration, or rubber enema bondage, or any of the other far-out delicacies the modern porn industry has made available to the general viewing public? Yes, yes, the mainstream porn biz is doing filthy, filthy things, and their marketing departments will natter at great length about how this week's release is pushing the envelope like nothing you've ever seen, totally extreme to the max. Whatever.

Yet as softcore as they obviously were, "Girls Gone Wild" looked like the real deal. "Girls Gone Wild" seemed way more transgressive than hardcore porn—because the girls themselves felt that way. The girls in the TV ads are crossing their own boundaries, breaking their own rules. They aren't "Wild Girls"—they're "Girls Gone Wild," emphasis on the "gone," on the idea that they didn't used to be slutty exhibitionists and you're getting to see them cross that line. They seem like they're probably fairly normal girls when they're not at Mardi Gras or spring break, and they seem to think that what they're doing is naughty and dirty and slutty and bad—and, therefore, way more fun.

And that's something the porn industry just can't give you. I don't care how many guys are jerking off in the actress' face or what she's putting up her butt—she's a professional. She's almost certainly done this before, and if she hasn't done this exact thing, she's sure done plenty of other things that aren't all that different. There's no way that she feels like a good girl breaking the rules, no way she's feeling that sudden exhilaration of stepping over a line and gazing into a bigger and freakier sexual world. She stepped over that line long ago, and she's been in that big, freaky world for a while. I'm not knocking it—I have a lot of respect for professionalism in the porn industry; in fact, I often wish there were more of it. And I like seeing people get nasty when they're comfortable with their bodies and their sexuality. But if what you want is the thrill of watching someone break their own rules and do dirty things they never imagined themselves doing, you aren't going to get it from the Vivid Girls.

Which leads me to the other very special thing that "Girls Gone Wild" seemed to offer...and here's where we start getting into some seriously fucked-up regions of my psychosexual geography. Because the other thing "Girls Gone Wild" appeared to offer was humiliation. Not faked, not acted, not a fantasy. When the girls in "Girls Gone Wild" stepped over that line, it seemed like you'd be getting to watch, real-time, while they shamed themselves: like you'd be watching them let go of their dignity, place themselves in a position of public debasement, offer up their bodies for the crude enjoyment of a leering public eye. While I certainly don't think flashing your boobs in public needs to be any of those things (God knows I've done it enough times, and it didn't feel that way to me), it seemed that these girls would feel that way. The girls in the GGW ads seem like fairly ordinary, non-sex-radical girls, "girls next door," if you will, girls who most of the time would have some degree of modesty and sexual shame. And what you get to see in these videos—or what it seemed from the TV ads that you get to see in these videos—was the moment when they let go of their modesty, and let themselves experience that tingly, twitchy, nakeder-than-naked blend of eroticism and shame. In my fucked-up and deeply kinked little libido, that had more oomph than almost anything mainstream porn could provide.

The more I thought about all this, the more it turned me on. The "Girls Gone Wild" ads went from an occasional bit of fleeting, guilty pleasure when the ads came on, to full-time masturbation material. Interestingly, I never imagined myself as one of the wild girls: I've been around way too many blocks way too many times, and not even in my most fevered sexual imaginings could I picture myself feeling embarrassed

"Girls Gone Wild" seemed way more transgressive than hardcore porn— because the girls themselves felt that way.

or naughty about pulling up my shirt for the camera. (For one thing, I've already done it more than once....) No, my typical "Girls Gone Wild" masturbation fantasy always put me behind the camera. I'm the one enticing the giggling girl to pull up her shirt, or pull down her pants, or take a shower for the camera, or fondle her girlfriend...and I'm the one who's then enticing her to pull down her pants and spread her butt cheeks, or get on all fours in the shower, or turn her naked friend over her lap and spank her while she giggles and writhes, or any of the filthy things I was hoping might be on the videos. And I'm the one making sure my leering eye caught every bit of it on tape.

So finally my curiosity (and my libido) got the better of me. Among other things, I wanted to know if the videos lived up to the promise of the TV ads. Would there, in fact, be more and wilder footage they couldn't show you in the ads? Or was that just a come-on? And my libido was dying to know: Would this actually be a turn-on? Wouldn't an hour or more of drunken, softcore amateur porn and girls pulling up their shirts get a bit dull after a while? Would "Girls Gone Wild" make me reach for my vibrator or reach for the remote? I decided I had to have the courage of my erotic convictions, that a woman of my stature in the sex-positive community shouldn't be afraid of a little bad taste and commercial hype. Besides, nobody but me had to know. (Unless I wrote about it in a big sex anthology or something....)

The Actual Videos

See, all this stuff I've been saying about transgression and humiliation and the moment of sexual revelation—that's just speculation. I've been telling you what's hot about the "Girls

Girls Who Like Girls has one of the sweetest, most touching, most genuine lesbian sex scenes that I've seen in any porn.

Gone Wild" TV ads. I haven't said a damn thing yet about the actual videos.

I wound up getting three "Girls Gone Wild" DVDs: *Girls Gone Wild: Uncensored*, a DVD collection of the first three videos they released; *Girls Gone Wild: Doggy Style*, the one with Snoop Dogg; and *Girls Gone Wild: Bad Girls/Girls Who Like Girls*, a two-DVD set that I hoped, based on the title and the description on their website, would be more explicit than the other videos.

The DVD with their first videos is very much what you probably think of when you think of "Girls Gone Wild": shot after shot of Mardi Gras or spring-break girls pulling up their shirts to show their boobs or pulling down their pants to show their butts and occasionally their pussies, with intermittent footage of moderately more explicit activity. Watching it was very much what I'd expected and feared: tedious, grating, marginally arousing but ultimately a grave disappointment. True, the girls aren't as completely hammered as I'd expected them to be—a lot of them definitely seem tipsy, but none of them are puking-and-falling-down drunk. But apart from that, *Girls Gone Wild: Uncensored* confirmed every nasty, uncharitable thought I'd had when I first rolled my eyes at their stupid TV ads.

Actually, in some ways it was worse. Whatever eroticism there might have been in the sight of girls showing off their goodies to the crowd was all too often disrupted by the sight of unwanted, groping hands reaching into the shot. Ugly, gross, upsetting. The prevalence of fake boobs was disap-

pointing, as well: It's always distressing to see young, attractive, healthy women who've cut their lovely breasts open and replaced them with ugly, plastic blobs. And the sound—a relentless, one-note cacophony of drunken frat-boy hollering and "woo-hoo"ing—was like a jackhammer going in the next room. Even turned way down, it gave me a headache.

And for all the supposedly uninhibited bacchanalianism, those first GGW videos have an odd absence of sexual pleasure. Sure, there's a certain amount of sexual activity along with all the flashing: tit-licking, tit-fondling, butt-smacking, dry-humping, even some brief cunnilingus—most of it girl-girl, with a few guys in on the action—plus pouring beer on tits and similarly idiotic spring-breakitudes. But almost none of it seemed like the girls were doing it to get off. It seemed like they were doing it for show, for the crowd and the camera and the shock value. The fondling and such usually didn't last very long, and it didn't look focused, and the girls didn't seem all that interested or turned on, and it typically ended with them collapsing in fits of "I can't believe I just did that" giggles.

I'm not saying they weren't enjoying themselves—most of them seemed to be. I'm saying that the pleasure they were seeking didn't seem to be sexual. Not physically sexual, anyway. I think they were enjoying the attention, the recognition of their beauty and hotness, the power they had to get the crowd worked up, the exuberant thrill of the forbidden, the triumph of going further than the other girls and being the baddest and bravest and hottest and most attention-getting of all.

Not that there's anything wrong with that. I'm not one of those puritanical feminists who think seeking sexual attention is an automatic sign of poor self-esteem. I think that's crap. We're social animals; we seek attention in a zillion different ways, and seeking sexual attention is no more screwed-up than seeking attention for your art or athleticism or intellect. I'm saying that there's a huge difference between sex done for sex's sake and sex done for show. (I used to work as a stripper, so I'm intimately familiar with that difference.) And the latter is a whole lot less interesting to watch.

In *Uncensored*, you could usually tell when it was real and when it wasn't, when a girl was letting another girl grope her to get the crowd screaming, and when she was doing it for the pleasure of a hand on her breast. The times that it seemed real were actually pretty hot, even kind of beautiful. But those moments were few and far between, and they didn't last very long (nothing in this video lasts very long), and if anything, they made the rest of the video that much more frustrating. (*Girls Gone Wild: Doggy Style* was much the same in all the abovementioned ways, only with better production values, a lot less spontaneity, and intermittent footage of Snoop Dogg irrelevantly wandering through the action and blathering.)

I'll admit there's a certain hotness to it all: for many of the reasons I mentioned at the start of this piece, plus a few more I'll get to later. After a couple of hours with *Girls Gone Wild: Uncensored*, I was definitely ready to head into the bedroom for a session with the vibrator. But the images in my head weren't the ones I'd just seen. They were the ones I'd hoped to see, the ones I'd wanted to see and hadn't. That's not what I want from my porn. Even my softcore, frat-boy reality porn.

Which is why I'm glad I got more than one DVD. Because *Girls Gone Wild: Bad Girls/Girls Who Like Girls* is a whole other kettle of wax.

I am still somewhat embarrassed to admit this in public, but this video is surprisingly hot. Like, really. Like, I thought about it obsessively for days after I first saw it. For one thing, *Bad Girls/Girls Who Like Girls* is rather more explicit than *Uncensored* or *Doggy Style*. The brief scenes of girls pulling up their shirts and making out in the streets are accompanied by longer, more elaborate scenes of girls in hotel rooms: seriously fooling around or even having flat-out, unabashed lesbian sex. It's much less of a titty show and much more something resembling actual porn.

This does make the video hot—but not just for the obvious reasons. It makes the video hot because it gives it some variety and some direction. *Bad Girls/Girls Who Like Girls* has an actual arc of arousal: The eroticism builds, unfolds, starts with a gentle tease, and gradually gets nastier and more serious. The flashing doesn't just go on and on *ad nauseam*; it starts somewhere, then takes you somewhere else, seduces you and draws you in, with increasingly greater delights and the promise of still greater delights yet to come. It's still a tease, but it's a fun tease, a tease with a purpose, a tease that actually results in something other than the repetition and frustration and "one note endlessly blaring" quality of *Uncensored* and *Doggy Style*.

But there's something else cool and special about *Bad Girls/Girls Who Like Girls*. It has the unique payoff of a documentary or really good reality TV: You don't know what's going to happen next. Nobody knows what's going to happen next. Not the camera guys, maybe not even the girls themselves. It's not like a standard porn movie, where you and everyone else knows that the blowjob will be followed by fucking, followed by anal, followed by the money shot. There's suspense, doubt about how far they're going to take it. As a result, there's sexual tension. Real sexual tension, the kind you get when you're making out with someone for the first time and you don't know how far things are going to go.

Of course, GGW isn't the only reality porn on the market. You can get "real couples having real sex" videos elsewhere. I've seen many of them—they're hot; I like them. But *Bad Girls/Girls Who Like Girls* is different from those; not necessarily better, but different in a way I appreciated. It has a spontaneous quality, with a sense of adventure and a spur-of-the-moment flavor that's hard to find in standard porn. Even with the most authentic, unscripted, do-your-own-thing "real couples" video, you know that the filming was scheduled and planned well in advance, that the couples thought carefully about what to wear and what toys to bring and maybe even what sex acts to do. There's a huge difference between that—between videos of long-term couples carefully choosing to explore their loving sexual connection in a public forum—and giggling party girls getting crazy with each other in a hotel room because a "Girls Gone Wild" camera guy asked them to and they decided, "What the fuck." These are both good things, but they're good in different ways, and the latter definitely has charms that the former doesn't.

Finally...I don't quite know how to say this, but the hotel-room scenes in *Bad Girls/Girls Who Like Girls* are just fun. Enormously and infectiously fun. The three girls in the hotel room in *Bad Girls*—Rachel, Amy, and Rebecca—are hilarious. Playful, giggly, trash-talky, vivacious, they're natural exhibitionists, into each other as much as they're into being on camera. They're clearly no innocents: They know their way around each other's bodies and their own, and they're more than just a tiny bit kinky. But they're not jaded or bored either, and they still have enough reticence and modesty to make it fun and nasty when you watch them overcome it.

And *Girls Who Like Girls* has one of the sweetest, most touching, most genuine lesbian sex scenes that I've seen in any porn—and that includes by-lesbian-for-lesbian porn. Michelle and Christine, the young women in the hotel room, are real lovers—Michelle has doofy argyle socks under her sexy black boots, and they talk during the lulls about their sucky job schedule that keeps them apart—with genuine affection and a few years behind them. For them, it's not about giggly exhibitionism: It's about deep love and pleasure. The raucous party you can hear outside the room only emphasizes the sweet, peaceful joy inside it, and the sex is so authentic it makes your heart stop. When they're giggling and wrestling, there's not even a hint of, "Oh my God, I can't believe I'm doing this," or, "Did the camera get that angle?" Their sex is stunningly real, with real kissing and real fingerfucking and real cunnilingus. You can tell the cunnilingus is real because they aren't pulling their heads back and sticking their tongues out and lapping away to give the camera a good shot. The footage is less explicit than most mainstream porn...but that's not because the sex is less authentic. It's because the sex is more authentic. It's because they're fucking for each other, not for the camera. And it's so fucking beautiful that it almost made me cry.

Now, before you run off to the GGW website with your drooling mouth hanging open and your credit card in your quivering hand, I should make something very, very clear: This is not nature's perfect porn. This is a seriously mixed bag. Even though *Bad Girls/Girls Who Like Girls* is nastier and more authentic by far than the other GGW videos I saw, there's still an element of doing it for show instead of for pleasure—not nearly as much as in *Uncensored* and *Doggy Style*, but still more than there should be. There's also way too much sameness among the girls: While the GGW videos aren't anywhere near as homogenous as a mainstream porno, the girls are still overwhelmingly young, slender—and white, white, white. And the unscriptedness means that tempting ideas often get dangled under our noses only to be dropped or ignored. I was so very titillated when Rebecca in *Bad Girls* said she had "dirty, kinky titties that need to be punished"...and so very disappointed when neither Rachel nor Amy picked up on this charmingly obvious hint and obliged her.

Worst of all, the camera guys in the hotel-room scenes are often annoying, even intrusive. You can hear them talking to the girls while they're taping, and thus you can hear them not being able to shut the hell up. They offer their own running commentary on the action, commentary that (for the most part) adds nothing to the *mise-en-scène* except yahoo-dude stupidity and annoyance. And their intermittent directions to the girls interrupt the spontaneity, imposing (or trying to impose) what they want to see over the natural flow of what the girls want to do.

I did enjoy *Bad Girls/Girls Who Like Girls*. I even enjoyed it a lot, certainly far more than I'd expected. But I can't be 100% sure that I would have liked it as well if my expectations hadn't been so low.

But What Does It All Mean?

What does it all add up to? Was my pre-having-any-actual-information analysis anywhere near on target? What is the place of GGW in the socio-sexual landscape? The politico-economic landscape? What do I think of these videos as a dyke, as a sex radical, as a radical feminist, as a porn aficionado? Were my expectations fulfilled? How would I rate them on a scale of one to ten? Would I recommend these videos to a friend?

Well, let's see. With a few notable exceptions, my pre-actually-seeing-the-damn-videos analysis wasn't that far off. The girls weren't nearly as drunk as I'd thought they'd be, so I

was definitely wrong there. And the whole humiliation angle pretty much dissolved as soon as I started watching. The girls seem perfectly happy to be showing their boobs or making out or whatever, and most of them are quite brazen about it. There is a certain glimmer of the humiliation thing which I'll get to in a moment, but for the most part, that just didn't pan out. (Somewhat to my disappointment, but mostly to my relief—I was actually pretty uncomfortable with the thought of getting off on real-life, real-time sexual shame, no matter how compelling the idea seemed.)

But the verisimilitude, the transgression, the moment of the reveal—all of these were there in trumps. Even in the crappy videos that sucked, they were there. If anything, I underestimated the importance of the reveal. The simple sight of naked boobs is definitely not the main point—the pulling up of the shirt, the moment of naked-boob revelation, is very much the point here. That's not just a lucky triggering of my quirky personal kinks—it's a decision on the part of the producers, an intentional triggering of what seems to be a lot of people's kinks. There's actually one scene in *Girls Who Like Girls* where the camera guy asks one of the girls to *pull her pants back up*, so she could pull them down again. (He was trying to get her coordinated with her friend, and it clearly wasn't enough to have two naked butts onscreen at the same time—he wanted the simultaneous reveal, the two naked butts being bared at the same moment.)

The GGW producers know that the reveal and the transgression are hot, and they market accordingly. According to Bill Horn, vice president of marketing and communications for Mantra Entertainment (the parent company of "Girls Gone Wild"), "There's something about watching that girl go over the line: go over from, 'Come on, do you want to, do you want to go wild, no no no'—and then you see, right there, she does go wild. That's appealing to people." That was a little distressing, actually: to find out that my brilliant, sex-radical, sex-theorist theory was actually part of their goddamn marketing plan....

But I can see why. If they'd shot, say, an hour and a half of footage at a topless beach in Italy or Spain, with half-naked women casually swimming or reading or sunning themselves, it'd be unbelievably dull. It's the moment of exposure, and the girl's own excitement at that moment of exposure, that makes it exciting. There are, in fact, a few scenes in GGW of girls just dancing around topless—and they're definitely less enticing than the flashing.

Interestingly, a lot of the flashing scenes end with the girl pulling her shirt back down over her breasts. (Or pulling her pants back up. Or whatever.) This lends credence to the whole "good girl crossing a line" theory: When she covers back up, you're reminded that she really is a girl next door going wild and not just your garden variety exhibitionist slut. And it's also where the faint glimmer of humiliation finally comes in. It's true that I didn't see much sexual shame when the girls pulled their shirts up to show off their boobs. But I did get a whiff of it when they pulled their shirts back down to cover them again. In that moment, you do see the return of modesty, the hyper-awareness of lost dignity seen in the attempt to regain it. Call it the "what the fuck did I just do?" moment, if you don't want to be so high-falutin'. It's subtle, but it's definitely there. And while I doubt they were purposely screwing around with kinky shame fetishes, the "Girls Gone Wild" editors clearly made a deliberate effort to include that moment—again and again.

Are the girls being exploited? Arguably. In the strict Marxist sense of being used to make money for someone else without being proportionately paid for their labor, certainly. They're being paid for their labor in T-shirts and Mardi Gras beads—that pretty much settles that. But it's also clear that the girls are getting something out of it: They like the attention; they get off on exhibitionism; they enjoy feeling sexy and wild; they like having an excuse to do dirty things they wouldn't ordinarily do. Money isn't the only thing you get out of being in a dirty video, and it may not even be the most important thing, especially if you're not a pro. I myself performed for an adult video for no money back in my salad days, for a small, indie, low-low-budget lesbian porn company (*Clips* by Fatale Video, if you want to look it up). If anyone said the producers were exploiting me, I'd be sorely tempted to smack them. I was a grown-up. I wanted to do it; I got what I wanted out of it, and I don't regret it. And I don't like being patronized by being told that I didn't know what I was doing.

For what it's worth, the GGW producers make the argument that they don't pay the girls because the whole point of the videos is the amateur vibe, and if they offered money they'd be sure to get pros in the mix. A strict Marxist would probably say they were full of shit, but having seen the videos (and not being a strict Marxist), I do see their point. There was one extremely dirty dirty-dancing scene in *Bad Girls* where I suspect that the girl was a stripper...and while I love and adore strippers, my suspicions did make the scene less hot.

Are the GGW producers taking advantage of the wild girls' drunkenness and poor judgment? Will the girls regret it later? Possibly. If a Girl Gone Wild wants to run for President or something, almost certainly. A lot of us have done things in our youths that we now regret and can't take back. (My entire first relationship leaps to mind.) That's part of how we learn, how we grow, what makes us who we are, blah blah blah. And telling people—especially women—that they can't make decisions—especially sexual decisions—because they're in-

experienced and impulsive...it's beyond patronizing. It's so far beyond patronizing that it moves into contempt. Besides, I saw way less flat-out drunkenness in the GGW videos than I was expecting. Tipsiness, yes. High spirits, yes. Impaired judgment, probably. Drunkenness to the point of obliterating consent—no. And anyway, according to that nice publicity man, Mr. Horn, any Girl Gone Wild who changes her mind can get her footage pulled, as long as she does it before the video is edited. (If she changes her mind after the video's been edited, she has to pay for the extra production costs of yanking her scenes. And if she changes her mind after the video's been released, tough beans—she's a grown-up, and she gets to live with her decisions.)

Now, Mantra was successfully sued in mid-2005 by a woman who gave them a verbal okay to being filmed for "Girls Gone Wild" but later said she was too drunk to fully understand the consequences. But the case didn't seem to be about whether she actually was too drunk to consent; the crux was that they filmed her in Virginia, where you have to get written permission to use someone's image commercially. So while the GGW folks obviously aren't as careful about consent issues (legal or personal) as they somewhat piously claim to be, I'm not sure this lawsuit really changes anything ethically.

So where am I now with all this? After spending I don't even know how many hours watching six "Girls Gone Wild" videos on three DVDs (plus one "Guys Gone Wild" disc—I swear to God, I thought it was just a joke on the *Onion*, but there really is one), what am I left with?

Weirdly enough, I'm very much where I was when I started. I'm still dismissive (although rather less so), still fascinated, turned on, embarrassed about being fascinated and turned on—and despite having seen several of the videos, still kind of curious. The whole tease thing is remarkably effective; if it doesn't leave you completely frustrated, it leaves you ravenous for more, hoping to be taken just a little further the next time. I'm disappointed and frustrated with most of these videos; in fact, I'm wondering what the hell I'm going to do with them now...and yet I'm finding myself seriously tempted to get one of the new ones. *Island Orgy/Daddy's Little Girls*, if you want to know. The GGW website promises that "you'll witness sexy 18-year-old Amber loose [*sic*] her virginity to another girl" and that "sweet young things corrupt each other when Daddy's not around," and I keep thinking that this could be another *Bad Girls/Girls Who Like Girls*, with the great, nasty scenes in the hotel rooms. I also know I can't get the thing in time for my deadline, so I can't even justify it as research or a business expense. So I keep trying to think of someone else I can write it up for, so I can write it off on my taxes...and so I can order it without admitting that I just want to use it to get off.

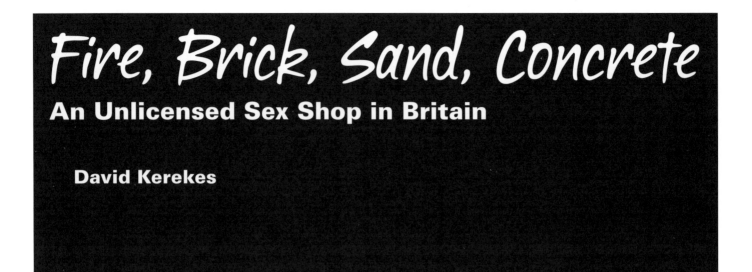

Fire, Brick, Sand, Concrete

An Unlicensed Sex Shop in Britain

David Kerekes

The legal availability of hardcore pornography in the United Kingdom is only a relatively recent phenomenon. Whether in magazines or on video, up until 2000—the year in which hardcore was effectively legalized in the UK—an erect penis or penetration constituted the loose benchmark for what was considered hardcore, and any depiction thereof or anything more gratuitous was taboo. Possession itself was not an offense, but the means of obtaining it generally were. Because of numerous statutes—notably the Obscene Publications Act of 1959, the Post Office Act of 1953, the Customs Act of 1876, and the Video Recordings Act of 1984—hardcore pornography under British law could not be imported, published, sold, or distributed.

As they do today, sex shops prior to the legalization of hardcore required a license, which meant that the stock had to

These tended to be watered-down versions of magazines available in more liberal countries like Denmark or the Netherlands.

adhere to the law or there was the risk of a police raid, prosecution, a fine, and possibly a jail sentence. Contrary to what the staff would promise in some of these establishments, the magazines lining the shelves may have looked like the real thing, with tantalizing covers bearing titles recognizable as the European trademark of porn quality (such as *Color Climax* or *Rodox*), but in reality it was often a deception: These tended to be watered-down versions of magazines available in more liberal countries like Denmark or the Netherlands, substandard reproductions that removed the hardcore altogether.

Worse still, sometimes the covers were the most hardcore

element of the whole deal, the covers having been removed from the genuine article in order to mask softcore magazines of a sort readily available from any high street news agent. Imagine the frustration and disappointment of dashing home, tearing open the shrink-wrap and finding that the promise of unadulterated hot, steamy sex was in fact a several-month-old edition of *Razzle*—having cost four or five times the price one would normally expect to pay for such a thing.

The videos in licensed sex shops bear the R18 certificate. As with most material released theatrically and on video in the UK, these were films passed by the British Board of Film Classification (BBFC). Despite the fact that the sale of product rated R18 was restricted to sex shops and therefore only available to a discerning few, their content still had to conform to strict guidelines, and in reality the tapes were only marginally more explicit than regular 18-rated films, which were available anywhere.

Prior to 1997, the difference between the two ratings was that R18 allowed the depiction of non-explicit group sex and came with the somewhat ridiculous category guideline: outer labia in, inner labia out. Films were submitted to the BBFC in accordance with this criteria (it would be foolish and expensive not to, given the cost of getting a film examined by the BBFC), whether they had been shot in Britain, like the "Ben Dover" series—available overseas uncut—or imported, like the "Buttman" adventures, cut accordingly.

These were the licensed sex shops. Unlicensed sex shops were an altogether different matter—they operated within a twilight zone that was outside of the law but carried a thin veneer of legitimacy in that they didn't exactly call themselves sex shops.

In order for a shop to avoid being branded a sex shop, it had to carry a proportionally larger stock of non-sex material. The ratio works out at around 10% of smut to the banks of dusty old novels, racks of discarded hobbyist magazines, and boxes of long-playing vinyl at the front of the shop.

The porn on sale in unlicensed sex shops was, and remains, the real deal: uncut, unrated, and unlawful. That's where their appeal lay. Unlicensed sex shops didn't have to conform, and the promise of hardcore and a diversity of it is what drew the customers.

This is where I come in.

✕✕

Sometime around the mid-1990s, I was asked if I wanted to earn some easy money in the run-up to Christmas. The job on offer consisted of working only one and a half days a week—Friday afternoon and all day Saturday—but the pay was exceptionally good. It had to be.

Hardcore pornography was illegal in the UK, but in the center of Manchester, on a busy intersection next to a takeaway café on the one side and a flash car showroom on the other, stood an unassuming bookshop.

Once an essential haunt for record collectors, comic collectors, readers of choice sci-fi, cosmic literature, and perusers of a broad assortment of zines, Bookchain was situated on Peter Street just off Deansgate, one of the main thoroughfares through the city. In its heyday it was a place that pumped loud rock music into the streets and boasted a clientele that included Manchester luminaries and misfits, movers and shakers, such as Mark E. Smith (of the Fall), Pete Shelley (of the Buzzcocks), TV presenter (and star of *24 Hour Party People*) Tony Wilson, and others.

Densely packed with books on the ground floor, as a regular visitor in the early 1980s, my own favorite part of the shop was downstairs with the boxes of comics (predominately b&w ones published by Warren), film magazines, and more esoteric fare. As the years rolled by, the stock seemed to stagnate and, its halcyon days in decline, my field trips became less frequent. Now its patrons consisted of passersby and the die-hards who steadfastly trawled a regular route through the city's dwindling book emporiums in the hope that something new and unusual might still be found.

But mostly it was those who came for porn. These people kept the place going.

For all intents and purposes, the place was now an unlicensed sex shop: 10% smut, 90% everything else.

Bookchain—along with other center premises, House on the Borderland and Orbis Books—was owned by Savoy, the Manchester-based publishing house responsible for the controversial "Meng & Ecker" comics (issue number one was found obscene and is now banned in Britain), with a long and cool history of fighting the Man. Their books range from an early volume on James Dean by a young Morrissey to, more recently, an unexpurgated edition of Colin Wilson's novel *The Killer* and *Fuck Off and Die*, a new volume of "Meng & Ecker" strips. Their book *Lord Horror*, written by Savoy cofounder David Britton, ended up in court on charges of anti-Semitism but was acquitted. Author Jon Farmer has described Savoy as almost single-handedly inventing alternative culture.

I accepted the job of working in Bookchain. It was common knowledge that the place was owned by Savoy, but no paperwork bound them to the premises. There was nothing to link them. The paper trail stopped dead with the guy who offered me the job—a young man whom, for the sake of argument, we will call "Bob."

There was good reason why Savoy didn't want a link between itself and the frontline. Its shops were raided by police and emptied of stock on a regular basis. At first it was bootleg records—Savoy was at the center of Operation Moonbeam in 1979, a sting described in the press as the "smashing of

Unlicensed sex shops were an altogether different matter—they operated within a twilight zone.

the biggest bootleg ring in the UK." This landed Savoy with a heavy fine that threatened to close it down. Then, when James Anderton—self-professed "God's Cop"—became Chief Constable of Manchester Police, there followed raids aplenty as Anderton made it his mission to clean up the city. The Chief Constable held a particular dislike for Savoy, and material that was readily available elsewhere around the country was targeted for seizure in Manchester.

All told, Savoy was raided something like 50 times over the years.

If it was going to be raided for paperback books and relatively innocuous fetish magazines, Savoy decided it might as well go the whole hog and stock harder material.

I can mention Savoy and the Bookchain shop now because the shop is no more, demolished as part of the rejuvenation scheme that is systematically wiping the heritage from the city. As David Britton told me: "It's a different time now, and the powers that be cannot touch us in the same way."

David Britton: It was only during the last six years

of our reign that we sold hard porn. The police, as I saw it, gave me no option. Mike [Butterworth, cofounder and business partner] and I had been taken to the Eleventh Floor (one floor down from Chief Anderton's office) in Stretford House and interviewed about *Lord Horror* and *Meng & Ecker*. The police greatly disapproved of these titles. We had a strong feeling that our time was up as proprietors of bookshops on the high streets of Manchester. Again, if you remember, my first prison sentence was in Strangeways, just for selling paperbacks. Now, the police told me, they were going to get me sent down one way or another. They had me in court two or three times on *Janus*-related material [a spanking magazine published in Britain].

I could see the writing on the wall, and I sold heavy porn under their noses and in their faces, unleashing a flurry of hard pornography on city center Manchester. This in turn encouraged other shops to do the same, so in the end the police only had themselves to blame for the cumulus of filth that dropped on them.

I got the job. There was no formal interview or any interview of any kind—my face was known because I used to visit the shop. I had no contract. Cash was in hand.

The shop was not a patch of its former self. The downstairs—once a comics emporium—was closed off to the public and no better than a tip, with rubbish and bits of furniture strewn about. All the stock was kept at ground level, the store stra-

"In the end the police only had themselves to blame for the cumulus of filth that dropped on them."

tegically divided by racks of books and revolving magazine stands. To the right of the counter was a small section where pornographic magazines were shelved. A handwritten note pinned to a wall warned that this section was open to adults only and that no browsing was allowed.

A good deal of the pornography on display was hardcore and imported from Holland (through various nefarious channels). Lining the shelves were copies of explicit straight and gay magazines sealed in plastic bags and given a price tag often in excess of £40 [approximately US$70]. It's a price that seems as expensive now as it did back then, but a price that people were willing to pay for a product not legally obtainable.

Hardcore videos were also offered, but the sale of these was somewhat more discreet, and tapes were hidden in the vari-

ous holes, nooks, and crannies about the place. As the building was very old and had a dilapidated basement, these hiding places were many.

None of the hardcore videotapes carried proper covers—or covers at all, for that matter. They were dupes created by whom I don't know. A couple of them were stored in the hollow beneath a loose slat of the wooden steps leading to the basement. Other tapes could be found behind loose bricks in the walls.

David Britton: If I remember rightly, you did Fridays and Saturdays with Bob amongst the dying embers of what had been a fantastic shop in its heyday. Do you remember all those video titles I used to think up? *Cuntsucking in Ackrington*, *Muffdiving in Oldham*, *Whorewives of Radcliffe*, even. Or didn't Bob carry on with that?

Unfortunately, Bob didn't. A less imaginative method of identification was utilized while I was there. Tapes were labelled *Fire* or *Sand* or *Concrete* or whatever—a seemingly random code that carried no obvious indication as to what films were featured on what tapes, nor what particular sexual peccadillo. Different tapes were geared towards specific tastes, but I can only assume that identification lay in the places they were stored around the shop.

Like all sex shops, customers were encouraged to return with a half-price exchange policy towards their next purchase.

I have several surreal memories about working in Bookchain, some of them relating to conversations Bob would have with confused customers pertaining to videotapes.

Bob: "Have you had *Brick*?"

Customer: "*Brick*? No, I don't think so. I've had *Slate*. I think."

David Britton: It had taken me years to work out that you could sell more porn tapes if you glossed them over with local references. The incentive for the punter was that he would perhaps get a raunchy sight of his next-door neighbour, or even his mother-in-law. If you sold this homemade, cottage-industry type of tape, you discovered they parted with their £35 with greater alacrity. These outsold all the *Color Climax*es and *Rodox*es ten to one. Of course, the tapes bore no relation to the title, but there was still some damn good action on them, all pervert approved!

Circumventing the need to carry a sex shop license, the "front" for Bookchain was the musty old pulp novels, true-crime magazines, and music papers. Some of the general stock was occasionally interesting but mainly decrepit. For instance, I found in the back of the shop a half-dozen sealed cardboard boxes covered in dust, which didn't look to have been touched or opened for about fifteen years. I pulled off the perished sticking tape that clung to the first box and found inside scrapbooks containing a collection of news clippings—all relating to music groups of the Merseybeat era. The scrapbooks were comprehensive and should have been in a library or museum.

"Who does this belong to?" I asked Bob. But he didn't know and wasn't particularly interested.

I didn't bother looking in the other boxes. They were filthy—I'd need to wash my hands, and there was no running water in Bookchain, so I let them be.

☖☖

There was a deep-rooted feeling of paranoia that came with working in the place. The feeling dispersed somewhat in the short time I was there but never went away completely. I was warned about this. According to Bob, in order to function you had to suppress the thought that you might get busted by the police at any moment.

If a bust did come, I was advised that I should pretend I was a customer.

The insidious paranoia was not helped by the fact that Manchester's central police station was situated over the road, a mere two- or three-minute walk from the shop front.

On more than one occasion, I thought the raid had come. Whenever police walked past the shop front—invariably with a "we've got you marked" expression on their faces—I half-expected them to make a dive for the door with a notice of seizure. One morning the outside of the shop was cordoned off, but it transpired that Frank Bruno, the boxer, was due to arrive in town to star in panto,* and the whole of the thoroughfare was being closed to traffic. Seeing as the police had started with the shop—which was neither at one end of the street nor the other, but in the middle—I figured it to be some kind of dark on-duty humor.

Did I really think that a raid would be telegraphed with the use of police cones? I wasn't thinking straight.

In the end, no raid happened while I was at Bookchain…although a priest did come into the shop once, and on another occasion someone spat at us in disgust.

Every few hours, into the basement Bob would go for a smoke. The place had noise blaring out the door, reeked of dope, and was a target for police harassment. It was a com-

bination that didn't make for an easy mind.

I decided I would stick the job out until Christmas. Any longer and I would have gone insane—not necessarily with the anticipation of being busted but out of boredom. The shop was never particularly busy. A dozen sales on a Saturday afternoon was pretty good going. On a bad afternoon, you might manage only a single sale. Most people who came into the shop came for pornography (I loved it whenever anyone bought anything else), and you had to watch that they didn't steal anything…or at least at first I thought that was the reason I was watching them. I later figured I watched them for something to do.

Other distractions consisted of a cassette player with which Bob listened to old rock'n'roll at a volume that positively invited trouble, and a temperamental TV set with built-in VCR on which we played *Two-Lane Blacktop* and filled the shop with the sounds of a revving Chevy. The Chevy noises and rock'n'roll made it difficult for customers to communicate with us, not that many ever did, but occasionally one would have a question or a complaint.

A good deal of the porn that Bookchain carried was of a fetish variety, in particular spanking material—that peculiarly quaint British relish. One day an unhappy gentleman returned a videotape.

"I like a bit of spanking," the customer said, "but this is ridiculous."

According to Bob, in order to function you had to suppress the thought that you might get busted by the police at any moment.

Bob asked whether there was a fault with the tape and placed the thing in the VCR. The screen came to life with a man bringing his palm down on a woman's naked bottom. Except the whole thing was played in slow motion, enhanced by an effect that gave the scene an audio and visual echo. It was annoying, to say the least. The hand would come down slowly, leaving behind a trail of hands. Impact. The sound of a slap-slap-slap-slap, fading. The hand slowly lifted. Down again. Slap-slap-slap-slap.

Bob hit the fast-forward button. It was a little further into the tape, but the same scene was still being acted out, only the audio and visual delay had gotten longer.

"Not a fault as such…" the guy said.

It didn't make good business sense to hand back cash to a customer, and it never happened while I was there. The guy went away with a replacement tape instead.

There is a pattern to the way that people buy pornography. Not counting the compulsive browsers (like the chirpy post-office worker who came in every morning to look at the magazine covers), most everyone slotted into one of two specific porno consumer types.

The first type would come into the shop and start with the sci-fi section—the farthest point from the porn—the impression being conveyed that they were having a casual, leisurely browse. Making their way around every single book, comic, and magazine, they would finally, inevitably arrive at—*hello, what's this?*—the porn section. A routine adhered to on each and every visit to the shop, this browser wanted to impress that he had no real interest in porn but bought it out of curiosity.

"I like a bit of spanking," the customer said, "but this is ridiculous."

The other type of customer would stride in with a sense of purpose, always stop to make small talk on his way to the pornography and stop again on his way back. These were folk for which pornography was clearly not a hang-up—and they wanted you to know it.

People rarely bought porn if there was a woman present in the shop, and anyone in the porn section would surreptitiously slip into another section—or out of the shop altogether—until the threat of woman had passed.

There were, of course, some nonconformists. But these were invariably customers who were illiterate or not of sound mind. One young man brought to the counter a video that carried an 18 certificate (e.g., it was a legit release) and asked me to read to him the blurb on the back cover (I hesitate to use the word *synopsis*). It was such a left-field request that I complied and read aloud the ridiculous hyperbole. On returning the tape to the shelf, however, he came back with a second tape and the same request. I told him I wasn't reading another sleeve blurb. He claimed he was illiterate; I claimed the blurb didn't matter.

On another occasion, another young man brought to the counter a videotape. He looked insecure, and I got the impression he was mentally challenged. The video was part of a series depicting *Playboy* models lounging around in swimsuits and looked tame even by softcore standards. I asked him if he wanted the tape in a bag. Without daring to look up

and without daring to speak, he nodded. I felt like giving him the tape for nothing.

Both Bob and myself were surprised when one day a smartly attired gentleman laid down cash for porn as a woman was standing at the counter. Not only that, he then pointed to a film fanzine on display that featured a suggestive image from Pete Walker's *House of Whipcord* on its cover and said, "I'll have that, too."

One of the curious things about my time working in a porn shop was that I never bothered to look at any porn. Of course, I saw the covers on display and flicked through magazines that were brought in for exchange to ensure that everything was in order, but I never felt the urge to look through the stuff for kicks.

On Christmas Eve, my last day of employment, I was sorry and relieved at the same time. Doing nothing all day was pretty taxing. But the job had its perks: Money was the biggest, and I cannot imagine there are many employers who actively encourage smoking and drinking (I didn't do the former but a lot of the latter—polystyrene cups of coffee from the café next door complemented with large shots of whiskey as protection from the cold).

Although I no longer worked there, I continued to pop into Bookchain from time to time—more often than not to drop off publications from Headpress, my own publishing outfit—until it closed its doors and got knocked down along with the rest of the block.

As unlicensed sex shops in Britain go, Bookchain was not a typical representation. Arguably, it wasn't even a sex shop—it never used to be, but that's how it ended up.

Every place around the country selling smut on the sly will have its idiosyncratic origins, its stories to tell. I've a few more myself with this one, the last of the Savoy shops, but they were crushed beneath the rubble on Peter Street.

David Britton: Wish you could have seen our shops in the seventies. They really were something else, and to see M. John Harrison wrapping up *Big Bouncy Ones From Jamaica* was an education. I do miss those days of piracy and excess in that square-mile center of Manchester we called Savoyland.

* A British form of pantomime theater often performed at Christmastime.

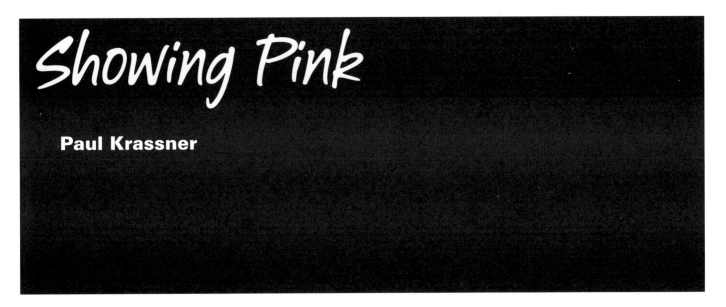

Showing Pink

Paul Krassner

As *Penthouse* magazine was on its way to bankruptcy, publisher Bob Guccione said, "The future has definitely migrated to electronic media." And *Hustler* publisher Larry Flynt—who eagerly joined that migration—has complained, "If you ever cruise the Net and see everything that's available, it's glutted with sleaze. It's a nightmare out there. This has to be affecting the revenues of people like myself."

But both have played pivotal roles in the evolution of popular pornography. Men's magazines had started out showing breasts but not nipples, buttocks but not anuses—and never, *never* a vagina. Nor did pubic hair used to be all over the place, only to eventually get bikini-waxed out of existence except for occasional exclamation points. Even nudist magazines had once airbrushed men and women into genitalia-free department-store mannequins playing volleyball.

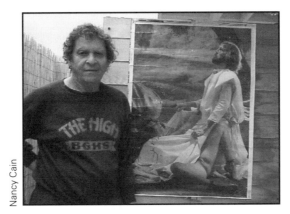

Paul Krassner stands beside his poster of the *"Jesus and the Adulteress"* shot that Hustler *never ran.*

The great pubic breakthrough occurred in *Penthouse* in 1971. A triangular patch of dark, curly hair eventually opened Pandora's box wider and wider until *Hustler* began "showing pink" in 1974. Even Flynt's own wife, Althea, showed pink. One issue featured a scratch-'n'-sniff centerspread. When you scratched the spread-eagled model in her designated area, a scent of lilac bath oil emanated from her vulva.

In November 1977, Larry Flynt was flying with Ruth Carter Stapleton, the evangelist sister of President Jimmy Carter, in Flynt's pink private jet, which, when it belonged to Elvis Pres-

ley, had been painted red, white, and blue. Up in the air, Flynt had a vision of Jesus Christ. Flynt's entire body was tingling, and he fell to his knees, clasping his hands in prayer. Thus was he converted to born-again Christianity.

The next month, at *Hustler*'s Christmas party, Flynt announced that I was going to be the new publisher. This was the first that I had heard the news. Before, I had been wondering how the magazine would change, and now it turned out that I was the answer to my own question. For Flynt to bring *me* in as redeeming social value was an offer too absurd to refuse.

Now that Flynt has evolved from a con artist into an authentic First Amendment hero—in July 2000, he spoke at the Commonwealth Club in San Francisco—I recall what a pariah he was in 1977. In Los Angeles, at the building in Century City which housed his office, *Hustler* was not allowed to be listed in the lobby.

At the time, I was writing a syndicated column for alternative weeklies. Specifically, I was working on my "Predictions for 1978," leading off with this: "Since Larry Flynt has been converted to born-again Christianity, the new *Hustler* will feature a special scratch-'n'-sniff Virgin Mary."

"Hey, that's a great idea," said Flynt on New Year's Day at Nassau Beach in the Bahamas. "We'll have a portrait of the Virgin Mary, and when you scratch her crotch, it'll smell like tomato juice." He was rubbing suntan lotion on my back. "I'll bet Hugh Hefner never did this for you," he said.

Flynt wanted to know who would be appropriate to write an article for *Hustler* that would expose the Pope as gay. I suggested Gore Vidal, who had already stated in an interview that Cardinal Spellman was gay. So much for our first editorial conference.

There was an unwritten agreement among men's magazines that human female nipples would not be clearly visible on a cover. I was also learning to accept certain arbitrary rules then governing the inside pages. An erect penis must not be shown. Semen must not be shown. Penetration must not be shown. Oral-genital contact must not be shown.

The next month, at *Hustler's* Christmas party, Flynt announced that I was going to be the new publisher.

A few months later in Georgia, Flynt was shot during a lunch break in his obscenity trial. I flew to Atlanta and went directly to the hospital. Althea brought me to Larry's room. It was extremely unsettling to see such a powerful personality so helpless, kept alive by medical technology, with one tube feeding him and another breathing for him. He appeared bug-eyed with painkiller. Althea lifted the sheet and showed me his gaping wounds, a truly awesome sight.

"Oh, God, Althea," I said, "he's showing pink."

"I'm arranging for a photographer to come in here," she said. "We're gonna publish Larry's wounds in *Hustler*. I want people to see what they did to him."

I sat down in a chair by Larry's bed. I didn't know what to say. We simply clasped hands for a while. Finally I broke the silence. "Larry, tomorrow is Good Friday. So, uh, you don't have to go to work."

I glanced toward Althea to reassure myself that I hadn't in-dulged in irreverence that was *too* inappropriate, but she said, "Oh, Paul, *look*," gesturing toward Larry—"he wants to show you something." Above the oxygen mask, Larry was blinking his eyes over and over again in rapid succession.

"He's *laughing*," Althea explained.

It was a moment of unspeakable intimacy.

Althea had transformed the Coca-Cola Suite of Emory University Hospital into her office, where she was studying the slides of a "Jesus and the Adulteress" photo spread, including a nearly life-sized poster in the form of a centerfold pull-out: There was a generic barbershop-calendar Jesus looking reverently toward the sky as he stands above the prone adulteress—almost naked, her head bleeding from the stones that have been cast—and, just as the Bible says, he is covering her, *but not quite*, and she is, inadvertently, still showing pink. Sweet, shocking, vulnerable pink. This was a startling visual image, unintentionally satirizing the change from the old *Hustler* to the new *Hustler*. The marketing people were aghast at the possibility that wholesalers, especially in the Bible Belt, would refuse to distribute the magazine with such a blatantly blasphemous feature.

Faced with a crucial decision, Althea made her choice on the basis of pure whimsicality. She noticed a pair of pigeons on the window ledge. One was waddling toward the other. "All right," she said, "if that dove walks over and pecks the *other* dove, then we *will* publish this." The pigeon continued strutting along the window ledge, but stopped short and didn't peck the other pigeon, so publication of "Jesus and the Adulteress" was postponed indefinitely. And the poster would instead remain on my wall as a memento of my six-month stint at *Hustler*. Maybe I should try to auction it off on eBay.

As for Larry Flynt's born-again conversion, he now attributes it to "a chemical imbalance in his brain."

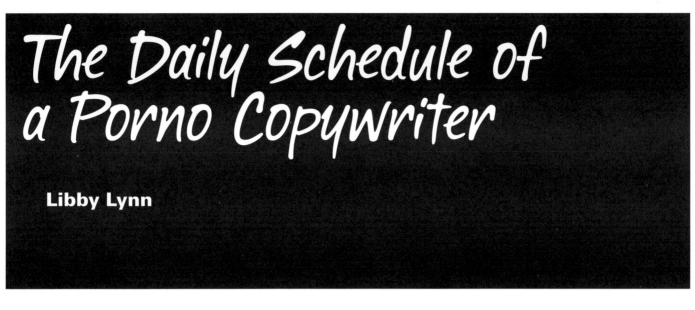

The Daily Schedule of a Porno Copywriter

Libby Lynn

6:00 AM: Welcome, Libby!

I wake up in a mortal panic. I'm 31 years old, and if I died today there'd be no proper documentation of my life, except for all the porn I've written. In the dazed layer between dream and wake, I weigh the meaning of my career. What if I died in a car crash? Or from an overdose of Lamictal, which I take to keep my bipolar noise at a low hum? Or from a seizure brought on by too much masturbation?

"Jesus," they'd say, gathered around my half-naked corpse.

"What a way to go," they'd say, staring at the panties tangled in my jeans. They'd gape at the bottle of lube in my stiff right hand, and the copy of *Ass Fucking Whores #2* in my left. Where in the world had my life come to?

Welcome, lovers, to my small adult world, where I have one singular and specialized duty: to write product descriptions for porn videos, sex toys, and all manner of erotic products. Welcome to the company I'll call Sex World.

My job is a mix of the *ennui* of marketing and the anomaly of pornography. I relate equally to wealthy mainstream art directors and their grossly underpaid staff, and to filthy-rich pornographers and their grossly overpriced pornstars. It's the greatest and weirdest job I've ever had.

Before this, I'd been writing copy at mainstream media companies for eight years. It was skull-numbing. Between bouts of actual work, I'd browse porn sites, masturbate in bathroom stalls, and search for other copywriting-job ads.

"FULLTIME ON-SITE COPYWRITER POSITION; MUST BE COMFORTABLE WITH THE ADULT ENTERTAINMENT IN-DUSTRY" was the ad that called me to Sex World. I started when I was 27 and didn't question entering the world of porn.

Four years later, I question whether I'll ever leave.

—

9:00 AM: Your daily schedule is as follows:

I unlock my office door at 9:08. I'm usually late two days a week. My boss, just outside my office, gives her Look. I turn on my computer and check my email: 247 spams and fourteen work-related emergencies, which I respond to immediately. Next, I check my dreaded Outlook calendar, and another meeting-jammed day at Sex World begins.

—

9:30 – 10:00 AM: Write copy for three porn videos that don't have screeners yet. It's doubtful that you'll ever get the actual videos, but at least you have the DVD cases.

After four years, I've learned to write video copy just from looking at its packaging. I used to thrill at coming up with synonyms for body parts and sexual acts. But I'm automated now. If a video merchandiser blindfolded me and yelled, "*White Chicks & Black Dicks*—GO!" I could finish an accurate seventy-five-word paragraph in five minutes.

—

10:00 – 11:30 AM: Attend meeting and bitch about the incompetence of the latest Team Scapegoat. Complaints include spending three days completing one 8x5-½" video ad flyer, flubbing deadlines, and badly managing time management. Remind those present that scapegoats are a necessary variable for the daily grind to function smoothly.

It would take 300 pages to explain the business structure of Sex World. I work with a team of graphic designers, product merchandisers, copywriters, and print buyers that sells every imaginable adult product to our appropriate demographics.

We work in porn, but we're primarily a marketing company. And like every other marketing company, we have meetings. Creative meetings and concept meetings and blue sky meetings and review meetings and results meetings and monthly employee meetings and feedback meetings and consultant meetings and—the mother of all meetings—team meetings.

This type of meeting is porn-free. This is the exchange of carnality for bloodshed. This is the platform where we discuss the progress and regress of our team. This is where we're trained to use euphemisms: Concern, not anger. Assumption, not gossip. Improvement, not complaint. Adult videos, not porn. Come, not cum. Great sex, not fucking.

At this point, I've watched at least 6,240 hours of porn, and that's just for work.

After ten years, I've spent $316,495 on psychotherapy for manic depression. But the team meeting is free. It's group therapy for the psychoses that arise from dealing with sex as a commodity. Although the team loathes these biweekly appointments, the sessions will prove invaluable for the rest of our lives.

Now I've become more functional as a Sex World employee than I ever was on the therapy chaise lounge. So I quit my shrink and started spending her $150 hourly fee on cocktails, computers, books, and clothes. I love the team meeting.

—

11:30 – Noon: Write copy for new lingerie products while continuing to observe the aggravating courtship between ex-boyfriend coworker and his latest girlfriend coworker.

A year into my job, I began a time-consuming affair with a fellow Sex Worlder. Our attraction was based on four crucial details:

1. We both had Todd McFarlane action figures of Leatherface on our desks.
2. We both wore Ramones T-shirts on the day we noticed each other.
3. We both were nursing heartbreaks with a lover's elixir of booze and barbiturates.
4. We both were raincoaters fostering our porn addictions with grudge-fucking.

It's impossible to keep illicit romances secret inside an office—especially when the office is stocked with more explicit material than any secular citizen should see. I've summed up this year and a half of interoffice drama in one universal chunk of wisdom: Kids, don't fuck your coworkers.

—

Noon – 12:30 PM: Scarf down your lunch while screening comp porn that makes your brain wince.

Ah, the power lunch: unmonitored excursions filled with sushi and roasted duck over a bed of baby bok choy, topped off with Grey Goose martinis and industry gossip. Glamorous café settings where Armani-suited pornographers negotiate exchanges of footage for funds. Where more ass is kissed than in any analingus video.

But, sadly, not so.

I eat ramen noodles at my desk, with a plastic fork in one hand and a remote control in the other. My lunch hours are spent simultaneously writing copy and watching shitty porn. These videos are called "comps," and they're the worst kind of porn: chopped-up footage from existing productions, badly edited and unworthy of masturbation. I save these comps for lunchtime to balance how much they suck with the pleasures of Cup o' Noodles. And that's my power lunch.

—

12:30 – 1:00 PM: Taste-test the new Spanish fly gels and try not to gag on flavors like Iced Tea and Mulberry Delight. Knock out nine descriptions for products like the White Poon Pecker and the Black Cock Dong. Admire the equal opportunities for jelly dongs at Sex World.

After twelve years of marketing, I believe you can bundle vomit in a pink satin bag and make people believe they can't live without it.

Be Sexy. Be Sick.
Lose Your Lunch in Our Heavenly Pink Puke Bag!

I used to feel guilty for writing copy that lied about how every dildo was unique, every comp was a high-quality production, every lingerie garment was as soft as Japanese silk, and how every liquid stimulant with an exotic blend of ginseng and L-arginine could make the most frigid clitoris reach orgasm at a whisper's flutter.

But when I saw how many stock dildos and comp videos and scratchy negligees and genital gels our customers purchased, I realized that writing copy isn't lying. Sometimes people believe more in the idea of the dildo than what the dildo actually is. No matter how foolish or unnecessary or cheap a product might be, it makes someone happy. And that's what matters.

—

1:00 – 1:10 PM: Receive call from father. Halfway into conversation, remember to mute the moaning and scream-

ing and *"Fuck my tight pink pussy, motherfucker!"* coming from your television. Say goodbye and hang up.

Any family asks, "So, how's your job?" You answer: "Great! Yeah, busy as always," or, "Same old stuff." My family asks, "So, how is the porn going?" I answer: "Great! Yeah, busy as always. Same old stuff."

This job goes over easy with my folks because they have four other children with equally unusual careers. One is a brilliant scientist who deals with some manner of chemistry. One is a bartender who makes more money than I do. One is a journalist at a respectable newspaper. And one is a missionary who made a career of Christianity. My parents are impossible to shock.

—

1:10 – 1:30 PM: Ten minutes later, receive troubling call from hysterical friend in need of advice you are not fit to give. Rearrange weekend plans for a consolation vacation.

My friends are another matter.

When I first started working for Sex World, I made sure everyone knew about it. *Everyone.* I'd pass out business cards to random people for no reason other than to yell, "I TOTALLY WORK IN PORN!"

I abused the power of these business cards in order to flirt with men or to get ten friends into the VIP section at every strip club in town. I was a big hit at my tenth high-school reunion. People loved my job.

It was novel for a year or two. But then my closest friends began to show concern.

"So you're still with Sex World?" they'd ask.

"Yep!" I'd say, with my most compelling grin.

"How long has it been now?"

"A couple of years."

"And you're still watching porn all the time?"

"Yep."

"How much porn do you watch, like on a weekly basis?"

"You don't want to know."

"Hasn't it warped your brain?"

I've thought about this a lot. My therapist and I had at least $1,200 worth of discussions about the effect of viewing an average of 30 hours of porn per week. That's 1,560 hours of porn per year. At this point, I've watched at least 6,240 hours of porn, and that's just for work.

You'd think I'd be sociopathic or at least burned out. But I still watch porn for pleasure. If anything, the only noticeable changes are that my empathy for people has actually improved, and my porn standards have skyrocketed. I have pretty stiff requirements these days:

1. I accept videos only from specific companies.
2. The production must be fucking excellent.
3. The female performers must be true sexual dynamos with no traces of breast augmentation.
4. The male performers must be engaging and aggressive.
5. I don't like features or storylines or dialogue or contract stars or comp videos.
6. There must be real heat in every scene.
7. I enjoy sexual humiliation, so long as the performers truly get off on it.

I'm not a big fan of shock acts like double anal or piss-swallowing or triple cocksucking, and I absolutely loathe cum- or spit-swapping. But I do enjoy domination, submission, odd sexual philias, rape fantasies, and unsanitary acts like ATP or ATOGM or PTOGA. I'll let you and my therapist figure those out.

I take some pride in the fact that I'm a female raincoater and an inundated sex writer who still enjoys porn. I like watching it fly in the faces of feminists who still believe that porn is man-made misogyny made for men. This information, however, doesn't impress my friends.

"But don't you still want to be a writer?" they ask.

Yep.

—

1:30 – 1:45 PM: Another phone call from your friendly bar owner, forgiving you for doing drugs in the bathroom and inviting you to the Wet, Hot & Wild dance party on Friday night. Politely decline this engagement because you'll be consoling your troubled friend. Consider dodging friend in order to attend party. Feel shame and continue writing copy.

Working in porn is a lot like dealing drugs: You gain a fine lot of fair-weather friends. The only difference is that my porn buddies don't need a fix every week. They come around at sporadic times like bachelorette parties, dry runs of monogamy, various sexual crises, and unemployment, when their need for stimulus beats off their energy for finding a new job.

I also get requests for gay porn, which is expensive, and from jaded Web junkies who are tired of paying memberships, short sex clips, or staining their computer desk chairs.

But sometimes I make friends with entire establishments—

especially bars and strip clubs—in need of promotional goodies, more patrons, and bigger bar tabs.

I like my porn buddies. Any savvy drug dealer will tell you that the goods all come back in the end. Bar owners let me drink for free before their doors even open. I get invited to all manner of events. People give me free passes to movie premieres and rock shows. I eat free meals. I get discounts at clothing boutiques, hair salons, and tattoo parlors. And best of all, everyone knows my name.

Well, at least the name on my business card.

—

1:45 – 2:00 PM: Leave the building to take a smoke break and proof your copy. Note four run-on sentences as you notice the new beefy salesman smoking a cigar around the corner. Note that his biceps and cheesy crew cut are not your type. Find his stature oddly appealing while pretending to proof remaining copy.

This is a heavy subject to tackle.

I've seen the good in almost everyone. Specifically, I've seen good reason to fuck almost anyone. There are three reasons for this:

1. I used to not know that hypersexuality comes with bipolar mania.
2. I used to entirely depend on porn for sexual gratification.
3. I used to indulge in meaningless sex with many one-nighters.

Let me try to explain.

First: I was born with a sexual birthmark in my manic genes.

Second: I saw my first porn video at the premature age of ten, and knew I was hooked.

Third: I'm on the left side of the 1:3 ratio of women who were sexually abused before the age of eighteen. In my case history, the files will tell you that I was six.

One common consequence of molestation is growing up without steady sexual boundaries. I've had more sexual partners than Jenna Jameson. But that's nothing to brag about, because I didn't get paid to do it.

It took me years of therapy to realize the difference between what molestation meant to the world and what it meant to me: With the help of an abused teenaged boy, I discovered my clitoris and how good it felt to be touched.

The sensation of being touched by a fresh finger or tongue or cock is a sexual rush that I still have to resist today. It also took me years of romantic disasters to understand the dif-

ference between sexual addiction and intimacy. Behold how I've terrorized:

High-school boyfriend: two and a half years. I tortured him with the terribly scarring things that fucked-up teenagers do to each other. He's a Christian minister now. There isn't a decade that goes by that I don't wonder if I'm the reason why.

College boyfriends: six months average. All are fathers, gay, married, or drag queens now, and there isn't a year that goes by that I'm not astonished by and proud of them for still talking to me.

The girlfriends: one or two weeks apiece. All of them are actual lesbians, and there isn't six months that go by that I don't wonder if or why I'm not.

First true love: eight years. Responsible for trying to teach me the purpose of sexual boundaries. There isn't a month that goes by that I don't wonder how things might've gone if I hadn't gone astray...eight or eighteen times.

Best sex: two years, one of which overlapped the true love. Fighting and drinking and fucking. There isn't a week that goes by that I don't wonder how we managed to last as long as we did.

And now, *my man*, where my terrors grew up, got old, and died. There isn't a day that goes by that I don't thank him for dating a 31-year-old bipolar pornographer who publicly celebrates her career and conquests in lieu of repeating past mistakes. I don't know if I'll ever understand why he chooses to be with me. He's beautiful, sexual, brilliant, tough, and best of all, he runs at full capacity.

Now, would I have ended up working in porn without all of these factors?

I'll always have to take a pill to calm my manic sexuality. I'll always have a porn habit. It'll always be a challenge to remember the consequences of standing face to face with the intoxicating mugs of temptation. My demons are everywhere, bowing to my body with their phallus-curved horns. Sex is my heroin.

So, the answer is, probably not. But I can say this: I've busted my ass to learn where my limits end and how to like my life within them. Plus, my job is more interesting than yours.

—

2:00 – 2:10 PM: Receive sweet phone call from boyfriend, who has planned an unexpected night on the town. Thank your lucky stars for dating a solid, secure, and understanding man.

I can't speak for the significant others of everyone who works in America's adult industry. But at Sex World, the employees' romantic partners typically fall into one of five categories:

1. The partners also work at Sex World. Aside from the ill-kept illicit affairs I've mentioned, many of my fellow cumrads met their partners at the company. These couples work together and go home together. I have no idea how they handle this, especially when they have children. What happens at parent-teacher conference night?

"Hello, Mrs. And Mr. X-rated!"

"Hello, Ms. G-rated!"

"How are things at Sex World?"

"Very sexy, thanks. Is our little Jenna doing well in her courses?"

"Well, little Jenna's English marks need improvement. But she maintains straight A's in business math, and she's the best gymnast on the entire team!"

"She has always been good with money, and also very flexible."

"Little Jenna is very popular. The boys and girls are very fond of her. She's going to be a heartbreaker some day."

"Ms. G-rated, thank you for keeping an eye on her."

"The pleasure is mine."

2. The partners don't exist. Being a bachelor at Sex World has its benefits. Anyone who's ever attended an adult-industry convention will wholeheartedly agree. Pornstars eager for a taste of cock that hasn't been tasted by a thousand other well-compensated lips. Private orgies in lavish suites at the Venetian. Blowjobs in bathroom stalls at the Bellagio. Fucking on the dancefloor at the top of the Rain nightclub.

These are all lies.

Adult conventions are unlike what you'd imagine. They're a claustrophobic feeding frenzy of incomprehensible proportions, where the porn industry and the public mix into a grueling blend of turmoil and mayhem.

These conventions are expensive, crowded, dissolute, and exhausting. Everyone's bushed from going to parties they don't want to attend and having client dinners with unsavory stereotypes. The lines—taxi lines, guest list lines, drink lines, convention entrance lines, and airport lines—are soul-killers. It's totally exciting the first night and total hell the next day.

The truth is that sometimes it's easier to be single when you work in porn, especially in regards to the #3 types.

3. The partners are prone to jealousy. Being romantically involved with someone who works in porn is not an easy job. You have to deal with the fact that your lover is surrounded by beautiful young girls and well-endowed men whose primary purpose is to arouse.

The porn world also depends on a revolving supply of new talent, so its employees stay the same age. Getting old is scary enough, especially in America, where ageism is rampant and youth and beauty are tossed into your eyes at every turn. But you can't turn your eyes away from the young and beautiful products of your partner's porn career. If you can't stand the sight of continuous sex, your easiest option is to find another vista that's easier on the eyes.

Honestly, if I were on the other end of the stick, I don't know if I could handle it. That's why I'm thankful that my partner is a #5.

4. The partners handle nonmonogamy outstandingly. I admire relationships that successfully revolve around primary and extracurricular partners. It takes years of trust and honesty to build an open relationship. A lot of people fantasize about it, some give it a shot, but very few can actually handle it. Polyamory is a rousing and dangerous place.

I tried it once, and it was a disaster. As much as my body loves fucking around, my mind requires monogamy. I'm mind over matter, and steering clear of attractive matter is a matter of my survival.

5. The partners are solid, secure, and understanding. Most of my coworkers' partners, and thankfully mine, fall into this category. After all, working at Sex World brings home the bacon. Our lovers realize that the world of porn is a fantasyland. It's not a pot you'd want to dip into.

Whether in front of or behind the camera, dealing with sex on a constant basis can be difficult, and it's nice to come home to someone who understands this.

"How was your day, sugar?" my boyfriend asks.

"Fucked up and busy as shit." I've spent the last six hours at a lingerie photo shoot. My hands are dirty from handling G-strings and panties that are soaked with what we call "model juice."

"I made dinner tonight," he says. The smell of chicken enchiladas drifts from the kitchen. He pours me a glass of wine. I make him a Crown and Coke. We go outside and sit on the patio. We listen to the evening and sip our drinks.

"So how was your day? Tell me about it," I say.

"Fucked up and busy as shit," he says, wiping his forehead with the back of his hand. My boyfriend works with power tools, dangerous chemicals, and heavy equipment. I suppose our jobs are equally hazardous.

He doesn't hold anything against porn. He isn't threatened by my job. And for that, I think I might be the luckiest girl in triple-X.

—

2:10 – 4:00 PM: Attend review meeting for an "out of the box" project that management suggested. Smile and take it up the ass when management claims the project strays too far from "the way we *do* things." Allot three hours into schedule for an entire re-do.

These aggravations are well known to all professional advertisers. It's the age-old battle of Corporate vs. Creative. Although it's mostly guesswork, there are proven tactics that help marketing campaigns succeed. Sometimes creative strategies are wrong. Sometimes corporate strategies are right. But most of the time, these battles are just fucking retarded.

If you're lucky enough to work on a creative staff for any company that advocates risk, your bosses have my blessings and you have my envy.

Here's an example of why.

Corporate says: We're doing too much of the same thing. We're getting lazy and falling back on formulas instead of expanding ideas. Let's have a blue sky! Let's think NEW. Let's think INNOVATION! Let's think **OUTSIDE THE BOX**.

Creative says: Okay! We've been aching, longing, and praying to do something new and different. Thank you! We accept this request with open arms, and we shall proceed beyond the box.

Corporate says: Excellent. Your deadline is in five days.

Five days pass, and the team reviews the project again.

Creative says: Look at this new ad! We totally got outside the box on this. See how the woman's legs are spread, with a decency dot that doubles as a call to action? See how we used blue and black on thick kraft paper, instead of pink and red on regular paper? See how we decided to use a curvy brunette chick with natural breasts? See how we wrote header copy that says, "Cum One, Cum All"? Isn't this different? Isn't this clever?

Corporate says: Let's start with the woman's legs. They can't be spread open *that* wide. It's too explicit. The call to action needs to be the headline, not a decency dot. You need to follow our existing layout template. The colors are all wrong. Why did you choose black and blue? Are you connoting a boxing match or an abusive relationship? You *know* we use pink and red as our color scheme. We're unclear as to why you changed this. And the kraft paper is too expensive. As far as the girl goes, you *know* that thin, big-breasted blondes have more visual appeal, which is why we always use them. And as far as the copy goes, no clever, and absolutely NO CUM.

Creative says: But you told us to think outside the box.

Corporate says: We always encourage new ideas. But this just strays too far from the way we do things.

I deal with every manner of box. Shaved, trimmed, hairy, young, mature, ugly, pretty, tight, loose, virginal, and veteran, and I love them all. The only box I don't love is the box I'm asked to get out of, then told to get right back in.

—

4:00 – 6:00 PM: Receive your latest round of edited product copy. Your editors, all 53 of them, disagree with both your copy and each other. Spend five minutes crying, ten minutes laughing, and an hour making revisions from all 53 editors.

After four years of writing product descriptions for Sex World's vast treasure of adult products, I've noticed that the copywriting cycle has four stages. First, we're presented with more porn and sex toys than anyone should ever handle. Second, we thoroughly research each item. This is the fun part. Third, we write "absolutely NO more than 75 words, Libby!" to describe the unique selling point of each product. And last, we print out each document and submit them to the painful process known as copy editing.

Taken out of context, these copy edits are funny to people who don't write copy for a living, especially when the editors' comments in the actual Word documents conflict with each other:

> Are we really sure our customers know what "DP" is?
> *Our customers know what "DP" is. We've been using that acronym for like 10 years.*

> I'm not comfortable with assuming they know what "DP" is. Please spell it out.
> *Not enough room to spell out "Double Penetration." The visual of the girl with two cocks in her holes will spell it out just fine.*

> ~

> Is there another adjective besides "chocolate" or "ebony" or "cinnamon" to use to describe black performers?
> *No.*

~

Tell me why this is the best new masturbator on the market.

~

No "deep doggie dump-humping."

~

No comma after strap-ons.

~

Is this vibe really shaped like a gerbil? Who made this? Please see me.

~

What are "these little pussies" so hungry for?

~

75 WORDS OR LESS, LIBBY.

~

A vibe CANNOT be shaped exactly like a G-spot.
Yes, it can. That's why we made it.

No one knows what a G-spot is shaped like!
Yes, we do. It was in development for three years.

Why did we develop this vibrator? Whose idea was this?
IT WAS YOUR IDEA.

~

Don't say "mouth hole."

~

Tell me my boobs and ass will look great!

~

Is she the Perfect Woman or the Ultimate Sex Machine?

~

DO NOT SAY, "This nurse knows a spoonful of semen helps the meaty shaft go down"!!!

~

Use "cock" instead of "man meat."

~

She is NOT cheap & EASY.
Yes, she is. She's a love doll.

~

Do we want to talk about church-going girls?
Catholic schoolgirls are fine. But don't mention anything about a church or a priest or a father.

~

$5.49 is too cheap for a vagina.

~

I think this is misleading; they're not "real" lesbians.

~

I'd rather not say "beaver."

~

Can we get extra stimulation in the headline?

~

Since this Spanish fly doesn't actually work, don't emphasize the "aphrodisiac" qualities.

~

Pussy cleavage is GREAT!!!

~

No beautiful blowjobs, please.

~

Do customers know what a box is?

~

They're not real hookers, but hookers are the theme of this video.

~

No one cares if the cyberskin cock has a pleasant smell.

~

You say "ass" too many times here. Try tush or buns or butt. Too much ass.

~

Again, too much ass. Please use a thesaurus. We can't have ass everywhere.

~

Your first sentence says that this will fit fat women very nicely.
Maybe we should address bigger gals as "voluptuous"?

~

Good couplet! Nice alliteration! Flows off one's tongue.

~

Do you realize you have six headlines here? Customers don't read the copy, so please choose one and stick to it.

~

Don't say it makes your dick hard. Some people who buy it won't even have a dick.

And, as always, my favorite:

Libby, we need to discuss your continual use of the words fuck, shit, bitch, cunt, whore, slut, man meat, mouth hole, and asshole.

—

6:00 – 6:45 PM: Watch four porn videos crammed with young girls whose fake tits make your gut cringe. Feel sympathy for these women as you note the scar tissue and asymmetrical placement of each implant. Feel empathy as you consider the similarities you share.

When I was eighteen, I was very angry at everything. I made sure everyone knew how pissed I was by marking up my body with angry tattoos. These souvenirs from my troubled youth were poorly executed. Not "apprentice at Wicked Ink" bad. Not "my friend Jason does tattoos" bad. Not "cheesy flash" bad. Not even "prison" bad. These tattoos were somewhere in the vicinity of "ink pen and Exacto knife" bad.

I recently decided to get my tattoos fixed. So far I'm satisfied with the results. But when my favorite tattoo artist, Mark Van Ness, told me, "They'll need to be continually touched up for the rest of your life," I realized that tattoos are just like breast implants.

I got my bad tattoo jobs when I was too young to understand their everlasting ramifications. And most of America's pornstars get bad boob jobs when they're too young to realize the same thing.

Fake tits and tattoos have so much in common. They're both body modifications that fit certain social paradigms. They can both be badly done. They both require continual maintenance. They both change the way that people look at you. They can both cause regret. They both wear with age. They're both costly and painful to remove. And we usually get them when our bodies are still blooming.

That's why I have empathy for young girls who get boob jobs in order to let the world know that they're hardcore pornstars. I can't judge these women, even if I think their tits look like shit. They'd think the same thing about my tattoos. If I could go back and choose not to get tattoos, I would. But they're marks of my past, and because of that, I'm fond of them. Sometimes I wonder if the porn veterans feel the same way about their old, bad boob jobs.

—

6:45 – 7:15 PM: Drive home and consider your day. Think about how weird your job is and how much you enjoy it. Think about the way your family and friends see it. Think about how much money you're not making and how much money you would be making if you decided to become a pornstar. Think about why you work in porn and how much longer you will. Think about how much porn you watch at work. Think about how much porn you masturbate to. Think about how fucked up the adult industry is, and why. Think about how sexually fucked America is and what it would take to change this. Think about coming home and writing about it. Then think about normal shit, like eating enchiladas, doing laundry, hanging out with your boyfriend, and talking to your friends and family on the phone.

I love this job. I love how weird it is. I love the challenge of selling something that simultaneously arouses and threatens people. I love being fascinated and appalled by the adult industry. I love the way that people react when I tell them how I've put my college degree to work. I love that my family and friends both support and worry about what I do. I love being a chick who gets off on watching and working in porn. I love learning about the history of American porn, and I love keeping an eye on where it's headed.

What I don't love is America's sexually schizophrenic attitude towards the people who work in sex. We can argue that the adult industry is misogynistic, belittling, sick, unnatural, violent, and completely fucked up. But we don't argue much while we're using its products.

What *really* pisses me off is that the adult industry—burlesque troupes, strip clubs, escort services, prostitution, sex clubs, porn, and every other business that revolves around compensated erotic service—is also the one that adults against selling sex as a commodity condemn the most. Even if their most adamant critics don't participate in any of these services, which I think they do, I guarantee that they're at least fantasizing about one of them.

That makes them hypocrites. But that doesn't make them entirely wrong.

If you look beyond the people fucking on your TV screen, you'll see the reality of what happens behind the porn scenes. The physical job hazards are high: HIV, herpes, warts, gonorrhea, yeast infections, vaginal bleeding, anal tearing, enemas and douche bottles, and lots of Viagra. Meth, coke, Vicodin, Valium, OxyContin, weed, and booze are popular self-medications for the mental stress that pornstars deal with on and off the set. Although it has great perks, being a good pornstar is actually a very tough job.

I have tremendous respect for the people who can handle it. I believe sex workers should be valued by the billions of people who buy their products. They work in a harsh cultural climate where they're belittled and denounced by the same people who jack off to their work. America's sexual schizophrenia is harmful as hell. This hypocrisy takes place inside the adult industry as well, which is even worse.

—

7:15 – present: Arrive home.

Oh, America. It's a good thing we're free. You know, to do as we please.

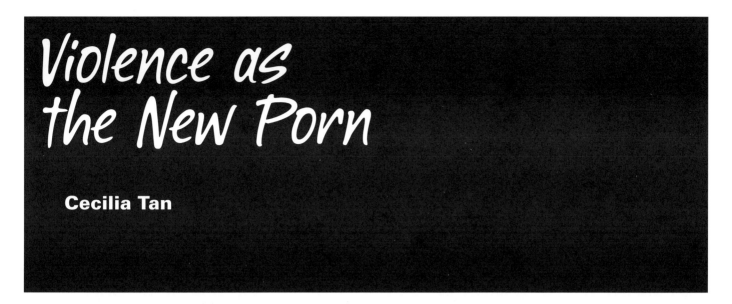

Violence as the New Porn

Cecilia Tan

I sat in a dark theater recently, at first stifling my mounting arousal, then lounging back, languid, giving myself over completely to the images on the screen. I know what you're wondering—you want to know what I was watching. Was it the theatrical re-release of *Deep Throat*? The latest from Jenna Jameson? It couldn't be modern porn, because all "those" theaters have been torn down, haven't they? Yes, they have. I was limp in my chair from a PG-13 action movie.

The world of films is the world of dreams, the world of the cultural hive mind ingrained in our brains. Freud knew this, and so did the Dadaists, and so does every Hollywood executive who wants to cash in on our subconscious needs. And, man, do I have needs. But fads, political correctness, and our ultramodern gestalt move quickly; what the audience wants, and what they can get, changes in a short time. What is taboo one year can be commonplace five years later. The opposite is also true—what was once commonplace, even necessary, in a film, is now shocking.

If we use the James Bond franchise as a barometer, it's amazing how *little* actual sex takes place in the current films as compared to earlier films in the series, given that Bond is supposedly a womanizer. Beyond the standard hottie silhouettes in the opening credits and the usual innuendo-laced dialogue, the Bond franchise has gotten remarkably chaste about what it will show. Then again, perhaps Grant Morrison had it right in *The Invisibles* graphic novels, in which a character says of the Bond filmic *oeuvre*: "Every scene is a sex scene." More on that in a moment.

Another indicator: Bare breasts, once *de rigueur*, are now out. Remember that Steven Seagal film *Under Siege*, where he plays the Navy cook who single-handedly saves the battle-ship from terrorist takeover? The meaningless but necessary boob shot appears when a stripper pops out of a cake. That film came out in 1992. In 1997 we had the coed shower scene in *Starship Troopers*. Here's another one from that year, *Universal Soldier*, starring Jean-Claude Van Damme. To shoehorn some boobs in here, the plot calls for our hero to use the computer...at a strip joint. What better way to get some girls on film?

Now tell me, when was the last time you saw some gratuitous titties in an R-rated action flick? I actually searched using

Perhaps Grant Morrison had it right in *The Invisibles* graphic novels, in which a character says of the Bond filmic *oeuvre:* "Every scene is a sex scene."

some of the Christian right's movie review sites (like ScreenIt. com), and disappointingly, I could find *no nudity* complained about in the dozens of recent action flicks I looked up. They moan about fishnets and a short skirt, so you can be sure any actual breasts that appear would be catalogued. The only R-rated action flick released from May 2004 to May 2005 that had any nudity in it was *Sin City* (most of it was germane to the plot, and really, what else would you expect with a title like that?). None in *Sahara*, *Hostage*, *Constantine*, *Blade: Trinity*...you get the idea. It looks to me like the free boob shot has disappeared.

Why? It's not that the filmmakers are going for a PG-13 rating. If you're going to have an action movie with a lot of ass-kicking, you're probably going to get slapped with an R rating anyway. Why not sex it up with more skin? I can think of three reasons.

One, in an age when high-ranking politicians feel that the bare breast on a statue of Justice is offensive, well, maybe this just isn't a good time for tits.

Two, maybe directors are maturing and have realized that something as gratuitous as a full rack nicely displayed but which does not actually advance the plot in any way should be left on the cutting room floor (or not filmed in the first place).

Three, maybe the tit shot doesn't come close to the sexiness of the actual "action" in action films these days. In fact, it might detract from the experience since nudity, so closely associated with pornography, may destroy the suspension of disbelief and force the viewer into an external, voyeuristic mode. I could speculate that the sex we can't show these days has been transformed instead into violence...but I'd be wrong. There are plenty of sexual themes and sex-related plotlines in the recent breed of action films, even if the nudity itself has been attenuated. There may be less nudity, but

When Wolverine reveals his claws in *X-Men: The Movie*, it's better than Rocco Siffredi unzipping his pants.

there is more sex and sexiness than ever, both in carefully choreographed "love scenes" and in the equally carefully choreographed action sequences.

Yes, "every scene is a sex scene" in a film like this (thank you, Mr. Bond), because action-film directors have figured out what I—the slobbering audience member—want: a visceral, physical experience which is *akin* to sex. We want to "get off" on the violence in these films—it's why we plunked down our $9.50 per person to see it in a dark theater with Dolby SurroundSound on a Friday night instead of renting the DVD later (or using BitTorrent to pirate it off the Net). We want to bleed with Mel Gibson, kick ass with Arnold Schwarzenegger, and angst with Keanu Reeves. We want to be completely sucked into the film, have our subconscious tossed around, and come out whole and refreshed.

If that sounds kind of like what people want out of a session with a dominatrix, that is no coincidence. I like that idea: the action film itself as dominatrix—the kind who gets right inside your head and can make you come without touching you. Ahhh. See, the regular porn film—even the snazzy, high-production-value stuff that is put out by Vivid and Wicked, even Jenna Jameson's fanciest offerings these days—relies on and even capitalizes on the fact that you, the porn viewer, are aware of the fact that you are watching professionals who fuck for a living. Not only are you aware of it, you accept it and even may be a fan of it. The shaved snatches, the extra

makeup, the vignette-style sex scenes and set pieces that have no connection to any plot or character, they all scream at you: You're watching porn! Now get off, dammit! For most people, that's all they need.

But maybe I'm not like most porn consumers. I'm a woman, and although we all keep saying that women are taking over the porn industry (mostly for politically correct reasons and our own wish fulfillment), the majority of the porn made and bought today is by and for men. You know the cliché: Men are supposedly more voyeuristic than women. And men like to be grabbed by the dick and jerked off, while women like to be seduced.

For me, seduction is all about getting inside my head, engaging my imagination, and getting those fantasy juices flowing. This is why I like S/M sex—sure, the bondage and spanking is fun for a sensation-whore like me, but it is the mindfuck, the role-playing, and the fantasy aspects that really get me. Your modern porn film does very little to engage the imagination—I'd say most of them discourage it. If you're a fan of modern porn, you're a fan of watching sexual athletes at the top of their game. This is not a knock on what they do; they do it very well, but I find myself all too often yawning in boredom because my head is not engaged. I'm not in the story. I'm not living the part of the characters. There is only one possible way to consume modern porn, and that is as a voyeur.

So if nudity is one of the triggers to voyeurism, maybe we ought to avoid it if we want to really get the audience to suspend their disbelief and make them feel like they're on the rollercoaster with us.... I think this is one of the rationales behind the disappearance of nudity in recent action films. Do I miss those pretty knockers? Not at all, because today's action directors have gotten better and better at satisfying me. Yes me, personally. I don't think I can speak for the general action-movie fan, since my erotic tastes can be pretty unique, but when it comes to getting me hot and bothered, give me a sword sliding out of its sheath any day. Sex used to ride gratuitously on the surface of these films (because really, who has time for an actual love scene when you're busy saving the world? *The Matrix: Reloaded* might be the one exception, and that was mostly an excuse to have an extended music video in the first act of the movie). Now the sexual images have been sublimated into stylized violence, and the plots of the movies are entangling our heroes, heroines, and, of course, villains in ever more lust-laden plots.

We partly have the buttoned-up Chinese to thank for this. Hong Kong action movies have been the pinnacle of non-English-language action cinema for decades now, and if you think there's little sex in American action movies, there's practically none in their Hong Kong counterparts. Do you remember ever seeing Bruce Lee in a love scene? Of course not. Even in his Hollywood incarnation, Bruce is all about loyalty, honor, and revenge. In *Enter the Dragon*, the black guy and the white guy get all the pussy they want, while Bruce's concubine is actually a double-agent helping him overthrow the evil overlord.

God, I'm getting hot thinking about it.

If I can be Freudian for a moment, can it be any more obvious that long swords and pointy knives and guns that spray bullets everywhere are phallic objects? (I am soooo into penetration.) I realized this some years ago when I discovered that the hottest thing on television was the *Highlander* television series, starring Adrian Paul. Maybe it was partly that the show was coproduced for broadcast in France, so it was by default sexier than your usual North American fare. When you're an Immortal, the list of ex-lovers who can show up in any given episode (and in flashbacks) is quite long, so there were plenty of opportunities. But really, what's not to like about guys who look like they just walked off the cover of a romance novel trying to kill each other with long, shiny swords? Every episode ends with a fatal duel, the "cum shot" being when one rival beheads the other, precipitating a magical transfer of power called "the Quickening." Oh, no, not sexual at all. And how Freudian that these rivals must behead one another, clearly a stand-in for emasculation/castration—especially when you consider that our hero, Duncan, pretty much never takes the head of the female Immortals he encounters. And he encounters quite a few, from a Catwomanish Joan Jett to beauty queen Elizabeth Gracen. Oo la la.

It's the overtly sexy themes that keep cropping up that make me think it isn't just me who gets off on screen violence. The filmmakers have to be in on it, too. Unlike porn, where the more stylized it is, the less arousing I find it, with swordplay and gunplay, the more stylized, the better. The highly stylized cinematography and improbable fighting moves succeed in transporting me into a fantasy realm. My imagination is engaged, and my heart starts to race. Maybe Freud was right about some things.

When Wolverine reveals his claws in *X-Men: The Movie* (which had a PG-13 rating, by the way), it's better than Rocco Siffredi unzipping his pants. Sure, he can flick them out switchblade-style ("snikt" is his sound effect), but he can also extrude them gradually, just like an erection emerging from the foreskin. If these things aren't phallic, what are we to make of the fact that Rogue and Wolverine don't estab-

lish intimacy and trust until after he penetrates her? With his claws, I mean. These two characters, who have had a sort of attraction/tension between them for much of the film, are put into a classic sexual set-up, in which she slips into his room at night while he is having nightmares. But instead of a compromising erotic situation, a compromising violent situation stands in—he stabs her.

Look at the classic "heroic bloodshed" films from John Woo's days in Hong Kong. The best are those in which he teamed up with star Chow Yun-Fat—Hong Kong's answer to Cary Grant—especially *The Killer* and *Hard-Boiled*. Both stories have a subtext of unrequited love and—being Chinese—these films have buried their emotions under an inscrutable mask of revenge and honor-bound violence. (Music-video director Antoine Fuqua does his best Woo imitation in 1998's *The Replacement Killers*, starring Chow. Although I enjoyed it, it was strictly softcore.)

Woo isn't having fun unless he's sublimating love, lust, or both, into some kind of symbolic gun battle or violence, which is why *Face/Off* is his best US film. When the bad guy (Nicolas Cage) swaps his face for the good guy's (John Travolta), each man enters the other one's life in intimate ways. One of the most symbolic scenes comes when the villain gives "his" daughter some fatherly advice after he witnesses her boyfriend trying to get into her pants against her will. After beating the boyfriend black and blue, and giving her a cigarette, he asks the daughter if she has "protection."

"You mean like condoms?" she asks. You're expecting him to whip a foil packet out of his jacket pocket and toss it to her. But no.

Her grip tightens on the hilt, and in ultra-close-up she slowly but firmly glides the blade several inches from its sheath.

The very next shot is a slo-mo on his right hand, unfolding a butterfly knife. The sides spread open sensuously, and then it clicks into place, the blade lusciously curved and glinting in the light. "Protection," he repeats. If you aren't lusting after the weapon after that cinematic treatment, you're dead from the neck down.

Then there is Woo's signature fight-scene move—the intensely intimate "Mexican standoff" in which two characters (or more) meet in the heat of battle, each with a gun pressed to the other's head. In *Face/Off*, Woo doesn't pass up the opportunity to make a kind of 69 out of it—when each man (who is having some sort of relations with the other's wife/girlfriend) "faces off" against the other, they end up on opposite sides of a two-sided, full-length mirror. This time the face each man sees is his enemy's, but also his own.

👸

Speaking of Mexican standoffs, the next director who seems to share my kink is Robert Rodriguez. Take a look at *Desperado*, his sequel/pseudo-remake of his own cult-indie hit *El Mariachi*. The weapon-as-object-of-lust theme translates easily from culture to culture in cinema. As one character says of the protagonist, who carries his guns in a guitar case: "He sat that thing on the stool beside him as if it were his girl." Rodriguez is not subtle in this film, and I love him for it. It stars heartthrob Antonio Banderas, described by his fan sites as "the Ultimate Latin Lover." Rodriguez pairs him with the sexy, sultry Salma Hayek, and I do mean pairs.

Here's how the major sequence of the first act unfolds. First, Rodriguez's camera lingers over Banderas' beauty, as our hero shaves, puts back his hair, and dons his best jacket. *Hot.* To go out and pick up a girl? Yes and no. His intent is to kill just about every inhabitant of a seedy Mexican bar. He does, with verve and oodles of choreographed, Woo-esque gunplay. As he walks away from the bar, the lone survivor stalks him unseen through the daytime streets. Or so we think.

The bad guy catches up to our hero just as sexy Salma enters, in a midriff top that causes a car accident as she crosses the street. She sees the gunman coming from behind, and at the last moment, our hero sweeps her out of the way, turns on the assailant, gets shot in the arm, and ends up on the ground

Action-film directors have figured out what I—the slobbering audience member—want: a visceral, physical experience which is *akin* to sex.

on top of him, with the bad guy's guns pressed under his own chin. The cum shot: Our hero shoots him, blood sprays everywhere, then Antonio swoons into Salma's arms. Honestly, if that isn't all an analog for sex, I don't know what is.

Act two opens with a beautiful S/M scene between the two of them, where she tweezes the bullets out of his wound in sadistic fashion, scalds him with hot water, and plays with needles, while they make repartee. In the next scene, she looks through his guns and finds one that looks remarkably like a strap-on dildo, and he says that she can have it. The list goes on. Did I mention I love Robert Rodriguez? There's even a sequel, *Once Upon a Time in Mexico*—check out Salma and her garter full of knives. Oh, baby. Rodriguez directed the aforementioned *Sin City*, as well. The next time I go to see one of his films, I may as well bring a Pocket Rocket vibrator in my purse. (Provided it isn't *SpyKids 4*, of course.)

No discussion of modern action would be complete without mentioning Rodriguez's *compadre*, Quentin Tarantino, a man so influenced by John Woo's work that upon seeing *A Better Tomorrow* he started wearing a skinny tie and trench coat like Chow Yun-Fat in the film. The look—though not the suppressed but inherent sexuality—of Chow's characters surfaces in Tarantino's *Reservoir Dogs* and *Pulp Fiction*. Tarantino, I think, appears to have some sexual hang-ups himself, and he repressed them deeply for his first several films, where he investigates violence as violence (what a concept!).

We get a taste of the lewd from him in the cheesy, over-the-top flick he and Rodriguez did together, *From Dusk Till Dawn*, which features Salma Hayek doing one of the hottest stripper acts on film (though note, again, no actual tittie shot). But despite that foray, Tarantino's gunplay and bloodshed don't read, for me, as sublimated sex, so much as an actual fascination with pain, humiliation, and violence.

That is, until his magnum opus in two parts, *Kill Bill*, in which every sexual impulse Tarantino probably has ever had comes exploding out like the snakes from a joke can. (The Pussy Wagon. The nurse outfit right out of a fetish fantasy catalog.) The film is structured as a kind of *Debbie Does Dallas* of violence, in which each fight scene (sex scene) involves more important characters than the previous, coming ever closer to the big finish in which yin meets yang, Debbie meets Mr. Greenfield, and the Bride confronts her former-lover/killer, Bill.

In one of the early sequences in the film, Uma Thurman's character (called "the Bride") fights another female assassin—this is the standard girl-on-girl scene in a porn flick, which is a warm-up for the guy-on-girl action. When the Bride visits renowned swordmaker Hattori Hanzo and he shows her his swords, the music that plays can only be described as a light love theme. A lilting, wordless vocal, this is the music that should be playing when a hero sees his love interest for the first time, or when they first fall into bed together. Instead, Uma stares lovingly at a rack of swords. She reaches hesitantly for one, shy, nearly fumbling like the eager *ingénue* at a man's belt, but then her grip tightens on the hilt, and in ultra-close-up she slowly but firmly glides the blade several inches from its sheath. She could just as easily be gliding down the jockey shorts of some young lover, letting his boner stand up.

There's more. The sexual themes run the gamut from the disgusting to the uplifting, from the apparently regular rape of a comatose woman by hospital employees to the life-changing experience that procreation can be, even for assassins. The action ranges from orgiastic, as when the Bride kills off the entire henchman population of the Crazy 88, to intimate, as when sultry teen assassin Gogo asks the man on the barstool next to her if he'd like to "screw" her. When he replies in the affirmative, she stabs him, asking again if he'd like to "penetrate" her. But these are all just warm-up scenes, akin to the ones in, say, *I Dream of Jenna* (a Jenna Jameson bestseller), where the climax of climaxes comes when Jenna does her lone boy-girl scene—at the end.

In the final part of the films, Bill (David Carradine) and the Bride meet and have some of the most bizarre ex-lover banter ever filmed, as it becomes clear that, like so many exes, they each have a mound of conflicting feelings for one another and they want to kill each other—literally. In his way, Tarantino takes the ultimate step in equating love/lust/desire with violence, where the kill is the consummation. He creates a fantasy world, one where people carry their samurai swords on airplanes and where "thieves' honor" has become "assassins' ethics." Bill and the Bride ultimately are meant for each other. They share a value system (unlike the Bride's rival, Elle), and they speak the same language. When they communicate, foreplay, flirting, and attempting to kill one another are all part of the same exchange. Since his arrival on the scene, Tarantino's films have been the id of Hollywood, the primal (some would say infantile) need for gratification, but with *Kill Bill* the sexual urge finally takes its place alongside the other themes in his work.

—3

Which brings us full-circle to Asian cinema. Here we have the newly emerging genre of high-gloss fantasy martial arts films, launched by the success of Ang Lee's *Crouching Tiger, Hidden Dragon* in 2000. This film's got it all, with a story of unrequited love between Chow Yun-Fat and Michelle Yeoh (an action star in her own right), plenty of "flying wire" action with swords, knives, furniture, etc...as well as some actual young love run amok as kung fu *ingénue* Zhang Ziyi plays an upstart princess who steals a near-magical sword and ends up having a passionate affair with a barbarian-in-exile. There's a "girl talk" scene in the beginning of the movie when Michelle shows the sword to Zhang, who gets breathless looking at it while the older woman waves it around and tells her stories of its prowess. Yep, everybody wants the phallic symbol.

"It must be exciting to be a sword fighter," the girl says, "to be totally free!" She believes that the ability to fight or use a sword is the same as the ability to love whomever you want and when—and for her it's true, as she has not only secret fighting skills but a secret lover. Ang Lee has never been afraid to tell deep stories about human desires (*The Wedding Banquet*, *The Ice Storm*), and in making a martial arts epic he

melds the love story with the fight scenes by making them thematically equivalent. In other words, the fight scenes *are* love scenes.

We find out about the princess' barbarian lover and then are treated to a long flashback about how they met. His band attacks her caravan. He snatches a jade comb from her hand, and she downs a man and takes his horse to pursue him. Their "flirtation" consists of her shooting arrows at him and them exchanging sword and spear blows as their horses gallop side by side. They end up having a nice hand-to-hand match, then wrestling in the desert sand. Since we already know that they end up lovers, this all serves as an extended love scene for the audience (or at least for me). This is the slow nibbling on the chin, the caress down the neck, the soft focus as the lovers throw their hair back and slide down onto the satin sheets...except in this case the nibbles are smacks with a sword, the caresses are spinning backfists, and the satin sheets are wherever they fall while fighting.

At the end of the fight, they both fall back exhausted and pass out. Hmm. Later in her captivity, when the budding erotic attraction between them has been revealed, they finally have

Penetration is penetration is penetration.

actual sex. But how does it start? She stabs him. His blood pours over them as their wrestling turns sexual. Penetration is penetration is penetration.

Later, she steals the sword and sets off to find her fortune. Her story reminds me in an uncanny way of the plot of *Behind the Green Door*. In this classic porn film, Marilyn Chambers' character is kidnapped for an erotic sex show. First, she is mentored by an older woman, as Zhang Ziyi is by Michelle Yeoh. Next, she takes on a group of people who all want a piece of her—in *Behind the Green Door* she's touched by many hands, pleasuring her on stage, while in *Crouching Tiger* she fights multiple foes who are trying to get the sword. Then comes a confrontation with the Big Man on Campus—in *Green Door*, a black man with sizable equipment, and in *Crouching Tiger*, swordsman-hero Li Mu Bai (Chow Yun-Fat again).

The parallels eerily continue. The princess has an orgiastic fight scene where she takes on all the kung-fu fighters of a whole village; Chambers does multiple men at once, including three on trapezes, whom she handles one in each hand, one in her mouth, while straddling another man underneath her. Then a man from the audience, who is sort of a narrator of the story, grabs her and runs off with her for an intense one-on-one "true love" scene. In *Crouching Tiger*, she ends up back in the arms of her true love, the bandit Lo. I am not making this up.

Follow Zhang Ziyi to her next big, international martial-arts fantasy hit and you find her in *Hero* (billed as *Quentin Tarantino Presents...*), where she stars with three giants of Asian cinema, Jet Li, Maggie Cheung, and Tony Leung. This could have been titled *The Complicated and Dangerous Love Lives of Assassins*. Like Tarantino's society of killers, but without the sarcasm, the characters here interact in a rarefied atmosphere of danger and violence, where swordplay stands in for not only sex but also love, insult, flirtation, confession, etc.

Told in a series of flashbacks with alternate versions depending on who is doing the telling, various characters love, cheat, kill, or sacrifice themselves for one another in a filmic orgy of

It's Romeo and Juliet *and* a double-headed dong scene all in one.

honor-bound action. In the first segment—which is all about passion, as a love triangle turns jealous warriors against each other—everyone sports tumble-in-the-hay hair, tousled and disheveled seductively into their eyes. In the next segment, the lovers spend one last night together before they go to what they know is certain death in the morning. Nothing is shown other than some symbolic pushing aside of curtains and a chaste shot of them lying, fully clothed, asleep while holding hands.

No, instead the true mark of their passion is shown on film when the lovers are walking to the fight, expecting death: Flying Snow stabs her partner—but not fatally—in order to spare his life. (He'll be too injured to fight to the death.) No final kiss—just a sword in the side. Snow stabs her lover, Broken Sword, in several segments of the film, sometimes killing him, sometimes not, and I find it...*interesting*...that the way the actor Tony Leung plays it, his first reaction is to pant. Surely I cannot be the only person who finds this hot? And then the consummation between the two lovers, their final passionate scene, in which they both die upon the same sword. Flying Snow, spooning Broken Sword, pushes the sword that has already killed him (which she put there herself) into her own body, as well. It's Romeo and Juliet *and* a double-headed dong scene all in one.

But *Hero* turns out to be just a warm-up for the truly passionate follow-up from director Zhang Yimou: *House of Flying Daggers*. Here's Zhang Ziyi again, this time paired up with the most gorgeous man in all of Asia, Takeshi Kaneshiro. This one has a love triangle, too, and if you thought the stabbings in *Hero* stood in for sex, this time you're sure. This is the film

that had me limp in the theater, breathless and waiting for more—and, get this, its rating was only PG-13.

The big opening sequence of the film has our hero, Jin, a cop, posing as a rich drunk at a brothel, and our heroine, Mei, an assassin and spy, posing as a blind dancer/whore. He's lounging on cushions on the floor, and she stands above him. He draws his sword on her, the tip to her neck, and when the camera shows a shot from above, down the length of the blade, it's like the slow pan up a porn star's legs. The shot, both the way it is filmed and the way it is played, reads essentially as if he whipped his dick out of his pants and caressed her face with it.

Am I the only one in the theater who got moist (or hard) at that point? I doubt it, and yet I don't think the directors can come right out and admit what they're doing, in much the same way that the packaging on vibrators has to hide the device's true intent, perhaps even deny it. (I kid you not, my trusty Con-Air vibe came with explicit instructions warning me not to apply the device to my genital area.) Zhang Yimou's commentary about *House of Flying Daggers* is mostly obscure. "The women in my films often personify a deeper allegorical meaning," he told one interviewer who inquired about the issues of sex and love in the film. Zhang is accustomed to having to dodge tough questions, though, since for decades he has had his films banned and/or censored by the Chinese government.

John Woo's first "heroic bloodshed" film, *Heroes Shed No Tears*, was shelved by the studio in 1983 for being too violent, but after his success with gunplay films, they eventually released it with an added sex scene. Woo reportedly hates the scene. Robert Rodriguez told reporters on his press junket for *Sin City* that the sex scenes were truncated not for MPAA purposes but because translating the sexual action of the graphic novels to film gave it too much weight and time. "They're single panels, but when you go to the movie, it just keeps going and going," he said at a press conference. "After a certain point, it would look like [we] were just filming for our own pleasure rather than telling the story at that point."

So maybe they are making films designed just to make me wet, or maybe it's all my oversexed imagination. If it is, well, that's cool by me, as long as I can get my itch scratched when I want it. With *Sin City* topping the box office and *Kill Bill* at the top of the DVD sales charts, I have a feeling I'll get what I need, for a few more years anyway. After that, I guess I'll be stuck looking for the sexualized undercurrent in Major League Baseball or something.

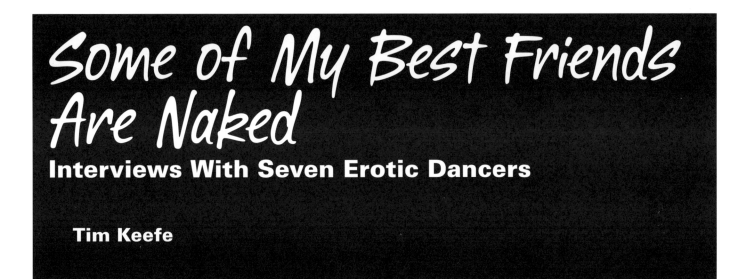

Some of My Best Friends Are Naked

Interviews With Seven Erotic Dancers

Tim Keefe

Editor's Note: From 1985 to 1991, former therapist, teacher, and manager Tim Keefe had a backstage job at a San Francisco peep show in which all the individual booths look onto a single, large stage occupied by several dancers (late in Keefe's stay, they added a single one-on-one booth). During his stay, he conducted long, epic interviews with seven of the women. The results were published in early 1993 as the 383-page tome Some of My Best Friends Are Naked, *which remains one of the best, most insightful books ever published about sex workers. Unfortunately, it was put out by the tiny, short-lived Barbary Coast Press and has never gotten the recognition it deserves. What follows are excerpts that present a sliver of this scarce, overlooked book.*

Minx Manx

Part of the promotion for your show says, "Live Nude Dancing, Lovely Lusty Ladies, Naked Naughty Nasty." Is this a good description of who you are and how you perform at work? ~ It's a good partial description. Certainly the "Lovely, Lusty, Naughty, Nasty" talk about fantasy, and at work I'm working off a fantasy. I guess for some folks it's just a job, but to me it's part of my erotic playtime. And I'm checking out who are the people and what are they doing on the other side of that window. It's my anthropology. There isn't anything on the sign that says, "Lovely, anthropological nymphet will be watching you as hard as you're watching her," although I suppose some folks know that. It's about a fantasy of women who want to show off for all the guys who walk in. And yeah, part of that's true for me. The role of the place is purveying fantasy.

Describe how you dance, display, and touch your body during your stage performance. ~ I start out actually danc-ing. It warms me up. There's a lot of posing, vogueing, show-ing off, and sticking my pussy up as close to the window as I can get it. I watch myself in the mirror—it's voyeurism and exhibitionism at the same time. That's fun. I pick customers to interact with, and, depending on their energy, I'll be some-what desultory and save my energy. I'll show pussy, pose, and do mostly eye contact interaction, or else get into pretty active masturbation. Partly because it's hot for me to be there and it makes time go more quickly to be actually erotic rather than potentially erotic, or to be an erotic subject rather than an erotic object. Because it turns me on to be an erotic object and an erotic subject, I go, more often than not, to the cor-ner booths where there's a ledge and I can do a lot of body movement. I kneel, lean back on one hand, and display my upper torso, arched back. I masturbate with my other hand till it gets tired. It's really bad for the spine, so I get up and do something else for awhile. I've learned how to get my whole body much more involved in my active eroticism and orgasm. I do come onstage, and it can be just from undulating and moving my hips rather than putting my finger there and wig-gling it. That's how I was masturbating when I first got there. A lot of times people have to remind me to take my break.

What sexual depictions do you perform? ~ Depictions of reality. I do masturbation. It's fun to spread my legs, bend my knees, and pretend to be on top during a fuck. I do it to the air or place my palm against my ass and fuck my own fingers. I key in to the men who are masturbating to make the situa-tion mutual. It turns it into an overtly sexual situation for me. I wanted to be an erotic performer to be erotic, more than to perform. More often than not, the sexual and orgasmic depic-tions and the actual orgasmic faces are the stuff that I go for, probably because if I was on the other side of the window that's the stuff I would like to watch. "Do unto others what you would have others do unto you."

I was quite surprised when I first heard that healing occurs here, women healing themselves, each other, and customers. Describe what you know about this. ~ It's profoundly healing for some women, me included, to take charge of their own eroticism in such a public way. To be able to say to yourself, "Me and my sexiness are going to get in a box and hang out there for all to see for several hours at a stretch," is a profound piece of work, and that really is how I have experienced it.

It has done worlds for my performance anxiety. I've learned to be sexually spontaneous in a way that I never was before. I've learned to come through visual stimulus, talking dirty, and humping the air. It's made me more orgasmic, which is always healing. None of us know what it would be like to have as much sex as we ever wanted because we don't have time, we don't have permission. I get a lot more time and per-

I do come onstage, and it can be just from undulating and moving my hips rather than putting my finger there and wiggling it.

mission in the booth than I get anywhere else. That's been real healing. Good sex is healing.

Any woman who steps across the line to do overt sex-industry work has gotten shit from somebody about it. Most probably from herself. We do a lot of "staffing" about that, as therapists would say. We help each other feel good about it. I don't know what we're all going to think twenty years down the line, but right now we can be together and give each other support for being nontraditional women, for being women outlaws truly. This culture has always thought of women who sell it and women who are slutty and women who want it all the time as not really okay. They idolize us and they want to chase our ass, but we are not okay.

Often women who come here have never been in a space that's so female before. We're surrounded by hard dicks, but we're onstage together and it's about tits and pussies and girl smell and women being erotic. It's funny to watch women who aren't accustomed to female sexuality start to get a clue. [*Laughs.*] There's a lot of lesbian fantasy that gets brought a lot closer to reality 'cause we are being sexual together, and how could you not notice? [*Laughs.*]

I think men come to places like the theater more than anything else to be in an environment where someone will tell them it's okay to have a hard-on. To want to look at it, and to want it. And there's no place in the world out there, including a lot of marriages and primary relationships, where people get the

signal it's okay to want it. It's okay to want it in the middle of the morning when you've got your business suit on, damn it. It's okay to want it when you just got done painting a Victorian and you're taking your lunch break. It's okay to want it when you're wearing your rubber slicker and you just got off a boat down at the Wharf and you stumbled in in your thigh boots. I had this fucking guy come in in his rubber slicker and thigh boots—I'm going, "Whoa, I'm jackin' off with Captain Ahab. This is amazing!" [*Laughs.*] "Hey, did you catch Moby Dick or what?" And so often what they want is not just orgasm, is not just jackin' off. It's not just to get their dick hard—it's to talk about eroticism and sex and feelings. To talk about the fuckin' weather, to just talk to somebody.

What are they in there for, if it's not about some kind of healing? Some kind that I probably can't even put my finger on. Something about just interacting with a woman, a person. A lot of guys come in to do just what the sign says, to talk to a live, nude girl. And I think all of that is healing.

This culture doesn't let us have our sexuality, and whether it's because of culture or hormone surges, guys get reminded of theirs a whole lot and feel like they have to get put down and shut down around their sex in order to be productive members of society and good husbands and not pester their wives too much, and, damn it, they want a place where they can go and just have it. And more than anything else, that's what the theater and places like it are about. That's what it's about for me. That's especially true of guys who have divergent sexual interests, who want to show off their lacy panties and garter belt to somebody. My favorite guy can stick his dick up his own ass. He wants to show off to somebody. He wears a wedding ring, and I bet his wife doesn't know he can do that. Just imagine bursting into the bathroom one morning to get your nylons drying on the towel rack and going, "Honey, uh, what are you doing?" [*Laughs.*] The guys who want you to watch them suck themselves off. The guys who want to play with submission and age-play and incest-play and want to call me Mommy. And women, too; occasionally, we get a woman who is there for the eroticism. Sometimes couples share that. All those people get told by our culture, their partners, by everybody that it's not real okay to be sexy and turned on the way they are, and so they've got to find a place where they can have that, where people won't turn them away and shut 'em down and tell them they're wrong and bad and sick and evil. I really think that these people use peep shows for a kind of healing, a kind of affirmation.

And I in turn, because I am obviously a sexually divergent woman, both in my exhibitionism and the fact that I am really turned on doing this stuff, because I'm a sex worker, because I'm a former overt out lesbian and still am quite queer in the *global*, queer, sexual sense, because I'm into S/M and dominance and submission, because I'm into watching and being watched, talking and being talked to and finding out all the little byways of sex that women aren't supposed to *know* about, much less practice and see if they can get good at—I'm just as divergent as those guys are. They're coming in to be with me and trust me with their sex, and their desire reaffirms me in mine. I doubt they know that they're doing that for me, but *I* know, and I know that I'm doing it for them. And every once in a while a man will be very clear, like the dominance guy who said, after he got off and stopped being nasty to me and calling me a dirty cunt, "It's so good that you people are here doing this." Just the kind of voice he would tell the waiter to please convey his compliments to the chef, you know? Same thing, same thing. "Please let everybody doing this know that we appreciate you for being here and giving us something that we can't get other places." I know plenty of people who have well-rounded sexual relationships who started out by understanding that they could get that by visiting peep shows, by seeing prostitutes and getting it that somebody would want to fuck them or talk to them or see them or let them watch.

Yeah, there's a lot of healing. I am very clear that I am like one of the priestesses of the Goddess back in the temples of the Middle East, way before Yahweh showed up and took over, whose spiritual gift was to be there for any man who walked in to see the face of the Goddess. We're showing the face of the Goddess in a culture that doesn't believe in the Goddess anymore.

Describe your performance at its best and worst. ~ At my best I give the customer total permission to be who he or she is and want what he or she wants. I consent to being a fantasy object in those desires, whatever they are. At my best I become just as erotically involved with the customer as he is with me. So that we really are having sex together. That often results in orgasms for me and almost always results in orgasms for him, although that's not all there is to it. Orgasm is just reminding us that, yeah, we're still connected to our bodies. I communicate total acceptance, joy, and enthusiasm for sex. Which I think is a communication that none of us get enough of. A lot of us haven't ever really gotten it all.

At my worst, just like in partner-sex, I'm too tired to really connect. I'm not with the erotic flow any longer. At my worst it's, "Where's the sex? I can't find it."

Describe the customers. ~ Well, most of them are men. That's about all you can say that's generalizable. They come from a great many walks of life. They are all races. They are

from all over the world. Some are travelers and tourists, and some live right in the neighborhood. Some of them come from far away to have their sexual fantasy. Some are quite young, probably too young to be there. They are men old enough to be grandpas, and you hope they're not going to fall over while they're jackin' off. And every age in between. Most are in their forties, I would guess. They are packs of boys, Latinos, Asian Pacific, black or white, or combinations thereof; out on the prowl, checking it out, having a little testosterone party amongst themselves. Those are the most likely to misbehave in the hallway and suddenly turn sweet and shy in the booth. That's a little piece of information I never expected to get about the way young men behave.

They are from all economic classes. A lot more upstanding citizens than I ever thought. I had some prejudices about, "Who would go to those sleazy places anyway?" Well, a little bit of everybody does. The only people that we don't have a good representational sample of are females. I'd love to have more of them visit me. It's a special case when a woman walks in, it's like, "Oh, my God, it's a *woman* and she's here to watch!" Sometimes her husband or boyfriend is hauling her in, and she's kind of trying to hide her eyes behind her hands and go, "Oh, not this, honey," and sometimes she is

I've seen guys hump the window, hump the wall.

unabashedly as much a pussy hound as anybody else there. I want to see as many different kinds of women as men feel free to explore sexual entertainment. It's cultural—it's just not okay yet.

Do customers leave their social roles and status behind when they come to see you? ~ Sometimes. In some respects, a hard cock is a great leveler.

Describe the variety of sexual behavior customers express. ~ Everything from open, lascivious looking, a looking that is so sexual that you just don't see it any place else, except occasionally in the eyes of a lover. To pawing at the glass to pretend to touch your body. Making licking motions—"Oh, that pussy looks so good I could eat it." Kissing through the glass. Guys jerk off and occasionally sploosh on the window. I try not to let them actually touch the glass with their mouths, but sometimes they do it. I explain that it's not safe. I've seen guys hump the window, hump the wall.

Lots of taking penis in hand and rubbing, stroking, petting, teasing, jerking. I don't know if I've seen every form of masturbation, but I've seen lots and lots and lots, and it's a ceaseless delight to see how different guys do it. There's some whole-body self-sexuality, too. Some guys will get completely undressed and rub their hands over themselves and play with their nipples and asshole; occasionally, guys bring dildos in to use on themselves. Fabric fetishists bring in fabric they like and either wear it or jerk off into a satin slip or panties or something like that. Occasionally, I see coupled-partner sexual activity. And I myself, I might add, have come in as a customer with my partner. We call it "entertaining the troops" when we're sexual together. The women tease us a little bit and cluster around to see what we do. It's always a treat for me and a lot of the dancers when somebody is being sexual in the booth with somebody else. It's fun to see what other people do.

Many customers show a great deal of interest in the dancers' genitalia. Why do you think there is such great interest? ~ It's forbidden, taboo. I think a lot of men, especially older men, started out being sexual with women in the dark, in cars, in bushes, underneath the football stadium, wherever they could cop a feel, and never really got to see except in those strange split-beaver pictures that even now, no matter how many pussies you've seen, still look kind of

"Can I just look at your pussy? My *wife* won't let me look at her pussy."

unreal. I had an old man, he must have been seventy-five, one of the real grandpa guys who makes you go, "Is he still pulling it out and doing that? Oh, isn't that wonderful?" He came in, and he didn't want to pull it out. He said, "Can I just look at your pussy? My *wife* won't let me look at her pussy." This guy's probably married to this woman for fifty years, and she won't let him look at her pussy. He just wants to see what it is, how all the parts look together.

Guys come in and say, "Which part's your clit?" I think part of it is sex education; I really do. An eroticized, sort of nasty, dirty sex education, like looking at those beaver shots. But it's about, "Now wait a minute—how's this piece of me gonna fit in there, exactly? Where does it go exactly when I stick it in?" [*Laughs.*] It's that as well as the mystical pussy, and the dirty, forbidden pussy, and the pussy that you just want to stare at while you think about a pussy that you miss. It's all of those things.

I love watching them pull their cocks out 'cause it's the part *I* wasn't supposed to look at. So it's like, "Oh good, oooh, this one looks different than the last one did." I can get why they want to look at pussies 'cause I feel the same way about them.

What do the customers want you to do? ~ A little bit of everything. There are gestures that they're not supposed to use. Occasionally, women will say, "You can't tell us what to do," but I don't care, personally. I think that's either erotic or neutral. I don't mind doing anything if they're not rude.

They want me to spread my lips, to turn over, bend over, show them my asshole. They want to look at all these little parts close up, often jacking off furiously while they do. They want me to look at them, talk to them, kiss them, or pretend I'm sucking them off. It's always been just phenomenal to me that the illusion of a blowjob was enough to pay money for. I got sophisticated after a while and started sucking on a dildo—without it I felt sort of like the fish in the aquarium, make my mouth into an *O* and bob up and down. [*Laughs.*]

Men in the booth want me to talk about anything and everything. One guy came in three or four times in one night, and the first time he wanted me to be his aunt; the second time, his Catholic school teacher; the third time, his mommy; then he went back to auntie again. Another man wants me to pretend to be his sister.

They want me to masturbate with dildos, occasionally use a vibrator. They want me to stick things in my asshole and pee in a cup, and a lot of them want me to tell them how much I like it. And that's easy for me, because by and large I do. I say, "I do. I'm having orgasms—what does it look like?" If they've seen me squirt, they want to see me squirt again. They want me to come right up to the glass and watch them squirt, to be unabashedly interested in their cock, or they want me to play along with funny games like telling them that their cock is really big or really small. One guy likes to be told that his cock is extremely short. He holds it into his body cavity a little bit, and then at the last minute he pops it out, and it really isn't two inches long after all, and, oh, aren't I surprised? I'm supposed to be surprised every single time. [*Laughs.*] I wonder where he eroticized that one, too. I wonder about these guys. They're like treats and enigmas and puzzles, trying to figure out where things got erotic for them.

They want me to talk to them and do therapy and tell them stories and make up lies and tell them the truth. And tell them about when I first lost my virginity. And how often I like to do it. One guy thought he was going to shock the hell out of me when I asked, "Well, gee, what do you like to talk about? What's hot for you?" He said, "Dogs. Doing it with dogs." So I started talking about doing it with dogs, and he got out of there really fast. [*Laughs.*] I don't think he thought he was going to get somebody to work with him on that one.

Just about anything that you can imagine that's an erotic possibility, somebody wants to see me do or talk about, which is one of the absolute delights of it. I mean, if it was only one thing all the time! Well, I suppose even orgasm would get old, but it's always something different, always something new. I think of those Mummers parades, where everybody dresses up in outrageous clothes and parades around with their psyches hanging out. Some people come to the theater with their psyches hanging out, and it's wonderful.

Describe your adolescent sexuality. ~ I started to calm down about what my body looked like, a little bit, by the time I was fourteen or so. I had gone to the library and found out what fucking was, and decided I wanted to do it. I was up against the dilemma of the unusual kid: "I'm weird—who's going to want to fuck me?" The boys I hung out with were the oddball boys who were less in control of, less proactive with their sexuality than the boys on the football team, who had discovered that they could fuck pretty much anybody they wanted. *They* didn't want to fuck me. I was getting extraordinarily horny, and I wanted to do something about this stupid virginity.

I would try masturbating, and I would get up to "T-1 and counting," and my hand would freeze. There was so much physical tension in me that I could not make my hand move the last four strokes that it would take to get me over to orgasm. So I was a maniac, like a monkey on a string.

And what I did was have an affair with one of my former teachers. That helped take care of matters. It took me out of the social fishbowl of high school, where I wasn't fitting in very well, and put me into another realm altogether, an adult sexual realm, essentially. I don't suppose it was an adult sexual realm the first couple of times, but after that, I was having a relationship, the way I have relationships now. And it made a great deal of difference. I still wasn't orgasmic, but at least I was getting all the other things I wanted from sexuality—the touching, the attention, the "yes, you're desirable" stuff, all of that. And then I got the vibrator and that fixed the rest of it.

After a while it got around that I fucked—that took care of a multitude of sins, as far as all the boys were concerned. [*Laughs.*] But having sex with guys my own age was always perfectly weird. The level of communication and body knowledge that I shared with my older lover never got replicated with people my age, not till I got to college.

Describe your sexual fantasies. ~ Wow. I spend so much time living so many of them I don't [*laughs*] have a real active fantasy life right now. Actually, I do. My partner and I play family sex games, brother-sister and other kinds of taboo sex. I've got some strong fantasy charge on that stuff. Maybe I'm taking my funny business with my dad into a place that's entirely safe to have the parts that did get under my skin erotically. I have a strong fantasy charge on dominant-submissive energy. I've been a bottom for as long as I've been in touch with that, which is ten, twelve years now. I'm just starting to, in my fantasy life most of all, move into a place where I can be on top, and that's a real exciting change for me. I always knew it would happen, but I never knew when.

When I fantasize I stop at *some* humans; I'm not willing to imagine having sex with either Jesse Helms or Andrea Dworkin. Currently, my favorite non-human fantasy has to do with going to Marine World and getting a job as an underwater mermaid and having the dolphins try to get me when I go in to feed them after the place closes. I majorly want to have sex with a dolphin, and I don't know if I will ever get the chance. That's my big quirk fantasy for the moment. They're so smart, they must be good lovers, you know.

At what age do you think people should be allowed to view pictures of human genitalia? ~ Well, they got to be out of the womb because they can't see in there. I'm serious. Maybe on the way out. There should be decorations on the walls of the obstetrics ward. People should be able to view pictures of human genitalia at every age. People should be able to view live human genitalia walking past, in the persons of the brothers, sisters, mommies, and daddies, and when they go out on weekends to the nude beach. Genitalia should be no more outrageous to view than ears, and until we get over that one, we will have certain problems associated with shame and guilt. And probably a higher level of adrenaline attached to our titillation around nudity.

What would a sexually positive society look like? ~ One in which kids weren't stigmatized and punished for their sexual feelings and explorations. It would be one in which gender roles were not strict and behavior by gender category was unknown. It would be one in which everybody was encouraged to make sexual pleasure a priority in their lives. It wouldn't be assumed that just because you found a partner that everything would fall into place easily, that sexual pleasure would have to be something that real compatibility was found around, and that would be honored. When you bring your potential spouse home to your mom, Mom wouldn't say, "Oh, how nice, dear, how much money does he make?" but, "Oh, how nice, dear, are you having multiple orgasms together?" [*Laughs.*] That would be healthy.

I think more people would try more kinds of sexual behavior so there wouldn't be so clearly defined sexualized groups of people. Maybe some people would settle in one particular kind of behavior, but maybe other people would just zoom up and down the range of things that they could do for their whole lives. I think there would be less heterosexual monogamous partnering, perhaps less monogamous partnering altogether, that jealously would be much less a problem than it is now. And for good measure, we might eradicate all sexually transmitted diseases.

How can we achieve that society? ~ Talk about sex a hell of a lot more and a hell of a lot more honestly and openly than we do now. Start to look at the fact that strict gender-role differentiation hurts people, doesn't help people, doesn't allow for men or women to achieve their best qualities and makes us feel like we're separate species, which we're not, even though we're trained to act like it. Start providing kids with space to be sexual and good sex education. Throw a lot more money at sexually transmitted disease-eradication research than is being thrown now. In the meantime, make free condoms available everywhere. Make sex okay, make it a cultural priority.

Ann More

What were you told was your job? ~ I was told that I was there to entertain men and to do what I wanted to do.

Now it's been proven to me that anything with tits and a cunt can do anything to a man.

Were you told that the men masturbate? ~ I was not told. I must have figured it out as soon as I got onstage. [*Laughs*.] As a matter of fact, as I watch other people get hired, it seems to me like it's something that's totally avoided. Women seem to be really shocked. [*Laughs*.] Management is kind of ignorant, so I think they just assume you know, or it's just part of the game now. Personally, I had no idea. People beat off—that's what happens.

What sexual depictions do you perform? ~ [*Laughs*.] None! God, I don't do anything now. I dance. I'll bend over. I play with my breasts, over and over and over again. I just move around. I'm more concerned about how far I can stretch my leg, how much I can suck my stomach in, where my cellulite is. I'm not worried about the customers or showing them anything. They might catch a glimpse of my labia, since I have a gold ring there. I'll play with that, but it's not for them—I'm looking at it. To bend over, to me, is basically an insult. But [*laughs*] they love it.

Do you test your power to arouse? ~ Not any longer. I did the first year and a half. It was a trip. You want to see what you can do, and now it's been proven to me that anything with tits and a cunt can do anything to a man. [*Laughs*.] I know they're desperate to get attention from me because I have no pants on. So there's no test. They walked in the door—I won. [*Laughs*.]

How much of your performance is you and your sexuality and how much is persona? ~ Basically, it is me. I am basically a negative, cold, non-sexual person. I think the world has been overloaded with all of it. I wish there were some-

where else to go, but unfortunately, there's no other world. Well, as far as my sexuality goes, the relationship I'm in now is wonderful. I'm very sexual with this person. That is very important to me because [*laughs*] my last relationship was very asexual. Nothing was happening. I saw cock all day and then went home to another ignorant cock.

Is there competition among the dancers onstage? ~ No, not at all.

Is the myth of the perfect body perpetuated here? ~ [*Laughs*.] No, not in this theater. [*Laughs*.] It's funny because I give myself a little credit or pride for trying to take care of myself and having one of the better, in-shape bodies there, and it doesn't matter. What matters is who has their legs open, who is sticking their asshole in some man's nose. [*Laughs*.] Who has tits hanging to their knees, who has the biggest is what it's all about. Whoever's giving a man attention is what it's all about. If you're anorexic, and you're looking at him, spreading your cheeks, then you're it to him. You're like a wallflower unless you are showing him your pussy, which is what he came to see. [*Laughs*.] I mean, please! [*Laughs*.]

Do you ever become aroused by what you are doing and what is happening around you onstage? ~ I remember three times, in the first year, when I was in heat right before my period, where I actually did get horny being with a pathetic man, using my power [*laughs*] and watching how he could just gawk and be so desperate. I just beat off and forgot about it. But it had nothing to do with them, you know what I mean? But now, nothing. [*Laughs*.]

Do you ever have sexual fantasies during your performance? ~ I have murder fantasies. Nothing sexual ever goes through my mind. Except maybe that I can't wait to go home and make love with my man, because this is so disgusting.

I was quite surprised when I first heard that healing occurs here, women healing themselves, each other, and customers. Describe what you know about this. ~ I don't know what you're talking about. This is news to me. [*Laughs*.] Healing? What are we talking—sexual, mental, physical healing? What are we talking about?

Describe the customers. ~ I have to find vocabulary—"pathetic" is getting old. They're like strays. It reminds me of being at the Humane Society and seeing a bunch of dogs in the kennel. But these you don't want to take home. These are the ones that you want to send away to be destroyed. Which is not fair to say, because you don't know them. But they're all so desperate, and they come there expecting so much. For a quarter, they expect a fucking prostitute. [*Laughs*.]

In our job there's nothing that you have to do. You're supposed to entertain the men, but you are not there to cash in on their whims. They think it's Burger King. They expect you to wait on them hand and foot. They're classless. They're just something that you want to be removed. With the exception of a handful of men who take the time to talk to you. They respect you; they're looking at you in admiration. They know that you're human and that you have intelligence, that you do other things.

But, basically, the men there are wrong. They're wrong, they're lost, they're lonesome, but they don't know how to deal with it. They're also afraid. I think there's a great fear that's going on. A window goes up, "Hello! You think you're Mr. Tough Guy? Here's five nude women; what are you going to do now?" They freak out, and I think out of fear, nervousness makes them act stupid. They say the wrong things; they do the wrong things. Should I be macho? Should I be sensitive? They don't know, so they do everything wrong.

I'm very intimidating. I go out of my way to intimidate them, which makes them slip even more [laughs] into the revulsion level, so...they acquire a lot of training. But that's what the whole theater's about, I guess—training. And I'm at a point right now where I don't even do that. They sicken me, and I go somewhere else mentally until they leave. Those are the male customers.

There are two kinds of female customers. The women who have never been here before, who don't know what to expect, women who have taken showers and never looked at themselves. They're out for the night, either with their boyfriends or other girls, and they don't know how to handle it, so they giggle. They come off very silly. Then there are the women who totally know what to expect. They're wonderful. They're full of admiration. They look at everyone in a very respectful way, watching how they move, like they're watching a ballet. They're very interested. They'll say hello. They're obviously in touch with themselves. Women are definitely cooler. There are no demands, no expectations.

There are lesbian and straight women. Straight women come in with their partners. Some of the couples are wonderful. The women are totally into their partners looking at these other women, and they're getting off on it. I can't imagine how it can be such an experience for them—they really enjoy it. [Laughs.]

Do you encounter violent men here? ~ Those are the kind of men that I attract, violent men. They'll be loud, and I've even had a couple of them threaten me: "I'll kick your ass." It can happen if you provoke them in the I way that they don't want to be provoked. Look, the men in there have hard-ons.

They think with their hard-ons. Their hard-ons aren't getting satisfied, they go off.

Describe some of the more unique encounters you've had with customers. ~ One I will probably remember until I die is the boy who came in and sucked himself off. I think that's wonderful. He rolls over, brings his hips up, and sucks himself off. Then he spits it out, which is a beautiful finish.

The businessmen with the lingerie totally kill me. They're the ones doing the "right thing," and then they strip down, and they're in women's lingerie and garter belts. That's just wonderful. I love the businessmen who get their dicks sucked by other men. [Laughs.] That's a real turn-on, actually! Because it's like they're allowing their power to be demoted in front of us. I love it.

Are you ever disturbed by the effect you have on customers? ~ [Laughs.] No, I enjoy it. I like to piss them off; I like to make them feel something else besides their fucking dicks. I want them to be in for a banger. It's like, you think you're here for a quarter, getting a fucking hooker? Hell no, you're getting a woman who's intelligent, a woman who thinks you're fucking pathetic, who can't understand why you have to do it. I've masturbated my whole life, and the idea of going to a place like that and putting myself on display—there's just some-

We run this whole fuckin' world. The world is based on pussy. Face it.

thing wrong about it. It's not wrong, it's just—it's pathetic. It's just pathetic that they have to pay a quarter and beat off. It's pathetic.

Do you ever abuse the customers? ~ [Laughs.] Yes! Yes, I abuse them. I find myself going out of my way to make them feel intimidated and insecure, and make it hard for them to achieve an orgasm. [Laughs.] I enjoy that, because it's not supposed to happen. You're supposed to make it easy, so I think they should be in for a little treat. [Laughs.] I'm so rude to them. I'm going to have to start being aware that when I laugh at people and they have sexual problems, they may go kill themselves.

Describe your family and its circumstances as you remember them during childhood. ~ My family was the perfect, all-American family. Mom and Dad were married, happy, and there was no abuse. They both worked, and I went to Catholic school and had the bike and the dog. I have an older brother, adopted also. Everything was just fine....

My family is middle class. My dad was always a truck dispatcher for major supermarket chains. My mom has been the secretary, computer analyst lady. I went to Catholic school, so I was always sheltered in regard to sex education. It's still taught in a sheltered way.

We always did what we wanted, the piano lessons, the ballet, everything. We always got what we wanted but had to work for it. They instilled that.

Has living in a male-dominated society played a role in shaping your sexuality? ~ Of course it has. I want a dick, you know. I want a dick to show them what it's like. I want a dick, and I want to drive it up their ass and stick it down their throat, and show them why I am cold and what I am feeling, to show them what they're like. Of course it's made me very angry when I look at the world, dominated by guys. Yeah! That's why I'm cold and bitter and angry. I don't like them. Fucked up.

Very few people have self-defenses, fronts, or attitudes when they're naked.

Do women play a part in the creation of male sexuality? ~ We run the whole show. We run this whole fuckin' world. The world is based on pussy. Face it. Obviously, we've made them dogs at this point. We have created that. We've made men really pathetic and desperate for women, for sex, for naughty sex, for infidelity. Yeah, we've made them macho. We have made you like you are, and now I think we're trying to reverse it all. We've lured them on to make money, to survive, so we've gone to our bodies. It started in the age of slavery when we were getting banged, but that was no choice, and we've just reversed it. We're basically making you the suckers. We've made you the dogs. Because we know that you want it and we've played on it.

Lilith
Describe the interaction and commentary among the dancers onstage. ~ It depends on who's onstage, how you get along with them, if they have the same musical taste as you, if you have things in common or not. I find I have different perceptions than a lot of the people because I'm not American. I'm not quite sure to what extent the Americans are aware of that.

There is a genuine level of warmth and support that's deeper than what's required for the job. Most of the women are very caring and empathic towards each other, even when they're being bitchy. There's a certain base level of support that doesn't disappear. I have been onstage very few times when there were incidents or bad feelings. It's one of the best work environments I've ever worked in.

Incredible levels of intimacy are reached because we're being

sexual with people. Upfront sexual with four other people. There's a lot more sharing about where people are at with their sexuality. There's advice, commentary, exchange of anecdotes, flirtation, right down to enactment of real-life sexual stuff. You hear about couples in the theater, plus crushes, fancies, and admiration.

I feel a very strong admiration for several of the women. For the warmth and compassion of their natures and how they deal with different situations onstage. These are traits not necessarily cultivated by the job, but traits that the women have themselves. It was very much an eye-opener for me to see some typically female qualities stronger here than they would be allowed to be in many other environments. Here we're dealing with the connection between female power and female eroticism, the forbidden, repressed secret not to be allowed connection—it's being forged, and that obviously empowers the women.

This is an excellent observatory of human nature and behavior. Very few people have self-defenses, fronts, or attitudes when they're naked. People are a lot more open and honest with each other here than they are in other fields. That's something that people want—partly this is what's on sale, the vibe between the women. It's pretty dead with four girls onstage who don't relate particularly well. When you are onstage with women who are possessed of high amounts of physical and erotic energy, it's a very strong power experience, very interesting. It definitely is a big part of the growth experience for me, having the opportunity to learn from some of the women. People make very sexual comments to each other, about each other, about their bodies, about how big or little their breasts have gotten; did it hurt when you pierced your clitoris and your nipples; oh, you've put on weight; oh, that looks nice on you, that doesn't; if you don't get along well with men, you should try it with women—everything.

I was quite surprised when I first heard that healing occurs here, women healing themselves, each other, and customers. Describe what you know about this. ~ I feel that I healed myself by deprogramming a lot of basic Catholic attitudes toward my sexuality, guilt, and the last vestiges of being unable to touch my own body. I've learned to feel proud about my vagina, feel that this is a good part of me. A lot of the final stages of my breakthrough went on in the theater by reprogramming out of patriarchal attitudes. Healing is happening on a physical, spiritual, and psychological level.

For a lot of women, it's a healing experience if it's the first time they come in touch with their erotic power. To feel their flow is definitely empowering and strengthening. It heals the whole space that women have between the nice girl and the bad girl. Reclaiming the bad girl, that's Lilith, makes a woman whole. It's healing finding and healing menstrual wounds, realizing that it's not a wound, it's sacred drops, the wonderful elixir of life. It took the healing process to realize that, and that I could dance and be so strong on my period.

I'm firmly convinced that what we have here is women healing men of the wounds that patriarchy has dealt men in relation to their own sexuality, and the general burden of sexual repression on all of us. The blocked orgone energy, the crossed neural pathways. The circuits where we should have pleasure and love and free sexual flow have been imprinted with violence, hatred, and freak-outs. There is a major chance here to uncross, reprogram. This can occur on a very unconscious level. A man can jack off and receive a healing experience, as well as an erotic one. In spite of the semi-sleazy environment, genuine, warm, human interchange occurs with compassion and a basic level of caring. For a lot of the men downtown, it's the only place in the city where they get to relate, at all. We are dealing with the most severely alienated society in the world.

In ancient Sumeria, Lilith went out into the streets and brought men into the temple, where priestesses of the Goddess made love with them and showed them how to love women and showed them the power of love. San Francisco is a long way in place and time from that culture, but certain elements of that experience continue to carry over. It has been a repressed part of the female psyche, and some of the women are living it out now. And even if they aren't conscious of it, healing is occurring. It's a general releasing of the blocks. You can see it with a guilty customer. How the dancer handles the guilty type of customer has a major impact on them slowly coming to terms with their guilt and how they received it. A lot of them may go out just as furtively as they come in, but there is a great potential for healing.

One of the big wounds to the collective psyche is Christian sexual guilt. There are a lot of energies interchanged through the window. If you have a good orgasm with someone who remains human with you to the end of it, it cannot help but be good.

Describe the customers. ~ All the men in downtown San Francisco. From fourteen-year-old Chinese boys (they just look fourteen) to ninety-year-old Chinese men to rude, white college students, incredibly rude, crude under-twenty WASP men. Lunchtime businessmen and sad, lonely men. Men in for fun and games or a party. Men who want to get rid of their work-related tension by jerking off. Some friendly, some aggressive, some gentle and shy and furtive and worried about their sexuality. Some adoring and admiring, "Wow," and some, "Spread it, girl!" and some normal, conversational. All looking for something.

Probably a lot of them are suffering from birth trauma. I think birth trauma is a big thing here—it's what draws people to vaginas. Something that went wrong on the way out, hopes to be cured by re-entry. [*Laughs.*] I've had friendly, warm, human, loving, erotic exchanges with people, plus some downright nasty, yucky, aggressive, horrible exchanges.

Women who dance in the theater come in to see a girlfriend's show or their favorite dancer. That's somewhat regular. There are women who are coupled. Some hover shyly behind their boyfriends, and he's urging them to look and maybe follow our example. Others are there to get off on the situation and make love with their boyfriends or indulge in foreplay. There are definitely women who come in to feel superior.

In spite of the semi-sleazy environment, genuine, warm, human interchange occurs with compassion and a basic level of caring.

There's a small number of lesbian women who come in. One memorable night, I had a really good exchange with four lesbian women in a corner booth. They were all loud and raunchy and really in to "see," very into explicit display, like show me cunt and masturbate for me. They were very appreciative and getting really turned on, starting to do stuff with each other, not at all putting any attitude over about "you girls shouldn't be here."

A lot of women point and don't engage in eye contact with the girls. They're sort of embarrassed, sometimes a mutual embarrassment scene goes on woman to woman. There's mutual condescension sometimes, too.

Phoenix
Describe how you dance, display, and touch your body during your performance. ~ I show and touch parts of my body that I really like. My ass is really gorgeous. [*Laughs.*] I can start out very seductive and sultry, letting someone in by my enjoyment of my body. I gradually open up by showing and touching and coming closer to him/her. Establishing eye contact is really everything. That's where something really electric can be communicated. That's not a cliché—that's what I experience. With eye contact, we're exchanging certain kinds of understandings or power. Sometimes I give shows where I'm not doing that, and that can also work, but it's a completely different kind of experience—it's more two-dimensional. I am being this visual, sensual machine for the

customer. Sometimes customers want to connect with me, and I'm not in a space where I want to do that. For the most part, eye contact is really enjoyable; the eroticism is much more powerful. No matter how much you talk about commercializing a sex transaction, you're still talking about two people with their own agendas and needs of the moment, and that shapes the interaction.

How much of your performance is you and your sexuality and how much is persona? ~ It's both. Sometimes I'm dancing as me, a lesbian enjoying my own sexuality. Other times I'm playing a straight woman and how a straight woman is being sexual.

What won't you do onstage? ~ I'd love to go farther. I'd love to screw women onstage. I'd love to be screwed onstage, but that's not permitted. I'd love to fuck myself onstage—that's the big fantasy. Oh, God! I would just *love* to do that, really.

Is there a difference in the customers' behavior when they are alone or in a group? ~ Men in groups should be banned from the streets. [*Laughs.*] They exhibit this animalistic behavior, boosting of each other's ego, and try to psych each other into believing that they actually are in control of the world. I find it truly offensive. More often than not we have them kicked out because they're behaving like little five-year-old monsters. Men in groups always, without exception, further foster their aggression. I've never seen men come in in groups and not be aggressive and derogatory towards women. It's infallibly that way. The only explanation I can

I was discovering that my body could literally make men stop their cars in the middle of the street.

come up with is that men...have been taught that they are constantly being examined by each other. So they are constantly trying to prove themselves when they are together, their prowess and their ability to command women, et cetera, et cetera.

When they're alone, that dynamic just isn't there. I see a lot of men being really shy when they come in alone. I think when a man is alone, more often than not, he's a little unsure of how to deal with the situation. Then it's my job to make contact and bring them out of their shyness and let them know that it's okay to communicate!

How did you first discover and use the ability to arouse? ~ It's weird because you learn it so early on; it's not something you discover when you're a teenager. You learn it in a variety of ways, at all these stages of development. I certainly

learned it with my father. I learned how to entertain and titillate him in a way that was emotional, sexual, psychological, intellectual. It all meshed. But way into my teens I was always putting down and trying to hide my ability to arouse.

When I ran away, I got a taste of a whole other culture. I met hustlers in Boston and became lovers with a boy who hustled men. That's when I became more aware of being sexually explicit. When I went back to Vermont, I was dressing much more provocatively in tight pants and shirts. I was extremely thin because I had been living on coffee and donuts, and I had gotten very sick.

In Vermont I gained a lot of weight and was very, very unhealthy. I had pneumonia for six months, and then I met this man who taught me yoga. It totally rehabilitated me and turned me into this voluptuous sex-bomb. I continued to wear fairly tight clothing; I don't think I was consciously trying to be provocative as much as I was discovering that I *was* provocative. I was discovering that my body could literally make men stop their cars in the middle of the street. It freaked the shit out of me. It felt powerful and yet terrifying. I felt powerful, but I couldn't handle it. I gained weight again in order to protect myself from their gaze.

Many people paint female sex workers as among the most obvious victims of male domination and declare that if you don't see yourself as such, you are suffering from "false consciousness" and "delusions of the oppressed." What is your response to that? ~ We're all oppressed; we're all part of the system. Men are oppressed because they are seen as the money-makers. They're not supposed to be emotional, and their sexual performance is separate from their emotional experience. That's pretty oppressive. Whether I participate in the sex industry or not doesn't make the dynamic that the sex industry is part of go away. I find it very empowering to be able to make money to pay my bills. If you are in a situation where you can't, you're oppressed. It isn't just about sexuality; it's about so many things. If sex workers are the most obvious, it's because the sexual power gender relations are *undisguised*. It's going on in every aspect of society. We are not any more victims—we're all victims of this situation. Sex workers are no more victims than their customers. I don't choose to use the word *victim* because I don't experience myself as a victim. I experience myself as accepting the situation and being empowered as best I can.

Lusty Lipps
Describe your first experience onstage. ~ It was kinda weird, all of these men looking at my naked body, but as they

was lookin' and enjoying it, I got with them and said, "Yeah, they like what I'm doing." I felt *goood* about it after about—five minutes. I did what would turn them on, and what turn me on is their smile and responses. It was great.

How much of your performance is you and your sexuality and how much is persona? ~ [*Laughs.*] All of it's for real. The only difference is where I'm at. If one of the guys was onstage, I'd say sure, why not? [*Laughs.*] It's nothing fake about what I do up there sexually, 'cause I'm actually showing them how I make love—it's me.

Why did you choose the stage name you use? ~ Because everybody used to talk about my lips! "God, you got big lips." So I said, "Shidd, I'm gonna call myself Lusty Lipps." My mom helped me pick out the name. Gotsta have 'em lusty. [*Laughs.*]

Do you ever become aroused by what you are doing and what is happening around you onstage? ~ Shit, yeah! [*Laughs.*] Oh, baby—don't leave. I look at them and say, "Mmm, hmm." If their ass attract me, I tell 'em to turn around. "Shit, let me see what you got." [*Laughs.*] Oh, yeah. Gettin' hot, it's nature. Shit, if I didn't, I think somethin' be wrong with me. [*Laughs.*] Shit, yeah, I likes dat. Men make me hot. [*Laughs.*]

What can you do onstage that you can't do offstage? ~ [*Laughs.*] Look at the customers and their dicks. Onstage you can take off your clothes, open your legs, and say, "Look at this—look what *I* got." You can't do this out in the street because *it's the law.* If it wasn't the law, I'm sure everybody'd be sittin' there with their legs open, "Hey, look at this, yeah." But that's just the way it is—somethin' that you have to accept. I would like to *change the goddamn law*! [*Laughs.*]

Many of the dancers who work here say that they prefer this closed type of stage and see it as safe and fun because of the absence of physical contact with the customers. How do you feel? ~ I like this, too, because a lot of men can get really abusive. If it was open, they could grab you. With my temper, I'd done knock one of the fuckers out. [*Laughs.*] They can touch on the window all they want, and I can touch on the window, too. It's in their mind—they actually think they're touching us, so it makes them feel better.

What is your favorite type of customer? ~ Erotic, exotic, and X-rated, along with me. One that can show me some motion. If he's gonna jack off, jack off right! [*Laughs.*] Show me some *motion.* Someone being there with a smile on his face, happy, showin' me some response.

I won't dance for the ones that always hollerin' 'bout, "Open up your pussy lips," and all that. I don't give them nothin', the time of day; they couldn't ask me for SHIT! [*Laughs.*] There's a certain way to ask. I make them say "please," and then I *think* about opening my pussy for 'em. I won't dance for people who laugh at the other dancers. Why should I give them the satisfaction of dancin' for 'em when they're up here makin' smart-ass comments about the other dancers? I say, "No, go dance for yourself and look in the mirror."

Describe the variety of sexual behavior customers express. ~ Oh, dear. [*Laughs.*] They bring their little tools and sexual things, such as dildos. One hand is holding his penis and the dildo is in the ass, which I think is totally their thing. It is great they can express themselves like that in front of us. It's no problem, doin' their own thing, like givin' theirselves head, and us bein' there supportin' them. "Yeah, baby that's it!" "Suck that bitch—wish it was mine you were suckin'." "You lookin' good down there." [*Laughs.*]

I guess some of them feel the need to wear women's clothes, to feel closer. Hey, if that's yo' thing, you like it, I love it. I don't have nothin' to say about that. One man likes to smell women panties, put panties over his head. I say, "Shit, yeah, baby, that's cool. I'm glad you did that." One man sucks the bananas and smash 'em against the window wit' his chest, and it turns him on. He turns me on, too, when he do it. [*Laughs.*]

So everybody has their little thang. Couples come in and make love in front of us. She'll give him head; he'll suck her—give

With my temper, I'd done knock one of the fuckers out.

us a show. I like it; I give 'em thumbs up. Shit, not too many people can express that. I think sex is a beautiful thing. I think it's great that couples are comin' in. Men get hot off'a us, and she gets off on us, too, by him touchin' her. They do their little business and they get on. Everybody's happy. They leave and we sit here—NEXT!

Describe your family and its circumstances as you remember them during your childhood. ~ I have three sisters, a brother, and Mom. My dad left early, which was good. [*Laughs.*] I knew him for about three years. He really doesn't matter. The circumstances of my family were good, as far as I'm concerned. Mom was Mom and Dad. She worked, and my oldest sister took care of me, before school. Mom worked with newspaper advertising, checking up, squaring up the newspaper. My mom's mom was German, and my grandfather is Navajo Indian. Mom's children are half black, a quarter German, and a quarter Indian. I don't know where my mom and dad met; I was never too interested in askin'.

What were you taught about human sexuality by your mother? ~ Everythang. My mother never hid nothin'—whatever we wanted to know, she told us. When I wanted to know how a woman got pregnant she said, "Well, a man's penis goes inside..." She just tells the whole thing. Instead of talkin' about the birds and bees, she talk about the dick and the pussies, 'cause that's what it actually is. She tried to explain orgasms to me, but she said you have to find out by yourself. She said, "I knew it felt good to me." And I said, "Well, yeah." I was all into it. She explained how a man ejaculates, what it looks like, how big the penises can be, how small they can be, how wide, how—all this. It's great; she didn't hide anything from me.

Were you sexually abused as a child? ~ Nope. I wish I was. [*Laughs.*]

Describe your high-school years. ~ I never dated anybody in my school, period. I didn't want a boy; I wanted a man. [*Laughs.*] I was basically goin' to school and comin' home, doin' my work, and playin' basketball. Never hung around female friends 'cause they wasn't 'bout nothin', always tryin' to steal somebody boyfriend.

When I was sixteen, I dated a thirty-three-year-old man. He was my first "piece." [*Laughs.*] It went on for a little while. I wasn't serious with him. It was just a nice friendship. I didn't

When I was sixteen, I dated a thirty-three-year-old man. He was my first "piece."

want a commitment at the age of sixteen; I just wanted to experience—fuckin'. It was nice. I also dated a thirty-two-year-old guy, and I screwed him, too. I had curfews and all that, but any time I could spend with him, I did.

Do you think your sexuality would be different if you lived in an egalitarian or female-dominated society? ~ No, it wouldn't be different. I'd still be the same way. I'd still look at the bodies, and thinkin' about the dicks inside the pants. I'd still be my own person regardless of who's runnin' what or whatever. I'd still have my own personality, my own mind.

Has dancing affected your politics? ~ I wasn't ever into fuckin' politics. Fuck politics! [*Laughs.*]

Attilla the Honey
What have you been telling the women to do to succeed at this job since becoming show director? ~ I tell them that I want them to be having fun, and if they don't like the work, or if they think there is something wrong with it, that they shouldn't be doing it. I tell them to establish lots of eye contact to establish a flirtation. We talk a lot about the pussy

show. Men will watch if you spread your legs; those little windows will stay open. But people don't have to do that. A lot of women find that erotic and powerful. I tell them to use facial expressions, play with your breasts and arms, kiss at them, use your whole body.

I also tell them that I want them to be responsible and reliable. People think that it's not a real job. I constantly hear that when I'm not there, people are fucking off. I stress that people should be responsible if they want steady raises. I tell them to experiment with costumes and characters. Try new dance moves, new aspects of your personality. Experiment and explore onstage. I tell them that I want them to participate and be active in the theater, but it doesn't happen that often. People tend to just check in and check out. I encourage them to be open with each other and communicate, especially around resentments. Be supportive, be gentle, don't be threatening, tell people how you feel about them, and if you can't tell them, tell me.

Describe your first experience onstage. ~ I was pretty excited and pretty nervous about returning to the sex industry after ten years. When I was nineteen, I started dancing topless and turning tricks. I worked in nude-modeling studios, and I ran a massage parlor in Arizona. I went through all that stuff and quit. I decided that it was bad. I should be a good girl, be normal. I did that for ten years, and I have never been so bored. I was shocked that that was what people wanted to do with their lives. You know, nine to five, predictable stuff. Everything's very safe; everyone pays attention to the rules. I did that for ten years, and I just couldn't do it anymore. But still I was wondering if I should be going back into the sex industry. Maybe there was something wrong with me, because I wanted to go back for ten years. I would stare at massage parlors and topless-dance places. I would always read the ads for dancers, escorts, and masseuses, and just long to be back in that environment, where people are really wild and open and in many ways more honest than folks in the mainstream. Especially the women. There are a lot of real strong women in the sex industry.

So anyway, I was onstage and sort of in a state of shock. Here I was, I had finally gone back. I don't get along with my family, but I had just begun a reconciliation with my sister. I knew that this was going to blow that. She would never approve, so I was sacrificing that. I had many, many friends who were so upset with me. It's a feminist issue, and I was like a traitor to the cause. This was terrible; this was exploitation. I thought I was going to lose all of my friends. That didn't turn out to be true, but it put a major strain on my friendships. I felt I had to do this to be true to myself.

I was taking the San Francisco Sex Information training and got complete support from those people. They said, If you want to do it, do it. You're not hurting anybody—go for it. It was the first time I had heard that from anyone. Everybody had been telling me for years, No, don't go back. Don't explore any kind of sexual issue that I was interested in, anything that was out of the mainstream. And since I come from a family that's very dysfunctional and sexually weird—I come from an incest family—it's a big concern. It's a major concern that I'm going to turn out crazy like Mom and Dad.

So, anyhow, I'm onstage going through all this shit, making this major decision, and there are all these guys around me jacking off. I always wanted to watch my boyfriends do that. They always wanted to watch me masturbate, but they would never let me watch them. So, suddenly, I can watch all these different guys, and it was really interesting. It was the first time I could just stare at a man doing that, stare at his body and his cock. I got very excited. There were definitely customers who really turned me on.

It was exciting and scary, a major decision, but frankly, it was really easy.

What criteria do you use in hiring women? ~ The first thing is, how attractive are they? Second, how comfortable are they onstage? Would they actually be happy working here? Do they have good rapport with the customers? Are they able to look at these guys? I look at whether they have high or low energy. They have to be pretty unattractive for me to not hire them. I think I've only told one woman that I couldn't hire her, and one over the phone because her application was unintelligible. I am certainly not one of the prettiest women here, and I still have a hot show. Looks do count in the business, definitely, and I pay attention to that. I would certainly love to hire lots of pretty nineteen-year-old college girls. It would be real good for the show, but I don't want people to just slide on their looks. It's sexiness that counts.

And I look for people who are intelligent. Women who I can talk to, women who think about things, who use their intelligence to question the world around them and do some exploring—that's important. I don't like bimbos, no matter how pretty they might be. I prefer having dancers and artists, actresses. Sometimes women from the financial district really cut loose.

What do the customers want you to do? ~ Consistently, most of them—not all of them—want me to show them my genitals. It's spread open and turn over so they can see my ass and genitals. Those are the requests most dancers seem to get. Sometimes they'd rather see me play with my breasts or just see my face. Sometimes they come in real depressed and just want some pretend contact. They'll put their hands up to the window and want me to put my hand up so we touch fingertips. Often I get requests from young guys to do some kind of insertion, which we don't do here. "Stick your fingers in," or, "Don't you have a dildo?"

The other night this little, short guy with a baseball cap and thick glasses, who looked like something out of a Gary Larson cartoon, said, "So, how much for the back room?" Some guys hold twenties or fifties or hundred-dollar bills up to the window. Most of the guys know that doesn't happen here, but there are requests for sex. "How much for a blowjob?" "How much to fuck you?"

They love to see me get wet; sometimes I'll fake that. I'll lick my fingers and touch my genitals. "Oh, she's getting excited." They never seem to catch on. They think, "I've still got it. I turned her on, this hardened woman."

In your experience are dancers more deprived, abused, and battered than other women? ~ No way. Not at all. Women always get harassed, shit on, pushed around, cheated, and gypped. Dancers are no exception, certainly, but we don't get treated any worse. And a lot of dancers make so much more money than other women and have so much more fun. In a lot of ways it's a real healthy job. Physically,

There were definitely customers who really turned me on.

it's very healthy. It's like you're exercising and getting paid for it. At the moment we don't make that much money, but it's still a good, high hourly wage, considering a lot of people in the financial district or the retail and restaurant business are making, five, six, seven bucks an hour. Here, it's real easy to get ten. In a lot of ways we get treated better, but we have to deal with the sexual stigma.

Since I was fifteen, stepping out the door, walking down the street, and being harassed by a group of men has been consistently a traumatic experience. I'm always loudly evaluated and aggressively pursued. That's how women get treated in this culture. I am certainly no more likely to experience violence than any other woman. That can happen to anybody anytime within a marriage, a family, a workplace, just walking into a bar. It's not women in the sex industry who get singled out for that kind of abuse—all women are. As far as sexual harassment on the job, clearly it's no worse in the sex industry than anywhere else. Even though you'd think it would be, it's not. One time the computer company I worked for hired a secretary who was an exotic dancer. She had her little dictation pad and would go in for a meeting with ten guys, and they would lock the door. When she got out, her dictation pad was blank. This shit goes on all over. The boss and his secretary—it's so common it's become a joke.

Do you recognize any characteristics common to those who dance? ~ A lot of the women are very bright and very rebellious. They tend to be artists, musicians, actresses, or just oddball people who have no desire to fit into the mainstream. The other type of women I've found tend to be not particularly bright. They tend to be drug addicts and people who don't want to work for a living. And for some reason they don't want to get into a committed relationship.

Have you lost self-esteem due to dancing? ~ No, I have absolutely gained it. I feel like I'm being myself now. Before, I had this terrible feeling that I was an imposter, a fake, that I was acting out this part, a recovered incest victim who is striving to make a better life. That I will have a monogamous, good relationship, children, a marriage, and a house in the suburbs and all that shit. It's something I never really wanted. I guess I felt like I had to prove that my family situation did not, in fact, destroy me, that I could be normal, that I could be like everyone else. [*Laughs.*] But I don't want to be like any-

Dancers talk about how much they're in love with each other and how they want to fuck each other.

one else. I think everyone else is kind of boring, I mean those normal types out there. I love eccentric people because I am eccentric. I'm feeling more and more free to be who I am. I'd say that dancing has really liberated me.

What do you consider to be the failures of the women's movement in the United States? ~ They've had a very rigid definition of what is okay for women to be. Exactly as males have had for centuries. They have taken a few traits and said, these are okay, but the rest are not. They have ignored those special concerns of women of color. They have ignored all kinds of cultural and religious concerns. They have ostracized women in the sex industry. They decided that they were going to save us without ever asking us whether we wanted to be saved. They have really trashed homemakers and people who want to stay home and bear children. They've alienated them and other large, important groups of women. They have adopted pretty much a male, patriarchal view of what is okay. They are very concerned with education and upper-middle-class, white, *male* values being transferred.

Jackie

What sexual depictions do you perform? ~ There are times when I feel like I'm actually making love with a customer. That's particularly when we're both turned on and mastur-

bating. I learned a great technique from this really hot little number who breezed in and out once in a while. She would pretend to lick the customer's cock and then look up into his eyes with these big, soft, submissive brown eyes, and he would go nuts! When I am tired of dancing for a customer I pretend to give him head, and he gets off quick and goes away. [*Laughs.*] I think most dancers know that, but we don't really talk about it. What she did looked submissive at first, which I was a little uncomfortable with, but now I see it as a whole other way to be incredibly accepting, erotic, and loving. There are times when I'm pretending that the customer is a voyeur and I don't know he's there.

Does your performance contain elements of dominance and submission? ~ Absolutely. There are customers who are very submissive—we tell them they have to lick the windows. One guy we called "Slug" loved to lick those windows!

Then there are the customers who really want to be in control of the show. They motion and say "turn around," "come here." I have a real hard time as soon as someone tells me what they want. Even when I'm willing to do it, there's still initial resistance. We always tell each other, "You don't have to do anything you don't want to. It's your show; you're in control." Sometimes we'll tell the customers, "This isn't Burger King—you can't have it your way." It becomes not fun, not ours, doing what somebody tells you to do. It's like being a waitress. It's really stressful to have a shift where that's all you get.

I've recently had a tremendous breakthrough in this area. I read *Slave Girl of Gor* [*laughs*], and I was exploring my submissive fantasies, being totally submissive. A lot of my fantasies when I masturbate are that I have absolutely no choice about it—I'm tightly bound. It's pretty clear to me that I don't want to let go unless I'm forced to. I don't want to take responsibility for letting go. So anyway, I thought I'd be a slave girl of Gor onstage, and it was so hot. The customers were so drawn to me. I had four of them for about an hour, nonstop. There was absolutely no room for them to tell me what to do; they just wanted to see what I was doing! I was making love to myself, really going for it. I was acting like I was totally theirs, that my whole purpose in life was to satisfy them. I had total control of them. It was really interesting to actually experience it, not just know that it's true.

From stage you see a lot of tongues. Describe this. ~ It's a way for them to be submissive, to say, "I would love to lick your pussy." "Your pussy is delicious-looking." "I would love to return this, to arouse *you*." It's a way of communicating, especially for the guys in the stand-up booths. We can't see the rest of their bodies, so they can't gesture with their

EVERYTHING YOU KNOW ABOUT SEX IS WRONG

cocks. Our pussies are right at their face level. Some men just *love* to lick pussy! I have fantasies that their wife or girlfriend doesn't like it, or they're not in a relationship and they just need their fix. For some men it's shorthand for, "You're doing a nice job." Some are trying to get you to their bedroom, and they're demonstrating their technique! [*Laughs.*]

Onstage the music plays almost continuously. Describe the variety and part it plays in your performance. ~ If it's a song I really love, I have a hard time doing my job. I just want to dance, not having anything to do with sex, just dance. The music has always been a huge issue for the dancers, the source of a lot of dissatisfaction. The management doesn't have anything to do with it. The rule is, if you have a complaint, buy some records, the theater pays.

Describe the interaction and commentary among the dancers onstage. ~ I've heard everything imaginable onstage. There's on-purpose commentary and off-purpose commentary. There's gossiping about life and what's new— girl talk. Dancers talk about how much they're in love with each other and how they want to fuck each other. They don't use those words, but that's the context. They acknowledge each other's sexiness. A lot of, "oh baby," a lot of stuff that if a man said it to me on the street, I'd be really pissed off. Sometimes a guy will have either a huge cock or a great physique, or maybe a pair of red undies, nylons, and high heels on, or he's doing something really kinky. We'll all start squealing and take turns looking and telling him we appreciate it. There's a lot of trying to manage the customers: "Smile," or, "Please don't do that," or, "Isn't she hot?"

At its most fun, the dancers are constantly enrolling each other in activities, and it can get really wild. An old Motown song comes on, we'll start doing a Supremes routine. The barriers go down, and we're "us" instead of "me and her." Dancers get into pretending to make love with each other. There's a lot about who's dancing for whom and are you interrupting them, or, "Can I take a break from this guy—will you please go dance for him? I'm tired," or, "I just can't dance for this guy—he looks like my father."

Is the myth of the perfect body perpetuated here? ~ Yes and no. Most of the customers still want to see the mythic female, and those women get the most attention. Quite often they make the most money. In this job, if you're beautiful, you can go far. You don't have to be a particularly good dancer; you don't have to work as hard. But the truth is, there are some hot women who wouldn't fit the myth, and they get validated as well. What's more accurate, every customer has their own myth and there is really, literally, a man for every woman's body on this planet! [*Laughs.*] I know from listening to the customers' comments. Things that the woman con-

centrates on as being the icky parts, the customers couldn't care less. They see the beautiful breast, the shapely ass, the incredible puss, or whatever. They're drawn to what they like, rather than being stopped by what the dancer thinks is not perfect—her stretch marks or her little roll.

There's not very much forgiveness for fat dancers at all; she has to have something perfect on her body, some redeeming quality. Our culture's just anti-fat. Our standard shifted to include heavier and heavier women. At one point we hired a woman who was between 250 and 300 pounds. She lasted about a day. We were really clear with her that it may not work, but we were willing to give it a shot. The owner was here for her first shift and said, "There is a woman big as a house onstage! But I'm just giving you feedback!" And the customers really didn't like her. The least forgiving in general are younger men. It was frustrating because I know there are men who L-O-V-E big women! Those chunky-ass magazines say it. The *Big Beautiful Woman* magazine and *Fat Is a Feminist Issue* are real breakthroughs. But it's not integrated into our culture yet.

Do you ever become aroused by what you are doing or what is happening around you onstage? ~ I couldn't believe how aroused I got by the width of this one man's cock. He's got the hugest, widest cock I've ever seen. I felt my body reacting like, just, aaahhhh, yes, please. I was astounded, I had no idea I was a size queen! It was very interesting to recognize that on some levels I have no choice about my arousal. It's programmed, and I just go along for the ride.

My fantasy is to be able to actually have an orgasm onstage. I have to move around a lot to have an orgasm, so I'd be too embarrassed, not in front of the customers, but in front of the other dancers. I think they would judge. It's a shame. One day Crystal said, "My God, I just had an orgasm. I have to go and wash off." I was so envious. It was like, right on for you!

It can be extremely arousing, exhaustingly arousing. It can ruin your sex life, because when you come home, you want to have some intellectual conversation, you want to go see a Woody Allen movie—you don't want to have sex! The lesbian dancers seem to be more comfortable exposing themselves as aroused to other women. It's harder to arouse me now; I've sort of reached a saturation point, but I am aroused by another dancer getting aroused, for sure.

What can you do onstage that you can't do offstage? ~ I get to be worshipped! [*Laughs.*] I get to be totally in control of men. I get to be the center of attention, the sex kitten. The fact that I don't have to deal with these men in any other regard gives me so much freedom, it's like the zipless fuck. Sex without strings!

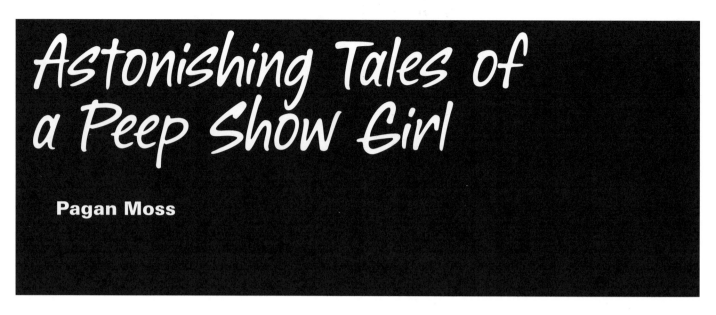

Astonishing Tales of a Peep Show Girl

Pagan Moss

Girl & I

It was first thing Tuesday morning, and I was already in the booth doing a show for one of my regulars—a Mercedes dealer on the hill. He was an ass man. He came in once a week, and today he was paying me $40 just so he could hunch down and do some poppers while he stared at my ass, wiggling through a pair of sheer black panties. Some days he paid me $60 to spread my bare cheeks, and some days he offered me more if I'd just slip a finger inside. But today it was only $40, and I was bored as hell, staring dumbly at the wall ahead.

My mind drifted toward the conversation taking place in the booth on the other side of the wall. I was working with Girl, a popular peep show girl who was twenty-three but looked fifteen and made a lot of money at it. She was freckled, five

"Ready for a two-girl show?" she said, still concentrating on the mirror.

feet tall, ninety pounds, and had the delicate features of a child. The name Girl suited her quite nicely.

I hadn't heard the grinding gears of her curtain rising or the unmistakable whir of the bill acceptor, signaling a new show, so I figured she must be workin' some poor guy, coaxing him doe-eyed with that wicked tongue of hers. Sometimes a guy doesn't know a good thing right away when he sees it.

The Mercedes dealer shot his load right on time, with five minutes still ticking off the clock. He was all business—not one to chat afterwards. There were luxury sedans to be sold, and there were important men with thick wallets who were waiting to buy them. He checked his watch, cleaned up, and was out the door in a flash.

I jumped out of my booth and found Girl gazing, squint-eyed, into the mirror, trying to tease something out of her long, strawberry-blonde hair.

"Ready for a two-girl show?" she said, still concentrating on the mirror.

"Yeah?" I said, adjusting my panties. "With the guy you were just chattin' up?"

"Yep," she said, flicking whatever was in her hair onto the floor. "I've done shows with him before. He's that young, straight-looking guy who's got all those crazy piercings and metal implants in his cock. I told you about him a couple of weeks ago, remember?"

I nodded, but I couldn't remember. My mind was too full with things from this place.

"Well...he said his grandmother died last month and left him some money. He just got the check in the mail today."

Girl reached inside her booth past an array of stuffed animals (which management said she couldn't have in her booth because they were "sick") and grabbed her moneymaker—a bright-pink, vibrating monstrosity she called Bob. She also snatched the tattered blanket she'd had since she was three—a pink baby's quilt with a white, satiny edge worn thin with love. She tossed her stuff into my booth, which was slightly larger than hers—better able to accommodate two girls rolling around inside.

The customer hit the ATM, and we ran to the bathroom to freshen up. We both grabbed baby wipes from the dispenser on the counter and went to work with a foot on the toilet seat—lips spread—carefully wiping between each crevice and fold, then the ass, until everything was smelling baby clean. Girl handed me a tissue, and I wiped off my bright red lips so I wouldn't stain her milky-white skin. We both popped a mint and jumped into the booth.

The customer was already back from the ATM. Girl had trained him well. As soon as he spied us, several twenties pushed excitedly through the makeshift tip slot—a small, barely noticeable crack below the bill acceptor carved by some unknown saint so that we girls could actually make some money around this place. The customer pumped a few more twenties into the machine, and the shade rose.

"Hi," Girl said, coyly. "Nice to see you again."

"Nice to see both of you," he said with a boyish grin.

"This is my girlfriend," Girl said, stroking my bare shoulder.

The customer's eyes turned big as plates.

"I mean, she's my real girlfriend," she went on. "We get together outside of here, too. I bet you'd like to see real girlfriends get it on."

He looked like he was going to pee his pants. "Whatever you girls want to do is fine with me," he said with a gulp. "You can pretend I'm not here if you want."

"Okay, baby," Girl purred, "we'll pretend we're in our bedroom, then...alone."

With that, I grabbed the bottom of Girl's tiny T-shirt and pulled it up over her head. She wasn't wearing a bra—she didn't need to. Her breasts were small and pink with puffy nipples looking ready to bloom. I reached out and cupped them, enjoying how small and firm they felt. I fingered her nipples and gave them a nice pinch, knowing how much she liked it rough. She smiled and writhed with delight and started clawing at my shirt. I helped her get it over my head, and as soon as she saw my bare tits, she pulled me into her, hard. We rubbed our tits together for a while, nipples bristling, then I pulled away and started kissing and sucking at her childlike bosom.

"Mmmm...I like that," she cooed.

"Stand up so I can take off your panties," I ordered.

When she did, I jammed my fingers down the sides of her white cotton panties, ripping them down to her ankles so that her bare little pussy was staring me right in the eye. It was one of those pretty pink pussies where everything fits neat and tidy between the lips.

I stood up and pulled my panties down myself. I stepped out of them and kicked them to the corner, where our clothes were piled high. We were both completely naked now...except for our seven-inch, strappy heels and Girl's white, knee-high stockings.

I sat on my heels and arched back with my hands behind me, thrusting my tanned, lean hips toward her. Girl was still standing, and I told her to straddle me so I could lick her pussy. She smiled.

I started at the back of her knee, licking and kissing ever so lightly, making gooseflesh form on her leg. I moved up the inside of her thigh slowly, stopping here and there to draw her flesh into my mouth so I could suck and savor her salty flavor.

When I got between her legs, her body tensed with anticipation. I paused, then stretched out my tongue—just grazing the very tip of her clit. She gasped, but I didn't stay there. I wanted to tease her. It made me wet knowing how much she wanted it. I started down the inside of her other thigh.

When I finished bathing Girl with my tongue, we laid down side by side, facing the customer with our vibrators turned on. Mine was lagging a little as the batteries needed changing, while Girl's hummed away at a cheery pitch. It wasn't long before she was moaning—a loud, lascivious moan like she was really enjoying herself.

The batteries in my vibrator were fading, so I tossed it aside and got behind Girl. I started kissing her below the ear—my bare pussy glued to her ass. I bit down on the lobe and held it as I firmly gripped the inside of her thighs, flattening my breasts onto her back. I wanted her to think of me—not the vibrator—fucking her. She sighed loudly. Our hips rolled in perfect sync as she worked the vibrator to a feverish pitch. Beads of sweat were running down her back, my skin was sticking to hers, and we became one sweaty mess.

It was one of those pretty pink pussies where everything fits neat and tidy between the lips.

I heard her say something under her breath. Her voice was all shaky. She started talking to herself like someone else was working the vibrator.

"Yeah, that's it...oooh, right there," she whispered.

My fingers slid toward the vibrator. I could feel her sweaty mound and her hand rocking back and forth. I searched for her clit, but she was already there, rubbing. I put my hand on top of hers and she pulled away, letting me take over. She leaned forward toward the glass, bracing herself with her free hand, while she continued to fuck herself.

"I'm gonna come," she gasped.

I tightened my grip and rubbed faster.

She threw back her head, eyes closed, mouth wide open, and arched her back sharply as she let out a huge moan. Then she collapsed forward. Her hands braced her fall, and her cheek came to rest against the glass. I laid on her for a moment. My hair stuck to the sweat on her back. I sat up and watched her back rise and fall as she caught her breath. It took her a while to move—when she finally did, her hands were shaking and her eyes were only slits. I knew she didn't fake it. I was happy.

The customer sat there staring, with his jaw practically unhinged. He hadn't said a word the entire show, and I'd almost forgotten he was there. The first words out of his mouth were: "How can I get a private show?"

I searched for her clit, but she was already there, rubbing.

After he wiped himself clean and left, we both rolled out of the booth with our cash—a mess of sweaty bodies, tangled hair, and smeared makeup. Girl walked sideways to the bathroom like a drunkard. She was still in her own world. I put my clothes back on and got ready for the next show.

I heard the toilet flush, then the faucet turned on. A couple seconds later Girl emerged, grabbed a cigarette off the counter, lit up, and sat on a chair, still naked. She took a long drag and exhaled. Her head hung down as she relaxed.

After a few more long drags, she turned to look at me and said in a very, very soft voice: "Thank you."

The Golden Boys of Kobe
I knew they were trouble as soon as they walked out of the theater. There were three of them—three Asian businessmen wearing nice suits, looking like they had just come in on a whim after downing a few at the nearest martini lounge.

I sat in my booth and watched them laugh and stumble down the hallway until they caught sight of me, sitting in a pair of trashy cut-off jeans and an obscenely cropped gingham top, which revealed just a hint of bare breasts at the bottom. I stood up in my seven-inchers and twirled one of my pigtails with my finger, flashing them a devilish grin. They all stopped and stared up at me.

The one in the middle was noticeably taller than the other two. He was strikingly handsome and stylish...c o o l. He reached into his jacket pocket and drew out a pack of ciga-

rettes. He tapped one out and promptly lit up. He took a hit and leaned back—giving me a long, hard look, then exhaled as he nodded.

The one on the right was short and round with plump red cheeks like apples. He seemed the shyest of the bunch—not able to look me in the eye.

The one to my left had round glasses and wore a serious look. I sensed he was the leader of the group. After a couple of minutes of them standing in the hallway, sizing me up, the one with the glasses finally came into my booth. I picked up my phone and peeked through the crack in the shade, trying to get his attention. He finally spied me and his mouth formed a slight smile. I showed him my phone and pointed to where his phone was, and said, "Pick up!"

He picked up the phone but didn't say anything.

"Hi, baby," I purred. "Ever been to a place like this before?"

"No," he said. His accent was thick.

"Where are you from?" I asked.

"Kobe," he said. "How much?"

"Twenty for nude."

"Okay," he said. He opened the door and waved in his friends.

The other two filed in fast, and the tall one closed the door behind him. He then pulled out a wad of cash and peeled off a twenty, which he promptly stuck into the machine. I closed the shade to the hallway and picked up the phone again. "I mean twenty for one of you." I pointed to the guy in the glasses, and he looked at me like he didn't understand. "Twenty for me and you, baby. Only one person in the booth at a time or I could lose my job," I said.

They all smiled, and the guy in the glasses replied, "We like to watch all together."

"Are you guys gay?" I asked.

They smiled blankly.

"Are you guys going to get it on?" I asked.

They looked at each other and started to laugh.

"No, we like you," said the guy in the glasses.

It was well past midnight and the management was long gone. The only clerk working was Keith, and he didn't give a fuck what we did. He was much too busy watching porn, which played on a TV mounted below the front counter. My biggest worry was the janitor. He was an old fart named Hank, and he was a regular ballbreaker—mad at the world for having to come out of retirement because his wife ran off with all his money with that "fuckin' neeegro" down the street. He hated this place...the whores who worked here and the pervs he had to clean up after. We would surely all be fucked if he caught sight of eight feet underneath the booth door. But fate had been set. The money was in the machine, and the time was ticking off the clock, and these lonely guys were hungry for a show...although for $20, they weren't gettin' much.

I did a little striptease down to my G-string and pressed my pink tits against the glass. They all moved closer to the window, but none of them took it out. When the time was coming to an end, the one with the glasses pointed to my G-string.

"You want me to take this off?" I asked. They all nodded vigorously.

I slowly took off the G-string and crawled around the floor like a sex cat, pausing here and there to flash them some more pink. The short and round one in the middle spied the time. He started searching my booth, anticipating what I might whip out for the grand finale. When nothing happened, he asked, "You like toys?"

"Mmmm...I love them, baby," I said. "But toys are extra."

The shade started to go down.

There was a long pause behind the closed shade. I heard a voice pipe up: "You pee?"

I wasn't sure if I'd heard right. "Do I pee?"

"Yeah, how much for that?"

I thought for a moment. I had always tried to avoid these type of shows in the past, but it wasn't because I thought it was gross or dirty, which I don't (unlike defecating on someone), but it was more about the fear and anxiety of going to the bathroom under the microscope.

I figured the worst that could happen is that nothing would come out or that I'd panic and stream a puddle onto the floor, both of which would be relatively easy to explain away. Besides, money and circumstance often trump one's will, and it just seemed to fit that night that I would pee for them. It was like I was a preordained player in a scene from a David Lynch movie, and they were my casting agents. It was practically theater...art, baby.

"Yeah, I'll pee for you," I said. "But it's gonna cost you sixty."

There was more talking, and I had to restrain myself from the sudden impulse to cry out, "Torah! Torah! Torah!"

I peeked through the crack in the shade again. The guy with the glasses took out the money, then handed it to the guy in the middle, who handed it to the guy at the end, who then pumped it into the machine. The shade went back up, and the time started counting down. I looked around the booth, forgetting I needed something to pee in. I had left my mason jar at home that day, much to my sudden annoyance.

"I'll be right back," I said, jumping out of the booth. I ran into the bathroom, praying to God that the clear glass vase was still under the sink. ("Dear God, I know I don't go to church much and all, and I make fun of all your fundie followers, but please, do me a favor and make sure this vase is there so I can pee in it in front of three Japanese men? Thank you, God. It's me, Pagan.")

I gingerly squatted over the vase and raised myself with one arm.

The girls kept the vase under the sink, just in case...just in case of a pee-show emergency. It was the perfect standing feminine peeing receptacle, practically designed for such purposes with a wide opening at the top and a long, clear shaft for optimum voyeuristic viewing. Plus, the tank at the bottom was ample.

I flipped on the light and bent over, and to my utter delight it was there. There was no time to check its cleanliness—I clutched it and ran. I was certain I had heard that urine was sterile, anyway, and that babies consume their own urine in the womb...or maybe I had misunderstood. Maybe it was only sterile for a short while after its initial release from the body.

Either way, I jumped back into my booth with the vase, and the trio greeted me with smiles. They watched in amazement as I carefully placed the vase in the middle of the booth. They were entranced as if watching a magic show—their eyes large, their mouths agape. I had some time to kill while I summoned the flow, so I danced around the vase feeling more like an Indian summoning the rains.

When the time clicked down to a couple of minutes, I gingerly squatted over the vase and raised myself with one arm. I used my free hand to spread my smooth lips and pulled back a little, aiming my urethra while simultaneously sticking out my clit like a tiny penis. I relaxed. I guess the dance had worked because the golden stream, weak at first, eventually blossomed and made its sustained way into the chosen destination.

Toward the end, the stream morphed into a dribble. I bounced over the vase a couple of times to shed the last droplets, then wiped my pussy clean with a baby wipe. The trio stood in silence as the shade fell. "Thanks," I said, putting on my robe. "You guys were fun."

One of them asked through the shade: "Do we get to keep it?"

"Keep what?" I asked.

"We keep pee?"

"You want the pee?"

"Yes. We want the pee. Please. Pee, please. We want your pee-pee, please."

Well, he was being polite.

"If you want the pee, it's gonna cost you more."

"How much?" he asked.

"Fifty?" How much was pee going for these days? Maybe I

"We want the pee. Please. Pee, please. We want your pee-pee, please."

shoulda looked that one up on the Net first.

"Okay," he said.

Damn! I could have got a hundred, I thought. "Meet me at the back door," I said. "It's the one right next to the theater entrance."

"Okay."

I tore out of the booth and scrambled to find something to pour the pee into. I found a large McDonald's cup in the corner, complete with straw and lid, and decided to use it. I emptied the vase into the cup as carefully and quickly as I could. Aside from a small pelt of urine on my arm, it went pretty well.

I opened the back door, and the three men were standing there, smiling. I handed the McDonald's cup to the man with the glasses, and he handed me the cash. "Don't drink it all in one place, baby," I said.

He nodded politely.

P**p Show

The clock had just inched past midnight when a customer walked up to my booth window. He was fairly clean-cut, average build, and looked to be in his middle to late thirties. He had a shy demeanor but seemed interested in getting a show, nonetheless. I thought maybe he'd need a little prodding, so I moved closer to the glass and yelled, "Hey, baby, would you like to get a show?" He just stood there, smiling blankly.

The glass is thick in the booth, and most of the time the customers can't hear what the fuck we're saying when we try to talk to them in the hallway, so we usually end up pointing to our booth door as we make the universal phone sign: head cocked to the side with hand held up to the ear—pinky and thumb extended. This usually does the trick, getting them into the booth, but some of the nervous ones run off when they see this.

This customer seemed a little skittish, and for a moment I thought he might run off, too, but he eventually went into the booth, put some money into the machine, and the show began.

"You been here before?" I asked.

He nodded yes.

"Are you a naughty boy?" I asked, taking off my bra.

His eyes darted toward the ground, as if he were guilty of something. He smiled and said, "Yeah, I'm naughty."

"What kind of naughty things do you like to do?" I asked, taking off my panties.

He pointed at my ass and said, "I like that."

"Oh, you like my ass." I smiled. "What would you like to do to it?"

He bit his lip and said, "Well...I would start by licking it."

"Oh, really?" I said, slapping my ass.

"Yeah...and once it was nice and wet, I'd stick my cock in it," he said.

At this point he had his cock out, and he made a thrusting motion with it toward my ass.

"Oh, I like it up the ass," I said.

He stopped masturbating and pulled his pants down to his ankles. "Do you want to see my ass?"

I really didn't want to see his ass. Normally, when a guy asks you this question at a peep show, what he really means is: "Do you want to see my asshole?" I'm never good at getting myself out of these situations. I tend to be too nice at times, so of course I responded: "Sure."

A huge smile spread across his face. He turned around and leaned forward toward the wall. He reached one arm around, grabbing his left ass cheek and spreading it.

Oh, my God, I thought to myself. I tried to avoid making eye contact with the sphincter surely staring back at me. He looked at me over his shoulder, checking for my reaction. The only thing I could get out was: "Nice."

He took his other hand and started messing with his bottom. I wondered what the hell he was doing. I didn't want to look, but unfortunately I focused unintentionally on his finger, which had now disappeared into his sphincter. He quickly removed it, but something else happened. I tried to deny it... made excuses for what it could have been. I mean, it was dark and my mind was probably playing tricks on me. But... I could have sworn I saw something dark push through the sphincter momentarily, then retreat back inside.

The customer quickly turned around and picked up the phone again. I acted like I hadn't seen anything, thinking he was probably embarrassed—had an accident. However, the customer didn't seem fazed at all. He started masturbating again, telling me how he liked it up the ass, too.

I saw him bring his free hand to his mouth. He held what looked like a Tootsie Roll. He started licking it. I quickly realized this was no Tootsie Roll but was what I feared it to be... a piece of poop. He licked it until the tip bent to one side so it now resembled a Hershey's Kiss. My eyes started to blur a little, and I tried to look past the customer's face.

I felt like I had witnessed some horrific event...like someone getting hit by a car. I thought this must be some internal protection mechanism kicking in, as I had seen too much. I consider myself open-minded, but I just didn't see how this could be healthy. I looked at the time and saw that it was just about up. The customer noticed this, too, and I saw him reach for more money. Fuck, I thought. I couldn't believe he was getting more time. My attention quickly shifted to the cash he was handling. Normally, at the end of our shift we get the money that comes out of the machine. My mind started racing, thinking about the bills he was pumping into the machine with his poopy hands, and what story I'd have to come up with to get the clerk to trade out my money. The clerk would surely laugh and tell me I was fucked if I told him the truth.

I wasn't able to interact much with the customer for the rest of the show. My brain felt like it had been wrapped in warm wool. I just shook my head when he asked me a question and smiled a lot. I don't think he noticed. I think he was just happy to share this side of himself with someone else. The second part of the show went by fast, and before I knew it, his time was up again. He cleaned himself up, thanked me for the show, and left the booth. I watched him leave without using the restroom.

I gathered my thoughts, put on my clothes, and opened the shade to the hallway. Standing there was an attractive young man. He looked like a student. He seemed excited to get a show and immediately headed for the door to my booth. I panicked, thinking what might be left over from the last guy. I held out my hand and yelled through the glass that the booth needed to be cleaned, and thankfully he understood, waiting patiently by the door.

I ran out of the dressing room and told the janitor what just happened. He didn't flinch. He was an old-timer around this place and claimed he'd seen it all. He grabbed the cleaning supplies and went to work. As soon as he was done, the boy went in. Seeing his young, innocent face made me feel better.

Keeping up With the Joneses

We were both asleep—I on the couch and Mistress Sativa on the floor—when the beep beep of the front door went off. Mistress Sativa pulled her blankets over her head and curled up in the fetal position. "You're up next, right?" she asked—her words barely audible under all the fluff. "I thought it was your turn," I said. "The last show was your regular, wasn't it? The guy who manages the Mexican dive down the street?"

"Oh, Ass Man," Mistress Sativa said. "You're right, he was the last custie." She poked her nude, wig-capped head out from under the blankets and blinked her false lashes madly at the light.

I sat up and squinted at the small black-and-white monitor across the room, trying to make out the dark forms standing in the lobby. It looked like a couple, but not the typical couple that walked into this "lingerie showroom" joint.

"They look like Ward and June Cleaver."

"There's something strange about them," I said. "I can't quite put my finger on it but—"

Mistress Sativa cut me off mid-sentence. "Yeah, they look like Ward and June Cleaver. They're probably from out of town and got lost trying to get back to their hotel after an exhausting day of shopping and sight-seeing. They probably think this place is actually a tanning salon," she said with a laugh.

"It would be our luck," I said.

"You take them," Mistress Sativa whined.

"I don't want to deal with them. It's your turn; you go."

"P-L-E-A-S-E! I don't feel well. I think I'm going to start my period any minute," she said, scrunching up her face. "Besides," she continued, picking up what looked like Strawberry Shortcake's scalp, "I rolled over my wig when I was asleep, and it's gonna take me at least five minutes to brush this thing out. And I can't go out there just wearing my wig cap."

"All right," I agreed reluctantly. "But you have to wash the cum-towels tonight."

"All right, whatever you say." She closed her eyes and retreated back into her warm nest.

I stood up and smoothed out my naughty nurse uniform. I put on my trench coat and reading glasses, slipped on a pair of flats, and walked out to greet the couple, leaving my seven-inch heels behind.

I opened the door to the lobby and found the couple standing patiently in the middle of the room. They were attractive, middle-aged, oddly perfect. The mister was dark, tall, and handsome with broad shoulders. He had a square jaw and perfect hair and teeth. He wore a dark suit and shiny black loafers. The missus was thin and surprisingly tall for a woman, almost matching his height. She wore her hair in a tight blonde bob, which curled under perfectly at the ends. She was strikingly beautiful with sharp features and piercing light-blue eyes, which eerily matched the color of her form-fitting polyester skirt suit, circa 1950.

"My wife actually thinks you're really beautiful."

I sat down behind the front desk. "Hi, can I help you?" I asked matter-of-factly.

They both smiled their perfect smiles and started walking toward me. "We were hoping you could tell us a little bit about this place," the man said. The woman kept smiling as she daintily clutched a large, white patent-leather purse just below her slight chest.

"Sure...of course," I said. I pointed to a pair of chairs next to the desk. "Why don't you have a seat?"

"Thank you," the man said. He took a step back and held out his hand like a gentlemen, gesturing for her to sit first. When they were both seated, they scooted to the very edge of their chairs and leaned forward as if eager to hear the good news.

"There's a folder on the table next to you," I said, pointing in that direction.

The man picked it up and laid it open across his lap for both of them to see. My nails dug into my palms as I watched them peruse the menu, waiting for their smiles to dissolve into shock and dismay. After a couple of seconds, the woman leaned over and whispered something into the man's ear. His face turned serious. "Are you the one who does the shows?" he asked.

"I can...or if you had another hair color or body type in mind,

there's another girl in the back," I said. "I'd be happy to bring her out."

"Oh, that won't be necessary," he said. He smiled and placed his hand on the woman's knee. "My wife actually thinks you're really beautiful. She just wanted to make sure you were the one." The woman laid her head down on the man's shoulder, coyly brushed a lock of blonde hair from her face, and gave me a wink.

I grabbed the paperwork and started to write. "So you want a couple's show, right?" I asked. They both smiled and nodded vigorously. "Okay, I just want to make sure you understand this is a non-nude show. You both can get as comfortable as you like in the room, but we can't touch each other during the show."

"But we can touch each other, right?" he asked, pointing to the woman, then back at himself.

"That's correct," I said.

"Sounds great." He opened his wallet and handed me several twenties. "The rest is for you," he said with a wink.

"Thanks," I said. "Now I just need your names to finish up the paperwork. It doesn't have to be your real names. You can make something up if you'd like. It's just this stupid little procedure we have."

The man immediately responded, "We're the Joneses, Frank and Betty." They seemed amused as they watched me write in the book.

"Nice to meet you," I said. "My name's Kate. Follow me and I'll show you to your room."

They eagerly followed me down the dark and narrow corridor. I opened the door, and they stepped inside. "Go ahead and make yourself at home. I'll be back in a couple of minutes wearing something a little more comfortable," I said, tugging at my jacket.

A couple minutes later I came back and knocked on the door.

"Come in," Betty said.

I opened the door and vamped into the room wearing my seven-inchers. Betty was lying beautifully naked on the couch with one arm draped dramatically over the edge. Her skin was creamy white, except for the pinkness of her nipples and the ample mound of dark, curly hair between her thighs.

Frank sat naked on the back of his heels atop a towel he had spread out on the carpet. His body rippled with aging muscles covered in dark, wiry hair that seemed to grow everywhere. He looked up to see my reaction. "We don't have a lot of time," he said. "So we thought we'd just get down to business."

"Of course," I said. I let my jacket drop, revealing a white lacy bodysuit with matching white thigh-high stockings.

"Wow," Betty said. "Doesn't she look beautiful, Frank?"

"Oh, yes, darling," he answered. "Just like a little angel."

"Thank you," I said. "You both are looking quite sexy yourselves."

"Really?" Frank asked. "You don't think we're too old?"

I laughed and said, "Too old? You can't be older than thirty-five."

He cleared his throat and smiled. "Try fifty, darling," he said.

"I don't believe you."

"It's true," he said, flexing his biceps. "Lots of exercise and sex...right, baby?" he said to his wife.

Betty smiled and nodded, then pointed to the floor. "Frank, darling, would you get my bag for me?"

"Of course, dear." He handed it to her and sat back down on his towel.

She opened the bag and pulled out a white hanky, which she neatly spread on the table. She then proceeded to take out an impressive collection of sex toys and lube, which she carefully arranged on the hanky.

"She wants you to watch her," Frank said.

I grabbed a chair and sat down right next to her.

Betty picked up a large hot-pink dildo from the table and started licking the sides as she gazed into my eyes. "What do you think of my husband's cock?" she asked.

I looked over at Frank. He proudly held it out for me to see.

"Isn't it perfect?" Betty asked. "It's the most perfect cock I've ever seen. He could have been a model."

Frank smiled and looked down at his cock. "I don't know about that, baby," he said with a laugh.

"No, I agree. It's really a nice one," I said. "I've seen a lot, and I'd have to say it's one of the nicer ones."

"Really?" he said. "You're not just saying that?"

"Of course not," I said.

"Wow, thanks," he said. "That means a lot coming from an expert."

I was no expert.

Betty grew bored of licking and sucking the dildo and decided to play with her light-blue, medium-sized vibrator instead. She picked up her lube, squeezed a generous dollop onto her palm, and reached between her legs, working the slippery mess into all her curves and folds. She gave the vibrator a quick suck and turned it on, filling the room with a low, steady hum. She teased each of her nipples with the vibrating tip before moving down between her legs. She closed her eyes and gently worked the vibrator back and forth over her clit, moaning softly. "Come here, Frank," she gasped. "I want to show Kate how I suck your cock."

Frank quickly got up from the floor and walked over to the couch. He took his cock in his hand and waved it teasingly over her face. Betty stretched her tongue and wagged it wildly, trying to reach it.

"You want this, don't you?" he said in a husky voice. Betty nodded. He lowered himself, and she greedily took his firm cock into her mouth, making him gasp and moan as his hairy ass forged onward in delight. Betty looked over to make sure I was watching. She reached her free hand between her legs and spread her hairy lips, revealing the soft, pink wetness beneath. She lowered the vibrator further and let just the tip slip inside her tight pussy, teasing herself...and me. She pulled away from Frank and said, "I think I'm ready, baby."

He paused for a moment, trying to catch his breath. "Okay," he said as if he knew exactly what she wanted. He reached inside Betty's bag and pulled out a pair of latex gloves and a small plastic bag. Anticipating my reaction, he immediately said, "Don't worry, we're not crazy. We just like to take precautions."

"Of course," I said, not totally convinced.

He kneeled at the side of the couch near her feet.

I slowly stripped off my bodysuit, letting it fall to the floor, and danced around the couch in my bra and G-string. "You have such a great body," Betty said. "I know you can't touch us, but I was wondering if you could sit over my face while I come?"

"Sure," I said, smiling. "I'd love to."

We all stood up and laid out clean towels on the floor. Betty lay down first and resumed with her vibrator. Frank followed, sliding between Betty's legs to lick up all her juices. I got on all fours and carefully crawled over Betty toward Frank until my pussy was directly over her face. "Can you lower yourself just a little more, honey?" Betty gasped.

I lowered my hips until I was just inches above her. "Perfect," she purred. I could feel her words.

I looked ahead while Frank's tongue feverishly darted against Betty's clit. I reached down and touched myself through my panties as I saw the muscles in Betty's thighs begin to tense. I watched the tension as it rippled downward like a gathering wave toward her feet, making her toes spread and curl as she yelled out: "Now!"

Frank skillfully reached down between Betty's cheeks with a gloved hand and pulled out a string of black anal beads as she let out a murderous scream. He quickly dropped the greasy beads and his gloves into the plastic bag, then proceeded to quietly finish himself off over Betty, coming onto her stomach. Betty didn't move—she just lay sprawled on the ground like the dead—her eyes closed, her mouth agape. The only hint of life was the slight rise and fall of her bare chest.

He seemed so vulnerable, and I felt special in a way...like he trusted me.

I stood up and put on my jacket.

"That was wonderful," Frank whispered. He looked at Betty, still lifeless on the floor. "Don't worry about her," he said with a laugh. "She just had a big one."

"Take your time getting ready," I said, walking toward the door. "I'll be back in a few minutes to show you out."

Five minutes later I knocked on the door.

"Come in," Frank said.

I found them still dressing. "Sorry, it takes us awhile," Betty said as she straightened her skirt. She put on her jacket, picked up her bag, and gave the room a final once-over. "I think we're ready," she said, smoothing her hair.

Frank checked his watch, and his brow furrowed. "Yeah, we better get going, honey," he said. "We told the kids we'd be picking them up from the movies around this time."

"Oh, dear," Betty said with a laugh. "I didn't realize it was so late."

The Man Who Lost His Penis

I was filling my bottle at the water fountain out front when the head manager caught sight of me from across the room. He was usually an asshole, always bitching and moaning to us girls about money and how he was going to lock up our tip slots if more of it didn't start rollin' in soon. So I capped my water quick and made for the dressing room, hoping to dodge the fat fuck. However, he was determined to talk to me, speeding up to cut me off before I could escape down the

hallway. He stood there in front of me with his arms crossed, smiling a sinister smile. He looked more like a gorilla than a man standing there like that, and I knew there was no way of getting around him, so I stopped.

"You on shift?" he asked, maneuvering a toothpick around in his mouth.

"Yeah, I'm headed back to the dressing room right now," I explained. "Just getting some water." I held up my bottle.

"Very good," he said—his smile getting bigger. "I have a special customer for you. He's a crossdresser, and for the past hour, I've been helpin' him downstairs pick out some lingerie. You wouldn't believe how much this guy just spent."

I nodded, uninterested.

"Anyway, now he says he wants to try out the peep show...said he'd heard how hot it was from a friend last night. Wanted to know who gives the best show here." He bit down hard on the toothpick and gave me a wink. "You know what I told him?"

I didn't say a word. I knew the answer...I was the only girl on shift.

"I told him how kinky you were," he said with a snort. "He said he'd be right up after settling his bill."

"Thanks, sounds like fun." I started back to the dressing room.

I got back in my booth, and a couple minutes later the manager came around the corner with the customer in tow. They stood in front of me, and the manager gave him the spiel. The customer smiled and nodded, then the manager waved goodbye and left.

The customer turned back to me and flashed a rugged, nicotine-stained smile. He looked like an old biker—the retired Hell's Angel type. He wore a thick, black leather jacket and a pair of old work jeans and steel-toe boots. He had a large, round, weathered face and a head of wild, salt-and-pepper hair. He also had a matching beard and mustache and a tuft of wiry hair that spilled out generously over the top of his button-down denim shirt. He pointed toward the bathroom across the way and held up the large plastic bag containing his recent purchases. I nodded as he rushed off to the bathroom.

He emerged a few minutes later. I half-expected him to vamp out wearing a slutty pair of high-heel shoes and a silky pink teddy, but he looked the same as before. He ducked into my booth and picked up the phone.

"Have you been here before?" I purred.

"No," he said in a soft, nervous voice.

I went over the various shows and prices. He decided on the basic $20 show. He put his money into the bill acceptor, and I closed the shade to the hallway. As his shade began to rise, he greeted me with large brown eyes, framed with thick, long lashes. I was struck by how kind they were compared to his otherwise rugged appearance. They revealed a sensitivity I rarely see around this place. I was immediately drawn to them.

"Hi," I said, jiggling my tits.

"Hi," he responded, looking away shyly.

I started to undress, and his smile widened a little. "Do you mind if I get more comfortable, too?" he asked.

"Of course not. It's better that way."

He started to undo his shirt, revealing a black lacy bodysuit underneath. He undid his pants, pulled them down to his ankles, and stepped out of them entirely.

"Oooh," I said, "you look so beautiful."

"Thank you. I just bought it downstairs."

"It's so sexy that you like wearing women's clothes," I said.

"I wear 'em under my work clothes every day," he said, proudly stroking the fabric of the bodysuit. "I like the way they feel against my skin."

"You have a girlfriend?" I asked, twirling a strand of my hair.

"Nope. I've got a group of guy friends I hang out with, though. Every Friday night we get all dolled up and go out on the town."

I gave him the once over, trying to imagine him and his friends making the rounds dressed up like women. He was short and thick, and his body was covered with thick, wiry hair. I just couldn't picture it.

I sat back with my legs underneath me...naked. He didn't seem so interested in me being naked, though. I imagined he was one of those types...the type of customer who wouldn't notice if you were wearing a canvas smock. He came to be watched...listened to. And for the most part, I was the type of girl who was happy to admire and listen.

His hands disappeared between his legs and started groping for the snaps to the bodysuit. It took him a while, blindly squirming and sweating, but he finally managed to undo them. He tucked the bottom flap under the top portion of the

bodysuit, so it looked like a sexy lace tank top. My eyes followed his hands back over his hairy belly, down to his groin. He had a large mound of thick, coarse hair down there, too. But something was wrong...terribly wrong. I searched and searched, but it wasn't there. The customer with the big, brown, sensitive eyes had no penis.

I wasn't sure how to bring it up. I'd seen a lot of things working here, but I'd never seen anything like this before. The customer had a large gut, so there was the possibility that it was there—just that it was small and hiding in that thick mess of bush underneath.

He seemed like the easygoing type, so I decided to bring it up. "Did you have the operation?" I asked.

He smiled and patted his mound. "No, I lost it in an accident."

"Oh, gosh, I'm sorry," I said.

"That's okay, it happened a long time ago. I've gotten used to it," he said. "Besides, I've decided to go through with the change. I started taking women's hormones a couple of months ago." He caressed his flabby breasts.

I didn't say anything to him, but I was thinking that those hormones didn't seem to be working very well. He was as manly as they come. Maybe it took a while for them to kick in.

"Can you still have an orgasm?" I asked.

"Yes," he said with a smile. "I'll show you."

He bent down and started going through his duffle bag. He

His hands disappeared between his legs and started groping for the snaps to the bodysuit.

pulled out a butt plug and some lube and squeezed a generous glob into his fat palm. He reached around and worked the lube into the crease of his ass. He squirted some more onto the plug and started working that in while his free hand rubbed his hairy mound like a woman. His eyes closed, and his mouth opened, and it looked like he was feeling something.

I lay back and watched in awe as my fingers glided up and down the inside of my thighs. He seemed so vulnerable, and I felt special in a way...like he trusted me.

His rubbing became intense, and his face tightened. A couple seconds later, his body lurched forward, then relaxed as he let out a long, quiet sigh.

Wow, could that have been it? I looked to see if there was

any cum. I wondered if cum came out anymore, or if that part was sealed off now.

I asked, "Did you come?"

"Yeah," he said, trying to catch his breath.

"Does it feel the same?" I asked.

"Nope, but it still feels good."

I had a million questions I wanted to ask but didn't. He did tell me, however, that pee comes out...but cum doesn't.

He started to dress and thanked me for the show. I thanked him for being so open, then he left. As I dressed, I thought about what I just saw. For some reason, I felt closer to humanity.

The Placebo Effect

He stepped into my booth, and I closed the shade to the hallway. He always came back too soon. I wondered if it was even worth the ten dollars I made doing his shows. The routine was easy enough, but I didn't like the things he revealed to me.

I slid off my silk robe and laid down naked on my side, facing away from him. He didn't say a word as he put the money into the machine. As soon as the shade began to rise, he turned around and faced the wall and started to undo his pants. I closed my eyes and waited quietly as he leaned back against the glass and emptied a small pillow of lube into his palm.

After a couple of minutes, he finally spoke: "Tell me about our life together."

"We live in a small cottage by the sea, surrounded by a beautiful garden," I said.

"We're married?"

"Yes, we just got married today...on the beach," I said. "Tonight's our honeymoon, and we're in Italy."

"Rome?" he asked.

"Yes, and we're lying in our bed ready to make love."

"Tell me how you love me!"

"I love you, baby...more than I've ever loved anyone else before," I said.

"I love you, too," he said. "You're the most beautiful person I've ever known. I'm the luckiest man in the whole world."

"And I'm the luckiest girl."

"You promise we're gonna be together forever?" he asked.

"Of course, baby. I couldn't be with anyone else."

"Really, baby? Promise you love me?"

"I love you, baby," I said. "I promise."

We went on that way for the rest of the show, blindly professing our love for one another until the curtain finally came down.

The customer wiped himself off with a tissue and zipped up his pants. He gathered his things and left the booth without turning around or saying goodbye.

I slipped my robe back on and lit up a joint. I left the shade to the hallway closed. I needed a moment to collect my thoughts. I didn't feel right lying about love. I lied about plenty of things around this place, but love wasn't one of them. But maybe for some people, I thought...fake love was better than no love at all.

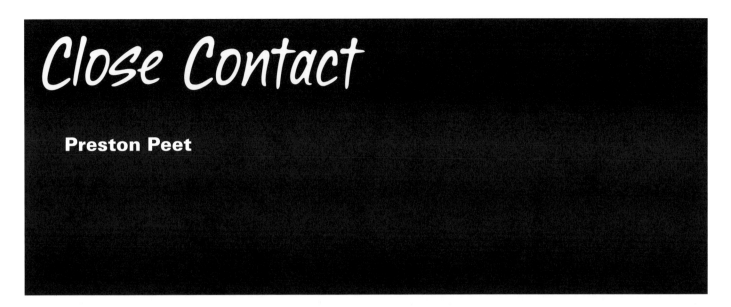

Close Contact

Preston Peet

"Need a ride?"

The first time I'd heard this from a passing car, I'd been mortified, letting the driver know in no uncertain terms that no, I did not want a ride and to get the hell away from me. As soon as the driver had pulled away, though, I regretted my quick response. Having smoked the last of my cash buying crack cocaine, I couldn't believe I'd just turned down what promised to be very easy money. At that point I'd not ever sold my body for cash to buy drugs, but from that moment on, I was on the lookout with the idea bouncing around in my head until I finally landed on Palm Avenue, downtown Sarasota, Florida's cruise strip, landing a ride in short order.

From that night forward I've hustled in every city I've lived in, both for drugs and simply for cash when on the streets trying to figure out where I was going next. I tried in Tampa but never had any luck, and Orlando was only slightly better. Atlanta, while not as dry as some places, was the only place I've ever been arrested on the prowl for a ride, garnering myself a misdemeanor civil disobedience charge for not leaving the area fast enough after some undercover cops told me to.

By the time I hit Amsterdam, I was busking for my cash, but in the midst of such a cold, brutal winter, it was hard, hampering my ability to make cash standing, playing guitar on the streets, what with all that ice and snow everywhere. Therefore, I did occasionally take the offer of a warm bed, companionship, and some easy cash. In London I'd stayed away from the hustling angle, managing to do pretty well just playing guitar and singing, but now in NYC and completely strung out, without a guitar, it was inevitable that I'd take the offers when they'd sometimes come.

"I know how to make some money," Sean leers at me as we sit in Tompkins Square Park by the kids' pool, regarding our now empty cookers and rigs.

"Oh, yeah? How's that?" I need my drugs and am willing to try almost any scam to obtain more.

"I know a guy who lives up on 14th Street, who'll pay to give you a blowjob and pay me for bringing you over there."

At first I hesitate, not having turned a trick for over a year, but completely without drugs, it doesn't take me long to agree to it.

After stopping at a payphone to make sure Jonathan is in and open to a visit, we walk to the West Side, meeting up with him outside a deli at the corner of 5th Avenue and 14th Street. Exchanging pleasantries, Sean introduces us, then Jonathan withdraws money from the ATM inside the deli. Sean takes a couple of proffered bills and leaves. Jonathan leads me in and up the elevator to his swanky sixteenth-floor apartment.

At this point I really only want to get this over with, whatever it entails. I want my cash so I can hit the road. I'm jonesing pretty hard for more cocaine and will need more heroin soon, as well, not having had more than a bag all night. But Jonathan is in no hurry. Unlocking his door, he holds it open, waving me into the air-conditioned interior. As hot and humid as the spring air is outside, I don't pay much attention, still thinking mainly of the next shot to come.

"What would you like to drink?" Jonathan walks to the bar set up by the windows, through which there's an incredible view of downtown Manhattan, the World Trade Center towering over it all.

"How 'bout a whisky?" I'm beginning to suspect this might

take longer than I'd been expecting, and I need something to sooth my jangling, coke-wired nerves if I'm going to get through this. Jonathan pours me a large glass on the rocks.

"Why don't you take this and jump in the bathtub," Jonathan firmly suggests, rather than asks, as he hands me the alcohol. Though I'd prefer to simply get my blowjob and go, I find the whisky and steaming hot bath relaxing, and soon the cravings for another shot subside enough to allow me to function and communicate more coherently without twitching and searching the room for something to steal.

Donning the oversized terrycloth robe Jonathan put in the bathroom for me, I walk into the bedroom of the spacious apartment where he's waiting, lying on the king-size bed. I'm unaccustomed to the feel of something so clean as this

"See, the deal is, I pay $25 for every orgasm."

robe, enjoying the sensation as it brushes softly on my naked body.

"Oh my, what a drastic improvement," Jonathan exclaims. I have to admit, the bath felt great. I'd been more than filthy, both me and my clothes, and I'm embarrassed when Jonathan notices the condition of my socks. "Remind me to give you a new pair of those when you go," he says.

I'm feeling the whisky, not being a drinker by habit, the warmth of the alcohol tingling in my skinny body. The cocaine jones further recedes.

"Come lay down." Jonathan pats the bed next to him, so I do, placing my glass on the nightstand next to the radio clock. I've never really been averse to making money this way, not since my initial hesitation. I figure if I can have fun and make money at the same time, no harm done and more power to me. Besides, life as a street-bound junkie can and often is a lonely existence. I'm starved for affection, for the touch of another human being. Though some of the tricks I've done in my time have left me feeling unclean inside more than out, those I usually put behind me quickly, choosing not to dwell on the particulars, even while engaged in the acts themselves. This time is rather nice already, so I allow myself to let go, to enjoy the moment.

"Let me take this off you." I lean forward so Jonathan can pull the robe off over my shoulders, raising my arms over my head and exposing my pierced nipples. "You are very beautiful," Jonathan tells me as I lean back against the pillows. "I'd like to give you a massage, treat you to something special." Jonathan picks up a bottle of baby oil and rolls me onto my stomach. The feeling is incredible, erotic and sensual, Jona-

than's hands caressing me gently where appropriate, firmly where needed. I float on the clean sheets, letting the fears and anxieties of living shot-to-shot fade into the dark recesses of my mind, relishing the rare contact with someone who not only turns me on but is going to pay me for this pleasure.

Jonathan eventually rolls me onto my back and continues the massage until I'm fully aroused, almost begging for release. He goes down on me, taking his time, gauging the reaction of me in his mouth and throat, pulling away each time I'm close to coming, prolonging the most intense sexual bliss I've experienced in years of difficult, isolated existence. Finally, it's no use and I explode, Jonathan swallowing every drop, wringing me dry. Exhausted, I lie there with my back propped on the feather pillows, sweat soaking the sheet underneath me as I smoke a much-needed cigarette.

"Did you enjoy that?" I can't lie, so I tell him I most certainly did.

"That's twenty-five bucks I owe you now. See, the deal is, I pay $25 for every orgasm. Feel up to another try, or should we leave it at that?" Jonathan smiles as he gives me another squeeze. This is the first mention of money between us, though it's been implicitly understood from the beginning that this is nothing more than business, that as nice as this is, I'm here for the money.

Immediately, I'm thinking about how much more cocaine and heroin I'd be able to buy with $50 instead of $25. Thinking only moments before that I'd been wrung completely dry of every drop of cum, I'm suddenly ready to go again. Besides, how could I really say no to such a pleasurable way to get paid?

"I'd love to try again," I smile, sliding down the pillows till I'm flat on my back. Jonathan sets to work. This time it takes much longer, slowing me to further enjoy the close contact, to close my eyes and imagine other places and times, with girlfriends I've loved and lost to my affection for drugs, to drift in the most base, carnal pleasures without guilt or shame. I finally come again, much to my amazement and glee. But tonight's sensations are brief respite from the daily grind of my life, a dream from which I now wake, knowing I can get paid. As soon as I realize I'm finished, the drive to score takes over, and I quickly climb from the bed, asking for my money as I look for my clothes. Jonathan sighs, then grabs his wallet. He hands me two twenties and a ten, along with a new pair of socks.

Dressed, I let Jonathan give me a kiss goodnight and goodbye, then head for the elevator, already envisioning the emotion-killing shots I'll be able to inject from this evening's earnings. Regretting nothing and feeling good for now, I hit the night sidewalk, to blow the money I just made, alone.

EVERYTHING YOU KNOW ABOUT SEX IS WRONG

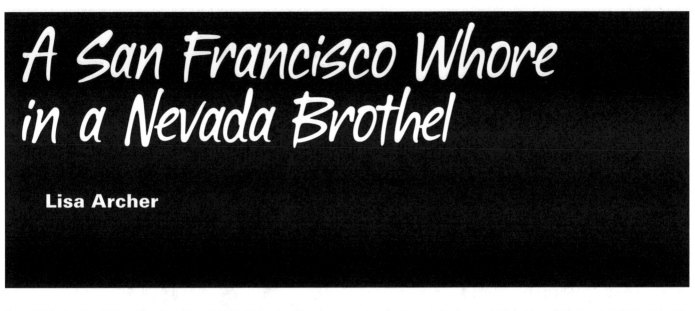

A San Francisco Whore in a Nevada Brothel

Lisa Archer

I'm sitting in the parlor of a legal brothel in Nevada. I'm the only one here who didn't get her nails done on Tuesday. Marta has red nails. Gina's are deep burgundy. They could be in a Lancôme ad at Nordstrom. When the bell rings, I scurry into the line-up with ten other girls. There are a few dark-haired women, a few with small breasts, but we're far outnumbered by tit jobs and platinum blondes. Some of the women look at me funny, because when we're not in line-up, I read or write email.

I've been working in this brothel for five days. Like many women, I started doing sex work to put myself through grad school. The inspiration for this trek to Nevada came from an acquaintance who made $10,000 in two weeks. I was sold. Plus, I didn't have to worry about being busted. In 1998, the San Francisco vice squad cracked down on middle-class whores like me who did in-call. They arrested consenting adults in the privacy of their own homes—and they targeted the key organizers and groups promoting prostitutes' rights. I was naked in bed with a client when a cop burst through the door and pointed a gun at my head.

I was one of thousands arrested in this crackdown. We each received an official-looking letter detailing our options: Fork over $1,000 cash or face charges. I didn't pay, but the charges were dropped. It was a scam. The vice squad lined their pockets with cash, and the press skirted the issue, aside from two pieces in a local weekly.

Here in this Nevada house, the threat of arrest is lifted, so I can shed the precautions and inhibitions I've adopted like a second skin. I can talk about sex and money in the same breath without worrying whether a prospective client is a vice cop hiding a microphone. This is a relief, but safety (and legitimacy) comes at the expense of some freedoms.

As an illegal, self-employed whore in San Francisco, I worked under a diffuse but constant threat of arrest. The Nevada brothel, by contrast, is saturated with its own set of rules and regulations. In this legal but tightly controlled laboratory, the intimidation tactics are more direct: I've been registered with the police, photographed, fingerprinted, and surveyed.

I fly into the Reno airport and meet the "runner" who will drive me to the brothel—a swaggering, poker-faced gent named Stan. Jogging beside him to the van, I ask if we can

The inspiration for this trek to Nevada came from an acquaintance who made $10,000 in two weeks. I was sold.

stop to pick up some baby wipes, antibacterial soap, and paper towels. "We'll take care of all that," he says, "but first, we're going to the doctor's."

The madam had told me over the phone that as soon as my plane landed, I'd go straight to the doctor, and it would cost $85. Stan pulls into the parking lot of a building that says "Fast Medical Clinic"—the McDonald's of health care. I fill out paperwork with my name, address, birthdate, person to contact in case of emergency, place of employment, and, of course, occupation. I've completed forms like this for numerous jobs, but this is the first time I've written "prostitute" on the application. I spend a good ten minutes agonizing over which of my friends would be least fazed by a phone call from a legal brothel saying that I'm hospitalized or dead.

Once I turn in the paperwork, the nurse takes me into a private room and draws my blood. Under Nevada state law, I must test negative for chlamydia, gonorrhea, syphilis, and HIV before I can register with the county sheriff and get my work permit. After the blood draw, I have the world's fastest and most painless gynecological exam. A man enters the room, deftly inserts a plastic speculum into my vagina, glances around inside, and says, "Thank you, ma'am." He leaves without ever having made eye contact, and I hardly felt a thing.

The brothel is on a ranch in rural Nevada. In 1971 Nevada legalized prostitution in rural counties with populations of fewer than 200,000—and only within state-licensed brothels. Prostitution remains illegal in the counties housing Nevada's main cities—Reno, Las Vegas, Carson City, and Lake Tahoe. City governments fear that too much tolerance of whoring might scare away tourists and detract from their main business,

San Francisco is known for its bright, witty whores.

which is gambling. Still, the women who work illegally in the cities far outnumber the brothel-workers in the sticks.

The ranch looks like a large trailer home with a fence around it and a few cows lowing in the backyard. The front door opens onto the parlor. When a client steps inside, the girls scurry into line-up, and the madam introduces us one by one. Most clients are too overwhelmed to choose right away and head for the bar at the opposite wall. To the left of the bar, a long hallway leads to the girls' rooms, where we sleep and turn tricks. The rooms are like any cheap motel rooms except for an emergency button and intercom system—so the women at the front desk can hear what's going on. As I'm filling out my paperwork, the madam suddenly comes barreling down the hall, belting, "Somebody's in trouble!" It turns out that one of the new girls pressed the emergency button, thinking she could order drinks that way.

I feel somewhat protected here—but at what price? I'm forbidden to work outside the brothel. I have to abide by their rules and give them half my pay. It doesn't feel that different from the classic trade-off, where "good girls" give up their sexual freedom in hope of protection from sexual violence.

Of course, the laws regarding prostitution are not primarily intended to protect me. The fact that we can only work in state-licensed houses keeps the brothel-owners in business and protects the neighbors from whores running loose in their streets and backyards. State regulations benefit everyone but the working girl. (This is why most politicized whores want prostitution decriminalized, as it is in Amsterdam, but

not legalized, as it is in Nevada.) Meanwhile, the brothels pay as much as 70% of the county's property taxes—hence, the friendly relations between the bordellos and their neighbors. I had no problem getting directions to the nearby brothel from a cheery housewife watering the plants in her front yard. Try asking the locals on the streets of San Francisco the way to the nearest whorehouse, and you'll see how unusual this is.

But the neighbors' friendliness is the benign face of surveillance. At nine the next morning, Stan takes me to the sheriff's office, where I present my test results to get a work permit. The secretary looks downright grandmotherly, but she doesn't take her job lightly. She orders me to stand on one yellow line while she photographs me, then another yellow line while she takes my fingerprints. During the fingerprinting, she yanks my hand—causing me to stumble across the line. "Don't cross the yellow line!" she barks, as if I'm a dangerously confused teenager behind the wheel for the first time. After fingerprinting each thumb, finger, and all four fingers together on each hand, she checks me for identifying birthmarks, scars, and tattoos, as if there were a high probability that I'd escape from prison or that she'd have to identify my mangled body. By the time she finishes, I feel like I've just been through an "arrest drill" for hookers.

Upon my return, the madam introduces me to Starlet, who will show me the ropes. There's something very prudish and schoolmarmish about her, despite her see-through red dress and platinum hair. She opens a thick, black binder and starts reading me the "house rules" one by one.

All new girls work from 8:00 a.m. to 8:00 p.m. You can stay in your room if you want, but as soon as the bell rings, you have to be up in the parlor and ready to go.

Never answer the door yourself. You'll be fined $100 each time you do. When the bell rings, you get in line with the other girls, and the greeter will answer the door and introduce you to the customer. You aren't allowed to talk to the customer while you're in line. That's called "dirty hustling." Some girls do it, but you're not supposed to.

Sometimes the customer picks someone right away, but most times they don't. They're too intimidated by all the girls, so they head straight to the bar. You aren't allowed to speak to a customer before he's ordered his drink. Once he's ordered his drink, you can come on to him all you want—but don't butt in while another girl's talking to him. That's "dirty hustling," too, although lots of the girls do it.

Never talk prices on the floor. When a guy's interested in you and wants to know your price, take him to your room. This is a classy joint. We don't talk in the parlor about what we do and how much it costs.

While it's perfectly legal to exchange sex for money here, it's not polite to talk about it. Politeness, delicacy, and "class"—in the sense of etiquette and "good taste"—replace the legal prohibitions against whoring. You still can't talk about sex and money in the same breath, only behind closed doors—hiding the raw economic relationship where you're working him for money and he's paying you for sex.

※

A lot of the women who work here come from middle-class backgrounds—like me and many of the whores I know in San Francisco. They chose whoring over straight work largely because they found that prostitution was less exploitative or more lucrative than many straight jobs. Some are students or have graduate degrees. But as I talk to them, I find they're much more conventional than the whores I know in San Francisco. They don't seem especially interested in challenging the codes of sexual propriety.

San Francisco draws a fundamentally different kind of whore than the Nevada brothel. Since the glory days of the Barbary Coast, the city has lured mavericks of all sorts, including sex radicals. For those with the temperament to enjoy the work, prostitution makes a lot of sense. It saves the creative and adventurous from nine-to-five tedium, offers good money and flexible hours, and allows one to go to school or to pursue other projects one simply wouldn't have the time or money for otherwise. San Francisco is known for its bright, witty whores. Like the Nevada brothels, we're a tourist attraction, and we provide a service that will always be in demand.

The Nevada brothel-workers are a different breed. There are some bright and witty whores here, too, but most are less invested in sexual freedom. Hence, they don't mind the highly regulated brothel system. Unlike some of the radical whores in San Francisco, many Nevada girls are more concerned with "class" in the sense of upwardly-mobile pretensions and refined aesthetic taste. The legalized brothel system reproduces middle-class values, such as the expectation of privacy around sex. The whores are confined to the brothel while working, and even in the brothel, they aren't supposed to talk about sex in the parlor, because it's "bad taste."

In short, "classiness" eclipses class consciousness. It's not that I think all whores should read Marx and analyze class conflict, but I like to see some effort at solidarity. One of the friendlier women mentions, "I'm here to work, not make friends." I feel the absence of women's solidarity more acutely because bisexual and lesbian women are in short supply.

I comfort myself by enjoying occasional glimpses of queer culture—unintentional drag shows by pornstars who dress like Liberace and wag their tits at the camera. One of the platinum blondes, Candy Curvature, dresses like a petite, hourglass-shaped Elvis impersonator—white polyester pantsuits, fringe skirts made of fluorescent-green latex, and stilettos that light up red and green in the black light of the parlor. Her bedroom eyes droop under mounds of sparkly gold glitter paint and false eyelashes.

She notices me quickly averting my eyes and starts flirting with me. The main problem with cruising these girls is that they're hypersensitive to being cruised, and most of them aren't lesbian or bisexual—just panseductive. As I unwrap my Quaker granola bar, the sweet strawberry smell wafts over to Candy, who coos, "Oooh, I want..."—knowing that she never has to finish a sentence before the basking addressee (me, in this case) places it in her hand like a mechanical doll. "Thank you," she mouths sensually—before I even realize she's taken most of my lunch—and plants a kiss on my cheek in slow motion. When I come to, I wonder why she worked me as if I were a straight guy. It's not like I could give her anything she'd want, not even an expensive dinner. Candy's not malicious, but she's so used to seducing men for money that she can hustle a granola bar from a coworker without realizing

While it's perfectly legal to exchange sex for money here, it's not polite to talk about it.

it. So much for sisterhood.

The lack of solidarity goes hand in hand with a kind of heterosexual orthodoxy. The first time a client chooses me from the line-up, Starlet comes into the room with us. She's there only for the very beginning—to teach me how to do "dick check." That's when I check the client's penis for visible symptoms of STDs. Once "John" and I decide on a price for a blowjob and intercourse, Starlet spreads a towel on the bed and asks John to drop his trousers. As he pulls down his pants and boxers, his erect cock springs up like a flagpole. Starlet puts on a latex glove and squeezes the tip of his cock, which eagerly emits a clear droplet.

"What you're looking for," she turns to me, "is anything greenish white—that's gonorrhea—or any blisters or sores on the skin."

She peels off the glove. "It's that simple. Now he can put his pants back on, and you take him to the cashier in the hallway, so he can pay."

"Wait a second—how much would it cost for the two of you?" asks John.

"I don't do doubles," says Starlet in her crisp, professional voice. "But if she's okay with a two-girl party, I'll take you out into the parlor and introduce you to another girl who does that." The client declines.

After the session, Starlet tells me a bit about "two-girl parties": "Some of the girls like it because you can make more money. There're more things the three of you can do together. Most of the girls," she says pointedly, "just fake it."

She's defending two-girl parties by saying I can make money without actually having to engage in lesbian sex. She repeats that I shouldn't feel this is something I have to do. This

But then I ran into mainstream America head-on in a Nevada brothel.

shocks me. It's never even occurred to me that some women would rather have sex with a client than with another working girl. I've always preferred "doubles" (another name for a threesome between a client and two girls). Frequently, I get to work with a friend, and there's camaraderie in turning a trick together. In San Francisco even the "straight" whores I know will do other women for pay. Once again, this brothel reproduces some of the most depressing constraints around sexuality.

Ultimately, this isn't surprising, since most of the sex industry

caters to people who are straight, or at least pretending to be. But there I was—presuming that all whores were willing to participate in bisexual activity. I'd been a whore all these years and had never come upon the stereotypical "straight girl" prostitute who can only talk about hair and nails. This place has shown me how thoroughly my assumptions about sex workers were based on a few exquisitely rare cultures in San Francisco. I had somehow acquired an irrational faith that all middle-class sex workers would be radical activists, committed to fighting for sexual freedom everywhere. I'd imagined that whores automatically flouted the bourgeois expectations of privacy around sex. But then I ran into mainstream America head-on in a Nevada brothel.

⌒

Despite the cultural claustrophobia, I'll probably come back here. The money and safety outweigh my complaints. Besides, I can live outside San Francisco for a week. (I've had lots of practice.) And there are some kindred spirits here. It just takes a bit longer to find them.

From what I've seen, legalized prostitution is extremely confining. In some brothels, the girls can't leave the premises. But we can ask for time off when we need it. After three days indoors, I can't stand it anymore, so I go for a walk in rural Nevada. A few motorcycle bars around, some houses, not much else. The wide-open spaces don't ease my sense of confinement. I wonder why this whole experience feels so familiar. On the plane out of Reno, I realize that it reminds me, strangely, of visiting my parents.

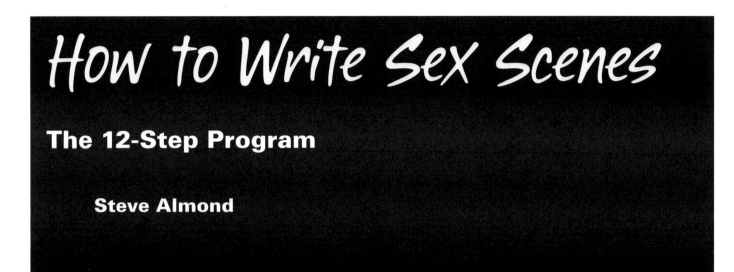

How to Write Sex Scenes

The 12-Step Program

Steve Almond

Now that I am an internationally famous author celebrated for my graphic portrayals of *amour* (see "A Pervert Among Us," *New York Times Book Review*, April 2002, and "How Low Will He Go?" *Us* magazine, January 2003), I am frequently asked how I manage to write such incredibly hot sex scenes. This usually happens at one of the many celebrity author venues I frequent, such as the Playboy Mansion Reading Room.

My general response to these inquiries is to laugh shyly and say, "Look, kid, ask Updike; he's even smuttier than me."

But I must admit that the question is being asked so frequently these days, and with such delicious sycophancy, that I feel duty-bound to respond to my public somehow.

Therefore, in the general interest of preventing more bad sex writing from entering the cultural jetstream, I am officially setting out this, my 12-Step Program for Writing Incredibly Hot Scenes:

Step 1

Never compare a woman's nipples to:
- a) Cherries
- b) Cherry pits
- c) Pencil erasers
- d) Frankenstein's bolts

Nipples are tricky. They come in all sorts of shapes and sizes and shades. They do not, as a rule, look like much of anything, aside from nipples. So resist making dumbshit comparisons.

> Note: I am guilty of the last.

Step 2

Never, ever use the words penis *or* vagina.

There is no surer way to kill the erotic buzz than to use these terms, which call to mind, my mind at least, health classes (in the best instance) and (in the worst instance) venereal disease.

As a rule, in fact, there is often no reason at all to name the genitals. Consider the following sentence:

"She wet her palm with her tongue and reached for my penis."

Now consider this alternative:

"She wet her palm with her tongue and reached for me."

Is there any real doubt as to where this particular horndoggle is reaching?

Step 2a

Resist the temptation to use genital euphemisms, unless you are trying to be funny.

No: Tunnel of Love, Candy Shop, Secret Garden, Pleasure Gate

I'd take a sweet, embarrassed pussyfart over a shuddering moan any day.

Equally no: Flesh Kabob, Tube Steak, Magic Wand

Especially no: Bearded Clam, Shaft of Manhood

I could go on, but it would only be for my own amusement.

Step 3

Then again, sometimes sex is funny.

And if you ever saw a videotape of yourself in action, you'd agree. What an absurd arrangement. Don't be afraid to portray these comic aspects. If one of your characters, in a dire moment of passion, hits a note that sounds eerily like Celine Dion, duly note this. If another can't stay hard, allow him to use a ponytail holder for an improvised cock ring. And later on, if his daughter comes home and demands to know where her ponytail holder is, well, so be it.

Step 4

Do not allow real people to talk in porn clichés.

They do not say: "Give it to me, big boy."

They do not say: "Suck it, baby. That's right, all the way down."

They do not say: "Yes, deeper, harder, deeper! Oh, baby, oh Christ, yes!"

At least, they do not say these things to me.

Most of the time, real people say all kinds of weird, funny things during sex, such as, "I think I'm losing circulation," and, "I've got a cramp in my foot," and "Oh, sorry!" and, "Did you come already? Goddamn it!"

Step 5

Use all the senses.

The cool thing about sex—aside from its being, uh, sex—is that it engages all five of our human senses. So don't ignore the more subtle cues. Give us the scents and the tastes and the sounds of the act. And stay away from the obvious ones. By which I mean that I'd take a sweet, embarrassed pussy-fart over a shuddering moan any day.

You may quote me on that.

Don't cut from the flirtatious discussion to the gag-defying fellatio.

Step 6

Don't obsess over the rude parts.

Sex is inherently over the top. Just telling the reader that two (or more) people are balling will automatically direct us toward the genitals. It is your job, as an author, to direct us elsewhere, to the more inimitable secrets of the naked body. Give us the indentations on the small of a woman's back or the minute trembling of a man's underlip.

Step 7

Don't forget the foreplay.

It took me a few years to realize this (okay, twenty), but desire is, in the end, a lot sexier than the actual humping part. So don't make the traditional porno mistake. Don't cut from the flirtatious discussion to the gag-defying fellatio. Tease the reader a little bit. Let the drama of the seduction prime

us for the action.

Step 8

Remember that fluid is fun.

Sex is sticky. There's no way around this. If you want to represent the truth of the acts, you will likely be required to pay homage to the resultant wetnesses. And I'm not just talking about semen or vaginal fluid. I'm also talking sweat and saliva, which I consider to be the perfume of lovers, as well as whatever one chooses as a lubricant. (Sesame oil is my current fave, but it changes from week to week.)

Step 9

It takes a long time to make a woman come.

I speak here from experience. So please, don't try to sell us on the notion that a man can enter a woman, elicit a shuddering moan or two, and bring her off. No sale. In fact, I'd steer clear of announcing orgasms at all. Rarely, in my experience, do men or women announce their orgasms. They simply have them. Their bodies are taken up by sensation and tossed about in various ways. Describe the tossing.

Step 10

Remember that it is okay to get aroused by your own sex scenes.

In fact, it's pretty much required. Remember, part of the intent of a good sex scene is to arouse the reader. And you're not likely to do that unless you, yourself, are feeling the same delicious tremors. You should be envisioning what you're writing and—whether with one hand or two—transcribing these visions in detail.

Step 11

Remember that, contrary to popular belief, people think during sex.

I know this is going to be hard for some of the men in the crowd to believe, but it's true. The body may race when it comes to sex, but the mind is also working overtime. And just what do people think about? Laundry. Bioterrorism. Old lovers. That new car ad, the one with the dwarf falling off the cliffs of Aberdeen. Sex isn't just the physical process. The thoughts that accompany the act are just as significant (more so, actually) than the gymnastics.

Step 12

If you ain't prepared to rock, don't roll.

If you don't feel comfortable writing about sex, then don't. By this, I mean writing about sex as it actually exists, in the real world, as an ecstatic, terrifying, and, above all, deeply emotional process. Real sex is compelling to read about because the participants are so utterly vulnerable. We are all, when the time comes to get naked, terribly excited and frightened and hopeful and doubtful, usually at the same time. You mustn't abandon them in their time of need. You mustn't make of them naked playthings with rubbery parts. You must love them, wholly and without shame, as they go about their human business. Because we've already got a name for sex without the emotional content: It's called pornography.

Bonus! Step 13

Read the Song of Songs.

The Song of Songs, for those of you who haven't read the Bible in a while, is a long erotic poem that somehow got smuggled into the Old Testament. It is the single most instructive document you can read, if you want to learn how to write effectively about the nature of physical love.

I am not making this up.

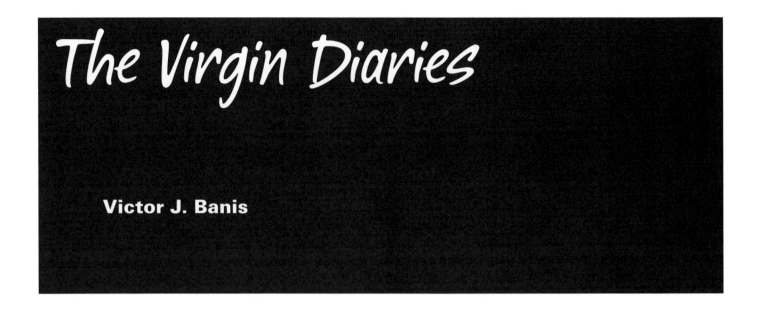

The Virgin Diaries

Victor J. Banis

I was a paperback virgin when first I met Earl Kemp, editor of big-time erotic-pulp publisher Greenleaf. Well, practically, anyway. There is a tale that lies therein, too, and it's not a pretty one.

My actual deflowering took place in Sioux City, Iowa, which is itself a sad thing to note, isn't it? I mean, there's glamour in a New York penthouse, luxury in a Beverly Hills mansion, but what does Sioux City have to offer beyond haystacks?

I cashed the check and waited to hear from the Pulitzer people.

But I am ahead of myself. The foreplay began, in fact, in Hollywood; no, not the Hollywood of stars and movie studios: the Hollywood of tawdry paperback bookstores. I strolled into one of these emporiums in 1963, leafed through a number of lesbian books—really, *faux* lesbian, the sort written by men for men—and thought, "Gosh, I could do this."

I read a dozen or so of them, after which, enlightened, I wrote my own, and sent it off to the publisher with the most variety: Brandon House Books, as it happened. In no time I had a letter back, saying that it was a bit on the short side (only about 20,000 words, and they needed more like 40,000), but if I cared to make it bigger, they would be pleased to buy it.

I'd had plenty of practice at making things bigger. I set to work, sent it off again, newly engorged and, in no time at all, I had my hot little hands on my first novel, *The Affairs of Gloria*, the uninhibited story of a free-loving, free-wheeling nympho (under the pseudonym "Victor Jay"), with a cover I thought quite stylish. I cashed the check and waited to hear from the Pulitzer people.

It was from Brandon House that I heard, however, a Mister Mel Friedman, who informed me that we had been indicted and were to meet the following day at the federal building for arraignment.

Arraignment? Don't forget, I was a virgin. "Indicted for what?" I asked.

"Conspiracy to distribute obscene material," was the answer.

Despite my virginity, I was not entirely ignorant. Sex movies weren't then available at your neighborhood shoe store, but you could find them if you knew whom to ask, and little stories on mimeographed sheets, and comic books with bizarre imitations of Flash Gordons and L'il Abners cavorting in sexual gymnastics.

Which, as I saw it, had nothing to do with my Gloria and her fondness for "manhood." There was nothing in *Gloria* that couldn't be found in her far less ladylike neighbors on the racks. Yes, she was frequently in and out of bed, sometimes with women, sometimes with men, but what was the fuss? The habitués of *Peyton Place* did not spend their time quilting and dancing polkas, and no one was dragging them into court.

In retrospect, I suppose that my innocence was criminal. I might point out, though, that I had not bought those initial paperbacks in plain brown wrappers or in any surreptitious manner, just strolled into a store in broad daylight, took them from the racks on the walls, and forked over my money. How could forking so openly be illegal?

Off I went for my arraignment, where I met for the first time my fellow "conspirators": Milt Luros, the owner of the publishing company; Bea, his wife and co-owner; Mel Friedman, who had called me the day before; Stanley Sohler, Harold Straubing, and Paul Wisner, who were editors; Bernie Abramson, head of their shipping department; Elmer Batters, a photographer; and two other writers: Sam Merwin and Richard Geis.

The "obscenity" involved a handful of books and nudist magazines. Mind you, the magazines were the *Sunshine and Health* sort of thing: naked people playing badminton, with here and there a bare bottom or a limp something—it was difficult to be sure what—flopping around. Nothing, I should think, to excite anybody, though admittedly I know people who get hot and bothered reading cookbooks.

The other defendants were named in numerous individual charges, plus the blanket conspiracy charge, but I was named only in the conspiracy, which would turn out to be significant in time.

We appeared before the judge to plead not guilty. I will admit, I was scared. And miffed. It was as we were leaving that I first met US Postal Inspector Donald Schoof, the mastermind behind our criminal case, who took me aside and whispered in a presumably seductive tone that he could make things easier for me if I would testify for the government.

Understand, I was no outlaw, no experienced criminal, but an upright, law-abiding citizen. My only prior legal mishap had been a distressing incident in which an unhappy wife named me as co-respondent in a divorce trial, one of the tamer episodes on *Oprah* today, but heady stuff in 1956 Dayton, Ohio, where it was guaranteed to get a laugh. And it did, but it did not carry the threat of ten years in the big house.

I was furious. Surely they knew from their investigation that I knew none of these people, and fondle where he might, Mister Schoof was not going to have his way with me. Besides, I felt sure they had only to reread *Gloria* to see their mistake.

They didn't, apparently. Our trial began in Sioux City in October 1965. Frankly, neither Gloria nor I would have set foot in Sioux City voluntarily—but federal law allowed charges to be brought where the material was shipped or received or anywhere in between. It would certainly be easier to get convictions in Sioux City than Los Angeles, but sad reality was, none of these books or magazines had ever been seen in Sioux City; even if they had, they would have been "under the counter." No overt forking in America's breadbasket.

I have to say that the experience was interesting, if only because book people are almost invariably interesting. It is not a business that attracts dummies—as, say, postal inspection might. Under other circumstances, I would have enjoyed spending time with these people.

Milt Luros was a graduate of New York's prestigious Hunter College, who set out to print quality art books, a not particularly profitable line. In short order he was printing sexy stuff—for others, initially, but eventually for himself. His field of business notwithstanding, Milt was a polite, soft-spoken gentleman of the old school. I liked him a lot.

I liked Bea too, but she was as loud and crude as Milt was polished. At lunch her fork was in everyone's plate, just in case you got something better. And while she ate yours and hers, she talked in a shout. Still, she was good-natured and took a Jewish Mama's interest in everyone's personal woes. Plus, she was very funny. I think she liked me because I always laughed.

The most fascinating of our group was Stanley Fleishman, Milt's longstanding lawyer, and probably the country's leading First Amendment attorney; certainly one of the profession's most colorful.

Having survived childhood polio, Stanley was left with nearly useless legs and walked all his life with crutches, which he sometimes used to advantage in courtrooms. Outraged by a prosecuting attorney's question, he would leap to his feet, forgetting those shriveled limbs. While everyone held their breath, Stanley swayed, seemed about to fall, and, at the last possible second, remembered to seize a crutch. By this time the prosecutor's remark had lost its sting or was forgotten altogether.

Milt hired a second attorney, legendary Texas criminal lawyer Percy Foreman, already known as another Clarence Darrow (he would in time represent Jack Ruby). A tall, folksy

He took me aside and whispered in a presumably seductive tone that he could make things easier for me if I would testify for the government.

man with a drawl and a mop of white hair in his face, he was scarcely any less dramatic. There were rumors that he drank. I never saw the bottle at his lips, but his breath once cleaned the spaghetti stains from my blouse.

Still, with ten years hanging over my head, I didn't feel much inclined to laugh. I was even less inclined as I listened to witnesses testifying falsely regarding meetings I had attended, phone conversations, etc. Frightening, and none of it true.

Had the jurors even looked at this material? I can say for sure, they did not in the courtroom, where they passed nudie magazines from one to another, gingerly holding them between thumb and forefinger with their eyes turned solemnly heavenward. Though I had no connection with those magazines, the charge against me was a conspiracy charge. A finding that the magazines were obscene could send me up that well-known creek without a badminton racket for a paddle.

A desk clerk at our motel whispered to me that our rooms had been bugged. I am sure he told the truth, because he whispered this from the next pillow, and by morning it was common knowledge that my night had not been spent alone. Yes, we were athletic, but not that athletic. Plus, my mail at home was left at the doorstep, the content displayed blatantly on

He was the first homosexual protagonist in fiction to be openly gay and proud of it.

top of the envelopes, so I could understand that it had been read.

The foreplay was over. I was on Mister Schoof's bed, and he misused me endlessly for four long months.

In the end, the forces of law and order did let me go, if reluctantly. I was acquitted on a technicality, when the judge tossed the conspiracy charge at the end of the trial (the only charge in which I was named, you will recall). The others were convicted, though those convictions were eventually overturned.

Free, then, but my innocence was gone forever. I had been screwed, and like any abused virgin, I felt sore and violated. I came home from Sioux City with a burning resentment for the callous disregard that had been displayed for what I considered some pretty fundamental rights. There's a reason the Bill of Rights mentions freedom of speech up front: Without that, the rest doesn't amount to beans, does it?

And all had been for naught. One would suppose that, in part at least, the indictment must have been intended to discourage me from further activity in the paperback business. Ironically, the result was exactly the opposite.

I'm not sure that, otherwise, I would have pursued a paperback-writing career. *Gloria* had been a whim, really, but I had no interest in writing of *faux* lesbians.

I was still hurting, however, and I felt practically compelled to write at least one more book, to show Mister Schoof that I was not intimidated. Besides, I quickly discovered I could write a book a week, and get paid, too. Better than leaning

against a lamppost on a rainy night, as I saw it.

I had acquired a long, hard passion for the gay male of the present and decided that he was what I wanted to write about. Problem was, gay males were *verboten* in the current publishing climate. The gay world wasn't just a "twilight world" anymore—it was darker than Sadie's backside, as someone used to say.

Our common travail notwithstanding, Milt and soon practically every other publisher declined my overtures. They all welcomed something from me in the heterosexual or lesbian vein. Fresno publishers Sanford Aday and Wallace de Ortega Maxey had recently been sentenced to twenty-five years in prison for publishing obscene books—that is to say, gay books, and tepid indeed, but the fact of their homosexual themes in and of itself rendered them obscene. Not even the bravest publishers would risk venturing into that realm.

Still, I remained stubbornly convinced that there was a large and untapped market for gay books. This was still five years or so before the Stonewall uprising, but gays were already coming out of their closets and dancing together in bars and clubs. The scene was jumping. The love that dared not speak its name was scribbling it on restroom walls:

"My mother made me a queer."

"If I buy her the yarn, will she make me one?"

I wrote my gay novel, *The Why Not*, and cast it into the waters, and who should fish it out but Earl Kemp? Prince that he was, Earl didn't even mind about my virginity. Anyway, I was still a "gay paperback virgin," which is what I started out to tell you originally.

I will confess, *The Why Not* was not a great novel, but it got good reviews (some of them may have been written by my mother, though she denied it), and it sold well enough that Earl welcomed more of the same. For an encore, I proposed a spy spoof, and *The Man From C.A.M.P.* (by "Don Holliday") charged boldly into bookstores in 1966—and caused a sensation.

"The Man" was Jackie Holmes, who made a mockery of every cliché regarding homosexuals. He was blonde, pretty, and effeminate, but he was also tough as nails and could outfight, outshoot, outrun the best of them. His white poodle, Sophie, was trained to kill with her razor-sharp teeth. Best of all, one could say that gay pride started with Jackie. He was the first homosexual protagonist in fiction to be openly gay and proud of it. Happily, he cemented the partnership between Earl Kemp and myself, as well as a friendship that has lasted until the present day, an unlikely coupling indeed, as we have both agreed often.

The gay world took to their new superhero with a passion—and so launched the gay paperback revolution that would change the publishing, and social, landscape of the 1960s and 1970s.

I considered that a good trade for my maidenhead.

♋

I have stated in other contexts that Earl Kemp is the Godfather of gay publishing, Il Capo de Tutti Frutti, notwithstanding the fact that he was as much a virgin to gay publishing as I was, and we lost our maidenheads together, so to speak.

To really understand this, you need to hearken back to the "swinging sixties": the sit-ins and love-ins and demonstrations in the streets. We were burning draft cards and bras and even jockstraps—well, admittedly mine wasn't having a blazing career anyway, but that's another story. The point here is, when one remembers the social and sexual revolution of the 1960s and 1970s, it is those dramatic goings-on in the streets and in public that one recalls.

Of course, it wasn't all so dramatic and not all so public. Some of the battles in that revolution took place in offices and at the desks of writers, publishers, and editors—at Greenleaf, in fact.

There's no disputing the impact of Greenleaf on gay publishing. The history of gay publishing divides cleanly into B.E. (Before Earl) and A.E. (After Earl). The few gay novels—and they were few—published before Greenleaf were mostly a dreary lot, in which we were generally portrayed as sickos, freaks, and monsters, living in guilt and angst, and soundly punished for our sins in the end.

To be sure, there was some good writing to be found if you looked hard. Jean Cocteau's *Le Livre Blanc* (*The White Paper*) from 1928 is wonderful indeed, but, after all, Cocteau is Cocteau. You can't say that about anybody else.

Der Puppenjunge (*The Hustler*), John Henry MacKay's 1926 novel, was originally published in German, and it wasn't until Hubert Kennedy's excellent 1985 translation that it could finally be enjoyed by the rest of us.

W. Somerset Maugham was gay and might have written "the great gay novel," but he grew up in an England still roiled by the Oscar Wilde trials and so remained in the closet throughout his life, though he did show a certain courage in including some gay characters in his books and stories. What is obviously a pair of male lovers appears briefly in *Christmas Holiday*, and in *The Three Fat Women of Antibes*, one of my favorites, the cigar-smoking Francis prefers to be called Frank and dresses "as much like a man as she could."

Robert Calder argues in *Willie: The Life of W. Somerset Maugham* that Mildred, the splendidly nasty "heroine" in *Of Human Bondage* ("every time you kissed me I wiped my mouth. Wiped my mouth!"), was in real life a young man. Maugham's custom of basing his characters on real people is well known, so the allegation is certainly credible, and it is interesting to reread the novel with that idea in mind, but of course, we can never know for sure.

Other writers sidled cautiously around homosexuality in their books. James Jones wrote a homosexual subplot into *From Here to Eternity*, though there was not a hint of it in the movie. Mickey Spillane's tough guy Mike Hammer has a serious case of the hots for the beautiful Juno in *Vengeance Is Mine*—until the very end, when her erotic striptease reveals the shocking truth: "Juno was a man."

Gore Vidal's *The City and the Pillar* (1948) exemplified the "sad young men" school of gay writing so common in the 1940s and 1950s and caused him to be blacklisted for many years, though the "frank" homosexuality would hardly get anyone's fist moving today.

Not all of those novels ended in suicide, of course. The heterosexual cure was a popular alternative.

I have said before that James Baldwin's *Giovanni's Room* from 1956 might better have been called *Giovanni Jones and the Temple of Gloom*, positively dripping as it does with gay self-loathing: "my sex, my troubling sex....(be it) ever so vile...." Not exactly positive reinforcement.

The real problem with most of these books is that, despite the sometimes fine writing, they are dishonest in their one-sidedness. Of course, in the 1940s and 1950s, gays lived with much harassment; they were beaten and robbed, sometimes murdered, with impunity; they were often blackmailed, sometimes by the police, and one can hardly wonder that they were often lonely, afraid, ashamed. Worse, the fictional mirrors these writers held up for us offered us nothing but bleak reflections.

Having lived through the era, however, I can tell you honestly that things were not as dire as these novels depict them. Some of us—most, I suspect—quite enjoyed our sexual activities. We made friends, found lovers. I know couples still together today who first met in that twilight world of the 1940s and 1950s.

We laughed, if often at ourselves. As anyone knows who's ever been around one of our street fairs or pride parades, gay boys know how to have fun, and they did back then, too.

Indeed, perhaps because it has always been somewhat underground, homosexuality often spawns a very special kind of camaraderie. Gay friends are often more like lovers than the buddies of the heterosexual world, sharing a peculiarly intimate kind of connection that at the same time is not in the least sexual in nature.

Not all of those novels ended in suicide, of course. The heterosexual cure was a popular alternative, in novels like Rodney Garland's *The Heart in Exile*, Lee Walter's *The Right Bed*, and Jay Little's *Somewhere Between the Two*. Indeed, it sometimes seemed the lowly pansy was an endangered flower.

I first encountered the word *gay* (in its homosexual context) in Nials Kent's *The Divided Path*, a novel that actually hints at happiness for its hero, until the finale when he is killed in a car accident—so much for that happy ending.

In James Barr's *Quatrefoil* and *Derricks* (obviously an inspiration for the Loon Trilogy that came later), macho men get it on with heroic enthusiasm but otherwise hardly seem to be gay at all.

Here, instead, was a book about happy homosexuals who spouted the gay cause and hopped blithely in and out of bed.

✕✕

In the years leading up to and including 1963, there were surely no more than another couple-dozen gay books, all much the same, with only a rare exception or two.

A decade later, there were at least a thousand gay books, maybe as many as four thousand. Even more surprising is that, apart from their homosexual characters and a new sexual bluntness, these books have little in common.

A gay man venturing into a bookstore in 1973 had whole shelves of gay books to pick from: nonfiction works, some of it scholarly, some nothing more than disguised porn; and, especially, an incredible variety of novels: mysteries, science fiction, adventures, war stories, gangsters, and cowboys, and even romances with happy endings. In those ten years a genuine and very dramatic revolution had occurred in gay publishing.

One other thing that many of these books had in common was Earl Kemp. By 1973 others were producing gay material: Sherbourne Press, Milt Luros' Brandon House Books, Lynn Womack's Grecian Guild. Maurice Girodias of Olympia Press fame in Paris (think such banned but worthy writers as Burroughs, Beckett, Genet, and Miller), launched an American gay-paperback series, "The Other Traveller." The first book with that imprint, my novel *The Gay Haunt* (by "Victor Jay"),

sold something close to 150,000 copies, an astonishing figure for a gay paperback novel in 1970.

These publishers, though, got on the bandwagon after it was rolling along and, not coincidentally, when they listened to the music of the cash registers ringing and realized that Greenleaf was making money with this stuff. The one who first got the bandwagon moving, however, was Earl, and he did it with my spy spoof, *The Man From C.A.M.P.*

I don't want to make myself out a hero, though I am proud to think that I made a difference, if only a modest one. I was mostly just having fun, making some money, and, yes, thumbing my nose at people like Donald Schoof.

Best of all, I got lucky. I got Earl.

I doubt that Earl had even read *The City and the Pillar* or *Giovanni's Room*, so he probably did not altogether grasp that we were supposed to be miserable and commit suicide or die in car crashes. He might well have thought that gays could reasonably be as happy as anyone else. A revolutionary concept in the early 1960s, to be sure.

It was certainly not, however, mere ignorance on his part. He knew of the convictions of Aday and Maxey; he knew, assuredly, that he was pushing the borders by publishing gay books at all, even "sad young men" gay books. Here, instead, was a book about happy homosexuals who spouted the gay cause and hopped blithely in and out of bed; and Jackie Holmes always got his man in the end. I am convinced that no other editor at the time would have risked publishing *The Man From C.A.M.P.*

Needless to say, once it's milked, you can't put the cream back in the cow. When Jackie Holmes made his debut, a new kind of gay hero was born, and the homosexual world adopted the baby as it own. A veritable flood of gay books followed, many from Greenleaf, and most of them were upbeat stories of gays who were no nuttier, no more unhappy, and no more likely to kill themselves than your average heterosexual. Which is to say, gay people just like the real ones.

Historians and scholars have opined that this boom in gay-paperback publishing first created for gays a sense of community, and I think they are probably right. In the past, we had been lucky to find any books about our world, and when we did, it was badly reflected. Often those few books were hidden under the counter, and we heard of them in whispers. Now bright sunlight chased away the shadows of that infamous "twilight world."

We felt a new kind of connection with the people in these novels, and, inevitably, with one another. We were less isolated than we had been before, more a part of a community, a "culture" uniquely our own, not one—those books told us in no uncertain terms—that we need be ashamed of, either.

Over the next several years, Greenleaf—and in time, others—published books about gay cowboys and Indians, gangsters, truckers, police and firemen, soldiers and sailors, detectives, and, yes, secret agents.

As we devoured these books, we began to see ourselves in new ways, not just as a group but as individuals. These novels offered us a whole new world of self-images. Macho images. Guilt-free images. Proud images. Come out, these books cried to us, share with one another who and what you are.

We began to feel a new spirit of togetherness, a spirit that would soon have us joining arms and marching together—and chanting, for the first time ever, "gay power."

—3

I've written so much about Earl Kemp's impact on gay politics that I fear I have almost certainly given a false impression. I don't want to suggest that Earl was, even latently, homosexual, nor was Greenleaf ever primarily a "gay publishing house." Under Earl's stewardship, Greenleaf published mostly heterosexual material, and that material, too, influenced the sexual and social revolution of the era, just as he had intended.

Others, however, were determinedly pushing those boundaries. Plenty of publishers, writers, movie makers, performers, et al., were willing to take on the puritan right on the heterosexual front.

Barney Rosset of Grove Press published an unexpurgated version of D.H. Lawrence's *Lady Chatterley's Lover* and created a sensation. Nabokov's *Lolita* and John Cleland's *Fanny Hill* were not far behind. Fellini's *La Dolce Vita* and Russ Meyer's *The Immoral Mr. Teas* were playing in movie houses, and Hugh Hefner published probably the most famous calendar photograph of all time.

There were plenty of gladiators, then, in the heterosexual arena. After the Aday and Maxey debacle, however, no one wanted to wrestle the fairy-tale dragon—until Earl jumped in and grabbed him by his lavender tail.

Earl has elsewhere called the sex-oriented publishing of the 1960s "a game." Yes, in a sense—scary though it was, it was exciting, too, and we found plenty to laugh about and cheer for—but it was a game with far more serious consequences than any Super Bowl, and none of us could ever afford to forget it.

In that revolution, some of us, as I have said, took to the streets and the demonstrations. I was there in those shouting, jostling crowds. It takes some courage, it's true, but you have the adrenaline rush and the group energy to keep you going.

It takes a different kind of courage to fight the war as Earl did, at his desk and, repeatedly, as the years went along, in courtrooms. In that one, as in any war, you sometimes lost a battle. Well, any Girl Scout can tell you, you have to crack nuts if you want to make brownies.

Sometimes you came home from the fight wounded, expecting a hero's welcome and found instead that people mostly didn't appreciate, hardly even remembered, your sacrifices. No medals, no monuments. Mostly, just the satisfaction of looking at the world around you, at how greatly it has changed,

Well, any Girl Scout can tell you, you have to crack nuts if you want to make brownies.

and knowing that you helped to make that happen. Gratifying, but you can't help wondering, in all modesty, if there oughtn't to be something more than that.

For what it's worth, soldier, there are some, mostly those who had been in the trenches with you, to whom you are indeed a hero. Who hold you in esteem and are grateful.

Which is what I said pages and pages earlier: Virgin or not, Earl Kemp is the Godfather of gay publishing.

Viva il Capo.

Beat Off 101

Earl Kemp

Masturbation is not only an expression of self-regard: it is also the natural emotional outlet of those who...have already accepted as inevitable the wide gulf between their real futures and the expectations of their fantasies.

—Quentin Crisp, *The Naked Civil Servant*

This is the graduate course. The prerequisites are "Pornography: Its History and Purposes" and "Propaganda: Its Use as a People Suppressor."

Very early in the life game, I became involved with dirty books, the kind men like, and I wasn't even one yet...a man...just a kid. Then, as quickly as I could and when I thought I was a man, I moved into the world of dirty-book publishing, all by way of setting the stage for what's going on here.

It was 1961 when I became a certified pornographer. I was thirty-one at the time, thought I knew it all, and couldn't say *fuck* without blushing. I signed on with Nightstand Books in Evanston, Illinois, which had been in business just over a year...almost like getting in on the ground floor. I was the third man hired to work side by side with science fiction cohorts Harlan Ellison and Ajay Budrys. In 1965 we made a massive move to San Diego, became Greenleaf Classics ("The Porno Factory" to insiders), and started ejaculating sleaze books in geyser fashion.

Those early years in sleaze-book publishing, in the USA anyway, found most of us involved with it floundering around and wondering what we were doing and how to do it just a little better. We were interested in profits to begin with, and not much of anything else, only over time that became much more about legality and moral issues and illegal activities by people beyond reproach but usually in it up to their sleazy, greed-stuffed assholes.

To offset that lack of knowledge, there were a lot of people conducting a lot of surveys trying to find out what it was that we should be doing, disguised as, "What is it about pornography that turns people on?"

Pretty early on, at the University of Copenhagen, Dr. Berl Kutchinsky was undertaking some groundbreaking research in just that. His studies involved interviews with a large number of people discussing the realities of their sex lives. I was fortunate enough to become involved with the fringes of the Kutchinsky studies during my frequent trips to Denmark during those days.

In 1968, President Johnson ordered up the big one, the Presidential Commission on Obscenity and Pornography, but that was a few years down the timeline. Because it eventually resulted in Greenleaf's *The Illustrated Report of the Presidential Commission on Obscenity and Pornography*, of which I am unreasonably proud, I can't pass up the opportunity to mention it again.

Then there's Donald H. Gilmore, PhD, the ultimate pornography connoisseur. He wrote fiction and nonfiction under his own name, "Dale Gordon, PhD," "Del Grayson, PhD," and others. Dr. Gilmore had been at it for years before me and was so saturated in it he could quote chapter and verse without lifting his carefully manicured hand or raising his voice even noticeably. It was uncanny to watch him in operation in the 1960s, because he was so smooth. He could've sold anything he wanted to, I suspect. He certainly sold enough to me. Enough to make me thank him and remember him and think of him forever, at least.

Gilmore was one of the first people I met when I moved with

Nightstand to San Diego. He did his best to impress upon me how very much I really needed him. He did it so well that he succeeded. He promised timely delivery of damned near anything I could ever think of wanting to see in manuscript form in any quantity. Complete with photographs and scholarly introductions suitable for reference in any First Amendment court proceedings going on anywhere in the country. He was *good*.

He was well underway during the mid-1960s establishing a vast, complex pornography empire operating out of Guadalajara, Jalisco, Mexico, with him as the head *jefe* and chief executive in charge of accounts receivable. It honestly involved a huge school of porno writers already in full operation, complete with a student body ready and willing to do the down and dirty on paper for a few pesos a day. Don had me flying back and forth from San Diego to Guadalajara frequently, smuggling in illegal typewriters. (And, on the side, we outfitted an entire electrical workshop/classroom for the local Salvation Army orphanage with all-smuggled equipment.)

At the time, the Mexican Customs people wouldn't allow tourists to bring any form of electrical appliance into the country. Only commercial importing could be done at duty fees frequently in excess of the retail price of the device in the States. Vaguely similar machines, of a very low quality, were for sale in Mexican stores at much higher prices than at home. The only answer was…smuggle. It was a national pastime for most expatriates. There were times when I would be driving my Blazer to Guadalajara (a thirty-six-hour, 1,300-mile, two-driver, nonstop fun run) with as much as $1,000 in small electrical appliances hidden inside it and large stereo speakers bolted into the floor as "my radio."

Needless to say, anything of an erotic nature, even copies of *Playboy*, was instant contraband. Stag films, beat-off books, naked people photo shoots, stuff like that, were all prohibited and had to be smuggled in past the border inspection personnel.

During those smuggling trips and on other pretenses when I would be a houseguest of the Gilmores, I learned what true luxury felt like. I could understand why literary agents would fly to Guadalajara from New York City just to be Dr. Gilmore's houseguests. It became a mark of status to have been so honored.

Walking down Gilmore's wide, curving, fairy-tale staircase like Rhett Butler coming directly from giving Scarlett a mercy fuck, her pussy flavor still on his lips and inside his mustache for later reviewing, tugging unconsciously at his period-piece trousers while buttoning up his fly. Those pants were so tight and clingy, they were almost transparent; you could

see everything that Rhett was so proud of…a tiny smear of afterlove clearly marking the place where his penis ended. Or, it could be Carol Burnett doing Vivien Leigh wearing the drapery gown and segueing into the Tarzan yell that bounced around backstage a bit as the reel ended and the houselights came up again.

On that movie-star staircase in Tara, walking tall and proud, looking gracefully ahead, and taking in that unbelievable 40x40x20 library/living room was reward enough all by itself. *Yes indeed, I **am** the King of Pornography, and these are my loyal subjects. All hail me!* It looked like acres of oiled and polished hardwoods in fifteen-foot-tall shelves filled in nice, orderly fashion with expensive display books. A room to lust after forever.

I seem to remember seven master bedroom suites alone, plus numerous other single bedrooms in that huge, old mansion, and that didn't include the servants' rooms on the third floor that accommodated a large number of people all wearing cute little matching uniforms. Someone's ultimate dreams come true….

Dr. Gilmore, as head instructor at Porno University, insisted that all his students have the best typewriters to work with. His choice was a portable electric Olivetti in a particular model. None other would do. (While I preferred, and used for years, a German portable Olympia.) Don would even occasionally fly in the Olivetti repairman from San Diego to enjoy a luxurious

> ## It honestly involved a huge school of porno writers already in full operation, complete with a student body ready and willing to do the down and dirty on paper for a few pesos a day.

vacation, all at Don's expense, just to keep those typewriters in top running shape, pounding out the porno. Don certainly had the house that would make any visiting dignitary think his station in life had suddenly escalated an enormous amount.

All of this was before word processors or personal computers made writing simple. You had to do it all on a typewriter then, fortunately an electric one. Just imagine the number and quality of manuscripts a true porno mill could turn out with today's computerized assistants. Thank God for copy and paste, for find and replace…the contemporary author at work.

Gilmore's Guadalajara porno complex also was to contain some elaborate sound stages with state-of-the-art recording and lighting equipment (that never got off the drawing board), a chain of retail bookstores (that did, with two of them open and operating), and on and on.

He was the only man I ever knew who could be actively managing half a dozen different kinds of enterprises that, eventually, would all somehow come together, while appearing to be bored out of his mind. But his thoughts never strayed too far from the fruits of his Porno University manuscript mill.

Toward that end, Don insisted, he had to know what it was about pornography that activated all the desired responses on the part of the reader. And, could the reader continue to read after one of his hands became occupied full-time in more gratifying pursuits?

He talked me into participating in this study with him. He might as well; he already had me smuggling things for his students and things for the Salvation Army Orphanage, his—

He had to know what it was about pornography that activated all the desired responses on the part of the reader.

and therefore Greenleaf's and my—adopted charity. I knew I could rely upon him to figure out a way to get me to pay for things, as well.

The actual classroom for his Porno University was a conveniently borrowed meeting room in the orphanage, set up with desks and outlets for all those smuggled Olivettis. Leave it to Gilmore to figure out multiple uses of facilities he could command for free. He taught the students how to follow the formula in the classroom, then sent them home with reams of typing paper and their Olivettis to do the "creative" work in private.

For years after Gilmore's Porno University closed down, some of the stellar alumni continued to write and sell many novels as full-time writers. Included among them were old western pulp hack Lee Floren ("Lisa Fanchon," "Matt Harding"), Leslie Gladson ("Kyle Roxbury," "Sebastian Gray," "Lee Gardner," "Genevieve St. John"), Vivien Kern ("Vivien Blaine"), and Peggy Winters ("Marta Summers"). In addition, Dr. Gilmore persuaded full-time professional expatriate writer Linda DuBreuil to join the Greenleaf writers group. While she was not one of his students, she was nevertheless the reigning Queen of Pornography. Linda ("D. Barry Linder" and numerous others), all by herself, wrote 300 novels during her sleaze-book career.

Gilmore, as instantaneous President of Guadalajara's 20,000-member Americas Society (no mean accomplishment, that), had all those expatriate US citizens delegated to be the guinea pigs for his experiments. For some reason I never understood—and there were many of them revolving around Don—those people really were his to command. They would do anything he asked, however improbable, like spending hours just looking at pornography and discussing their reactions. After all, they were practically your average Americans anyway, weren't they? What he wanted from me wasn't so much participation as financial backing. He wanted Greenleaf Classics to pay the printing costs for his test papers, course material, etc—everything that was involved with the studies.

The tests were divided about evenly between written pornography and visual pornography. This was because, at the time, Greenleaf was producing a number of photo-illustrated novels and nonfiction books requiring lots of really close-up and intimate color photography…so good you could smell the action and feel the warmth it was generating all by itself. We were also producing more than one naked people magazine a day.

Dr. Gilmore said that he was going to sell me most of the manuscripts that came out of his Porno University anyway, so I might as well help pay to get them done right. It made a sort of sense to me at the time, so I gave him the green light and arranged the financial backing he had requested.

At first there was a frantic period of gathering up materials to use with the test subjects. These included numerous 8- and 16-mm hardcore films, and hundreds of still photos of naked people alone and in doubles and in groups, and all of them doing things most people had never seen being done before. All kinds of books from classic pornography to the best of the 1960s sleaze paperbacks. And I was somehow expected to smuggle all that contraband from the point of origin to the place of use…a frequent touch-and-go proposition.

It took two weeks to train the staff that would be conducting the studies at Porno University. Several different elements were crucial to the study, and it was necessary that every staff member be prepared to cover more than one of them if necessary. For instance, they kept running score sheets of every test subject in the classroom. On those sheets, in code symbols, they indicated things like facial expressions, visible aggression, body language, etc. One very important element was to indicate the viewpoint of the subject to see if it was consistent or if it switched around and why. Were they bonding through reader identification with the fucker or the fuckee? Were they lover or beloved? Doer or done? Somewhere in between? All those things were given value points in arriving at Dr. Gilmore's conclusions and recommendations.

The testing itself, involving a long line of handpicked expatriates that seemed to be unending, required three full weeks to complete. Then it took another month to correlate and evaluate those studies and come up with The Lost Chord...the ultimate answer to the ultimate question...*What turns me on and keeps me going the best and why?*

The test subjects were divided into groups of twenty by age, with males and females included in the same group, and each group repeated the same tests at different times. As I remember—and I was only an onlooker, not a participant (forty years ago)—the tests themselves were divided into three categories: written pornography, hardcore photographs, and live-action sex films. The test subjects in each group were all given copies of the same books and sent home to read them in private.

In the classroom, as a group, the subjects were given hardcore photographs to examine and pass on to the next person. And, in the classroom again, using borrowed projection equipment, the subjects watched a number of hardcore sex films.

After each of these three tests, the subjects wrote their reactions on a special form listing the things that most turned them on about that test and the things that most turned them off. In many cases, the latter was much more informative than the former.

Finally, back in the classroom as a group, the subjects analyzed each other's written test reactions and discussed them considerably. That was a phenomenal time because the subjects didn't hold back a thing; they were all vocally expressing in public their most secret, personal, sexual reactions to the various test materials. While that was going on, the staff, on their individual score cards, was making a lot of those little code marks dance around.

I recall one test subject, a slightly repressed middle-aged housewife, who kept insisting that the aggressive female types should be allowed to be a bit *more* aggressive and dominant in the books and magazines. *I'm on top! Now it's my turn. I'm going to show you how to use that—oh,* nice— *cock, Studbuns....*

Greenleaf Classics was an equal-opportunity masturbatory aid provider. A female reader of our books or magazines was as entitled to her vibrating dildo and heavy-duty batteries as a male reader was to his conveniently placed bottle of hand lotion and box of soft, absorbent facial tissue.

In almost every respect, the results of those tests and interviews conducted by Dr. Gilmore proved to be as he had predicted they would be before the studies began. *Damn him!* He was always doing that, being right and much too right most of the time. Otherwise, he could never have been my best friend for over a decade. For years after that we managed to hang on to each other before we evaporated from each other's existence.

Wish he was here, setting all of us straight about everything.

⌒

Nine-tenths of the appeal of pornography is due to the indecent feelings concerning sex which moralists inculcate in the young; the other tenth is physiological, and will occur in one way or another whatever the state of the law may be.

—Bertrand Russell, "The Taboo on Sex Knowledge," *Marriage and Morals*, **1929**

Only the center 90% of the study conducted by Dr. Gilmore counted. The other 10%, containing all the extremes, the nut cases, the deliberate differents, was routinely discarded. What we had left, in terms of demographics, was our baseline market area. A full 90% of the test group, equally divided among males and females, among age and background characteristics, all responded in exactly the same manner to exactly the same degree.

There is a difference in the way males and females perceive certain aspects of pornography, but the response to the same stimuli is still almost identical. Females are noticeably more sensual than males and tend to want to dwell on that and the more sentimental aspects of intimate relationships. Males don't require anywhere near the same amount of attention as do the females, however good it feels while it's going on.

With 90% of the population backing up the data, exactly what is it that Mr. (and let's not forget Miss, Mrs., and even Ms.) Averageman needs to have included in his pornography to best serve his individual requirements, however pressing and however often and thoroughly served?

"Built like a brick shithouse" served well enough.

The reconciled data from the test groups concluded that Mr. Averageman wanted to read about himself when he read a book. Then, when he looked at a magazine or watched a porno film, he wanted to see himself in action. Only, he had a very highly idealized image of how he looked...much better than in reality. Not a one of the test subjects saw themselves or thought of themselves as being overweight, out of shape, sedentary, or just sitting there with the book open to the right passage and whomping down the homestretch.

When they thought of themselves, those Averagemen, they saw themselves with women with fine bodies and big, bouncy tits. They saw themselves with muscles and a waist and a dick that had somehow miraculously taken on some impressive dimensions. But all of that was okay, because they were exactly Mr. Averageman…just like the beholders.

They had a long list of don'ts, headed by "non-human bodies," described as steroid freaks. Also, no body piercings, no visible marks of any sort. No scars, no body sculpting, no birthmarks, no tattoos. No exotic, fashionable, or seasonable people…just ordinary, everyday Mr. Averageman. And, much to my surprise, they singled out smoking cigarettes…in 1966…as being very offensive to them and an intrusion upon their reading, viewing, or intimately involved enjoyment.

(Because of this, we issued immediate instructions to all model agencies, photographers, etc. working for us that all those things, especially tattoos, were forbidden in the future. Similar instructions went to the writers regarding the use of cigarettes and smoking by the characters in their books. We were years ahead of the times in producing "no smoking" books.)

We used those results to formulate what became the basic background formula for all our sleaze paperbacks and visual publications.

In the novels they wanted to read about people exactly like themselves, doing the same things they really wanted to be doing but for some reason weren't getting anywhere close to, not within blocks, and with them living in the middle of the hottest hooker marketplace in town. They wanted real people in real situations with things like bills and responsibilities that they could somehow set aside for a bit, just long enough to escape into a fantasy of steamy, smelly sex and lurid expectations that ended, inevitably, with splurts of blessed relief, *thank you, Jesus!*

We gave the writers new guidelines stressing the need to write down to the lowest possible common denominator. We encouraged them to use stock clichés and to never strive for a new way of doing or describing the same old thing. "Built like a brick shithouse" served well enough.

We asked for a certain amount of tease and anticipation, almost like foreplay, before the foreplay began, and to at least let the characters say something to each other before the first blowjob ends and the money shot splewies all over her nicely made-up face.

At times, the tease can be much better than the final resolution.

The writers of the heterosexual novels were required to focus upon the penis at all times. Regardless of what was ongoing in the narrative, within the central character's head—locked by reader identification with the reader—all of his thoughts—therefore, the reader's—were always to be centered on his penis. This was to help maintain the essential reason for the novel: to get it up, keep it up, and exercise it regularly or as prescribed by the family physician except in states where prohibited by law and common decency and don't forget to *lave sus manos.*

Then, by way of reminding the writers of reality, we quoted the immortal D.H. Lawrence, who said, "What is pornography to one man is the laughter of genius to another."

I am very glad that I accepted Don Gilmore's offer to back his study of the effects of certain sexual stimuli on the test subjects. We used those results to formulate what became the basic background formula for all our sleaze paperbacks and visual publications.

There was one more overriding criteria, of course, the legal one. Every time there was a new ruling in a major First Amendment court proceeding, we received new legal guidelines from our guiding light, Stanley Fleishman, who knew the route better than any other man. Then, with those constantly changing legal guidelines overlaying the basic formula, our paperbacks and skin magazines were ready to do their duty as none other had ever done before.

The result of the moves made to accommodate Dr. Gilmore's psychological and sexual studies within our manuscripts, and within our naked people magazines, was incredible. The sales proved the worth of the studies several times over and never stopped proving it until the whole merry-go-round broke down about fifteen years later.

Scattered within the debris and beneath the hooves of those brightly painted and exquisitely carved carousel horses were the remains of millions of copies of disintegrating pulp paperbacks. They were all that remained of the 5,000 novels and uncountable skin magazines produced by Greenleaf under my direction, and the additional thousands that followed after that. Fading into dust, disappearing into the past, and becoming all too quickly extinct.

And at the same time, for an increasingly large number of devoted sleaze-book collectors, they are the single most sought after and expensive (hundreds of dollars for single copies) masturbatory aids ever created for the ultimate blessed erotic benefit of all mankind….

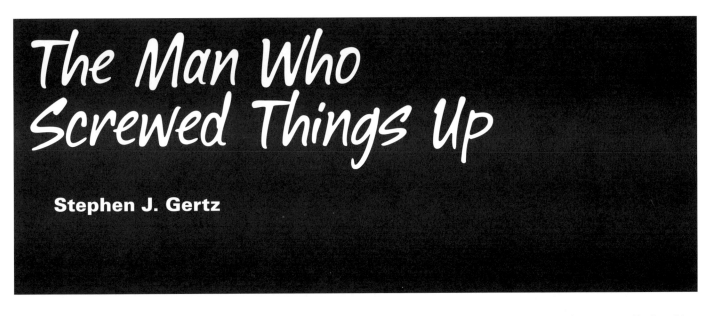

The Man Who Screwed Things Up

Stephen J. Gertz

Given the ubiquitous nature of pornography in contemporary American culture, one could easily assume that obscenity is legal in this country. It is not. Legally, the notion of what is obscene in the US has been muddy from the get-go, but by 1966 the Supreme Court had loosened censorship with an awkward yet liberal heuristic. In 1973, one man threw a monkey wrench into that formula, with dire results predicted. He was **THE MAN WHO SCREWED THINGS UP.**

But the long-term result of his actions and the Court's ruling would allow technology to make a mockery of the Supremes and usher in the modern universe of porn. Who was this forgotten, unlikely hero?

> "He [was] a paranoid schizophrenic."
> "[He had] very little sense of right and wrong."
> "He [had] a violent temper."
> "He [was] tricky in business."
> "I held him in great contempt."
> "He didn't care about anything except making money."
> "A thief and a *gonif*!"
> "He's a creep."
> "I think he worked out of a phone booth."

These are some of the nicer things that have been said about 1960s pornographer Marvin Miller, one of the more colorful individuals in a business bursting with them, a man who, if he'd been known to nineteenth-century British philosopher Herbert Spencer, would have been Exhibit One in his case for social Darwinism. For Miller—the first of the porn fast-buck artists of the era, impresario of Collector's Publications, for a few years a leading porn house—was a fierce survivor who, no matter what degree of material comfort he would gain in his adult life, would forever be haunted by a Dickensian youth. He was the Oliver Twist of the porn business, albeit Oliver

Twisted, an Artful Dodger who grew into a porn-Fagin with a fondness for silk underwear.

He was born in the slums of Chicago to a widowed mother who was mentally ill and on relief. He and his older brother often went hungry. Stability was a foreign concept. Marvin was an erratic, wild kid, raising himself, but five-year-olds make lousy parents. His violent temper was already manifesting itself. He hated to be crossed. His first experience with law enforcement occurred when he was six: He robbed a bakery shop for something to eat. Busted, he became the responsibility of Jewish Welfare, which arranged for his placement in a foster home. His first. He was sent to school. Nightmare time for the faculty. He was, to be charitable, a difficult child.

"It was like this," he remembered to journalist and novelist Carolyn See. "If a teacher would ever hit me, I'd hit her back. I'd scream and holler, I'd kick the wall and I'd kick her."[1]

His behavior in the first foster home set a pattern for the rest of his life. "I was an angel as long as I got what I wanted."[2] The couple that took in Marvin subsequently grew attached to him, and for a few years he experienced some degree of stability and affection, a modicum of family life. He got what he wanted. He was an angel. But the woman grew sick, and the couple had to give him up. He was ten.

Next stop, the University of Chicago's showcase boarding school for underprivileged kids, where it was discovered that Marvin possessed an almost idiot-savant-like ability in math. He was intellectually precocious, a boy-genius, and the recognition he gained focused him. He became a learning sponge, absorbing everything the faculty threw at him, spending nights and weekends at the school, often all by himself, reading, listening to the radio. He was a loner, his only regular interactions with the other kids being fistfights.

Sent by Jewish Welfare to another foster home at age thirteen, he remained there for five years. He went back into the public school system. He attended Chicago's Hyde Park High School, remained a good student. Summers were spent as a camp counselor. During the school year he worked at Sears and—this is key to his future—at Donnelley Printing, one of the largest such facilities in the US. He graduated, barely seventeen, and enrolled in the University of Chicago. But he was now used to having money in his pocket and, despite the workload from school, got a job.

The Miller legend now begins, a legend based on fact.

He went to work for Reynolds Aluminum. At the time, Cuba was responsible for manufacturing 25% of the world's supply of party *tchotchkes*—hats, noisemakers, etc.—the vast majority of which required aluminum foil in their making. But Cuba had a big problem: Reynolds, due to a strike, couldn't fulfill its contracts to Cuban party-supply factories. Marvin,

He was the Oliver Twist of the porn business, albeit Oliver Twisted, an Artful Dodger who grew into a porn-Fagin with a fondness for silk underwear.

already possessed of a keen eye for financial opportunity and a survivor's grit to pursue such tenaciously, made a brilliant move. Who in all the world could supply the Cubans with the aluminum foil they needed? Marvin knew: Hershey's Chocolate.

What?

Hershey's has to wrap all its candy bars in something; as a matter of course, it bought giant rolls of aluminum foil, but the candy bars are specifically sized, and Hershey's routinely had to trim the excess foil. The company had a shitload of trimmed ends sitting around that it would just toss out.

Marvin, independent of his employer, made a deal with Hershey's for all its foil remnants. Then he went to Cuba and made a deal to sell them to the *tchotchke* manufacturers. They gave him a letter of credit from Chase Manhattan Bank. With that, he bought Hershey's foil remnants. He quit Reynolds, shipped the foil to Cuba. He got paid. By the time the Reynolds strike was over, Marvin was a millionaire. He was seventeen.

Flush with success, he married his high-school sweetheart, invested his money in a home-appliances venture with a connection from the old neighborhood, a man twice his age, and went on a three-week honeymoon. When he returned, his partner—and his investment—had disappeared.

As Carolyn See wrote, "[B]y the time he was eighteen, then, Miller has not only chosen his life's partner, but earned and lost his first million, and been educated in the best schools—from the street to the University of Chicago to respectable Big Business itself—to every nicety of rip-off."[3] He had learned the value of a dollar at a tender age. Like Scarlett O'Hara in sharkskin after the Civil War: "As God is my witness, I'll never be hungry again!"

In the late 1940s, Marvin pulled up stakes and with the little money he had left, moved with his wife to California. He neglected to tell Ms. See about one of his early business ventures in the Golden State: managing a large linen-supply business and being convicted and incarcerated for falsifying its corporate records and embezzling over $35,000.[4] Prison counselors regarded Marvin "as a born-hustler, a man with a certain charm but also a limited sense of how the social system work[s], and even less awareness of what might get him in trouble."[5] Upon his release, he invested in carpets, becoming something of a carpet king via innovation, offering, as he recalled with the pride of a merchant prince, "the first tufted carpet ever introduced into the state of California."[6] Unfortunately, his factory blew up. "Too much viscose in the air," he explained to Carolyn See.[7] He next opened a doll-manufacturing factory. It blew up, too.

Not coincidentally, Marvin acquired a nickname, a moniker that on the surface appeared to reflect his incendiary temper: "The Torch." But a fiery temper was not the inspiration behind this sobriquet; it was Marvin's incendiary activities, for he had decided to take a few shortcuts toward his next fortune. He got into the flame-'n'-claim game. Yes, Marvin became a larcenous arsonist, a master of insurance fraud, and did very well. Until he got busted. In 1959 Marvin went to jail for the third time, doing two years in California's Chino State Prison on the flaming doll-factory rap before his parole.[8]

When he got out in 1961, he went to work for a finance company headquartered in Chicago. A trained accountant, Marvin became a turn-around whiz. When companies fell into financial straits, enter Marvin, whose financial acumen would bring them back from the brink. Marvin was now running a few businesses for his employers, two of which, significantly, were a publishing company and a print shop. His experience working for printers during high school had given him an unofficial degree in the mechanics of the trade; he knew the ins and outs, how to make a printing press print money. He took a shot at men's magazines: *Reel*, *Now*, and *Sports Review*. He was getting his feet wet, kinda thrashing around, seeking a niche. He knew printing, but publishing is another matter, and he'd soon learn another lesson that would only sharpen his survival skills and increase his already well-developed sense of do unto others before they do unto you.

But at this moment he did something that might be considered courageous in any other individual but in Marvin was just an example of brazen recklessness. In the immediate aftermath of the Kennedy assassination, he was approached by a CBS photographer who put together a "quickie" event book on the tragedy—amongst the first, if not the first, such quickie event books that would become standard over the years. But now, in late 1963, early 1964, a wholly controversial, some might say tasteless, opportunity. To make money. Which, for Marvin, obviated any objections or other considerations.

The CBS guy had shopped it around. Nobody wanted anything to do with it. Marvin? He published the book, *Four Dark Days in History*, in magazine format with a huge print run. According to his son, Ron, it sold 30 million copies and earned Marvin a small fortune.[9] But what was really controversial about the book was not its opportunistic tastelessness—Jackie and the rest of the nation were still grieving—but its immediate status as a political bombshell. For while everybody and his mother in the government had embraced the lone-gunman theory, the CBS photographer had the only shot that blew that scenario out of the water: the Mary Moorman photograph of the grassy knoll, clearly defining a person standing where alternative theorists claim the fatal shot originated. The photograph disappeared soon afterward, so the Warren Commission had to buy a copy of Marvin's book to see it. This was Marvin's first unlikely entry into American political-cultural history—a footnote to be sure, but a bona fide credential and by no means his last.

Marvin now had some publishing experience under his belt; he made money, a lot of it, by going out on a perilous limb. Another lesson learned. The books Marvin published afterward, however, were of a decidedly different character, and while they never matched his Kennedy book in sales, they were enormously successful. Marvin was the man responsible for such immortal novelty titles as *It's Fun to Be Jewish!*, *It's Fun to Be a Mother!*, *It's Fun to Be a Monster!*, *It's Fun to Be a Beatnik!*, *It's Fun to Be Offbeat!*, etc. It's fun to be a publisher: Marvin was making money hand over fist. He also published *Extremism U.S.A.*, a view of the far right and left; *The Official Polish Joke Book*; *Mrs. Goldberg Uncovers Hollywood*; *The Ugly Book*; and a host of other literary gems.

In 1965 he published what for him must have been the Bible (though he issued a magazine-format edition of that other Bible, you know, the Old Testament): *Justice Be Damned!*, with a cover featuring a gothic-looking electric chair and the tagline, "You Could Be Executed For A Crime You Didn't

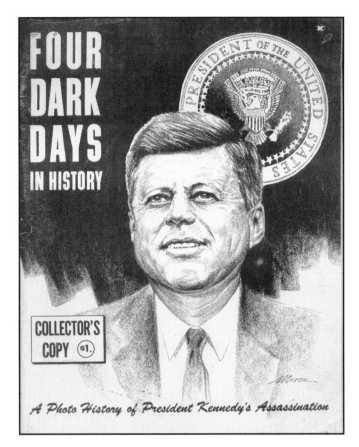

Commit!" His ad for the book read: "Every year 15,000 Americans are unjustly accused, tried and sent to prison. You or someone you love could be next!"

To gain a foothold in the burgeoning sex end of publishing, in June of 1965 he issued Daniel Defoe's 1724 novel *Roxanna; Or, The Fortunate Mistress* ("Another Searing Boudoir Saga From the Author of *Moll Flanders*!") and his 1726 *The History of the Devil, as Well Ancient and Modern; In Two Parts*, under the title *Devil* ("A Spine-Chilling Exposé of Evil Incarnate!"). These were sex-lite titles, classics; they'd never run afoul of the law since their original publication. Marvin spiced them up with suggestive covers and *galante* text illustrations.

Marvin learned a few new tricks. His edition of *Devil* was a photo-offset reprint of the first edition (London, Printed for T. Warner, 1726), which is to say he photographed the book and printed it from the photographic transfer plates—no typesetting involved and a major expense avoided. And—forget for the moment the public's wet dreams—he'd discovered the publisher's wet dream: free content! For the Defoe books were, and are, in the public domain. *Free content, no typesetting* became his publishing mantra. At this point, Marvin was working out of an office at 7046 Hollywood Boulevard, and these books were issued under the imprint APS (Associated Professional Services), with Marvin Miller Enterprises, Inc. as the copyright holder.

In February 1966, in advance of the Supreme Court's obscenity decisions, APS officially morphed into Collector's Publications, with an entirely different wrapper design. As its maiden publication, Marvin wanted to issue the massive Victorian erotic classic *My Secret Life* but was immediately sued. Grove Press was issuing its own edition of the classic, and news of Marvin's impending release was bad indeed.

There have been conflicting stories about the affair over the last thirty-five years. According to Grove's owner and publisher, Barney Rosset, in the fall of 1965 he asked the Kinsey Institute for its copy of *My Secret Life* but was turned down, despite offering a generous fee for the privilege of reprinting it. He next traveled to Hamburg, Germany, and made a deal with distinguished collector Karl Leonhart to reprint his copy from a photo-negative that Leonhart provided in exchange for $50,000 plus royalties. Grove then devoted an enormous amount of effort to editing the book, not to expurgate but rather to correct spelling, smooth out the narrative, and make it more readable.

When Rosset heard about Marvin's upcoming edition, Barney wasn't happy about it. How did Rosset find out about Miller's plans for *My Secret Life*? Even though Marvin owned his own printing presses, he farmed out work to other print-

To say the stock Marvin used for his books was suitable only for bathroom hygiene would ignore toilet paper's prime requisites.

ers for insurance; if he were to be busted, other printers are on the job. But Marvin was notoriously slow in paying his bills; hell, stiffing his creditors had become standard operating procedure. According to Marvin, his printer—expat Canadian Saul Simpkin, whose Offset Paperback Manufacturing would ultimately be bought by Bertlesmann, but at this time Simpkin was just starting out and would print anything, no questions asked—ratted him out.[10] Rosset took Marvin to court. It was, according to Rosset, simply a measure to stall for time so Grove could get its edition to market first. Barney knew perfectly well that he had a weak case; you can't claim copyright on public-domain material on the basis of making editorial changes.

To this day, Marvin's initial defense brings tears of laughter to Barney Rosset's eyes. "He claimed in court that the book was obscene—remember, this was before the Supreme Court's decision in March [1966]—therefore, in the public domain and had no copyright protection. Can you imagine anything more stupid? The judge tells Marvin—I actually liked him when we first met; we were both from Chicago—'Well then, if you're right, you're going to jail. Think about it. You've got a week.'"[11]

A week later, Marvin saw the light and changed his defense. No mention of obscenity; the book was simply in the public domain and not eligible for copyright. The judge ruled for Marvin, but it was an empty victory. The Grove edition was handsomely produced and issued in hardcover. Marvin issued his edition of *My Secret Life* in eleven volumes (as was the original, clandestine edition) in a cheap, cheesy, double-columned magazine-size format. It didn't sell anywhere near the numbers of the Grove edition. Though he'd won the case—he crowed to Carolyn See about it—completely lost on Marvin was the object lesson: Don't stiff your printer. Miller would pay for this, big time, in just a few years.

Now, Marvin's dash for cash began in earnest.

At first, he bought classic erotic books from dealer/collector J.B. Rund in New York, works that, because of their classic status, would avoid prosecution under the Supreme Court's 1966 *Memoirs/Fanny Hill* decision. Rund recalls meeting Marvin in Miller's New York "office," his suite at the Essex House hotel in toney Central Park South, where he noticed silk boxer shorts lying about. Miller "was a rather dapper dresser," Rund recalls.[12]

Marvin purchased manuscripts that had been privately commissioned during the 1940s and 1950s. But the free-content mantra was soon humming in his head once again. Marvin had been doing his homework, boning up on US copyright law. With few exceptions he reprinted virtually every book that Maurice Girodias had originally published in Paris, as well as many other erotica-in-English French publishers' books. All were photo-offsets with a wrapper design suggestive of, but clearly distinguishable from, those of Olympia Press, ultimately nondescript and without illustration.

"Girodias was a fool," Marvin said. "He could have come in with me if he'd wanted to; he'd have been a rich man."[13] Marvin taking on a partner? After his sorry experience in the home-appliance business? Preposterous. This bizarre statement completely ignores the fact that Miller didn't need Girodias or his permission to reprint the Olympia Press catalogue, which under US copyright law at the time was in the public domain. That Girodias didn't want to come in with Miller (there is no evidence that Miller ever offered Girodias a deal or that Girodias ever proposed an alliance, making the whole issue moot) only demonstrates good sense in a businessman otherwise lacking such; it's likely Girodias would have wound up as frog legs, filleted on Marvin's dinner plate. In any event, Marvin became a peripatetic traveler, going all over Europe buying up copies of erotic books for their cover price, filling suitcases full of 'em, never getting caught by Customs.

Learning long ago that the secret to printing money is to keep your presses running 24/7/365, Marvin took work from whomever, wherever. There is evidence that he printed books for pornographer Reuben Sturman, based in Cleveland.[14] He printed for notorious Gambino family associate Robert "Di B" DiBernardo of Star Distribution in New York.[15] And he printed magazines and books for "Jules Griffon," pseudonym of Edward S. Sullivan, a journeyman porn editor-publisher, owner of Jules Griffon Enterprises, a publisher of skin mags and erotic paperbacks that operated under the imprint Classic Publications.[16]

You can tell a lot about a publisher by the quality of his production. "He prints the shoddiest books of all of us," says Brian Kirby,[17] famed editor of 1960s porn-magnate Milton Luros' Essex House imprint, and truer words have never been spoken. To say the stock Marvin used for his books was suitable only for bathroom hygiene would ignore toilet paper's prime requisites: that it not chafe your ass and crumble while in use. Marvin used ground pulp, the lowest-grade paper available and high in acids; as soon as it's exposed to oxygen, it begins to brown, practically before your eyes.

Marvin was, to put it mildly, parsimonious. He not only refused to pay his debts on principle, he bounced a check to his star witness for the defense, Carolyn See, who, as a PhD in English literature, provided the requisite redeeming social value during his obscenity trials. (At the time, providing redeeming social value in obscenity trials had become something of a cottage industry for scholars.) Marvin called her "venal" for insisting that he make good on the check. She threatened to provide redeeming social value for the D.A. He sent her another check, this one good.

Perhaps experience as a turn-around whiz taught him that the best way to run a company was on a shoestring, keeping operating expenses to a bare minimum. He was a one-man band. He worked out of his house, a comfortable suburban tract home in Covina, east of Los Angeles. Woke up every morning at four, edited manuscripts and texts all by himself before dropping them off at the printer.

In his APS/Marvin Miller Enterprises venture, Marvin distributed through John F. Hayes' Kable News of Cleveland and New York. Periodicals distributors are pretty sharp operators, and it appears that Marvin met his match—or Kable News theirs. The two parties soon locked in a virulent fight over $600,000 in receipts. Miller appears to have decided that he couldn't trust distributors anymore, not an irrational conclusion. So, while continuing to move mountains of books through established distributors like East Coast-based Al Druss' G.I. Distribution and Robert DiBernardo's Star Distribution,[18] his friend Art Kunkin reports[19] that Marvin maintained a long list of in-

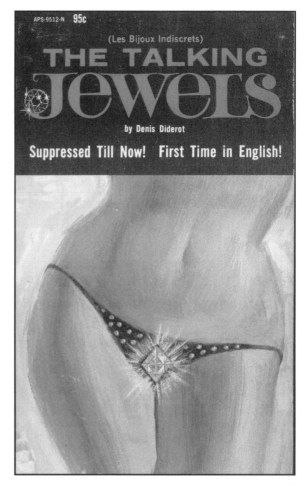

dependent distributors all over the country handling his stuff, including the legendary Shelley Wilson of New York, a "cigar-smoking, tough as nails, fun, good-time gal"[20] who had the moxie to stand up to wiseguys who tried to mess with her.

Marvin loved mail-order distribution, soliciting, and fulfilling all orders in-house, no middleman. He would send four employees to the post office to pick up orders, one to take them out of the post office box, the other three to keep an eye on the first and each other. He claimed to have movie stars, politicians, professionals, even the mayor of a large Western city on his mailing list. On this, we can probably take his word, for porn had become somewhat hip, and—though it may come as a shock to the innocent—even politicians have secret sexual desires, and, gee willikers, tend to be hypocritical about them.

Just because Marvin issued cheaply produced, cheesy editions, don't think that he didn't reprint some truly outstanding or unusual material aside from his Olympia Press knock-offs. Not that he had any idea what he was doing. He issued *The Sixty-Niners*, an offset-photo reprint (natch!) of a Continental Classics photo-reprint, their retitled edition of *Queenie*, a portion of a longer Victorian work known as *The Adventures of Lady Harpur*. Shortly thereafter, Marvin issued *Queenie* by

Lady Harpur from another source edition. He hadn't read either. Same book.

In May 1968 he issued *Orgy of the Young Virgins* by Sandra Jameson, a photo-offset reprint of E.L. Publishing's book of the same name. Five months later Marvin issued *The Debauched Maiden* by Kittin Haywood, a photo-offset of another source edition. Again, same book; both reprints of the classic *A Town Bull*.

Marvin put out the only openly published edition of *The Lascivious Hypocrite; Or, The Triumph of Vice*, originally published in 1890, an English translation of *Le Tartuffe Libertin*, an 1845 French erotic novel often erroneously attributed to Sade due to its false eighteenth-century issue date. He issued the only open edition of Samuel Putnam's rare, masterful clandestine manuscript-only English translation of Antonio Vignale's sixteenth-century classic of gay erotic facetiae, *La Cazzaria* (*The Book of the Prick*). He published the first American edition of *A Diary of the Senses* by Helen Tucker, originally issued in Paris by Oceanic Press in 1958, the first book in the English language and perhaps any language to deal with transsexuality. He issued a godawful translation of Denis Diderot's 1748 ribald classic of loquacious labia, *Les Bijoux Indiscrets*, under the title *The Talking Jewels* (from his APS imprint; he'd later reissue the novel as a Collector's Publication under the title *The Talking Pussy*).

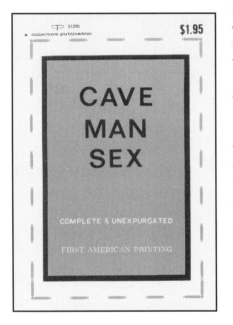

Hungry for fine literature...with hot parts? Marvin issued a photo-offset reprint of Joyce's *Ulysses*, apparently reasoning that the erotic aspects of Molly Bloom's soliloquy would more than offset the overwhelmingly nonerotic text. This is the paperback Doorstop Edition, collating to 933 pages of text plus 43 pages of ads.

Marvin commonly offset-reprinted books already offset-reprinted by smaller publishers, merely changing the title and author, cutting the other publishers' introductions, or leaving the introduction intact but cutting the name of its writer. He did all the editing himself, not for content so much as a little change here, a cut there to economize on the printing or provide a legally distinguishable edition. He wasn't very good at it. For instance, he cut the name "Allan Saunders, M.A." from the introduction to a book from Continental Classics, a small publisher out of Long Island City, New York, but neglected to cut the first line from the last paragraph: "Continental Classics is proud to present..." He issued photo-reprints of photo-reprints published by Classical Novels and Collector's Editions, two small publishers of which we know nothing, their copyright pages providing no identifying information save for a date. He also found E.L. Publishers, a small operation out of New York that published *The National Registry Official Swingers Publication*, a great source for material. He offset-reprinted a slew of their titles, many the first open editions of American clandestine originals from the late 1940s and early 1950s.

All porn publishers during the era had high spots in their catalogue; all had low. There were many in between, oftentimes so outlandishly ridiculous that it's difficult to know whether the author was unintentionally comic or deliberately so. By way of illustration, we proudly present Collector's Publications' *Cave Man Sex*. Please, bear with me:

Mongoon stood in front of his dirt cave and couldn't for the life o' him understand what those crazy signs his wife was making meant but he figured she wanted his cock inside her again, even though he had balled her four times already this morning. "Oo. Oo," he said, scolding her for being so bothersome. But then his cave man instinct brought his cock up real high and real thick, so he hit her over the head with his wood club, and fucked her good and hard while she was still unconscious.

That was how Mongoon liked taking his fucks, with the women quiet like a sleeping dinosaur. Mongoon's wife was called Ah-ha-oh, a name that sounds strange, but is really exciting and sexual when grunted passionately. For Mongoon and Ah-ha had no language as such....

Nor did the anonymous writer, who, though fitting somewhere between hack and imbecile, provides a Joycean touch. When we first meet the characters, they speak in a sort of Chinese/Native American pidgin: "Itchy-ook no sleep with Mongoon." "Come, fuckie." "No fuckie with Mongoon." As the story progresses, their language, like Stephen Dedalus' in Joyce's *Portrait of the Artist as a Young Man*, becomes more sophisticated:

"Listen, Omer, you come up here immediately. If she doesn't think Mongoon's son is good enough for her, then she doesn't deserve to be deserted by you. Now, I want you to stop being a fool and I

want you to be a man. You must simply snub her from now on, and I will tell Bish-mar that you have found his daughter repressed."

Thus the prehistoric origins of pretzel-logic, Don Corleone's advice to godson Johnny Fontaine, and Freudian theory are established.

All the cultural byways of cave-man civilization are presented, including the preferred method of suicide when grieving—stoning oneself to death. This would seem a less dependable method than merely throwing oneself off a cliff, but what do I know? I wasn't there. Judging from his Cro-Magnon way with words, the author apparently was. And so we learn that fucking was the primary form of communication, although it is admitted that one learned very little about a partner's inner life that way. There is even talk of exterminating the humans who have recently come onto the scene, are fucking like bunnies, and threaten cave-man existence.

The entire sweep of prehistoric man's development is compressed into a single generation: Mongoon (French for "My Goon?") emerges from his dirt cave to desert his wife, Ah-ha-oh, for the mountain whore, Itchy-ook (add an "n" to the second part of her name and her character is revealed), founds a dynasty, lives in a palace, keeps slaves, and—here's the topper—sires children who will later be worshipped by the Egyptians as Isis, Osiris, and Horus. Finally, the mystery of the Egyptian deities decoded. Not by some learned, namby-pamby, ivory tower Egyptologist/archaeologist but by a real, honest-to-goodness pornographer desperately in need of Haldol, the psychotic's anodyne.

Within eleven months, Marvin had issued 170 Collector's Publications titles.[21] Other publishers routinely published twice that many within the same time frame, but they had a staff; Marv did it all by his lonesome and earned his second million. And then some.

"I printed the dirtiest ones first. Apollonaire's *Autobiography of a Flea* [actually, Apollonaire did *not* write that English classic of a bug's-eye view of human sexual behavior], Pierre Louÿs' *She Devils* [*Trois Filles et Leur Mere*]. The government wasn't even on me yet. They hadn't even noticed. I kept putting the money I made back into the business. If I kept the millions I'd made in the first eight months, before the government got on me and I had to pay it all out in fines and lawyers, I'd be...I'd be a *millionaire*, that's what."[22]

Don't cry for Marvin. Though smut appears to have comically affected his reasoning powers, he still had plenty of dough.

Has it become clear that Marvin was a sociopath? "He doesn't have much sense of the human emotions the rest of us have," a business associate said. "He gives a pretty good imitation, but there's no conviction in it. He's been watching people all his life to find out how he's supposed to act. People talk about his temper, but he even gets angry on cue. He has no feeling; he has great charm. He can look straight at you, and smile, and tell you—he can tell you anything."[23] The rules applied but not to him. He had to get what he wanted. He was going to be fleeced if he wasn't hyper-vigilant. He had to survive.

Yet he appeared to revel in litigation and infamy. He was, as often as not, under one federal indictment or another for conveying obscene material. "Here, look at this," he told Peter Collier of *Ramparts* magazine, holding out a mimeographed page listing a series of porn titles and their publishers. As Collier relates, "It is headed, 'Books On Which Complaints Should Be Filed,' and is handed out by Citizens for Decent Literature, the national censorship organization that is particularly strong in Southern California [run by that paragon of civic

"Mongoon's wife was called Ah-ha-oh, a name that sounds strange, but is really exciting and sexual when grunted passionately."

virtue, Charles F. Keating, who in the early 1990s became the fraud poster-boy for the national savings-and-loan debacle]. With something akin to pride, Miller points to the fact that Collector's leads the list with 49 Books on Which Complaints Should Be Filed; his nearest competitor, Greenleaf, is a poor second with seven."[24]

Earl Kemp, then VP and editorial director for Greenleaf, was concerned that operators like Miller gave the business a bad name. "Mr. Marvin Miller has done things that bewilder me—and gotten away with them. Not only does he pirate books with perfectly valid copyrights [*Ulysses*, for example], but he deals in strange stuff like dildos and the like—in his mail-order business. I've been trying to get our attorneys to tell me how he gets away with it."[25]

Marvin didn't sell merely any ol' sex toy—he sold "A Revolutionary Sexual-Aid for Men, The Amazing New Improved UTHAID!"

This unique prosthetic device is designed to help married men with certain sexual problems recapture the joys, bliss, and harmony which only happy sexual relations can bring to husband and wife.

• Life-like texture.

- **Continuously Adjustable Fastening for left or right handed users [!?] and those with special preferences.**

- **Odor resistant.**

- **Grease resistant.**

ORDERING INSTRUCTIONS

In order to obtain your proper length, hold organ between thumb and forefinger and stretch gently away from the body until a slight tension is felt. WITH A RULER, MEASURE ON TOP IN INCHES FROM THE BODY TO THE END OF THE ORGAN. MEASURE ORGAN IN LIMBER STATE.

Marvin understood that escalation is the key to long-term success in hardcore porn; strong medicine to begin with, the dosage must be regularly titrated upward to keep the reader involved and aroused. The analogy to drug addiction, while not entirely false, is, however, weak. The stronger analogy is to the movie-going public's consuming passion for increasingly sophisticated, unusual, and elaborate...Action! Special Effects! Wild Stunts! To this end, in mid-1968 he schemed to broaden his catalogue, getting away from novels and into nonfiction. He told Peter Collier: "Now your homosexual novel isn't what it's cracked to be.... In fact, I think that the homosexual market is highly overrated. Take us. We put out a book of male nudes [*All Male Nudes*] in various poses a little while ago, and its sales took a nosedive."[26] The fact that the production values for that gem of a book were excruciatingly poor escaped him; the most avidly horny gay man would've been hard-pressed to get a hard-on looking at those lousy, grainy black-and-white shots.

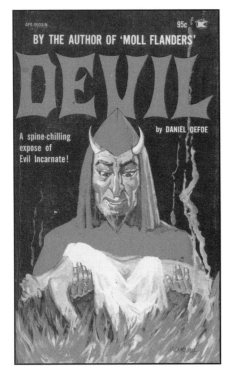

Marvin continued: "Right afterwards we put out one of females nudes [*Female Photographs*] and, frankly, we can't keep enough in print."[27] Marvin was out-of-the-ballpark wrong regarding sexually explicit gay pulp fiction. It was, in reality, a booming part of the business: More gay-sex titles were issued and sold during the era than at any other time in history. As for the success of *Female Photographs*, this only demonstrated that most straight, middle-aged men of the era were so desperate for a peek at the palace that they'd buy anything. The book was sleazy (no, that gives *sleazy* a bum rap; *tacky* and *shoddy* are more appropriate adjectives), one black-and-white split-beaver photo after another. One can only conclude that gay men in general do indeed possess a greater aesthetic sense than their straight brothers.

To further his profits—there was an industry-wide sales slump beginning in 1968 that apparently was the motivator for ratcheting up the raunch—Marvin issued *Intercourse*, a title that thirty years later might've been released under the title *Fucking for Morons*, a self-help guide providing—of course!—grainy, cheesy b&w photos of men and women demonstrating various sexual positions. "Believe it or not," Professor Marvin Miller, renowned sexologist and purveyor of the Uthaid, asserted, "some people don't know how to screw."[28]

✕✕

In 1969 Art Kunkin, publisher and editor of the *Los Angeles Free Press*, at the time the West Coast's premiere alternative/counterculture newspaper, was in trouble. As a public service, he'd recently published the names and home addresses of 80 local police and federal narcotics officers, and the city and feds had come down on him like a pile driver. He was being prosecuted for obstruction of justice, and his printer was being intimidated. Included as part of the indictment against Kunkin, the printer was offered a deal: Drop Kunkin, we'll drop you from the case. Kunkin became *persona non grata* with his printer and every other shop around town. The *Free Press* was being forced out of business. Kunkin heard about a plant in City of Industry. He visited the owner.

Just a few days prior to Kunkin's appointment, Marvin was sitting at home, watching evening TV. Former LAPD Chief Ed Davis, then a commentator on a local station's newscast, had recently blasted Kunkin on-air for revealing the identities of the narcs. On this night, Kunkin was provided with the opportunity to rebut Davis. Marvin watched Kunkin, and the seeds for a mutual love-fest were sown, for Kunkin demonstrated to Marvin that he was a true brother-in-arms, or rather fingers, specifically the middle one, in the struggle against authority.

So, when Art visited Marvin and asked if he could rent his printing plant for a few months with an option to buy (the *Free Press* had, with its recent addition of sex ads, become something of a cash cow, and Kunkin had ambitions toward a publishing empire), Marvin—without any discussion of terms whatsoever—reached into his pocket and tossed the keys to the plant to Kunkin, who was stunned by Marvin's generosity. "Just get the paper printed; we'll talk later," Kunkin recalls Miller telling him. Much to the frustration of the authorities, the *Free Press* survived. Kunkin ultimately bought Marvin's printing plant.[29]

Later in 1969, Marvin began another in a series of massive mailing campaigns. This time he had to assign the job to an outside printer; typically, he didn't pay his bill, and, once again, a printer took matters into his own hands: Legend has it that the printer included the mailing lists for the Cub Scouts and Boy Scouts of America in the solicitation. There is no evidence to support this. (In a statement released October 11, 1968, regarding a similar situation, the BSA declared that it never sold mailing lists to anyone, Scout's honor, especially to pornographers.) The reality was that Marvin bought a mailing list of 30,000 prospects at a dollar a name. But outsource mailing lists were notorious for inaccuracy, containing names of people who might possibly be interested in receiving sexual material but were not positively so, a risky roll of the dice Marvin could live with. Apparently, the printer added a few unlikely prospects of his own to Marvin's list as vengeful sport. As a result, Marvin's advertisements wound up in the hands of people who hadn't asked for them.

And so, shortly thereafter, Marvin experienced this: He walks out of his house at seven o'clock in the morning and is immediately arrested by the Covina police. He's booked, arraigned, and bailed out. As he walks down the courtroom steps, he's arrested by a new set of cops, schlepped to another jurisdiction, booked, and bailed. In a coordinated effort by authorities, Marvin goes through this procedure a total of *six* times in six different jurisdictions during the day before finally getting home at 11:30 at night, unkempt, exhausted, and starving. Just in time to enjoy his fortieth birthday surprise party before the clock strikes twelve.

The state prosecutor dropped the charges on all but the City of Orange offense—a complaint by the mother-and-son owners of a restaurant in Newport Beach that had received five (!) of Marvin's mail-order ads for books such as *Intercourse, Man-Woman, Sex-Orgies Illustrated*, and *An Illustrated History of Pornography.* Mom opened them. She definitely was not interested, nor was son amused. Marvin was convicted. He appealed.

By this time in his life, Marvin had been arrested for theft and sent by authorities to foster care; he'd been incarcerated on embezzlement and arson/insurance fraud raps; since issuing *My Secret Life* he'd been, as outlined by Carolyn See, "plagued by a special investigation from Washington, in which Miller's attorney was informed that Miller was to be the object of an extensive, extended investigation, primarily for the purpose of discovering whether Miller had ever con-

sidered evading his income tax.... [He] was the recipient of a 'special assessment' from the state of California to the tune of $180,000 in the form of a 'sales tax.' When Miller (naturally) didn't pay, the state seized one of his printing plants, and put up notices that there would be an auction for every stick of his printing equipment. Miller took it to court. The state of California settled for five thousand in back sales tax...but it took several months and $30,000 of Miller's money in legal fees."[30] The IRS put four men on Miller full-time for a year until they finally had to give him a tax clearance. "He owed the government $130," See reports.[31]

His telephone lines had been tapped. He was served with a barrage of subpoenas on a steady basis. "At any one time he might have representatives from the Treasury Department, the Secret Service, the Bureau of Internal Revenue, the Department of Justice as well as state and local police parked in front of his house.... [He] was once forced to close out his very substantial account in a local bank because his friends from the Treasury Department, the IRS, and the Department of Justice had a total of ten men constantly in the bank going over every check which Miller either drew or deposited."[32]

If you're in the pornography business, it's not paranoia when you think people are out to get you. It's reality. However, Marvin, with all that he'd endured and perhaps with a bit of the mental illness his mother possessed, now went over the top: He began to experience paranoid delusions. One day he frantically called his lawyer, Burton Marks. Cops had surrounded his place; he couldn't get to a window to count how many without letting them know that he knows they're out there. Marks sent an assistant to Miller's to report on the

As a result, Marvin's advertisements wound up in the hands of people who hadn't asked for them.

situation—a major bust might be brewing. Not a cop in sight. Nowhere. Marks has one of Marvin's secretaries scope out the grounds. Nicht, nada, nothing. Marvin calls Marks back. He "sees at least thirty cops outside his door in full uniform, brandishing their guns, and they're about to come in."[33]

Nineteen sixty-nine is turning out of be one hell of a year for Marv. It's not all bad, though. The year gives Marvin an opportunity to doff his dapper duds and drape himself in the flag and First Amendment.

SPECIAL FORWARD
The following pages have been inserted at the last minute, as this book goes to press. We believe

it is of prime urgency to bring to the immediate attention of members of THE COLLECTOR'S CLUB [Marvin's mail-order Dirty Book of the Month Club] and our other readers, the latest landmark decision of the United States Supreme Court, in the field of so-called pornographic publications and films.

On April 7, 1969, the U.S. Supreme Court reversed the conviction of a Georgia Citizen, who had been sentenced to jail for possession of "obscene" movie films in his home. The Supreme Court struck down the Georgia statute banning private possession of material classed as obscene, declaring it to be in clear violation of the First and Fourteenth Amendments. The Court's opinion, as delivered by Mr. Justice Marshall, stated: "...We agree that the mere private possession of obscene matter cannot constitutionally be made a crime..." and denied "the assertion that the State has the right to control the moral content of a person's thoughts." [Bravo!]

Inasmuch as Mr. Marvin Miller, President of COLLECTOR'S PUBLICATIONS, has been in the forefront of the winning battle to affirm and preserve the constitutional rights and freedom of citizens to read and/or view any material they chose, we have seen fit to print the full text of the Supreme Court's epochal decision in these pages.

A noble statement. And completely self-serving, disingenuous, ultimately grandiose. Marvin Miller never won a criminal case for any reason whatsoever, much less one involving First Amendment issues.[34] He couldn't have cared less about them unless they helped him in some way. Now, he elevated himself to defender of the faith. Miller had other reasons for reprinting *Stanley v. Georgia*. First, the reprinting saved money. Located prior to the text in many of his books at the time, its pagination dovetailed with the text's pre-existing collation; Marvin wouldn't have to spend money to reset the text's pagination before photographing it. Secondly, Miller had begun to get into film—initially for public exhibition but with an eye toward homes and hotel rooms via closed circuit and the emerging cable and videocassette platforms.

"He was one of the founding fathers of that part of the business," Miller adjutant and self-described "Asst. Everything" William Landes reports. "He was into *everything*. He was so far ahead of the industry it was *unbelievable*. He was building an entertainment conglomerate long before we thought of that kind of business structure."[35]

An unlikely prophet, Miller, in a vision of the future, foresaw the coming home-entertainment revolution and it was this:

No Postal Service to fuck with him, no distributors or exhibitors to rob him, no government to make his life miserable. He could deliver the smut legally into your home if you so desired.

At this point, Marvin was, for all intents and purposes, out of the porn-book business. He'd been legally enjoined from publishing dirty books. The business was being run by his wife, Jeanine (for legal reasons, the business had been in her name for some time, but the cops were well aware of who was in charge and mercifully left her alone), while Marvin pursued dreams of skin-flick moguldom and coped with his legal problems, which were consuming his fortune. Mrs. Miller didn't much care for the dirty-book business, and much to Marvin's chagrin, she allowed it to die on the vine. By 1970, Collector's Publications ceased to exist. But Marvin's story was far from over.

Deep within the womb of the Adult Education Institute of Covina, California—an organization that had absolutely nothing to do with "adult education" and everything to do with "adult" education—after passing through a series of hymenal security measures, you reached Marvin's inner sanctum where, on this day in late 1969, he was screening rushes from his newest venture, a skin flick called *Man and Wife* directed by Matt Cimber. Shot on a $32,000 budget, it ultimately grossed over $4.5 million,[36] though his son, Ron, and William Landes claim the figure to be considerably higher, near $30 million, in which case it was the highest-grossing skin flick prior to *Deep Throat*'s fabulous success. Because he partnered with Marvin in the closed-circuit/cable/videocassette venture, Vaudeo Inc.,[37] Cimber would eventually become embroiled in a major fight over money with Marvin.

Marvin converted his backyard barn into a film studio, and the crew was comprised of amateurs, including his son. According to Ron, the movie was shot in the barn while his mother and grandmother sat in the house; embarrassed, Marvin kept them completely ignorant of the sex circus close by. But now, the rushes. Marvin was transfixed. He was basically shy about sex, somewhat abashed by what he was viewing, and, when all was said and done, was blushing: "That guy was really *hung*."[38]

Man and Wife was the first of many skin flicks that Marvin released. With Cimber directing, Marvin produced *Sex and Astrology*, *He and She*, and *Calliope*, a production that Cimber nearly broke the bank with, his visions of art overwhelming Marvin's acute sense of commerce. Other films in the Miller *oeuvre* include *Sex in the Comics*, *Black Is Beautiful*, and what would appear to be a porn–Marlin Perkins' *Wild Kingdom*/Margaret Mead study of serious anthropological exploration, *Africanus Sexualis*. Alas, it was merely *He and She* with a black couple *in flagrante*, and how! From 1969 through 1971, Marvin produced and/or packaged upwards of twenty-five stroke films. He'd moved his offices and studio to Hollywood Boulevard, to a complex behind the Adam & Eve porn theater, which he'd bought along with the Tiffany on the Sunset Strip.

Curiously, though, Marvin had little interest in sex.

"I don't think Marvin has had one thought about sex with anybody. He's too busy counting his money and bouncing his checks and stealing change from blind newsboys," a business associate remembers.[39] And it's true. In contrast to many of his peers, Marvin wasn't a player. He was in the dirty-book business, the skin-flick business in LA during the late 1960s ferchristsake, and he didn't care about sex. A porn actress acquainted with him stated: "I wouldn't know much about him—he doesn't like girls."[40]

Marvin wasn't gay; he just didn't get hot for anything that didn't have the Secretary of the Treasury's signature on it in black on green. He was, by all accounts, a very handsome man, but a swinger he wasn't. He was, in fact, a homebody, and, given his closeness with a dollar, it should come as no surprise that he was not extravagant. Evenings were spent, for the most part, with his wife, daughter, and two sons. He enjoyed a fine meal at a fine restaurant, which, considering his childhood, is no shock. He didn't drink. While a dapper dresser, he didn't go in for sartorial splendor, silk boxer shorts aside. His home was relatively modest; no mansions for him. The backyard barn had been converted into office space; later, his film set. Milton Van Sickle, an editor who has worked for almost all the major porn publishers, was wrong: Marvin didn't work out of a phone booth.[41] But there was a pay phone in the offices of the Adult Education Institute. Visiting and need to make a quick local call? On your dime.

It's late 1970, early 1971. Art Kunkin's dreams of a publishing empire are evaporating before his very eyes. In addition to Marvin's printing plant, he'd bought two new, very expensive Mergenthaler printing presses and shipped them to Los Angeles from their home in England. But he had no place to put them. Idle printing presses with huge debt. The IRS on his ass for back taxes. The *Los Angeles Free Press* was once again about to go under. And Art was *persona non grata* with every bank in town. Time to visit his benefactor and friend.

Marvin generously offered to cosign a loan for Art, up to $150,000, the *Free Press* as collateral. Art told Marvin he needed only $60,000. So, signing a note pledging the paper, Art got his $60,000. Two months later, he ran out of money.

Marvin had asserted that "some people don't know how to screw," but Marvin knew how to screw royally. He foreclosed on the *Free Press*.

Within two months of leaving Milt Luros' American Art Agency, Brian Kirby went to work for Kunkin as associate editor—later managing editor—of the *Los Angeles Free Press*. Within a year, he and every employee walked out on the same day. They'd just learned that Marvin Miller was the new owner of the *Freep*, and though Kunkin would hold the title executive editor, they wanted nothing to do with Marvin, a man Kirby knew all too well from the porn trade.[42] The incident, however, earned Marvin another footnote in American cultural history: He made the cover of *Rolling Stone*. "Does Porn Call the Shots at *L.A. Free Press*?" read the headline of the September 16, 1971 issue. By now, Marvin had set up another corporation to umbrella his activities. Printed on the *Freep*'s masthead without a trace of irony (readers are encouraged to provide their own) was the new publisher's name: "Therapy Productions."

Kunkin doesn't blame Marvin at all for foreclosing on the *Freep*; they, in fact, remained friends. So, when Marvin decided to enter publishing again—under his Therapy Productions imprint—he hired Art to write the text for a couple of magazine-format books in his new series on the Mob, particularly a title on the Mob's influence in politics. Kunkin was concerned. "Won't that bother the boys in Chicago?" he asked. Marvin told Art to step outside so he could make a call. Five minutes later, he asked Art back in. "It's okay," Marvin reported. "No problem." While this was clearly showmanship (though because of his background on the streets of Chicago, he had many friends whose career paths strayed from the straight and narrow), it does raise the question of whether Miller was Mobbed up.

The answer appears to be a qualified no: Marvin—as with virtually every other pornster of the era—by need had to deal with Mob-affiliated individuals. Ron Miller recalls an incident when two Mobsters from San Diego paid Marvin a shake-

Man and Wife was the first of many skin flicks that Marvin released.

down visit. Marvin calmly picked up the phone, explained the situation to his listener, hung up, and confronted the two Mafiosi, who, upon hearing the name Robert DiBernardo, blanched, apologized, begged Marvin's pardon, and beat a hasty retreat. Di B made a fortune distributing Marvin's books and most certainly didn't want anyone to threaten the supply of golden eggs from his goose; protecting him just made good business sense, nothing shady about it. This was an example of what has often been described to me as a "courtesy connection." Had Marvin truly been in deep with organized crime, he would have solicited funds from his "courtesy connections" to fuel his rapid expansion, and he might well have succeeded in his grandiose plans, as Reuben Sturman did. Marvin was a rogue maverick; there's no way he would have jeopardized his independence in that manner.

Marvin's dream of skin-flick moguldom via production and exhibition through theaters, cable, closed circuit, and videocassette played a major role in his undoing. He suffered from classic entrepreneur-osis, a condition all too common to visionaries with gold in their eyes. He expanded far too rapidly in too many directions without adequate cash flow to finance his dreams. A primary reason seems to be that porn-theater owners were/are experts par excellence at underreporting box-office receipts, working every con imaginable to short-

Marvin's dream of skin-flick moguldom via production and exhibition through theaters, cable, closed circuit, and videocassette played a major role in his undoing.

change producers. Marvin worked every angle there was in negotiating terms directly with theater owners. With *Man and Wife*, he "four-walled"—bought out theaters for a fixed time at a flat fee, then exhibited and kept all the proceeds. But with *Man and Wife*'s success, distributors begged for his movies. And then robbed him; the theater owners were certainly robbing them. He was, according to William Landes, owed money from everyone, was selling off this to pay for that, constantly juggling his various bank accounts to make payroll, was seriously overextended; too big, too fast, and way too far ahead of the marketplace.

Ultimately, Marvin's dream collapsed because he didn't grasp what 1960s porn magnate Milton Luros and 1970s-1980s porn emperor Reuben Sturman so keenly understood in establishing their empires' own distribution infrastructures and becoming fabulously wealthy: Distribution is everything. You stand in the middle of the money river and let it flow into your pockets. But distribution is a dull, plodding business; a restless spirit like Marvin would have gone nuts.

Another reason Marvin's hopes evaporated was most certainly because his legal fees were astronomical. Since his bust in 1969, he had been supporting Burton Marks and an army of legal eagles full-time while the case wended its way through the appellate process.

❧

On June 21, 1973, Marvin Miller made the front pages—or,

at least the editorial pages—of every newspaper in the country. He finally had his day in court. The Supreme Court. And for the first time in its history, the Justices were in unanimous agreement on a legal issue, judging it impossible to determine a national standard of obscenity. Their agreement ended there.

After four years in the appellate process, *Miller v. California* had come to that august body for final adjudication. Marvin had been charged with violating California Penal Code ss311.2(a): "Every person who knowingly: sends or causes to be sent, or brings or causes to be brought, into this State for sale or distribution, or in this State prepares, publishes, prints, exhibits, distributes or offers to distribute, or has in his possession with intent to distribute or to exhibit or offer to distribute, any obscene matter is guilty of a misdemeanor."

The trigger had been the five brochures featuring explicit ads for Miller books sent to the mom-and-son restaurant in Newport Beach.

Carolyn See was present in Washington for the argument phase. She reported that Associate Justice Rehnquist asked questions of each attorney, then asked to view the obscene material in question. He fell quiet. Preternaturally so. "He seemed to be hypnotized by smut," she recently recalled to me. Thank goodness for long robes and high benches! It's all rather comical, and it was only because it's forbidden that laughter didn't spontaneously burst forth in that historic chamber. The Justices themselves had a difficult time restraining themselves during the arguments. (There were actually three obscenity cases decided by the Court, collectively known as *Miller*.)

See wrote: "The case was *The Entire Respectable U.S.A. Against Twelve Films*. One of the learned justices had opened the brief and read the name of the first of the films: '____ing and ____ing.' The learned justice broke out in a delighted grin and nudged his colleague who rolled his eyes, who nudged his colleague who glowered and flushed, and so on! The brief zipped down the bench and back; the justice's chairs began to rock—and stopped. But with a couple of exceptions, the faces of these wonderful old men looked more clear, more merry and bright, if you will, than they had the minute before."[43]

High comedy had, in fact, been an everyday occurrence during obscenity trials throughout the era. See, who attended many such trials during that time as an observer and witness for the defense, recalled: "[B]y late afternoon the judge, defendant, witnesses, attorneys and jury find themselves increasingly possessed by vagrant gales of laughter as the most harmless statements in the language are discovered to spring directly from humanity's horizontal positions; the room turns golden and time is redeemed while strangers laugh together at the absurdity of it all—the defendant is found guilty, but that's later."[44]

Famed Chicago First Amendment and civil liberties attorney Elmer Gertz recalled that when the *National Tattler*—a tabloid owned by Joe Sturman (brother of Reuben)—was tried on obscenity charges in the mid-1960s, he manipulated a key witness—an elderly woman—into admitting that she thought Jayne Mansfield's breasts were obscene. The courtroom erupted in peals of laughter. This scene brought down the house, and later, brought acquittal.[45]

But Marvin was not so lucky. No laughter, no acquittal. Of course Marvin lost.

Marvin had appealed the California court's conviction on the grounds that the brochure passed the Supreme Court's 1966 *Memoirs* test according to the national standard set therein but that the state had its own standard, in violation of *Memoirs*. "This case," as the Court stated in its 5-4 opinion, "was tried on the theory that the California obscenity statute sought to incorporate the triparate test of *Memoirs*. This, a 'national standard' of First Amendment protection enumerated by a plurality of this Court, was correctly regarded at the time of trial as limiting state prosecution under the controlling case law. The jury, however, was explicitly instructed that, in determining whether the 'dominant theme of the material as a whole…appeals to the 'prurient interest' and in determining whether the material 'goes substantially beyond customary limits of candor and affronts contemporary community standards of decency,' it was to apply contemporary community standards of the state of California." The Court rejected Marvin's assertion that a national standard could not be determined by conflation of a local standard.

Basically, the Court gave up trying to determine a national standard of obscenity despite the fact that the Comstock laws regarding the mailing of "obscene" material across state lines dictated the necessity for such. The Burger Court rejected the Warren Court's prior interpretation of *Roth* in its 1966 *Memoirs* case, which they asserted substituted a higher threshold for obscenity than the spirit of their *Roth* decision allowed. In *Memoirs* sexually-oriented material had to be "utterly without redeeming social value" for it to be proscribed. The Court correctly determined that that formulation made it impossible to prosecute; you can't prove a negative. But rather than just throw in the towel and admit that obscenity laws were unworkably vague and thus unconstitutional, Chief Justice Burger, speaking for the majority, rejected his colleagues' dissent that obscenity laws should be abolished secondary to their vagueness, and asserted that the federal government had a continuing interest "to maintain a decent society."

Considering that the Court was now stacked with Justices considered to be strict constructionists of the Constitution, this was odd indeed: A mandate to "maintain a decent society" is nowhere to be found in the Constitution in enumerating the functions of each of the three branches of government. This is aside from the fact that the concept of "decent" is wholly subjective. Since the Court's 1957 *Roth* decision, "contemporary community standards" meant that the nation as a whole devolved to every local jurisdiction in the country, not just to fifty state jurisdictions but potentially to every burg, hamlet, and village in the US.

In its new formulation, "The guidelines the Court composes to regulate obscene speech must be: (a) whether the average person applying contemporary community standards would find that the work, taken as a whole, appeals to the prurient interest, (b) whether the work depicts or describes, in a patently offensive way, sexual conduct specifically defined by the applicable state law, (c) whether the work, taken as a whole, lacks serious literary, artistic, political, or scientific value."

In his perceptive dissent, Justice Brennan strongly observed that the "new" test was as vague as the "old" test, since both tests relied on subjective concepts: prurient interest, patent offensiveness, serious literary value, and so on. Further, he stated, the majority of the Court "makes no argument that the reformulation will provide fairer notice to booksellers, theatre owners, and the reading and viewing public" that they may be selling, exhibiting, reading or viewing something illegal. Brennan's point is that there is a violation of an underlying constitutional protection, "that no man shall be held criminally responsible for conduct which he could not reasonably understand to be proscribed."

Justice William O. Douglas also dissented from the majority, asserting that the obscenity laws were unconstitutional due to their ambiguity, and that the idea that an individual could go to jail for violating a standard difficult to understand, interpret, and apply "is a monstrous thing to do in a nation dedicated to fair trials and due process."

The Court's decision received virtually universal condemnation in newspapers across the country. "Back to the Dark Ages With the Supreme Court," declared the New York *Daily News*.[46] The *Washington Post*, in an editorial, stated that the *Miller* decisions "have the double failure of loosening the check on zealous censors, while giving them different but no better, guidelines as to what is obscene."[47]

Within two weeks of the *Miller* decision, the Supreme Court of Georgia banned Mike Nichols' film *Carnal Knowledge* under the new Miller test. Reviewing the case a year later, the Supreme Court fortunately instructed the State of Georgia that they'd gone too far: *Carnal Knowledge* was legal.[48]

The good news for Marvin Miller, that paragon of publishing honor and honesty—Carolyn See reports that when she asked Marvin if there was an honest man in the dirty-book business, Marvin "stops, looks incredulous. He smiles. His tiny silver goatee dances on his chin. He looks like Dashiell Hammett's description of Sam Spade—a pleasant, blond Satan. 'An honest man? Why, Carolyn! Why me, *me*, of course.' His son, who is listening, falls over laughing"[49]—is that his name is attached to a pivotal Supreme Court decision of the twentieth century. The bad news? Marvin Miller went to jail, sentenced to five years, eight months (for a misdemeanor!).

The *Miller* decision remains the law of the land, and obscenity, as the Court has reiterated time and time again, continues to lack protection under the First Amendment.

Fortunately, his lawyer, Burton Marks, sprang him after eight months.

In retrospect, June 21, 1973, the date of the *Miller* decision, was significant as a corollary to the Court's regressive stand on obscenity. On that date, the 1960s—a spirit more than a decade—officially came to a close.

The high hopes of those who expected the porn industry to wither and die under local assault were ultimately dashed as local prosecutors found it just as difficult as state and federal authorities to successfully try obscenity cases. That damned, pesky Constitution kept getting in the way, and authorities, always three steps behind the public on social issues, were surprised to learn that to local juries, with Vietnam, Civil Rights, Watergate beginning to metastasize, increasing violence, drugs, economic inflation—the whole laundry list of American social and cultural concerns of the period—this obscenity thing was small potatoes, a mere wrinkle in the fabric of American life. As a culture, we had become inured to literary and visual depictions of sex. Sex had become an overtly accepted part of life.

The *Miller* decision remains the law of the land, and obscenity, as the Court has reiterated time and time again, continues to lack protection under the First Amendment; it remains illegal. The Court's devolution of any kind of federal rule down to local community standards, however, created a giant loophole through which Internet porn sped. The Internet makes local communities irrelevant.

As legal scholar Jeffery Rosen observed, "The exploding demand for Internet porn and the impossibility of restricting it to any geographical area makes the Supreme Court's traditional tests for defining obscenity [the *Miller* formula] incoherent."[50]

⚗

Sometime later, after his release from jail, Marvin decided to become a philanthropist. He got involved with the American Diabetes Association and, in a bid to raise money for the group, hatched a whacked-out free house giveaway sweepstakes scheme that got him into trouble once again. Convicted of securities fraud, grand theft, and other violations, he spent three years in prison. Poor guy, he never met a corner he didn't cut. He died in 1992, before realizing the enduring legacy of his legal screw-up in 1969: The Man Who Made America Safe For Internet Porn.

Endnotes
1. See, Carolyn. *Blue Money*. New York: David McKay, 1974: 19. I am deeply indebted to Ms. See for allowing me generous use of material from this book. **2.** Ibid. **3.** Ibid.: 21. **4.** Talese, Gay. *Thy Neighbor's Wife*. Doubleday, 1980: 408. **5.** Ibid. **6.** Op. cit., See: 21. **7.** Ibid. **8.** "The Millionaire Pornographers." *Adam* magazine, Special Report 12, Feb 1977: 58. **9.** Phone interview with the author, 29 Apr 2005. **10.** Ms. See is more polite. She reports in *Blue Money* (p 23) that Miller's printer "tattled" to Grove Press. **11.** Interview with the author, Aug 2000. **12.** Email to the author, 15 May 2001. **13.** Op. cit., See: 24. **14.** In the author's possession is a paperback titled *Moral Decay* by T.S. Palmer with Edw. S. Sullivan's autograph note: "Printed for Sturman." **15.** According to his son, Ron. **16.** I am thankful to publisher Richard N. Sherwin for this insight. **17.** Collier, Peter. "Pirates of Pornography." *Ramparts*, 10 Aug 1968. **18.** According to son, Ron. **19.** Interview with the author, Sept 2000. **20.** Interview with William Landes, 9 May 2005. **21.** Op. cit., Collier. **22.** Op. cit., See: 24. **23.** Ibid.: 22. **24.** Op. cit., Collier. **25.** Ibid. **26.** Ibid. **27.** Ibid. **28.** Ibid. **29.** Mr. Kunkin's recollection of this incident differs slightly from Ms. See's account in *Blue Money*. **30.** Op. cit., See: 14. **31.** Ibid.: 15. **32.** Ibid. **33.** Ibid.: 13. **34.** Grove Press' suit against Marvin re: *My Secret Life* was a civil action. **35.** Interview with the author, 9 May 2005. **36.** Op. cit., Collier. **37.** An ill-fated venture: right idea, wrong man. **38.** Op. cit., See: 17. **39.** Ibid.: 18. This sounds suspiciously like 1960s porn magnate Milton Luros, but Ms. See cannot recall her source for this quote. **40.** Ibid. **41.** Interview with the author, 11 Oct 2000. **42.** Interview with the author, 16 June 2000. **43.** See, Carolyn. "My Daddy the Pornographer." *Esquire*, Aug 1972. **44.** Ibid. **45.** Elmer Gertz was the author's great-uncle; over many years prior to his death he shared as many of his experiences working obscenity defense cases as he could recall. **46.** New York *Daily News*, 13 July 1973. **47.** *Washington Post*, 24 June 1973. **48.** *Jenkins v. Georgia*, 418 U.S. 152 91974. **49.** Op. cit., See, Blue Money: 25. **50.** Rosen, J. "The End of Obscenity." *The New Atlantis: A Journal of Technology and Society*, No. 6 (Summer 2004)

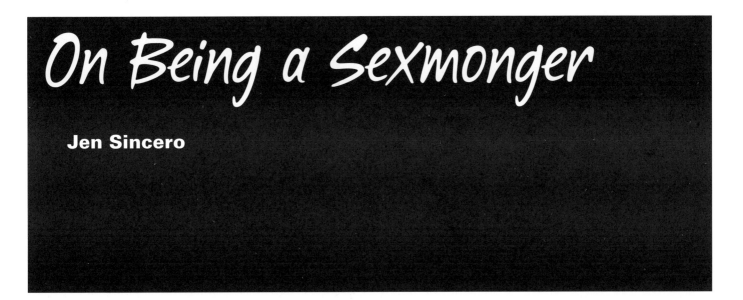

On Being a Sexmonger

Jen Sincero

Here's a special moment: I'm sitting at the dinner table next to an older, respectable lady in her seventies, whom I've hardly spoken to other than to tell her I like her cardigan. We're at a writer's retreat in the middle of nowhere, Wyoming, where I'm working on a new book and eagerly awaiting the release of my last one, *The Straight Girl's Guide to Sleeping With Chicks*. As we're about to leave the table, one of the staff walks in with the mailbag and hands me a bulging, padded envelope from Simon and Schuster. My book! I haven't seen it in its final, published form yet, and so it's with much excitement that I tear into the bag and behold my fabulous new work *d'art*. My neighbor is all aflutter (she really was a very cute lady) and asks if she might have a look, dear, as she pulls it out of my hands and opens it right to page 178.

Page 178 is the one that gets my vote for the raunchiest page in a substantially raunchy book. It boasts a large photo of a naked, Barbie-type doll bent over a bed, spread-legged and ready, while another doll pulls her hair and services her up the ass with a huge dolly strap-on. My new friend lets out a gasp, claps the book closed, and mumbles a congratulations as she shuffles out of the room, never to look me in the eye again.

It's times like these that I wish I was my married-with-children sister, a maker of muffins, or perhaps an elementary-school nurse. It's not that I'm not proud of my book, or that I've become un-enamored with the path I've chosen—it's just that every once in a while, lugging the old freak flag around gets a bit overwhelming. And although I was pretty much wrapped in the flag at birth, this whole sex thing has me flying it at full mast all the time. Because unlike my drunken bouts with nudity on-stage with my punk band in the 1990s, or that time I fucked a guy dressed like Pipi Longstocking on a trampoline at Burning Man, being a sex author/educator/pest is a much larger part of my identity. For one thing, you don't have to show up at CBGB or the Nevada desert to catch my act—you can go to your local bookstore or get it online. For another, it's now my job, meaning it can be brought up anytime, anywhere, and people, especially nosy grandparents, tend to need details. Then there's the severe tunnel vision people develop when the topic of sex enters the picture, and, just like all the lesbians and queers who are seen as homos first, people second, my sexpertise precedes me.

This all took a bit of getting used to, especially since I didn't set out to be a sex person—it just sort of happened, like most of the other sex-related events in my life. The book came about because I'd had a couple of experiences with women, found little out there to answer my questions, and decided I should write about it myself. With that began the research and the discussions, and soon I'd made the joyful realization that I'd stumbled upon something that gave me a big, fat boner. Sex is large, Marge, and it's relevant to everyone who's survived puberty. It's political, psychological, controversial, emotional,

Did my dad read the part in my book where I talk about how much I love buttsex?

and physical—it's such an important topic that, especially at this alarmingly conservative time in American history, I'm thrilled and honored to join the ranks on the front lines.

I took to it like a pig to mud but quickly discovered that while it's totally worth it, it can also be totally weird. Do all my friends think I want to fuck them now? Did my dad read the part in my book where I talk about how much I love buttsex? Things were definitely going to change, some for the better and some for the worse. And I figured I could handle most of it, but there were a couple things that were going to be kind of difficult. Like all the icky male attention I would now be inviting into my life. I knew that there would be a select portion of the male population who would suddenly feel entitled to discuss my body parts or tell me what their thick, hard cocks had done for fun during the past week. As women we have to deal with some version of this all the time (until we get older, of course, then we often have to deal with no male attention!). But being a sexually vocal woman would take it to a level that made walking by a construction site in a miniskirt seem like a skip through the park. Because now I'd be opening myself up to engage in discussions, not just whistles and howls, which would make it more interesting, but also more personal and invasive.

The DJ must have seen the look on my face because she slid over a note that read, "This is Texas."

So one of the first things I did when I got my book deal was disconnect my phone and get an unlisted number to keep the lechers at bay. The next thing I did was accidentally call one of them up to chat. It was a guy from one of those glossy men's magazines who'd sent me an email about how well my girl-on-girl tome would go over with his readership. It was to be my very first interview about my book, and I was feeling kind of stuck up and excited about it. This was a big-deal magazine. I was a big-deal sex expert.

We said our hellos and he launched right into the interview, starting out with three insightful questions about my book: "So, you hot? You got big tits? How old are you?" In the old days, I would have responded by utilizing one or all of the following words: *asshole, dumbass, fucker, shitfucker, motherfucking prick*. But I was too surprised to speak. Plus, I wanted him to do the interview, so I heard him out as he went on to explain his idea for the story. He suggested we meet, throw back a few drinks, then hit the titty bars. I'd follow the suggestions in my guidebook to pick up a couple of strippers and take them home to fuck them while he watched. He explained that he was used to writing stuff like this, that he considered himself somewhat of an authority on female sexuality, actually. As a matter of fact, he was at that very moment writing a piece about all the porno chicks he'd banged and how he could tell which ones were faking it and which ones weren't. Somewhere along the way I lost interest in the interview and told him, among other things, that I found him and his ideas offensive, to which he replied, "You want in on the sex game, honey? You better get used to it."

But I'm pleased to report that I haven't had to get used to it. Not in the capacity I thought I would, anyway. Much to my surprise, those with intent to humiliate and degrade have been few and far between, save for the occasional email, a few sweaty-palmed freaks at my readings, and a run-in with Howard Stern. I also made the earth-shattering discovery that all men who have the audacity to speak to me inappropriately aren't necessarily being malicious—some of them are just a little clueless. The more I thought about it, the more I realized that of course they are! All these women are out there being sassy and outspoken and hoochie-mama-ing up a sex storm of conversation, then when some poor guy comes loping up, all excited to play along, he gets smacked in the snout. Not really fair, I'd say. It's certainly not the same response we'd give a woman should she choose to chime in.

But then there are few fair things about the male/female power structure, and I don't blame the angry ladies, either. Because there's an unfortunate connection between sex and violence that women tend to be on the receiving end of (I don't know about you, but it's always in the back of my mind when I go hiking alone). I'm constantly amazed by things like the porn industry's focus on degrading all us stupid, cumsucking bitches as we get rammed up the ass by monster cocks. Because porn is about making money, so obviously this is what a lot of guys want to see. I'd be lying if I said this didn't kind of bum me out. And I'd also be lying if I didn't say I love rough sex and heartily salute those with the courage to let their filthiest fantasies run wild. So where do we draw the line? Is all fantasy okay, no matter how violent it is? Fuck if I know! All I know is I need to feel like a guy is somewhat sensitive to the female plight before I can get potty-mouthed with him. Or that he's at least game to understand it. Otherwise, his overtly sexual comments can feel like a slap in the face.

Another thing that's been a real trip has been dealing with all the horrified God-lovers and self-righteous conservative folks. Since I tend to live in cities and other liberal-type places, I sometimes forget that the country is crawling with fatheads. But now that the book is out in the world, and I'm out in the world promoting it, I've had the bizarre experience of interacting with these people. And the fact that we're all being brought together on the topic of raunchy girl-on-girl sex never ceases to amuse me.

One of my first radio appearances was on an afternoon talk show in Dallas. Some woman called in demanding to know, "What if my twelve-year-old daughter goes into a bookstore, sees your book, and becomes a lesbian?" The DJ must have seen the look on my face because she slid over a note that read, "This is Texas." I'd heard a lot of good ones, but never that you could catch homosexuality, like a cold. From an inanimate object, no less. No amount of explaining would calm her down, so we eventually hung up on her, but it was an alarming reminder of just how stupid people can be.

Another humdinger was an email I got from some guy in Nebraska the day after I appeared on the Howard Stern show:

I heard you on Howard Stern the other morning. The book you wrote and your lesbian experiences sounded ridiculous and terrible to me.

Your last name is interesting. Some people may see "sincere" but all I see is the "sin" part.

I pray for you that one day you will see that God never meant for girls to sleep with girls. He gave us bodies to respect and cherish and you are doing neither when you use your body that way. I hope some day you find the shame in what you've done. Imagine, writing a book about it! That's horrible.

True, we are all sinners. But the point is to ask forgiveness for our sins and ATTEMPT to live a wholesome life. Your life will be nothing but pain and heartache if you keep living this way.

The thing that really struck me about this guy was that he listened to Howard Stern—talk about pain and heartache! He must love being upset all the time. Which is one of the most notable differences, I quickly realized, between us and them. They just love to crash our parties, while we can't be bothered with theirs. We're not spending our precious time hanging around fundamentalist churches or calling into Christian talk shows to explain how liberating a really good blowjob can be. Not only would it put me in a deep sleep, but it's terribly rude.

I managed a few emails back and forth with Mr. Nebraska and learned that he was listening to Howard because he believed Howard could be saved (and because Howard has hot, big-tittied women on his show, I suspect). He prayed for Howard daily, and now me too apparently, and was unreceptive when I suggested he instead pray for himself to be less judgmental.

All this obviously goes way beyond bad manners and kinky, voyeuristic tendencies, to much more serious things like hate crimes and laws that strip us of our rights. But as I try to do my part in fighting the powers that be, I take some solace in the knowledge that people are their own worst enemies. The "moral majority" will no doubt contract a slew of stress-related diseases by constantly worrying about who is sticking their what into whose hole, and the more we shamelessly talk about it, the more powerful we are. I mean, they're so easily distracted by it. Isn't there some way we could use that to our advantage—"Look, George! Buttsex!"—and then take back the country?

Regardless, I think it's fascinating. And terrifying. And I know part of the reason I have the *cojones* to be so loud-mouthed about it is because my family, and my mother in particular, has always been there cheering me on. Although I have to say, this last stunt really put us all to the test. Because no matter how wild I'd been in my past, this was the first time I'd played the sex card. I knew we'd all somehow rise to the occasion, but I suspected we'd probably do it with a lot of fumbling around. Because not only were we WASPs, which meant we never, ever, discussed the S word, but we were family, and up until now, the only proper response to the thought of, say, Mom and Dad doing it, was to gouge our eyes out. I couldn't imagine telling them all about my new gay sex book!

In the beginning we were all quite happy to just breeze on by the details, but the more excited I got about my project, the more I not only wanted to tell them about it, the more I wanted to involve them in it, too. I wanted to be open with them, to free us all from guilt and repression, to see each other as whole, sexual beings who could freely talk about sex without incestuous shame standing in our way!

Mom was unamused. We were in the car on the way to visit my sister, Jill, and I was blathering on about all the fascinating research I was doing and all the inspiring women I was interviewing. "Don't think for a second you're getting an interview out of me for that thing," she announced, as I put new batteries in my tape recorder, seconds away from asking her for

She was obviously drawing the line at telling me how she felt about eating another woman's pussy.

one. "I wasn't about to ask you!" I shot back. My mom is a sweet potato. She supported me through the punk years, even brought friends to a couple of my shows, but she was obviously drawing the line at telling me how she felt about eating another woman's pussy.

My sister, on the other hand, was all over me like a baby chimp. "I've always wanted to try being with a chick!" she said, demanding to know everything. She dragged me off to her son's room so we could be alone, and I got my first familial interview. Here's how it went:

Me: Have you ever been with a woman?

Jill: No.

Me: Why not?

Jill: I don't know. I wasn't ballsy enough, most likely.

Me: Would you have had the balls to make the first move if the situation presented itself?

Jill: Probably. I've done it with men before.

At this point our mother walks into the room. Jill and I stop talking and look at Mom while she hovers near the doorway and fiddles with something on the table.

A year later Mom was manning the merch table at my New York reading, selling smut, lube, and panties.

Me: Can we help you?

Mom: What are you guys doing?

Me: I'm interviewing Jill for my book.

Mom: Oh.

And she just stands there!

Me: Mom.

Mom: What?

Me: Get out!

And she leaves. Jill and I look at each other with raised eyebrows.

Me: Okay, so what about the experience intrigues you?

Jill: Probably that it's taboo. And that women are sexy.

Me: Does the thought of eating pussy freak you out?

Jill: Mom's back.

I look over to the door and there she is, fiddling with whatever the hell she was fiddling with on the table before.

Me: Mom, what do you want?

Mom: Nothing.

Me: Mom, would you get out? We're trying to have an interview!

Mom: I will! I just want to know what this is.

She holds up a little plastic box with a hole in it.

Me: It's a pencil sharpener. Now get lost.

But she just stands there holding the damn thing. I look at Jill, who shrugs. Then it occurs to me.

Me: You want me to interview you, too, don't you?

Our mother nods her head and puts down the pencil sharpener.

A year later Mom was manning the merch table at my New York reading, selling smut, lube, and panties, and no doubt doubling my sales by adding the kitsch value of "I bought lube from Jen's mom!"

Needless to say, I feel very blessed. After a while, even my 800-year-old Italian father came around to give me his weary nod of approval. "I don't know if you get older and wiser, or older and just more tired," he explained. I don't know either, but I really do believe that time is a magical thing and that people have the capability to eventually see the light. My worry is that we don't have the kind of time it would take for the likes of George W. Bush and Mr. Nebraska to grow brains between their ears, which means all us perverts and freaks have to be out there together, loud, proud, and unyielding. Even if it means we make a couple little old ladies blush in the process.

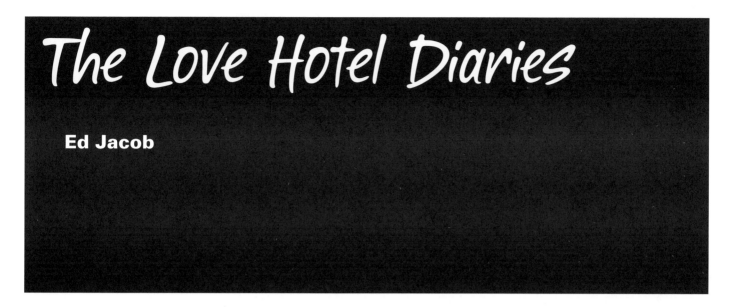

The Love Hotel Diaries

Ed Jacob

The love hotel is a uniquely Japanese institution, a sexual space for rent that is used by everyone from young teens in love to parents getting away from their children. Known for its over-the-top architecture and kinky theme rooms, the love hotel takes forms as diverse as Cinderella castles or luxury cruise ships, using everything from giant Santa Clauses to Statues of Liberty to attract customers. Inside, there are rooms filled from floor to ceiling with Mickey Mouse memorabilia, boxing ring beds, glow-in-the-dark jellyfish aquariums, and Marquis de Sade sex dungeons.

Walls in Japan can be paper-thin (literally); most Japanese parents sleep with their children until well into elementary school; the Japanese concept of *wa* (harmony) means that people go to great lengths to avoid upsetting their neighbors. Having an anonymous place for a romantic escape can be a godsend.

The first love hotels as such appeared in the early 1970s, but their ancestors date back to the age of the samurai. Originally places for assignations with prostitutes or settings for adulterous love affairs, they have evolved into an institution that's not just for sleazy sex.

The modern love hotel is a highly sophisticated leisure facility where couples go to spend quality time together, indulge in a little pampering, and enjoy each other's company in a love space with a romantic atmosphere and the latest in entertainment technology. The typical room is equipped with a widescreen TV, karaoke system, DVD player, video-game console, sex-toy vending machine, jet bath or Jacuzzi, and a wide variety of toiletries. On the pillow or headboard, there is always a condom.

Although the majority of guests are couples, newer love hotels offering afternoon tea, flower baths, and aromatherapy kits during the day are also becoming increasingly popular.

Japan's love hotels are found all over the nation and are said to receive more than two million visitors *a day*. According to calculations by University of Michigan professor Mark D. West, about half of all sex in Japan takes place in love hotels.[1] Think about that for a second. If this figure is accurate, you'd expect that half of the 1.65 million Japanese babies born every year are conceived in one.

With all the neon and strange rooms, it's easy to overlook one of the most fascinating aspects of love hotels—the *rakugaki chou* (literally, "graffiti notebooks"), guest books in each room in which customers write messages to each other or to the hotel's management. They contain jottings by teenagers sharing their first sexual experiences, messages from salarymen and office ladies having afternoon trysts, older married couples getting away from the kids for a romantic night, and other patrons.

About half of all sex in Japan takes place in love hotels.

Leafing through the pages, mostly pictures drawn by high-school or university girls with cute messages about how wonderful their boyfriends are, you will find some of the most interesting reading material you've ever seen. The following messages come from popular love hotels all over the country, found both in actual love hotel rooms and on love hotel-related websites.

Written by a female visiting the hotel with her boyfriend:

Today I came here with my boyfriend. He looks like Teru, the vocalist from the glam rock band Glay.

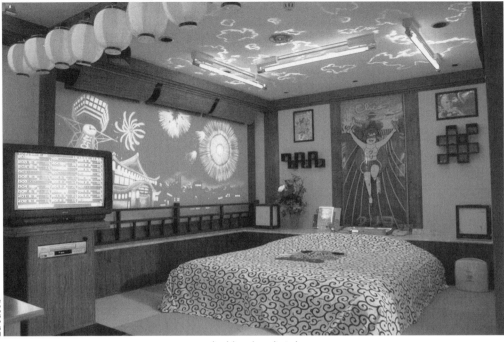
Inside a love hotel.

He was arrested by the police right in front of my eyes. Do you know how hard being arrested was on him? Do you know how terrible that must have made him feel? And do you know how hard it is on me to be alone? And how much harder it must be on him? Can you imagine how much more terrible his suffering must be, even than mine? No matter how hard you try to imagine it, you can never understand unless you go through it yourself.

But now I'm trying all the time to imagine just a little bit of what he must be feeling.

He's going to be away for at least five years. That's a long time. Everyone is telling me not to wait for him. Five years certainly is a long time, all right.

Maybe I won't be able to wait, but what other choice do I have?

Written by a woman staying in the hotel alone after a fight with her boyfriend:

Of all the hotels I've been to, I've never found one I liked so well as this. It's easy to check in, even for a woman alone. Of course, the rooms are clean, too. It's not so cheap, but the rooms are so nice that it's worth it.

I owe a lot to this hotel. I've come here with my boyfriend about twenty times, and when we have a fight, I come here alone to get out of our house. I come here a lot. And I'll probably come here again, too.

Written by an anonymous female:

My husband is still sound asleep. Yesterday we had wild, screaming sex for the first time in ages. We've been married for two and a half years. This is my first visit to a love hotel! Yay! Love hotel sex sure is good, isn't it? You can really go at it and get excited. Sometimes you have to be animals in bed. I love, love, love my husband! There are four hickeys on my neck, though, so I wonder if they'll be noticed at work. I was so excited yesterday that I didn't even notice them. I'm so embarrassed! You

He's sooo cool and handsome. And he's so good in bed, he makes me tingle all over. He's so lovely that I don't want to lose him to another woman. I'm going to marry him soon. I'll be the happiest person in the world.

This is something I can't tell anyone, but I'm dating three other guys. Tomorrow I have a date with another guy that I really like called M. We're really hot for each other. I'm really careful to keep him secret from my darling, though. I might be fooling around with your boyfriend too....

Written by a twenty-eight-year-old woman:

Dear Maria Theresia Hotel,

How have you been? We've been using your hotel a lot since we started dating. Thanks to you, we got married and have been blessed with a baby! Today is our first "Maria Theresia day" since we got married! We brought our ten-month-old baby to stay with us. Maria Theresia is a theme park paradise for a couple with a baby like us. We had a great time eating, drinking, watching a movie, and singing karaoke from our soft bed. Thank you so much. We'll be back!

Written by an anonymous female:

K's technique is so good that I came twenty times! And he's still horny! He actually made me faint!

Written by a female visiting a hotel alone:

have to come to a love hotel with your husband! Promise!

Written by a female office worker:

The truth is, I'm a really cute girl. Since I started working, I've had a lot of fans at my office. Even though I try to lead an ordinary life, I get hit on, given phone numbers, and ambushed all the time. Being popular with men isn't a problem, though. Right now my popularity is letting me play hooky from work to come here with H. He must be happy. Ha ha ha.

Written by a twenty-two-year-old female university student and addressed to her boyfriend:

I want to have a baby soon.

I've already chosen a name.

I'm happy that my first sexual experience was with you.

Thank you. It always *always* feels so good. You're so well hung!!

Written by an anonymous female who came to the hotel after being dumped by her boyfriend:

Fuck off and die!!! S***** H*****. You should never have come to Osaka, you fucking bumpkin! Hurry up and get back to the sticks of Kyushu where you came from. You're a spineless coward, but you're so arrogant you pick on people even more spineless than you so you can feel like a man.

Written by two female high-school students:

#1. We came from Nagoya, and we didn't have any money, so the two of us decided to stay in this love hotel.

Anyway, I wonder if there's any chance Koji will fall in love with me. But I'm sorry for lying to him and telling him that I'm twenty. Oh well, that's life. He looks like Issa from the pop band Da Pump. *Please* don't let him have a girlfriend. Please God, don't let him have a girlfriend.

There's only one week of summer holidays left so I'm going to have a lot of fun.

#2. While we were singing karaoke, the TV set broke. It's awful. I wish they had another packet of bubble-bath powder. The shower's water hurts because the water pressure is too high. The water seems salty somehow.

Written by a female:

Recently not one single good thing has happened to me. The sex is lousy, too. I don't even masturbate. Ahhhhh. I hate being a nineteen-year-old in this situation. I want to meet someone I can be happy with. All my friends have boyfriends. I've got to find someone!

Written by a lesbian office worker involved in several open relationships with other women:

Today one of my bosses asked me to sleep with him. What in the world am I going to do? He's married. I told him I liked him as a joke, but he took me seriously! What am I going to do???

Written by a twenty-two-year old Japanese university student studying in Beijing who came with a thirty-three-year-old man who was cheating on his wife:

You can be happy even if your partner is someone else's husband.

Written by a young woman involved in an enjo kousai *relationship with a married man.* Enjo kousai *literally means "compensated dating" and is a euphemism for prostitution. Women in these relationships often call their partner "Papa," a term similar to the English "sugar daddy":*

Papa is a prince, and I am a princess. This is the story of two people at the beginning of summer, who are fed up with their hectic daily lives.

"K's technique is so good that I came twenty times!"

Papa came to play at my castle. I cry every day because I want to escape from my castle. When Papa goes home, I want to escape with him. Papa seems annoyed with me.... This is the most thrilling, happiest time of my life!

Papa is a prince, and I am a princess. Papa's castle is smaller than mine and a little dirty, but it's more comfortable so I plan to stay there forever.

Written by an anonymous female:

My boyfriend has been eating me out since this morning again, excitedly licking my crotch like a thirsty cat lapping up milk. Lately my pussy hasn't been enough, so he's been licking my butt, too. He can hump for hours. But he also likes the clitoris. I want him to lick me till I come. Kinky sex is okay, too!

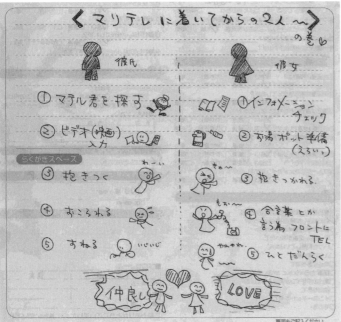

A page from a love hotel diary.

Ed Jacob

We didn't bring any ropes today, so he couldn't tie me up. They should sell rope in the vending machines!

Written by a twenty-one-year-old male university student:

It's been four months since we met.

We can't meet often because we're in a long-distance relationship.

But today we did a lot of hugging.

And a lot of kissing.

And of course we had sex.

Written by a woman in her early thirties staying at the popular Osaka hotel Maria Theresia with her husband:

In the spring of 1999 I was approaching the age of thirty, so my mother registered me at a marriage agency without my permission. By the fall of '99, they hadn't introduced me to anyone, so I got angry and went down to talk to them. Soon after that, I started dating a guy who had also been registered at the marriage agency by his parents without his permission. And I got lucky the first time.

I got seriously ill just before our marriage and some other things happened, but we got married in the spring of 2001. Now we're trying to make a baby (we started last year).

Today is our first visit to Maria Theresia, but we really love it. We want a "Made in Maria Theresia"

baby. We'll definitely be back again.

Written by a male:

I came here today with my friend's grandmother. It was the first time I had ever come to a hotel with a granny, so I don't know who to blame. I was doing the best I could, but when I looked at her, she seemed disgusted, and I lost my mojo. The most shocking thing was her underwear. Not only was she wearing giant panties that came up past her navel, but they had strawberries on them. Anyway. I want to get out of here. Damn! But the hotel was so expensive....

Written by a twenty-year-old woman and a thirty-nine-year-old married man working as a civil servant in Osaka who are involved in an enjo kousai *relationship:*

Her: I went out for a stroll with Papa. After we said goodbye, I got an email on my cellphone saying, "Don't go home." I didn't go home, which is why I'm here. We ate strawberry ice cream! Papa was embarrassed to eat it at a café, but you can hear him happily crunching and munching away on the wafers here. If we hadn't stayed together again, we wouldn't have been able to eat ice cream. Papa didn't want to go home either, so we stayed together a second day.

I'm so happy. We played pachinko [a combination pinball/slot machine], but only Papa hit the jackpot and I lost money, so I felt down. I'm not going to the pachinko parlor anymore. I love Papa. He's my favorite. But...but I want to meet him more often and do more fun things with him. Papa, thank you so much. You're always so nice to me. I'll always give my all to follow my dreams with you. Let's go to India soon, soon, soon. I wub you.

Him: Okay, it's my turn to write! Since last night Ayu has been all sparkly and lively. She seems like a different person. I think she's wonderful. Ayu has given me a dream, so I'm going to go all-out to make it come true, and, Ayu, you should go all-out to make your dreams come true, too! But, Ayu, your dreams and goals have gotten bigger, so I guess you'll be really busy....

Ayu, if you could spare me just a little of your time, it would be enough for me.

Because I love you so much!

I love you more than anyone.

You're the only one for me, Ayu!!

Together we will achieve the greatest happiness...

I weally, weally wub you!

Written by an anonymous female:

I just used a vibrator for the first time. It went *vroooom*. It felt really good. I've never been able to have orgasms, but I felt like I was about to have one (although I didn't quite come). I could get addicted to this thing really easily.

Written by an anonymous male:

My girlfriend is sleeping beside me right now. It's going to end tomorrow morning. We're going to break up. It's really hard. I'm sad.

The reason is me. I get angry easily, and I got angry just a little while ago. She seems sick of me. I don't want to break up. I really don't like breaking up. In my heart, I wanted to marry her. I really, really loved her. She was my reason for being. I'm going to be all alone, and I'm lazy at work. It's over. I don't have the will to do anything. But even if she breaks up with me, I will still love her, even if it's one-sided.

I want to see how much I can love the woman I loved more than anyone I've ever loved before. I'll do my best to show her.

I hope that the person who dates her next will be kind to her and make her happy.

Written by a female office worker:

That idiot keeps sticking his head up my skirt. What a pervert.

Tonight I drew a big nose around his nipples while he was sleeping. It made me really happy. Okay, time for a bath.

Written by an anonymous female to her lover:

A word to Papa. Your feet stink, you're stupid, you're ugly, you're nerdy, your eyebrows are too thick, your ears are strange, you have bad breath, you have a disgusting mole under your nose, your beard is too thick, your armpits smell, your legs

are short, and you're fat. That's you, but I like you. I know we fight a lot, but I hope we stay together, now and forever.

Written by a married couple:

We're married. It's been about two and a half years since our wedding. Even though we're a married couple, sometimes we want to get a taste of the feeling we had when we were dating, so we come to this love hotel. It's Saturday night, so we thought the hotel might be full. But our timing was good, and there was a vacant room. What luck! Even if you're married, you should still go to love hotels, everyone! But we haven't been able to have a baby. Anyway, until we have our baby, we're going to keep coming to this hotel. Be happy together, everyone!

Written by a female office worker:

"If I took some sleeping pills, I wonder if I'd die."

I broke up with a guy I'd been dating for a year and a half. Two days have passed, but I still can't believe it. Dying is all I've been able to think about since yesterday.... I just want to go somewhere else and be by myself. Today I played hooky from work and went for a drive. And I met my boyfriend by chance. He just ignored me. I went into a rage and broke into a sweat. When I'd calmed down, I came to this hotel. We often used to come here together. I want to die. I haven't eaten for more than two days. If I took some sleeping pills, I wonder if I'd die.... I just want to feel his arms around me one more time.

Written by an anonymous male:

My honey is so c-u-t-e. I love giving her hickeys. I look forward to the nighttime. Because I love having sex with my honey. I want to be with her forever. She's my treasure. She doesn't mind if I cover half her body in hickeys, but I overdid it a bit today, didn't I? I want to marry my honey soon.

Endnote
1. West, Mark D. "Japanese Love Hotels: Legal Change, Social Change, and Industry Change." University of Michigan, John M. Olin Center for Law & Economics, 22 Nov 2002. Working Paper #02-018.

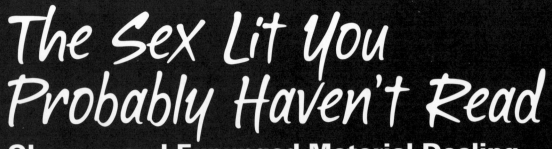

The Sex Lit You Probably Haven't Read
Obscure and Expunged Material Dealing With Everyone's Favorite Activity

Russ Kick

The Forgotten Sex Books of Charles Atlas

Charles Atlas has been transforming skinny runts, scarecrows, and bags of bones into muscle-bound he-men since 1924. "Hey! Quit Kicking sand in our faces!" shrieks weakling Joe (later rechristened "Mac") in one of the most famous ads of all time. After bulking up thanks to the Atlas program, he bitchslaps "that big bully." But becoming ripped wasn't the only change Joe's body was undergoing. He was becoming a "real man" in more ways than one, and Atlas wanted to teach him about that, too.

Thus it came to pass that in 1928 Charles Atlas published a series of ten books about sex. These odd publications—at 4x7 inches and 150 pages each, they are at the border between book and booklet—have been utterly forgotten. They are mentioned only in passing online, and the official Charles Atlas website doesn't acknowledge them at all (yep, the com-

He was becoming a "real man" in more ways than one, and Atlas wanted to teach him about that, too.

pany is still around, even though the only things Atlas himself is pushing up are daisies). I accidentally stumbled across these long-lost treasures when I searched the Advanced Book Exchange (the world's best used-books site) for sex-related books published before 1940. Running my bleary eyes across hundreds of titles and descriptions, up popped a complete boxed set of these beauties, decking me almost as hard as the newly buff Joe. What could Atlas possibly have told young men about sex in the 1920s?

Actually, Atlas didn't write these books; he didn't even pretend to via a ghostwriter. He published them under the im-

print "Roman Publishing Company"—evidently a nod to his homeland of Italy—with a notice that the copyright had been assigned to Charles Atlas, Ltd. The books were penned by Dr. David H. Keller, a psychiatrist who was then the assistant superintendent at a sanitarium in Bumfuck, Egypt (technically, Bolivar, Tennessee, with a current population of 5,800). Around the time these books came out, Keller was breaking into the world of pulp science fiction and supernatural tales. Hugo Gernsback would later praise him highly. If only Keller had stuck to writing stories and novels like "The Thing in the Cellar" and *The Human Termites*, a lot of boys might've been spared the guilt and psychic trauma of reading his largely sex-negative, crypto-Christian eugenics tirades.

The series kicks off with *Sex and Family Through the Ages*, in which Keller begins at the beginning, citing the appearance of one-celled organisms ("whether we believe it came from another planet or that it was created by a Divine Hand makes little difference as far as the fact of its existence is concerned"). Surprisingly, Keller believes in evolution and traces the history of sexual reproduction through groups of cells to sea life to cave people to the good, white, married Christian couples of 1928. Along the way, he gives us the money quote, the passage that informs the entire series of books:

> **The young people of the past chose their mates by a process of natural selection, just as the lions and humming-birds do today. Back of sexual desire, behind the thought of conquest and being conquered was the constant one of founding a home around a fireside and in that home there were to be children. In fact a home and marriage without children was intolerable and not to be**

thought of. **The very language shows this idea even at the present time, for a married woman is called a bride when she becomes pregnant and gives birth to a child and only then is she called a wife, and with the word wife is so often associated the word house that the common name for a married woman with children is house-wife which speaks plainly of the connection of home, wife and children.**

When this connection is lost sight of society is in danger.

Keller will hammer this point home again and again and again throughout the series. In the next volume, he wrote, even more forcefully and succinctly: "Happiness is the ultimate desire of every human being, and, no matter what happens to a man and a woman, they cannot be happy without children."

You must reproduce, understand? Breeding is not only your biological imperative but your duty to your race, God, and the State. That is what sex is all about. As a man, you are allowed to have fun while you're doing it (with your wife only), but only because that makes you more likely to get it on, which ups your chances of conceiving.

Keller believed that the federal government should give money in the form of pensions to young married couples, in order to encourage people to get hitched early in life. "The present social habits render early marriage difficult, and when a man marries at thirty or thirty-five he has spent the best years of his life in illicit sex relations, not only harming himself, but helping to degrade and ruin many young women, who, had they the chance, might have been happy mothers and contented housewives."

Yet pinning down Keller is not an easy task. He constantly chides male-supremacist attitudes, even while expressing various forms of them. When he speaks of the raw deal that prostitutes have gotten through the ages, he says: "It was simply the ageless habit men had of blaming the woman for everything bad and taking the credit for everything good." Then he turns right around and chillingly refers to the existence of mixed-race children as a "disgrace" and a "problem."

In volume two, *Sexual Diseases and Abnormalities of Adult Life*, Keller laments that one of the chief causes of unhappiness is ignorance regarding "sexual hygiene." Luckily, the good doctor is here to straighten us out! His info about syphilis and gonorrhea is pretty straightforward and unremarkable (and obviously very dated. Luckily, it no longer takes three to four years of intensive therapy to threat syph). He rails against

abortion, "one of the great disgraces of our modern civilization." Then we get to the long chapter on masturbation, and, boy, is it weird. To his great credit, Keller pooh-poohs the idea that whacking off leads to insanity or other mental problems. The deeply conflicted shrink calls the activity "abnormal," then immediately discusses its universality among humans and its appearance among other primates. But the best part is when he presents the most bizarre yet intriguing theory of jerking off that has ever assaulted my gray matter. He starts by noting that the masturbator is fantasizing about getting it on with another person (of the opposite sex, of course):

In other words, the actual physical body of one sex has intercourse with a mental body of another sex, but both of these sexes are contained within the same body. That body for the time being is bisexual. During that time, in its combination of a physical and spiritual duality, it is hermaphrodite. The ego of that person goes back to a previous stage of existence where the two sexes existed in one body and were able to reproduce without the aid of another animal.

Sure thing, Doc. So what's the problem with spanking it?

"It must never be forgotten that the urge in women is for reproduction and the act of sexual intercourse is only a means to that end."

Once the habit is established, a complete cure in adult life is doubtful. It is a poison as dangerous and insidious to the soul as opium is. It weakens the powers of resistance, destroys the best of the personality and leaves the habitue satisfied to remain in his world of dreams. In many ways there is a deadly resemblance between the two conditions of the opium habit and auto-eroticism.

One can imagine Atlas nodding his beefy head as he reads the manuscript he eagerly wants to publish.

Keller then tut-tuts those "unfortunates" who are attracted to the same sex. These "homosexuals" simply cannot achieve happiness, he argues, because they can't marry and start a family, which is the one and only path to contentment.

But there are even worse things, "the dark corners of life." The only two that Keller can bring himself to discuss, even to name, are male prostitution and bestiality. "Others that are worse are deliberately omitted."

In the next chapter, Doc looks at some practices that aren't strictly abnormal—because they don't interfere with spawning kids—but are somewhat unusual. He actually discusses S/M (while he doesn't name it, he describes "the relation of pain to the sexual act as a means of intensifying it and increasing the pleasure of the two participants"). More than that—don't let your jaw hit the table—*he approves of it.* But only within marriage (of course) and only with the husband doling out the hurt. "When the condition is reversed and the woman inflicts the pain, it would appear that the act is abnormal and is only saved from being pathological by the fact that the inflicted pain ends in normal coitus."

Keller says that some women simply need pain in order to be passionate and as long as both spouses are digging it, it's normal. Have we uncovered the earliest mainstream medical proponent of S/M, at least of the male dom variety?

Expanding his point, Keller argues that married couples must avoid monotony at all costs by engaging in a wide variety of (unnamed) acts that might seem kinky. He warns women that if they primly refuse to engage in such fun because it makes them feel like whores, they may well lose their husbands to actual whores. He recommends that both spouses fearlessly tell each other all their sexual desires, then bring them into reality.

"In many ways there is a deadly resemblance between the two conditions of the opium habit and auto-eroticism."

The book ends with Keller yelling in all caps:

> **THE RULE BRIEFLY STATED IS THIS: THE HUSBAND IS ALWAYS TO BE RECEPTIVE TO THE SEXUAL DESIRES OF THE WIFE AND ALWAYS READY TO GRATIFY HER REQUESTS FOR LOVE. THE TIME, FREQUENCY AND VARIETY OF THE SEX LIFE IS TO DEPEND ENTIRELY UPON THE INSTINCTIVE FEELINGS OF THE WIFE. IN OTHER WORDS, SHE IS TO TAKE THE INITIATIVE IN ALL THE LOVE LIFE, LEAVING ONLY THE ONE RESPONSIBILITY TO THE HUSBAND, AND THAT IS, SATISFYING HER DESIRES.**

The ease with which Keller switches from reactionary Cro-Magnon to progressive radical to babbling fruitcake truly boggles the mind.

The next two books are *The Sexual Education of the Young Woman* and *The Sexual Education of the Young Man*. In the former book, Keller gives a remarkably detailed, frank recounting of the physical changes that a lass experiences during puberty, takes a stab at girl psychology, declares that she

needs to be obsequious to her father, and recommends a soap suds enema during her first period. But the whole thing really is summed up in the third sentence of chapter seven: "The entire effort of her first twenty years should be devoted to the task of so caring for herself so that when she marries she will be a happy gentlewoman." The companion book is pretty much note for note the same, except casting things in male terms, of course. The point is to prepare the boy to be a wonderful husband/breadwinner. Among many other things, this means not reading "the sex magazines that are at present time covering every newsstand." (In 1928?)

As the title indicates, *Companionate Marriage, Birth Control, Divorce, Modern Home Life* is a grab-bag, which nonetheless has only one message: Breed! In Keller's most forceful statement yet, he graciously allows that not cranking out kids is acceptable only for prepubescent girls and "the old maid" who chooses caring for her parents over having children. "All other women, who, married and living with their husbands, continually and steadfastly refuse to perform their duty to the race and themselves by becoming mothers, are to be classed with some lesser form of creation. They are certainly not the women God created." Each unused ovum that gets flushed out every twenty-eight days is the same as a murdered baby. Is this what Mac thought about during his long workouts?

Love, Courtship, Marriage presents a *Leave It to Beaver* vision of the married couple, from puppy love to the "perpetual honeymoon" of marriage—with babies, of course.

If you thought Keller might hit a different note with volume seven, rest assured that he doesn't. *Mother and Baby* gushes on and on about pregnancy, childbirth, and taking care of the bawling infant.

After detouring for three volumes, Keller returns primarily to the matter of sex with *Sexual Life of Men and Women After Forty*. At this point in their lives, women typically aren't going to be having any more children, and many or most of the kids they did have may already be grown and on their own. With brats out of the picture, what on earth will Keller talk about? He urges women to take care of their physical appearances so their husbands don't end up with hookers. Men are warned to put less effort into screwing, which now can be "a fatiguing and even deadly act." There follows a fascinating chapter on admittedly worthless techniques to keep men sexually vital (such as monkey-testicle transplants), followed by Keller's advice: Don't shoot too much of your seed in your younger years, so you'll have reserves left in middle age.

Despite being part of "The Sexual Education Series," in *Diseases and Problems of Old Age*, Keller spends 95% of his time talking dryly about senility, constipation, retirement homes, card-playing, and so on. Only two short chapters deal with sex. He warns old men 1) not to confuse boners caused by an enlarged prostate with a return of sexual vigor and 2) to keep their mitts off little girls. Geezers should just smoke cigars and read.

Sex and Society is the final volume in this sad decalogy. Keller realizes that it's his last chance to make points about sex, and the man goes bonkers. This is by far the most outlandish and weirdly entertaining book in the batch. He covers a lot of the same ground as the previous nine books—rephrasing it in the strongest possible terms, sometimes contradicting himself—and makes a few new points. Among the choice passages:

If we can imagine a womanless world, where would be the incentive for doing ninety-nine of the hundred tasks of life?

~

He may be taught masturbation at this time of his life [age six to adolescence], but if he is well trained and educated in time, he will be able to avoid this unpleasant part of life.

~

Finally, these children grow up and there is a sexual relation between parents and child. This, if it is kept with normal bounds, is in every way a healthy thing, but if it sweeps past the bounds of normality, it becomes a threatening disease and vice. [Keller doesn't elaborate on this freaky declaration.]

~

So, the only sexual intercourse that is legal is that between husband and wife. This is such an important truth that it must be repeated. Its purpose is to establish the permanency of the home, give the children a respectable and legal paternity and fill the state with a multitude of moral families.

~

When a woman has been married five times and divorced four times and has never been pregnant by any of her husbands and is not yet thirty years of age, we can well ask ourselves if this is not a form of legalized prostitution rather than marriage in the true sense.

~

Consider the fact that some specialists in sexual diseases estimate that as high as seventy or eighty per cent of all males are infected with gonorrhoea before the age of twenty-one!

~

If three generations of boys can be properly educated and guarded till they marry, then in that length of time the entire evil [i.e., prostitution] can be wiped out.

~

It is well known that the colored race is unmoral rather than immoral and that sexual promiscuity is the rule and morality the exception.

~

The first abnormal sexual practice which threatens society is auto-eroticism.

~

[T]here are many evidences that distinct sexual perversions are practiced in the cities, especially among the wealthier class of women, and these perversions include the use of pet animals who have been specifically trained to give satisfaction to their fair but frail owners.

~

Every man should apply to himself the test as to whether his conduct is for the good or for the bad of the state.

~

[I]t must never be forgotten that the urge in women is for reproduction and the act of sexual intercourse is only a means to that end, but with man the primitive urge is for the use of a woman's body...

~

It is believed that much of the present immorality is due to the fourteen ounce dresses of the modern flapper, and her willingness to allow the varying forms of caressing, known under the collective term of petting.

~

The past history of all races has shown that the amount of clothing worn by the women, the degree of eroticism developed by contact, especially in dancing, and the two, combined with alcohol, are all powerful excitants of eroticism. In past ages these factors were always the prelude to the destruction of the nation.

~

The recent flood of pornographic literature, posing under the name of art, has even a more powerful force for the promotion of erotic in life.

~

Lacking the courage of normal men, they take their dope before killing, in order to stimulate their flagging lust for blood. Especially among the negro race is cocaine a precursor to crime. The negro will take a few sniffs of "snow", and at once he is a

"bad nigger", capable of murder or rape.

About two-thirds of the way through, Keller basically abandons the subject of sex and starts screaming about society's "unfit" and "undesirables."

The feebleminded man and woman always have more children than the superior man and woman.

~

It has only been recently that the code of society has promulgated the thought that all men are created free and equal. Of course, they are not and everyone realizes down at the bottom of his heart that this is not the case, yet, the law provides equality, and whereas in former days the weakminded were treated as so many cattle, now they are accorded practically all the privileges of normal members of society, especially the right to marry.

~

The imbecile is capable of having sexual relations; usually it is necessary for him to find a woman as mentally inferior as he is to have such intercourse volitionally. Lacking this, he often attempts rape, or failing to find a willing love object, turns to auto-eroticism or the use of animals. The higher types of imbecility are frequently not satisfied with rape, but go on to murder and mutilation.

~

The breeding of the unfit continues. What is to be done about it?

As an answer to this question, the book reaches a crescendo with Keller advising the forced sterilization and segregation of criminals, retarded individuals, "psychopathic personalities" (this, Keller informs us, includes the members of the Industrial Workers of the World), "the insane," and epileptics.

Not only did Charles Atlas publish a series of books about sex, he also put out a full-blown racist eugenics screed. Way to go, big guy.

Official Documents About the Mile-High Club

The flights I'm on are always pretty boring, which is actually fine with me. But the Federal Aviation Administration's flight incident reports reveal that things occasionally get pretty interesting and kinky at 20,000 feet.

Some passengers try to hook up with other flyers or the crew. In December 2001, a woman "drank, and tried to entice 3 male pax [passengers] in same row to have sex. Pax continued to talk sexually explicit with those 3 gentlemen in same row." Apparently, none of them took her up on her offer, at least not on the plane.[1]

When such approaches don't work, some passengers resort to force. "Pax, a man assigned to a seat, moved to another seat in same row and started to fondle and then bite the breast of pax seated next to him." A guy behind them restrained the shit-faced, puking perp, who was taken to a hospital for a possible overdose.[2]

Somewhat less vigorous was the eighteen-year-old woman on a San Francisco flight to JFK who walked around while the 767 was taxiing out. "When confronted by a female flight attendant the pax stated that she was going to 'slap the bitch.' The female pax also grabbed a male flt [flight] attendant's buttocks."[3]

Sometimes people get naked onboard. In November 2001, a drunk woman was on a flight from JFK to Santo Domingo. "Our pax took off her clothes and was belligerent. Thank God she was an older woman who we could ctl [control]!"[4] Also that month, a female passenger drank an entire bottle of rum that she had brought with her. The report notes: "She was incoherent, took her panties off in front of everybody, screaming." A flight attendant reported: "Later on in the flt, the pax urinated on the floor in front of her seat."[5]

One poor guy evidently had a nervous breakdown after his wife left him. On a February 2000 flight, "Pax took clothes off, refused to put them back on. Sat in seat reading the Bible." He was arrested upon landing.[6]

In other cases, though, not all the clothes came off—just enough to expose the naughty bits. "I noticed his scrotum and penis were completely exposed.... The man was wearing shorts, and that, when she [one of the female flight attendants] observed his genitals hanging out, it was because he had lifted his shorts up, so the genitals would be exposed. This he did deliberately." Two male attendants told the guy that his behavior "was inappropriate and not tolerated," but he refused to put away his goods. Air Marshals arrested his ass when the plane landed in Boston.[7]

Then there was the flight from Port au Prince International to JFK in March 1999:

When the male pax came out of the lavatory, he stopped in the aisle L-hand side and he fondled his genitals and he kept saying over and over "It's a Haitian thing." We all told him to sit down and fasten his seatbelt, it's turbulent, but he just stood there fondling himself and telling us "It's a Haitian thing."[8]

Diddling yourself in the air may be a Haitian thing, but actually fucking onboard would appear to be a Texan thing. In August 2002, on a Texas flight, a man and woman wearing sunglasses went into the lavatory together. Not at all suspicious, right? The crew made a special announcement that the seatbelt light was still on and all passengers should be seated. When the couple still hadn't come out seven minutes later, the captain told a flight attendant to open the bathroom door.

Finally, as she was opening the door, they came out of the bathroom. Still needing to know why the 2 of them were in the bathroom at an inappropriate time during the flt, I asked the flt attendant if the man appeared to be sexually aroused when he came out of the bathroom. She replied that she had noticed that he was.... The bottom line is: a couple had sex in our bathroom...[9]

Now we come to the *Fanny Hill*, the *Tropic of Cancer*, of FAA reports. In this masterpiece—which is pretty explicit for a government document—we find out what happened during a night flight from Dallas-Fort Worth to Manchester in October 1999. This report can best be appreciated in its entirety:

Flt attendant #1 rpted [reported] pax in seat X had taken her clothes off and she and pax in seat Y were engaged in sexual activity.

I apched [approached] the pax and told the man in seat Y that their behavior was unacceptable and they must refrain. I returned to the business class galley and seat Z (lady) requested that we please stop the couple from their sexual activity, as it was causing her distress. I rpted the couple to the purser and she spoke to couple also about their sexual activity.

They did not stop and continued until breakfast svc [service] was presented and light was emitted into the cabin. Pax seat X put her clothes on just prior to lighting in cabin. I observed pax seat X sitting in seat in bra and panties. She was masturbating in seat and pax seat Y was manipulating her and putting his hands in her panties and on her exposed breasts. They were kissing and writhing in their seats.

Purser repeatedly asked seat X and Y to stop their persistent sexual activity and they would not. She told the crew security would meet the flt.

Callback conversation with rptr [reporter, i.e., the crew member who made the initial report] revealed the following info: The rptr stated the

couple didn't start their sexual activity until after dessert was served, and not the whole trip, as it said in her original narrative. This was about 4 hrs from Manchester, England. The couple would not stop their sexual activity after repeated requests from the crew and the purser. The plts [pilots] would not come out of the cockpit for fear of being slugged.

The woman took all her clothes off, except for her bra and panties. She would not put her clothes back on, when ordered to by the crew, and in fact, became quite loud and profane when asked. She slung her legs over the seat in front of her. She was performing fellatio on the man and masturbating both of them.

At one point, one of the complaining pax was a 65 yr old woman on her first flt, who asked if this was a regular occurrence on flts!

The rptr strongly feels that alcohol was not a factor, because they didn't have that much to drink, and they both got completely dressed for lndg [landing], and she had replenished her makeup and hair. The Manchester police arrested the woman first, because she put up a loud and profane fight. They then decided to arrest the man.[10]

"She was performing fellatio on the man and masturbating both of them."

The Deleted 9/11 Sex Scene

Windows on the World by Frédéric Beigbeder is among the first novels—if not *the* first novel—to deal with 9/11. Originally published in Paris by Éditions Grasset & Fasquelle in 2003, an English-language translation reached US shores in March 2005 thanks to Miramax Books. But some of it was left in France. Specifically, Miramax eviscerated the sex scene between two doomed yuppies on an upper floor of One World Trade Center. Already treading on thin ice with a novel about the attacks, they apparently decided that such blasphemy would be too much for our delicate nature. And they were probably right.

The two lovers are never identified by name. In the English-language edition of the novel, we learn: "They both work for Cantor Fitzgerald: a blonde who is sexy despite her Ralph Lauren suit (do girls really dress like that anymore?) and a stocky dark-haired man who seems cool in his Kenneth Cole suit." They're never identified by name, always being referred to as "the blonde in Ralph Lauren" and "the guy in Kenneth Cole." The handful of scenes featuring them are comprised almost entirely of their staccato, emotionally flat dialog. They alternate single sentences, during which we learn that they're each married to someone else. The woman wants the man to ditch his wife, but he doesn't want to, nor does he want his coworker to divorce her husband.

The chapter "10:15" (each chapter covers one minute of that morning) contains only a dozen sentences in the US version. It's apparent that the adulterous lovers are having sex, but not one crumb of it is described. Graphic dialog is completely absent. The first paragraph describes the conference room. Then comes the only action, such as it is, with them "clambering" onto a conference table, the guy removing his pants, and the woman doffing her blouse. Suddenly, they're whispering sweet nothings to each other (which, as we shall see, indicates that the sex is over). The brief chapter ends with purple silliness: "In heaven, there were no thousand virgins, but there were once two. It's not only in hell that passions blaze."

She continues in French, with the translation being: "I would have loved to have your father whip my pussy good."

I got a copy of the French edition to see what we're missing. The complete chapter is very graphic, deliciously nasty in spots, although it doesn't exactly qualify for the Sex Scene Hall of Fame. As with the other scenes starring these hollow yuppie caricatures, it's mostly dialog, with little action described. Problem is, it cries out for explaining because the lovers' exchange is extremely disjointed. The action that can be inferred is confusing, making it seems as though they're simultaneously having oral and anal sex. Quite a neat trick.

You have to admire their willingness to go at it. The conference room is littered with purple corpses, filled with smoke, and water comes up to their thighs. During the course of their boffing on the conference table, fax machines boil and iMacs fry because the temperature is "a thousand degrees Fahrenheit." Yet still these asbestos lovers soldier on.

So here's my translation of what's missing from the US version. The French chapter opens with:

"Show me your breasts," said the dark-haired man in Kenneth Cole.

Instead of complying, the woman non-sequiturs: "I depilated my pussy with a laser for you."

You'd think this would warrant a response, but the man just tells her: "You will empty/drain [vider] my balls one last time."

She responds: "I will swallow you. I want to feel your hot cum squirt my tonsils."

He specifies: "Really stick out your tongue so that I can feel your piercing on my penis head." (The guy tends to use the more formal, clinical terms.)

In the fragment of the scene that also appears in the US edition, he drops trou, while she takes off her blouse. Beigbeder kindly informs us that "in spite of the odor of the dead and the atrocious heat, they are very exciting to look at" ("... ils sont très excitants à regarder.") Then the action once again becomes French-only.

Strangely, the blonde asks, "Do you feel my three fingers in your ass?" The man doesn't respond, but we can only hope that the answer would be yes. Instead, he commands: "Raise your skirt and impale your anus deeply on my dick." (Yes, he actually says "anus" (anus), not "asshole" (trou du cul). Not even hot sex and imminent death can rattle this guy.)

As usual, no action is described, though if we read between the lines, they seem to switch to anal action at this point. The very next sentence has the blonde cooing, "Twist my tits; grab my breasts."

Apparently, the guy's hands travel a bit lower, because he asks, "You like it when I pinch your clit, you slut?" As always, no answer.

Apropos of not much, the blonde starts in with Story of O-style talk: "I would've been gangbanged for you. I belong to you, so you can give me to others."

Her loverboy immediately picks up on the sentiment, replying: "Oh yeah, I should have tied you up and punished/disciplined [punir] you for strangers, and I should've buttfucked your little sister in front of you, you cunt." (Cunt is written in English, rather than as con, apparently as an example of what Beigbeder earlier referred to as "Franglais"—the amalgamation of French and English.)

The blonde's next utterance is also in English: "MM fuck me deep." I guess sometimes only Anglo-Saxon will do. She continues in French, with the translation being: "I would have loved to have your father whip my pussy good."

"I'm going to fill your ass with hot cum," the studmuffin suddenly announces.

"Wow, I'm getting there, too," the blonde intones, sans exclamation point. Then: "Afterwards, I WANT to drink your piss." (In the text, WANT (VEUX) is in all caps. See, she really does want to.)

Now the guy tells her, "Wait, I want to fist your soaking cunt all the way up my arm. I want to hurt you while I juice." Then he commands: "Really stick your tongue out so that I can come on it." Hmm, this would seem to imply that they've switched back to oral at some point, perhaps as he's fisting her in some acrobatic variation of the 69.

The blonde bottom starts yelling, "Spit in my mouth; claw me with your teeth; rip out my hair; eat my feet." Again, she switches to *Anglais*: "OOOoh, I'm comiiiing, I feel your cock in my ass." (If they're still doing it in the booty, what was that stuff about coming on her tongue two seconds ago?)

As he's spunking, the guy gets a great line linking sex, death, and birth: "I will torture you to death, kill you, disembowel you to fuck your entrails, stretch your vagina in order to get my whole body into your insides and die in the place where I was born."

We're then told: "They shout together. They French kiss with a mouthful of sperm." So he did shoot in her mouth, despite her crying in ecstasy about feeling his cock up her ass? Is Beigbeder trying to be quasi-surrealistic, or did he just lose track of the holes? I vote for the latter.

The blonde says: "I've died of pleasure. I've died loving you."

The man then gets the best line: "Death is better than Viagra," followed immediately by sappy pop-ballad lyrics: "You were my reason for living; you are my reason for dying."

The chapter ends with the French equivalent of the final two sentences in the US version, mentioned above.

Admittedly, the world of English-language erotica didn't lose much by having this scene completely bowdlerized in the translation, but at least we now know what we weren't supposed to see.

The Sex Fantasies Missing From
Our Bodies, Ourselves

Our Bodies, Ourselves is an undisputed feminist classic and perhaps the most important women's health book ever published. It's gone through numerous incarnations: published as *Women and Their Bodies* by the New England Free Press in 1970; reissued the next year with its current title; picked up by Simon & Schuster in 1973; published in its eighth edition in early 2005.

The Boston Women's Health Book Collective has made a lot of changes to the Simon & Schuster editions of their book over three decades. Obviously, the photos of 1970s women—with their perfectly straight hair, big glasses, and bell-

bottom jeans—were jettisoned, as was the photograph of a hairy vagina in a mirror. There's no trace of the chapter "In Amerika They Call Us Dykes."

And something else is missing. In the section on women's sexual fantasies, only two of the original fantasies remain. The other ten have disappeared or have been replaced. Not surprisingly, half of the missing dealt with highly forbidden sex acts. Though the newest edition mentions that it's okay to have taboo fantasies, it can no longer work up the nerve to actually present them.[11] Here are some of the deleted fantasies from the 1973 edition of *Our Bodies, Ourselves*, presented in the women's own words:

I've had fantasies of having to drink urine from a man's penis while he was peeing.

~

When I was a kid, every time I masturbated I imagined my parents spanking me as I climaxed. When I got older it changed to my parents making love, then to my being kissed by someone, then to my making love.

~

I used to have a recurring fantasy that I was a gym teacher and had a class full of girls standing in front of me, nude. I went up and down the rows feeling all their breasts and getting a lot of pleasure out of it....

~

I fantasize about sleeping with my brother, who is nineteen and groovy and looks just like me.... I acted on it by sleeping with his best friend.

~

I fantasize about making love with horses, because they are very sensuous animals, more so than cows or pigs. They are also very male animals-- horse society is very chauvinist.

Endnotes

All reports used for the mile-high section are National Aviation Safety Data Analysis Center (NASDAC) Brief Reports retrieved through the Aviation Safety Reporting System (ASRS) database at [www.nasdac. faa.gov]. The number of the Brief Report is given in endnotes one through ten. **1.** 553584 **2.** 617360 **3.** 463530 **4.** 530720 **5.** 529806 **6.** 464598 **7.** 447750 **8.** 434818 **9.** 559044 **10.** 453232 **11.** The 2005 edition does contain a single semi-taboo fantasy, which isn't in the first edition. After the text mentions rape fantasies, it presents a woman's verbatim fantasy, leading us to expect a rape scenario. Instead, the willing woman is tied up while a man and woman "make love" to her. This, plus her subsequent explanation, makes it clear that she's having a bondage-threesome fantasy, not a rape fantasy.

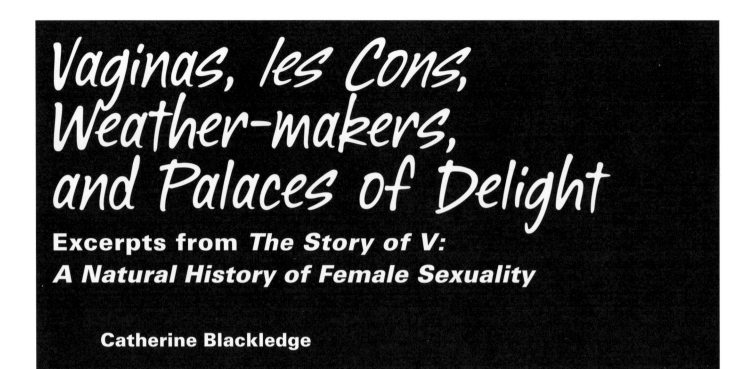

Vaginas, les Cons, Weather-makers, and Palaces of Delight

Excerpts from *The Story of V: A Natural History of Female Sexuality*

Catherine Blackledge

There is a Catalan saying: "*La maresposa bonasi veuelcony d'unadona*"—"The sea calms down if it sees a woman's cunt." This Catalan belief in the power of the vagina is, in fact, the source of the good-luck custom of fishermen's wives displaying their genitals to the sea before their men put out on the water. The flipside of this faith is, logically enough, that a woman can cause storms if she urinates in the waves. Moreover, according to folklore, it's not just the oceans that are soothed by the sight of a woman's vagina. A flash of female genitalia has the power to calm other forces of nature, too. For example, women in the southern Indian province of Madras were known to subdue dangerous storms by exposing themselves. And Pliny, the first-century historian of the

A flash of female genitalia has the power to calm other forces of nature.

ancient world, writes in his work *Natural History* of how hailstorms, whirlwinds, and lightning are all quieted and dispelled by a face-off with a naked woman.

Remarkably, the ability to mollify the elements is far from being the only capacity that folklore and ancient history ascribe to the act of a woman revealing her vagina. For many, female genitalia also present a potent apotropaic package. That is, the sight of a woman deliberately exposing her naked vulva is deemed to be capable of preventing evil from occurring. Driving out devils, averting vicious spirits, frightening carnivores, and scaring opposing warriors and threatening deities

away—all these heroic and dangerous deeds are reputed to form part of a woman's genital might. As a consequence, tales of women's vaginal derring-do are found in various cultures. Take Pliny and his fellow ancient historian and philosopher Plutarch (*c.* 46–*c.* 120 Common Era). Both these men described how great heroes and gods will flee in the face of female genitalia. Elsewhere, the report of a sixteenth-century traveler in North Africa records the belief that lions will turn tail and run from this sexual sight. At funerals, women were hired as mourners, with the express aim of exorcising demons via vaginal display. Delightfully, Russian folklore relates how when a bear appears out of the woods, it can be put to flight by a young woman raising her skirt at it. It seems that in the face of adversity, the best option open to a woman is to lift her skirt. For a man, it would be to make sure you're standing next to one of the sisters.

This view of the vagina may seem startling, disturbing even. Vaginas can calm the elements and drive out devils? It's certainly the case that this is a way of looking at female genitalia that is atypical in most cultures today. In the Western world of the twenty-first century, the idea of women showing their genitals tends to be inextricably bound up with sex, pornography, or images of women in accommodating positions rather than ones of power and influence. Sadly, for many, the idea of a woman revealing her vagina is seen as offensive, and seldom positive, let alone something to be welcomed or to hide behind. For women themselves, the idea of deliberately displaying their vaginas in public is more likely to provoke emotions of shame and embarrassment than feelings of respect and authority. And adding to the modern-day negative associations surrounding the naked vulva is the fact that a number of cultures put great effort into ensuring female genitalia are rarely viewed, and never publicly. At present, the most potent concept associated with the naked vagina is probably that of childbirth—the moment when a woman's vagina stretches wide and, miraculously, provides a baby with a safe gateway into the world. This parturition picture, it could be said, is also the one "acceptable" public face of female genitalia. The one vaginal image people are comfortable observing, without too much shame or embarrassment.

Yet it's apparent that women around the world have been lifting their skirts to full effect for centuries. From Italy—where folklore from the Abruzzo region tells of the power of a woman raising her skirt to display her genitals—to India, where the gesture was also understood to dispel evil influences, tales of deliberate female genital exposure abound in history, folklore, and literature. One eighteenth-century engraving by Charles Eisen for an edition of the book *Fables* by Jean de La Fontaine beautifully depicts the ability of the exposed vagina to dispel evil forces. In this striking image, a young woman stands, confident and unafraid, confronting the devil. Her left hand rests lightly on a wall, while her right raises her skirt high, displaying her sexual center for Satan to see. And in the face of her naked womanhood, the devil reels back in fear. In this way, the story relates, the young woman defeats the devil and saves her village, which Old Nick had been attacking. A couple of centuries earlier, the French writer Rabelais had his old woman of Papefiguiere rout the devil in the same manner, and reproductions of this vivid confrontation between the vagina and the devil can be found on seventeenth-century drinking mugs. A delicious sight to sup from, I'm sure.

The belief in the power of the exposed vagina to repel foes or expel demons is also, it seems, an enduring and widespread one. Significantly, accounts of women revealing their vaginas in order to achieve a particular effect are not rooted in any one historical period or any one culture. Instead, they span millennia, from the ancient past through to the present day, and cross continents, too. In his essay "Bravery of Women," Plutarch recalls a vulva-displaying incident where a large group of women lifting their gowns together changed the outcome of a war. He describes how, in a certain battle between the Persians and the Medes, the Persian men, losing heart against the strong, advancing Median forces, turned tail and attempted to flee from them. However, their way was blocked by a group of their own women, calling them cow-

ards. These Persian women proceeded to raise their skirts, exposing their nakedness to their fellow men. Shamed by this vaginal display, the Persian men returned to face their enemies, eventually defeating them.

Fast-forward 1,900 years or so, and the Western press describes similar incidents. In the *Irish Times* of September 23, 1977, one Walter Mahon-Smith contributed the following item:

> **In a townland near where I lived, a deadly feud had continued for generations between the families of two small farmers. One day, before the First World War, when the men of one of the families, armed with pitchforks and heavy blackthorn sticks, attacked the home of their enemy, the woman of the house came to the door of her cottage, and in full sight of all (including my father and myself, who happened to be passing by) lifted her skirt and underclothes high above her head, displaying her naked genitals. The enemy of her and her family fled in terror.**

At present, the most potent concept associated with the naked vagina is probably that of childbirth.

Outside the Western world, anthropological data collected during the last century regarding the people of the Marquesas Islands reveals a similar reverential attitude to female genitalia, albeit with a slight twist. This Polynesian culture credits female genitalia with supernatural influences. And these vaginal forces, Marquesans say, are strong enough to frighten gods or to drive out evil possessing spirits. Hence, exorcisms carried out in this part of the world consist of a naked woman sitting on the chest of the possessed. For this society, the belief that women have extra mysterious powers courtesy of their unique sexual anatomy extends elsewhere. For instance, Marquesans also consider that a woman can curse an object or person by naming them after her genitalia. I haven't yet tried this one myself.

So, according to many individuals and communities, the vagina is an extremely influential organ—and one possibly to be feared if you're on the receiving end of a vulval flash. However, there is another aspect to the gesture of female genital display. Some genital practices highlight how the protection provided by the displayed vagina is not only about preventing harm. Just as important, vaginal protection can encompass a more nurturing, nourishing influence. Indeed, historical evidence suggests that female genital display can also be about promoting fertility, such as causing plants or the earth to flourish. Up to the twentieth century, in many Western countries, belief in this vaginal ability can be seen in the custom of peasant women exposing their genitals to the growing flax, while saying: "Please grow as high as my genitals are now." And as strange as it may seem, the fairy tale of Snow White, or Biancaneve, is suggested to have arisen from an ancient Italian ritual designed to enhance the fecundity of the earth itself. A beautiful, noble girl would be sent down a mine which was running low in iron ore in order to expose Mother Earth to her vital female essence or energy. Biancaneve, so the theory goes, came from the Dolomites region of the Cordevole river north of Belluno in Italy, an area which was known for its magnesium-rich iron mines.

The fertility effect of the displayed vagina can work in more subtle ways, too. In ancient Egypt, women exposed their vaginas to their fields in order to bring about a double whammy effect, if you will. First off, the gesture was designed to drive evil spirits from the land, but the consequence of this apotropaic action was desired, too. With no evil spirits around, the women would increase the yield of their crops. Hence, the act of deliberate vaginal display is both evil-averting and fecundity-enhancing, as the former function promotes the latter. This double aim is also thought to lie at the heart of the custom recorded by Pliny, who noted how a woman can rid

The belief in the power of the exposed vagina to repel foes or expel demons is also, it seems, an enduring and widespread one.

a field of pests by walking around it before sunrise with her genitals exposed. Giving thanks for a bountiful harvest and asking for the same fruitfulness next year may well lie at the heart of one of the concluding parts to Marquesan harvest festival celebrations—the ko'ika to'e haka, the clitoris dance. Significantly, this traditional dance features young women in wrap-around skirts, which they raise to expose their vaginas and clitorises and the ritual tattoos emblazoned around their genitalia.

First Impressions
A view of the vagina by taking a tour of its lexical history would not be complete without considering cunt. And although a remarkably direct expression, cunt has multiple meanings, depending on the country you find yourself in. In Spain, if you wish to express your delight in a delicious experience, a suitable comment might be that it is como comerle el coño a bocaos ("like eating cunt by the mouthful"). If you're in Britain, though, this phrase would not go down so well. Cunt, one of the oldest words for female genitalia, is also the most taboo.

Yet in Spain, it's not. In fact, coño is so common a word in Spain (albeit an expletive) that just as the English have been dubbed les fuckoffs by the French, in Chile and Mexico, Spaniards are known as los coños. The Spanish seem to have had fun playing with their coño phrases. Otra pena pa mi coño—"another pain in my cunt"—is said when one is faced with something extra to contend with. If you're fed up with something or someone, you can be estoy hasta el coño, "up to your cunt with it." And if you want to get across the fact that a place is completely out of the way (i.e., it is the back of beyond), you can use the common Spanish expression en el quinto coño—"the fifth cunt." It remains a mystery as to why a particularly remote area should be described as "the fifth cunt."

The dichotomy of the significance of cunt is visible elsewhere across Europe. In Italy, figa (cunt) is not an insult or an ugly word. Rather, it is a common expletive (after cazzo, prick, it is probably the most used). Figa is the spoken form, fica the more common written term. Che figa! is actually a lighthearted expression. It can be applied to people—"Che figa," "What a looker!"; to objects—"Che festa figa!"—"What a great party!"; and to situations—for example, "Che figa!" can mean, "What good luck!" And although at times men can use it in a sexist way, akin to English men saying "chick" or "pussy," Italian women have reclaimed the word, making it applicable to men as the masculine noun, figo. So if you fancy an Italian man, go ahead and say, admiringly, "Che figo!" If something is excellent, it is figata.

However, in Germany, like Britain, cunt, or Fotze, reigns supreme as an extremely taboo word. Yet Fotze is also an old word for mouth, and in expressions such as "Halt dei' Fotze!" ("Shut your trap!") and hinterfotzig ("two-faced"), it loses some of its impact.

Like Italian and Spanish, the French equivalent of cunt, le con, is not taboo. Rather, it is used as an affectionate insult, as in vieux con ("old fool") or "Dais pas le con" ("Don't play the fool"). Con to the French isn't necessarily any stronger than calling someone a fool or an idiot. Le roi des cons ("king of cunts") implies a total idiot, while "Quelle connerie!" means "What rubbish!"

In Danish the word for cunt, kusse, has acquired no additional emotional baggage. The word conveys merely what it describes—female genitalia. In Finland, while vittu is still considered a strong expletive, it's flexible and various in the ways it is applied. You can tell someone to go get lost in Finnish by saying, "Vedä vittu päähäs!" ("Go pull a cunt over your head!"). It can be used as an adjective, as bloody is in English, in the form vittumainen ("cunt-like"). And there is a past participle, *vituttaa*, meaning "to be annoyed."

In England, *cunt* has been considered taboo in print and speech since the fifteenth century. Prior to this, though, it was an accepted enough part of English vernacular that it featured in the names for public thoroughfares. In about 1230, Gropecuntelane was a London street; other cities, too, including Oxford, York, and Northampton, possessed Gropecuntelanes in the thirteenth and fourteenth centuries. In Paris, there was rue Grattecon (Scratchcunt Street). Today, all that remains of the too-lewd lane names are truncated versions—Grove Street (Oxford) or Grape Lane (York).

Yet from 1700 to 1959, *cunt* was considered so obscene that it was a legal offense to publish the word in its entirety. This meant that lexicographers had a problem. The first edition of Francis Grose's *Dictionary of the Vulgar Tongue* (1785) bleeped it out with four stars, ****. Three years later, the second edition, incredibly and offensively, defined *cunt*, or *c**t*, as "a nasty name for a nasty thing." Amazingly, the *Oxford English Dictionary* did not permit *cunt*'s entry into its hallowed pages until 1976. The entry then read: "1. The female genitals, the vulva. 2. A very unpleasant or stupid person." In the twenty-first century, *cunt* is still not a word that "authorities," be they media-based or political, allow an individual to say freely. It remains the most taboo and insulting word in the English language.

When considering the etymology of *cunt*, it's hard to ignore the tone of the word. Whether it begins with a hard *c*, *k*, or *q*, the sound of *cunt* is particularly distinctive. A quick trip around old and modern Europe gives a veritable concerto in C, as well as an impressive history. As well as the *cunt*s listed above, there are: *cunte* or *counte* (Middle English); *kut* (the Netherlands); *kunta* (Old Norse); *queynthe* (Middle English); *qwim* (sixteenth-century England); *cunnus* (Latin); *cona* (Portuguese); *cont* (Wales); *cunnicle* or *cunnikin* (nineteenth-century England); *kunte* (Middle Low German); *cut* (eighteenth-century England); and *chuint* (Ireland). Outside Europe, this refrain continues. There's the Sanskrit term *kunthi*; the Indian words for cunt, *cunti* or *kunda*; and also Arabic and Hebrew, where *cunt* is *kus*. In these latter two languages, the word for cunt is said to be related to those for cup and pockets, making it some kind of receptacle. This idea of a vessel or container ties in with the suggestion that *cunt* is linked to the Old English word for womb, *cwithe*.

Other etymologists cite the root *cwe* (*cu*) as the connection between the words *cunt* and *cwithe* and a host of other words, such as *queen*, *kin*, *country*, and *cunning* (which derives from the Old English *cunnende*). This *cu* root, it is said, signifies "quintessential physical femininity." It's certainly the case that the basic term, *kuna*, meaning woman, is found in a startlingly large and geographically widespread number of languages and language families. Some of the language families *kuna* is represented in are the Afro-Asiatic (for example, in the Cushitic language Oromo, *qena* means lady); the Indo-European (in the English word *queen*); the Amerind (Guarani *kuña* means female); and the Indo-Pacific (the Tasmanian for wife/woman is *quani*).

Does *cunt* derive from a global word for woman—*kuna*? Some scholars suggest it does. They point to ancient Egyptian writings, such as the maxims of Ptah-Hotep, where the word for cunt is synonymous with that for woman. However, it should be made clear that for this culture, *cunt* was in no way an insult; rather, it was a word of respect. The Egyptian for mother, *k-at*, literally "the body of her," also means the female genitalia or vulva. An ancient Indian goddess provides another link between words for woman and words for cunt. *Kunthi* is both a Sanskrit term for the vagina and the name of an ancient Indian mother goddess. Kunti, a goddess of nature, was said to be able to take innumerable men into herself without altering her essence, just like the earth. She features in the epic Sanskrit poem of India, the *Mahabharata*. The ancient Anatolian goddess Kubaba, the "Creatrix of All," also shares the *cu* root.

Although the etymology of *cunt* is disputed, the most accepted and cited explanation again ties it to words for woman. This explanation is also the one that seventeenth-century Dutch anatomist Reinier de Graaf gives in his treatise on fe-

You can tell someone to go get lost in Finnish by saying, "*Vedä vittu päähäs!*" ("Go pull a cunt over your head!").

male genitalia. However, in order to understand how de Graaf viewed the word (*cunnus* in Latin), a question needs to be asked: What is cunt? In the twenty-first century, according to the dictionary, *cunt* refers to the female genitals (collectively), or a very unpleasant or obnoxious person. However, when de Graaf was writing, *cunt* had another meaning, that is, it was perceived in another way. And it is in de Graaf's view of *cunt*, I feel, that the true etymology of the word can be found. This meaning also explains why *cunt* wasn't always heard as a swear word, as it was merely a way of describing a specific part of female anatomy. For de Graaf, *cunnus* was the word used to describe "the great cleft." But what is "the great cleft"?

Well, this great cleft is simply the area of a woman's genitalia that is visible to an onlooker when she has parted neither her outer nor inner labia. Looking face on, what is visible is a pubic triangle, with a line running down the middle. Amazingly, *cunnus* just describes what you can see when you first look at female genitalia. This is what de Graaf meant by the great cleft, and he explains this clearly in Chapter II: "Concerning the Female Pudendum," when he says: "The great cleft is called...the cunnus, because it looks like the impress of a wedge (cuneus)." *Cuneus*, the term for the impress of a wedge, is, I feel, the true origin of the word *cunt*. Moreover, this etymology is underlined by ancient Sumerian pictorial writing, cuneiform (*c.* 3500 BCE). In cuneiform, the impressed word symbol for woman or female is the image of cunt—a downwards-facing triangle with a line cleft down its middle. It seems it's hard to separate cunt from woman. Woman with her cleft cunt and horned uterus. Devil-woman. Is it any wonder then that *cunt* went on to be considered such a wicked word?

Does *cunt* derive from a global word for woman—*kuna*?

The Palace of Delight

Looking at the various systems employed over the centuries to classify and understand the interior of the vagina, it's hard not to get the feeling that genital measurement isn't perhaps a particular male métier, as some vaginal dimensions are somewhat startling. Chinese sexual manuals, such as the Taoist text *The Wondrous Discourse of Su Nü*, detail how vaginas come in eight different varieties—each determined by the depth of the vaginal interior, and each 2.5 cm [approximately one inch] longer than the previous. However, some, such as the Zither String, seem surprisingly short, while others, like the North Pole, are somewhat on the lengthy side. In ascending size, the Eight Valleys, as they are known, are:

1. The Zither String or Lute String (*ch'in-hsien*), 0–2.5 cm
2. The Water-caltrop Teeth or Water-chestnut Teeth (*ling-ch'ih*), 5 cm
3. The Peaceful Valley or Little Stream (*t'o-hsi*), 7.5 cm
4. The Dark Pearl or Mysterious Pearl (*hsüan-chu*), 10 cm
5. The Valley Seed or Valley Proper (*ku-shih*), 12.5 cm
6. The Palace of Delight or Deep Chamber (*yü-ch'üeh*), 15 cm
7. The Inner Door or Gate of Prosperity (*k'un-hu*), 17.5 cm
8. The North Pole (*pei-chi*), 20 cm

Chinese sexual manuals also classified the relative position of the vulva—be it high (in a forward/upward location), that is, placed more ventrally or towards the belly, to the middle, or low (lower on the perineum).

So what is the average length of the vagina? Importantly, what the above ancient measurements do not articulate is that the interior of the vagina cannot be calibrated in this way—with just one length. For every woman, the ventral or anterior wall of her vagina—the belly side—is shorter than the opposing, posterior, wall (adjacent to the rectum). This is because the cervix, which sits at the apex of the vagina, projects down into the vagina, making the ventral vaginal wall shorter than the other. (The twin arch-like spaces that are created between the vagina wall and the curving cervix are known as the anterior and posterior fornices—singular, fornix—a word that is said to derive from the habit in Roman times of prostitutes renting vaulted or arched basements for them and their clients to fornicate in—the Latin word for arch being *fornix*).

And the average length from vaginal entrance to fornix and cervix? Most recently, average vaginal length (when not sexually aroused) has been placed anywhere between 7 and 12.5 cm [2.7 to 5 inches], with the posterior length of the vagina from 1.5 to 3.5 cm [0.6 to 1.4 inches] longer than the ventral vaginal wall. Importantly, just as all penises vary enormously in size, so too do all vaginas. There is no standard. And just as all penises lengthen when aroused and erect, so too do all vaginas.

Seeing in the Dark

We've already seen that the vagina is an incredibly intelligent organ—capable of sorting and selecting sperm with a remarkable specificity. But can you credit that the vagina has extra sensory perception (ESP), too? Startlingly, the discovery of the role of the vagus nerve in human female orgasm suggests that it does. In the studies investigating how women without functioning genitospinal nerves (complete spinal cord injury, SCI) perceived genital sensations and orgasm, two distinct groups emerged. The first were women who stated that they could consciously feel the genital stimulator in their vagina or against their cervix, and it was this sensation, transmitted by the vagus nerve, that then triggered their orgasms.

However, there was a second group of SCI women who were orgasmic, too. And orgasm in these women was more perplexing. These women experienced orgasm with the genital stimulator in their vagina or against their cervix, despite the fact that they did not consciously perceive any physical sensation from the genital stimulator or their genitalia. Somehow, though, their vaginas sensed the applied vibrating genital stimulation (even if they didn't consciously) and responded orgasmically. How can this be so? One suggestion as to how this might occur is that the vagina may be capable of experiencing the phenomenon known as "blindsight."

Blindsight is the term traditionally applied to the ability of some people with lesions in the visual cortex to respond appropriately to visual stimuli without having any conscious visual experience. That is, they respond as though they can see, even though they cannot see. And in some of the women with SCI, they respond as though they can feel the genital stimulation, even though they cannot feel it. So is this female orgasmic experience the equivalent in the female genital system of blindsight in the visual system? Moreover, is it the input of the vagus nerves that produces genital blindsight? With research into vaginal blindsight still at a very early stage, perhaps it's not surprising that the jury is still out on these questions. Other questions remain to be answered, too. Vaginal blindsight appears to suggest that the female genital orgasmic response is particularly robust. Why should this be so? Is female orgasm or the ability of female genitalia to respond in a characteristic muscular fashion essential for evolution or successful sexual reproduction?

Curiously, the human capacity for orgasm is not limited to arousal stemming from stimulation of genital nerves, be it the pudendal, pelvic, hypogastric, or vagus nerves. Orgasm can also be triggered as a result of stimulation of non-genital nerves, too. Non-genital orgasms—orgasms resulting from erotic and rhythmic stimulation of the breasts, mouth, knees, ears, shoulder, chin, and chest—all these have been recorded in a research setting. Pioneering sex researchers Masters and Johnson observed back-of-the-neck, small-of-the-back, bottom-of-the-foot, and palm-of-the-hand orgasms, and chose to view the whole body as a potentially erotic organ. Both

The woman added how her "whole body feels like it's in my vagina."

women and men with spinal cord injuries anecdotally report that stimulation of the hypersensitive skin zone that develops at or near the level of the injury to the spinal cord is capable of eliciting orgasm.

Laboratory investigations of these orgasmic episodes reveal that orgasm is indeed occurring. In one case, use of a vibrator on a woman's hypersensitive skin zone at her neck and shoulder resulted within several minutes in a characteristic increase in blood pressure, and an orgasm described as a "tingling and rush." The woman added how her "whole body feels like it's in my vagina." And while such non-genital phenomena demonstrate that orgasms can be produced by sensory stimulation of the rest of the human body, as well as the genitalia, other studies involving women show how, incredibly, imagery alone can be sufficient to trigger orgasm. For this group of women, physical stimulation was not needed to induce orgasm; their minds alone, thanks to fantasy, could take them there—despite being in a laboratory.

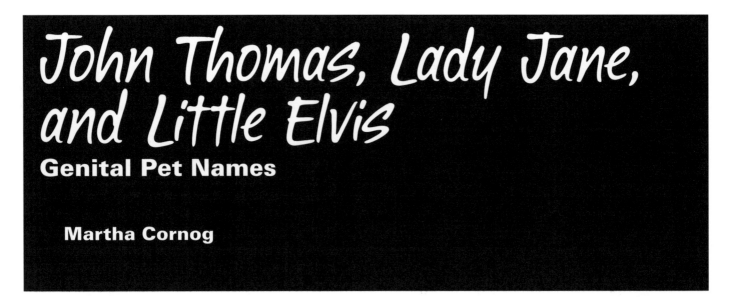

John Thomas, Lady Jane, and Little Elvis
Genital Pet Names

Martha Cornog

I am sitting in a room with about thirty women. The conference is billed as "A View Through the Speculum,"[1] and we are all attending a workshop on vaginal consciousness-raising. The group leader, a beautiful and vibrant woman of perhaps fifty, asks us each to say the word we use for our genitals. Going around the room, we speak in turn.

"Vagina."

"Pussy."

"Pussy. Vagina."

"Cunt."

"Mama's box."

"Henrietta."

Henrietta? Really?! Hmmm. In *Lady Chatterley's Lover*, Mellors the gamekeeper referred to his own erotic equipment as *John Thomas* and to Mrs. Chatterley's as *Lady Jane*.[2] Seems like D.H. Lawrence wasn't making this up.

Or was life imitating art?

Just about every language has dozens, even hundreds, of col-

orful slang expressions for the penis and vulva/vagina. Old friends in English include *cock*, *dick*, *hog*, *one-eyed wonder worm*, and *trouser snake*; *bearded clam*, *box*, *cunt*, *panty hamster*, and *pussy*.[3] But *John Thomas*, *Lady Jane*, *Mama's Box*, and *Henrietta* are clearly different in that they are used to refer to the genitals of one person only. Thus, they are not terms or expressions—they are proper names.

Indeed, our trusty Webster's confirms that a proper noun or proper name is a noun that designates a particular being or thing. We name people and pets, of course, real and fictional. As for things—well, we name places, movies, works of literature and art, songs, vehicles, and buildings. Sometimes we name weapons, like Aragorn's sword *Anduril* or the atomic bombs *Fat Man* and *Little Boy*. Oddball objects may get names, too, like a dancer's tap shoes or a favorite chair. Yet we don't name our ears, elbows, or legs.[4] ("Doctor, I just fell down the stairs, and I think Fred is broken.")

Naturally, I got curious. Did *Henrietta* and *Mama's Box* have much in the way of onomastic company in real life? Or did two very unusual women just happen to show up for that workshop? Eventually, I found out that that, yes, a fair number of actual humans do give pet names to sexual parts of the body: mainly the penis and vulva/vagina, and occasionally the clitoris, breasts, testicles, buttocks, and anus. I ended up collecting over 150 such names from adults in the US and Canada.[5] It was cheaper than collecting teapots, and, boy, did it make for interesting conversations at parties!

A fair number of actual humans do give pet names to sexual parts of the body.

But it's not like kids get a piece of paper from parents or teachers that says, "You can name your genitals if you want." You sure don't see chirpy little booklets in supermarkets next to those name-the-baby guides, say, something like *1001 Nifty Names for Naughty Bits*. Genital pet names are private names in more ways than one. Indeed, most people I talked to didn't know of anybody else who ever did this, and only a few had read *Lady Chatterley's Lover*. What kinds of names did they pick? How did it happen? And why? What did they think they were doing, anyway?

Patterns in Privates

Most of my name collection did sort itself into categories. About 6% somehow come from the name of the person whose body it is—let's call them the "owner." For example:

Penis

Chuck – owner's middle name is Charles

Goolie – short for *Guillermo*, "William" in Italian; owner's name is Bill

Hank Junior – owner's name is Hank

Little Willy – owner's name is Bill

Peter J. Firestone – Firestone is the surname of the owner

Maxwell's Silver Hammer – from the Beatles' song; Maxwell is the name of the owner

The Wilder Williams – Williams is the surname of the owner

Vulva

Little Joanie – owner's name is Joan

The largest group, about 51%, corresponds to normal person-type first names other than the owner's. Not a few sound unusual or old-fashioned:

Penis

George

Mortimer

Zeke

Vulva

Eunice

Miranda

Breasts

Jackie and *Jill*

Myra and *Myrtle*

A few people borrow names from celebrities:

Little Elvis – penis

Little Richard – penis; owner's name is not Richard or Dick

Sophia – vulva, after Sophia Loren, "the most beautiful woman in the world"

About 11% of the names are based on some characteristic of the genitals, real or attributed:

Penis

Sniffles – while examining a genital discharge, the doctor said that "maybe it had caught a cold"

Gnarled Tree Trunk – penis is heavily veined

The Little Mushroom – from the shape of the glans (the head of the penis)

Mexican Hairless – owner had little pubic hair

Vulva

Furry Rabbit

Fur

Hot and Juicy

Pink

Wonderland

Clitoris

Sweet Pea

Another large category, about 32%, comes from jokes or catchphrases, usually alluding to erections or sex:

Penis

Chunky – "open wide for a Chunky" was a slogan for a brand of candy bar

Lazarus – it rises from the dead

You sure don't see chirpy little booklets in supermarkets next to those name-the-baby guides, say, something like *1001 Nifty Names for Naughty Bits.*

Omar the Tentmaker – makes tents out of sheets

Owl – stays up all night

Winston – from the cigarette ad jingle: "Winston tastes good/Like a cigarette should"

Vulva

Fancy – as in, "tickle your..."

Rochester – city where owner lost her virginity

Virginia – from slogan of the state, "Virginia is for lovers" (also: similarity to the word *vagina* and play on the word *virgin*)

About 11% are variations of common terms for genitals:

Penis

   Dickie

   The Great Waldo Pecker

   My Favourite Member

   Putz

Vulva

   Coozie

   Honeypot

   Mama's Box

   Miss Muff

Testicles

   Ping and *Pong* ("balls")

I collected about twice as many penis names as vulva names.

In those conversations at parties, I was sometimes asked what the most common names are. Actually, I found few repeats. Only *George* and *Virginia* turned up as many as four times each; *Fred*, *Hank*, *Herbie*, *John Thomas*, *Peter*, *Winston*, and *Henrietta* all appeared twice. There's a reason for this that I'll get to shortly.

Who and How?

Who names genitals? Certainly not everybody, or I wouldn't have sat up at attention when I heard *Henrietta*. On the basis of no hard data whatsoever, I estimate that 5-10% of the population (maybe more) has either used a pet name or knows about somebody who has. Both men and women name genitals—not necessarily their own—and apparently most often when they are young and in an early or new sexual relationship. Here's how they talked about "the christening":

A quiz show was on the TV, and a couple had just been asked to name the dullest person they know. They replied, "Wilbur," and my husband promptly referred to his penis as Wilbur.... He's not always dull!

~

We were lying in bed and having fun, and the conversation had come up somehow to whether or not my penis was named, or her genitals were named, and she volunteered the name *Mortimer*. And I thought, "All right." And as quickly as I could, I volunteered a name for her, *Eunice*. So that just sort of became the pattern.

~

He had a large penis, with big veins sticking out all over it. And I guess I was playing with it. And for some reason, he made some kind of disparaging remark about it—the veins, somehow. And I said, "I don't know—I think it's really neat. It looks like a gnarled tree trunk." He was really taken by that. And he adopted it as a pet name and even shortened it to *GTT*. He'd say, "Old GTT here..."

Yet names could appear independently of any bed partner:

I remember I was in high school—I was on the football team, and one of the guys started naming everybody's male genitals as different dog names. And the reason I remember it is that one guy wasn't maturing as rapidly as the rest of them—he was a Mexican Hairless.

I collected about twice as many penis names as vulva names. But a good many came in pairs, two per couple:

Penis/Vagina

   Alice/Wonderland

   Baby/Home ("Does Baby want to go Home?")

   Butch/Little Place

   Calvin/Fur

   Darkness/Sunset

   Fred/Harriet

   George/Miranda

   George/Harriet

   The Great Waldo Pecker/Fancy

   Gruesome/Twosome

   Little Willy/Little Joanie

   Mortimer/Eunice

   My Favourite Member/Hot and Juicy

   Peanut Butter/Jelly

   Pedro/Virginia

   Snuffy/Katie Cooter

   Thurston/Sylvia

   Wilbur/Willeen

My favorite names were those supplied anonymously by a

couple who signed themselves only "Grampa and Gramma," taken from the characters in the kids' book *The Tale of Peter Rabbit*. Cute to the max, but so uncannily apt!

Flopsy and *Mopsy* – breasts

Cottontail – vulva

Peter – penis

The man who called his penis *Little Elvis* got it from Albert Goldman's biography—it seems that the King himself had a now-not-so-private penile moniker. Another man took penis/vulva names chosen by a teenage girlfriend and carried them over into his marriage, to somebody else. A couple of men adopted *John Thomas* from *Lady Chatterley's Lover*.

Since D.H. Lawrence was British, I wasn't surprised to read about a British guy-stripper who gave his business card to a woman reporter. The name on the card was "Jason."

"What's the name again?" asked the reporter.

"Brian."

"Then who the hell is Jason?"

"That's me penis, sweetheart. He's the one's got all the talent, you know."[6] (Was Jason looking for the Golden Fleece?)

Apparently, the impulse to name genitalia extends beyond English-speaking countries. A polyglot colleague collected several Arabic, Austrian, Hebrew, and Serbo-Croatian names known to linguist friends of his.[7]

So What's Going on Here?

Why do some people give names to body parts relating to sex?[8] As they told me stories about the names they came up with, I gradually got a feel for why they were doing this.

Secret Sex Codes. First, the names can serve as a deliciously secret language between lovers and sex partners or among other groups of people who know each other well. The chosen few can have a high old time talking about sex in public, with outsiders (including parents) completely clueless.

He was a very strong Catholic—very strong Catholic background. So we would be able to joke about this in front of his parents. "What are we going to do tonight?" He calls up on the phone. "I don't know, but let me ask Peter [his penis, *Peter J. Firestone*] about what *he'd* like to do." Or we would be sitting at dinner, and he would gratuitously toss off this comment, "Maybe we could double-date with Peter tonight." Then we'd

have to go, "Ha, ha, ha," and hope that his mother didn't see me turn red.

~

My friends, the Millers, Helene, always called Bill's cock *The Senator*. There was always a chance to make references in normal conversation; you see, they lived in Washington, DC.... Well, I know Helene and Bill very, very well, and years ago...Helene just somehow made a comment about this. And I said, "The Senator? What *is* all this?" And she said, and she sort of smiled a little bit and said, "Well, that's what I call Bill's penis."

Similarly, one of the *Winston* men and his girlfriend took sly pleasure in referring to "Winston's good taste" in front of friends.

Private Language, Private Games. Many people who supplied pet names used in a sexual relationship spoke of a sense of specialness and intimacy associated with the names, some adding that they were very much in love at the time.

We feel at ease when we use our pet names. It makes us feel closer.

~

We seldom use the "correct" words like *penis* and *vagina*. I guess *Calv[in]* and *Fur* are special names with their own special meaning, and that's why we use them.

"My friends, the Millers, Helene, always called Bill's cock *The Senator*."

The large percentage of genitals named jointly ("It just evolved in the course of our relationship.") seems to support the importance of this intimate language function. One sex manual advises genital-naming for this purpose:

Pat your man's penis during nonsexual moments. Give it a pet name such as "John Thomas," used by Lawrence's Lady Chatterley, or name it after its owner, calling it "Junior"—"David, Junior," "Mark, Junior," etc. A girl I know has long hilarious conversations with someone named Penis Desmond—P.D., for short—who answers her in a high-pitched falsetto voice. This little act is a fun way to humanize a woman's relationship to a man's penis.[9] [Note *Hank Junior* above.]

"Fun" is a good way to describe the way people use the names in intimate, joking conversations and games. I remember talking to the couple who use *Baby* and *Home* for penis and vulva. With much laughter and side glances, they told me about a card he had drawn for her showing a small house with a path leading up to it and a baby crawling up the path. Here's another story:

> **When I went up to visit him at college, he said, "I'd like you to meet the new Peter."** [*Peter J. Firestone*; see quote above.] **And I said, "Aw, c'mon." Standard joke. And he came back from the shower...with a pair of sunglasses on the suspended penis, hanging out as if it were a nose, and then of course he's got hair down there and his smiling scrotum underneath, and it was the funniest thing I ever saw in my life!... [T]hat was "the new Peter"—the new look.**

Talking and Not Talking About Sex. Genital pet names can also help people talk about sex in the broader sense. Many kids are not taught the "correct" terms for genitals. They may grow up with only expressions like *dickey bird* for penis or *muffin* for vulva—or with no words at all.[10] Girls especially may not know *vulva*, *clitoris*, or *vagina*. Or the youngsters may know the words but not be able to use them. I heard one story from a teacher in the Midwest about an eighth-grade boy who told dirty jokes and used four-letter words, but who became very upset when the teacher used *penis* in normal conversation.

Even when adults know all the words, they still may be uncomfortable with both correct and slang terms. Certainly, *pe-*

"He calls mine *Hot and Juicy*, while I call his *My Favourite Member*."

nis, *vulva*, and *vagina* can be associated quite unpleasantly with doctors and textbooks. But genital slang conjures up those dirty jokes. One woman in her late thirties expressly told me that she was uncomfortable with all four-letter words. Another admitted, "Because of the kind of people that we were [when she was twenty, in the 1950s], it was awfully hard to talk about sex directly." Sex educators working on college campuses have told me that although the students in their twenties may be using dirty words, they don't like to mix them with intimacy and romance. One educator said that nearly 50% of her classes in New York City gave some sort of idiosyncratic synonym or name when asked for terms for genitals:

> **I said [to the classes], "What are the advantages of these names? Why have another name for it?" [The names were] very similar to the street language, except the street language has no lovingness in it,**

and doesn't have that personalization that a pet name has.... They associate a lot of those [street] words—they're not positive words all the time. They're used to insult someone. And they're too common. I think most people feel special about the body. They don't want to use one word used by 87 million people.

The following comment in my files echoes this:

> **He calls mine *Hot and Juicy,* while I call his *My Favourite Member*. When I first met him I simply referred to it as Peter, but I soon wanted a name which would be unique and original in that it probably isn't used by anyone else.**

So here is why I found so few duplicate names. Nearly everybody wants something special and different. Thus, even if *1001 Nifty Names for Naughty Bits* were published, it would be more likely to inspire readers to come up with original names than choose any from the book. Because genital pet names are private, owners and their intimates have ultimate freedom in choosing them. They can pick *Agamemnon*—or *Happy Fella* (real examples). They don't have to keep up with the Johnsons' johnson.

A colleague of mine, a marriage counselor for several years, told me:

> **One of the things we frequently encountered were people who were having a great deal of difficulty verbally communicating about sex, and the reason was that they were extremely...uncomfortable with what they considered to be profane words, and they were uncomfortable with the official Latin terminology. And what was typically going on, then, was just nothing. With lack of a label, people weren't talking.**
>
> **So...after playing around with it for a while, I thought about the possibility of using made-up words. So we started doing that in therapy, and we found it to be very successful. A lot of couples who had had trouble before really got into it, found it very enjoyable, and developed a whole new vocabulary for sex organs and sexual acts....**
>
> **From a therapeutic point of view, it was a very good idea, because, in addition to giving them a label that they could use to communicate and increase the effectiveness of what they were doing,... it [also] created a very nice thing for them to do together. The process of thinking up names and developing this whole new vocabulary was a**

very enjoyable process of sharing for most of the couples that tried it.

Threesomes and Foursomes in Bed. Finally, the pet name bestows an identity upon the genitals: They seem to have a personality independent from the owner:[11]

Pet names do add to the intimacy of the relationship. It's as if they take on personalities all their own.

~

Since then, *Me Too* [her husband's penis] has his own personality and really adds to our sexual relationship with each other.

Much popular writing about sex and psychology describes the alienation and love/hate relationship men sometimes have with their penises. A hard-on in the subway that won't go away. An erection that collapses despite a hot date. As one men's lib book puts it, "He curses his penis for not performing, as he sweats and strains and informs his partner that *he* really wants to, even though something is wrong with *it*."[12] And a veteran of the gender wars recapitulates a skirmish:

My penis: I don't want to get turned on here. This bed is not safe for me.

My mind: Shut up! Perform! Don't let me down!... You're humiliating me in front of Rosalie![13]

A *Playboy* journalist writing about the penis quotes a man she interviewed:

"My penis is attracted to certain types [of women], falls in love, but these women and I never get along." [This man] is annoyed by, but affectionate towards his member, which he thinks is extremely demanding.[14]

Not that man vs. penis is new. As early as 426 CE, Saint Augustine wrote:

[A man] could wish that, just as all his other members obey his reason in the performance of their appointed tasks, so that organs of parenthood, too, might, too, function in obedience to the orders of will and not be excited by the ardors of lust.... [But] sometimes their lust is most importunate when they least desire it; at other times the feelings fail them when they crave them most, their bodies remaining frigid when lust is blazing in their souls.[15]

A man having some of these feelings who gives a pet name to his penis can thereby wash his hands of what "it" does

and at the same time diffuse his anxiety through humor. Lawrence's Mellors illustrates this:

The man looked down in silence at the tense phallus, that did not change. – "Ay!" he said at last, in a little voice, "Ay ma lad! tha'art thee right enough. Yi, the mun rear they head! Theer on thy own, eh? An' ta'es no count o' nob'dy! Tha ma'es nowt o' me, John Thomas. Art boss? Of me? Eh well, tha'art more cocky than me, an'that says less. John Thomas! Does want *her*? Dost want my lady Jane?... Tell Lady Jane tha wants cunt, John Thomas....[16]

People talk like this in real life, too:

Little Willy—he talked about *Little Willy* as being a separate entity totally. He was standing up at

"My penis is attracted to certain types [of women], falls in love, but these women and I never get along."

attention wanting *Little Joanie*.... [T]he most interesting thing [was that] he hated to have anyone call him Willy. His name was Bill.... [But] so far as his penis was concerned, he adored it.

~

My guess is, I first heard this from my father—this would have been around 1958 or '59,... after my mother stopped coming to the cabin [a vacation fishing cabin], and it was at a time when, as a regular occurrence, he would drink approximately a fifth of Governor's Club a day. During the week he wouldn't drink at all,... but in the weekends, he'd really lay into it. But this was up at the cabin... probably on the Saturday night of opening day [of trout season] I can remember vividly. He was drunker than a warthog. He was railing and ranting around...sing[ing] his songs, play[ing] his record player. And I remember the song in particular that he would play and still plays to this day, is "I Took My Organ to the Party, but Nobody Asked Me to Play."

And having played this song over and over again about 25 times, it came time when he had to relieve himself...and I had to relieve myself at the same time. I can remember being fairly sober at the time—this is too vivid a memory for me to have been too drunk. But we get out on the porch and he's saying, "Oh, what a wonderful time we're

having—" and sort of between that and singing, "I took my organ to the party," he's fumbling around with his fly.... He takes this rather large tool out of his pants, and he starts to relieve himself—a fairly steady stream—and he starts talking to his organ and, by God, he calls the thing *Hank*. He says, "Aw, look at old Hank here, poor, poor old guy." And he says, "You and I, we've been in a couple of tight places together and we've had our ups and downs, but I want you to know, you old sonofabitch"— and this is where he starts shaking it off—"that I outlived you!"[17]

And about a woman:

This woman called her clitoris *She*. Apparently it began when she became sexually liberated—she found her own moral beliefs somewhat at odds with what her newly awakened body wanted to do, so that it was convenient for her to explain her behavior as a result of physical urges that she now felt very strongly in her clitoris. Remembering that somewhere she had read that adolescent males were led around by their penis, she decided that that was what was happening to her; she was being led around by her clitoris.... [She would say things like:] "She made me do it; I had nothing to do with it" (in describing or accounting for how she had gotten involved in a number of sexual incidents).

Women sometimes name their dildos and vibrators.

Sometimes partners join the dialog:

I always talk to the penises of my male partners. That's something I always do. I've never stopped doing that. As if, you know, "*You* go away—I'm talking to *him*."

When we name something, what are we doing? Besides humans, we name pet animals, vehicles, weapons, and other special objects. We use these names to indicate a particular relationship with us and to say that we find whatever-it-is unique, even an "honorary human."

He had brought columbines and campions, and new-mown-hay, and oak-tufts and honey-suckle in small bud. He fastened fluffy young oak-sprays round her breasts, sticking in tufts of bluebells and campion: and in her navel he posed a pink camion flower, and in her maidenhair were forget-me-nots

and wood-ruff.

"That's you in all your glory!" he said. "Lady Jane, at her wedding with John Thomas."

And he stuck flowers in the hair of his own body, and wound a bit of creeping-jenny round his penis, and stuck a single bell of hyacinth in her navel.[18]

Like lovers and friends, the genitals seem to deserve special names because, like lovers—and alone among body parts!— the genitals can provide a very special pleasure, comfort, and satisfaction. Lovers and friends are very close to us, but yet not-us; so, too, our pelvic partners in life seem to be "us" and "not-us." And, like lovers and friends, our genitals sometimes disappoint us. But we always remain attached to them and they to us, part of us always, yet somehow...unique.

Endnotes

An earlier version of this article was published as "Tom, Dick, and Hairy: Notes on Genital Pet Names," *Maledicta*, 5.1+2 (Summer+Winter 1981): 31-41.

1. "A View Through the Speculum: A Workshop on Vaginal Health and Politics." Sponsored by the Elizabeth Blackwell Health Center for Women. Philadelphia, 17 May 1980.

2. Lawrence, D.H. *Lady Chatterley's Lover*. New American Library, 1959: 196-7, 212-4, 283. *John Thomas* is defined in slang dictionaries as "the penis; a personification of the penis" in British colloquial speech. (See Spears, Richard A. *Slang and Euphemism*. Middle Village, NY: Jonathan David, 1981; Healey, Tim. "A New Erotic Vocabulary." *Maledicta* 4.2 (Winter 1980): 191.) Thus, a man could refer to his own John Thomas or someone else's. But Mellors uses it as a proper name, parallel to *Lady Jane*.

3. For additional terms and expressions for genitals, see Tim Healey's article in note 3 and Hankey, Clyde. "Naming the Vulvar Part." *Maledicta* 4.2 (Winter 1980): 220-2.

4. However: "There once was a man from Montrose/Who diddled himself with his toes/He did it so neat/He fell in love with his feet/And christened them *Myrtle* and *Rose*." Here the feet become the vulva/vagina, thus in a sense, *Myrtle* and *Rose* are analogous to genital pet names. So too, the hands when used for masturbation: Basketball star Dennis Rodman has admitted to "an ongoing relationship with Judy (his right hand) and Monique (his left)" (Segell, Michael. "The Sex Men Lie About." *Esquire*, Sept 1996: 68). Indeed, pud-pulling slang in a number of languages personifies the hand, e.g., *go see Mary Fivefingers* or *estar casado con la viuda de los cinco hijos*. (See my *The Big Book of Masturbation*. San Francisco: Down There Press, 2003: 16-22.) Genital pet names carry over to artificial genitals—women sometimes name their dildos and vibrators. (Perhaps men name artificial vaginas, but I've never seen any examples.) In addition, some sex-toy catalogs use human names to refer to particular dildo designs. I have occasionally read about amputees who named their prostheses, and studying this is on my to-do list of neat projects. But I have never heard of anyone naming such common and nonerotic implements as false teeth or hearing aids. A phenom that could be related to genital pet names is the fact that expressions for menstruation sometimes personify it, e.g., "My Aunt Flow is coming from Redfield, Pennsylvania"; "I've got my friend"; "Grandma is here from Red Creek." See Ernster, Virginia L. "American Menstrual Expressions." *Sex Roles*, 1 (1975): 1-13.

5. Pseudonyms are used for informants' surnames. All informants were Caucasian. One woman self-identified as lesbian; the remainder, when information was supplied, described heterosexual relationships. I don't know of any research into genital pet names used by ethnic minorities or GLBT-identified people. More neat projects—anyone interested?

6. "A Big Gland for the Little Ladies." *Oui*, 4.3 (March 1975): 13.

7. Aman, Reinhold, and Friends. "What Is This Thing Called, Love? More Genital Pet Names." *Maledicta*, 5.1+2 (Summer+Winter 1981): 41-4.

8. Private sex slang between lovers can extend far beyond genital pet names. For one couple, "Do you need to get a sweater?" meant, "Let's leave whatever we're doing and go back to the house and have sex." I ran across many other expressions like *wiener roast*, *whoopee time*, *waffles*, *hoot-nanny*, *go play*. Proust's characters Swann and Odette use the phrase "do a cattleya"—a cattleya is a type of orchid, and the couple's first sexual encounter began with Swann adjusting her corsage. Proust's description underscores the intimacy and specialness of the phrase for Swann:

> **...and the [sexual] pleasure which he had already felt [with Odette]...seemed to [Swann]...a pleasure which had never before existed, which he was striving now to create, a pleasure—as the special name he gave it was to certify—entirely individual and new. (Proust, Marcel.** *Swann in Love.* **Trans. C.K. Scott Moncrieff and Terence Kilmartin. Vintage, 1984: 66-7.)**

9. Hollander, Xaviera. *Xaviera's Supersex: Her Personal Techniques for Total Lovemaking*. New American Library, 1976: 134.

10. For a list of "pseudonyms for sex organs" collected from children in several countries, see Goldman, Ronald and Juliette. *Children's Sexual Thinking*. London: Routledge & Kegan Paul, 1982: 210-1. Families and kids can find these terms fun, useful, and convenient. But everyone also needs to know terms like *penis* and *vulva* and use them when necessary, such as with health professionals.

11. Personifying the genitals goes much further than simply giving them proper names: it encompasses themes of talking genitals, genitals spoken to, genitals acting on their own volition, genitals drawn as independent beings, and genital gods. These themes show up in sexual humor, literature (*The Satyricon*, *Lady Chatterley's Lover*, *Tropic of Capricorn*, *Portnoy's Complaint*), mythology (Priapus worship), and graphic arts. Particularly striking are a delightful series of Japanese prints showing a Sumo wrestling match between a penis and a vulva—ending with the penis being engulfed by the vulva—or perhaps diving in (Kronhausen, Phyllis and Eberhard. *The Complete Book of Erotic Art*. New York: Bell, 1978; see the reference in note 1 for more examples). A waggish friend once gave me a "Jumping Jolly Pecker" wind-up toy, made in Hong

Modern erotic-themed Japanese manga comics may show personified genitals.

Kong and looking remarkably similar to these drawings. Modern erotic-themed Japanese manga comics may also show personified genitals. In Haruka Inui's *Ogenki Clinic*, a raunchy and hilarious send-up of sex therapy, clinic manager Dr. Ogekuri's penis looks just like him, with moustache and miniature glasses. One of the clinic's patients turns out to be a *shiimaru*—a woman with a penis. And *her* penis looks just like her as well, down to the sultry eyes and long blonde hair, making it indeed a female penis! (Studio Ironcat, 5(6), 1989; 7(2), 1989.)

12. Goldberg, Herb. *The New Male: From Self-Destruction to Self-Care*. Morrow, 1979: 120.

13. Rubin, Jerry, and Mimi Leonard. *The War Between the Sheets*. New York: Richard Marek Publishers, 1980: 120.

14. Schor, Linda. "Some Perspectives on the Penis." *Playboy*, July 1980: 151, 179, 183-9.

15. Saint Augustine. *The City of God* (abridged ed.). Garden City, NY: Image Books, 1958: 315-6.

16. Op cit, Lawrence: 196-7.

17. This story is quoted almost in its entirety to provide the background leading up to the father's rueful monolog. His wife no longer came to the cabin to make merry with the group—sexual and emotional relations had deteriorated almost completely between them. This was substantiated in other conversations with the son of "Hank's" owner.

18. Op cit, Lawrence: 213.

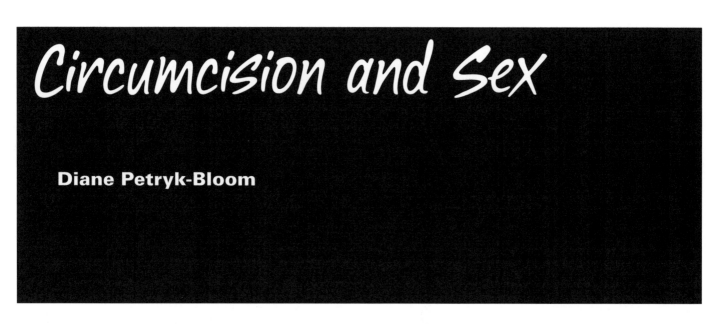

Circumcision and Sex

Diane Petryk-Bloom

Want her to *totally* want it, *totally* need it, and *totally* love it?

Want to have her thinking of you instead of thinking of England?

Men who want more sex, listen up. She needs to like it better, and she'll like it better if you realize what's missing—your foreskin.

As you read this, at least 100,000 men across America are taping, tying, and tugging their penises to stretch new foreskin.[1] Most lost their foreskins in infancy when they were circumcised, but somewhere along the line they discovered that sex without a foreskin just isn't what nature intended.

In the uncircumcised man, the sexually aroused penis peeks from foreskin, then bursts full-out, sending ripples of skin back on the shaft. Those waves of stretching and retreating foreskin give the male one the most exquisite sensations in all sexual experience.

That's because the foreskin is the most important sensory tissue of the penis.[2]

Pleasurable sensations provided by a foreskin are "so incredibly great," in fact, that "no man should miss out on them," says author Jeffrey O'Hara, a circumcised-but-restored—as far as can be—male.

That, in itself, isn't enough to motivate most men to worry about developing new foreskin. Here's what is: She needs it. It's the key to pleasuring your woman. Get it, get her more often.

Here's why: Circumcised men have lost considerable sensory tissue. Important nerve endings—gone. Some hate the idea. But many still say they have all the pleasure they can stand, so what's the problem? They have perfectly serviceable erections. They have orgasms and ejaculations. The problem is

how they get there. Researchers have recently discovered that the mechanism of arousal and intercourse is entirely different for the circumcised man and the foreskin-intact man.

Whether or not a circumcised male has any problems, recent anatomical studies show that his partner probably will.

In 1996 Dr. John Taylor and colleagues in the Pathology Department at the University of Manitoba decided to assess the type and amount of tissue missing from the circumcised adult penis. (Incredibly, humans have been trimming penises since 2000-something BCE[3] and no one had yet assessed the damage!)

Taylor found an elastic-like band of mucosal tissue at the tip of the foreskin. He calls it the ridged band.[4] It teems with specialized nerve endings—similar to those on the fingers and lips. The head of the penis, or glans, by contrast, and contrary to popular belief, is fairly insensitive.

When the penis is relaxed, the ridged band narrows over its tip like a drawn duffle bag. Sexual arousal dilates the band, sliding it back past the glans and onto the shaft, where it rolls up and down during intercourse. The rolling and stretching stimulates the erogenous nerves in the band to fire off sensations of pleasure.[5]

From an evolutionary perspective, the object of sexual stimulation in the male is to build up contractions in the genital musculature. Kristen O'Hara, with her husband Jeff O'Hara, explains in her 2001 book, *Sex As Nature Intended It*, that it is these alternate tensing and relaxing actions that lead to orgasm and ejaculation of sperm.

They point out that Josephine Lowndes Sevely's seven-year

study comparing male and female genitalia revealed that highly erogenous tissue equivalent to the female clitoris is located in the core of the penis throughout the entire length of the shaft. Only the foreskin is positioned to stimulate it by natural massaging action.

The circumcised man has to reach for equivalent stimulation in an awkward, unnatural way. Sometimes he has difficulty reaching orgasm. Other times he may not be able to extend intercourse more than a few seconds. In either case, his female partner suffers.

"It is important to understand how muscular contractions can bring on orgasm because the intact (natural) man and the circumcised man induce them differently," the O'Haras write. "[T]he means they use to create these contractions affect their thrusting movements and rhythms.

"The design of the natural penis indicates that nature intended for pleasure and orgasm to be induced by actions taking place mostly in the upper area of the penis. However, for the circumcised penis, the upper penis mechanisms and responses have been drastically altered and do not function the way nature intended. Consequently, the circumcised male is left to improvise alternative or supplementary means to attain orgasm. It is use of these odd varieties or orgasm-building (pleasure seeking) techniques that causes him to thrust much differently from the intact man, and which his female partner finds frustrating and disrupting to her pleasuring needs."

And sometimes downright painful.

Marsha Goudreau (name disguised), a Michigan woman whose late husband of more than twenty years was uncircumcised, later experienced sex with circumcised men and said she now knows her husband's foreskin was a blessing for both of them.

"The nice thing that happens is that the gliding back and forth stimulates the head of the penis without irritating it," she says.[6] "The shaft moves in and out of that glove, which pleasures the woman without painful friction. And if you're not having intercourse for some reason, the foreskin makes a handjob a lot easier."

In technical terms: "Mucosal surfaces of the glans and foreskin move back and forth across the mucosal surfaces of the labia and vagina, providing nontraumantic sexual stimulation for both male and female.

"This mucous membrane-to-mucous membrane contact provides natural lubrication necessary for sexual relations and prevents both the dryness responsible for painful intercourse and the chafing and abrasions which allow entry of sexually transmitted diseases, both viral and bacterial."[7]

✕✕

Yet couples with a circumcised man need not despair. Foreskin restoration offers reparations. Re-covered glans will soften again. Jeff O'Hara's message for circumcised men: "Restoring your foreskin is the best thing that's going to happen to you in this lifetime."

Kristen's message: "From the woman's sexual perspective, the restored penis is virtually equivalent to the natural penis in every respect."

There are surgical and nonsurgical methods of restoration. O'Hara opted for a graft of skin from his scrotum. It has the advantage of having muscle tissue that's able to provide the thrill of stretch upon erection. Nonsurgical restoration involves pulling what is left of flaccid skin at the base of the penis when it is not erect, to stretch it. Several simple devices have been invented for this purpose.[8] One consists simply of taping drawn-up skin, with a clip attached to the end of the tape and a tugging force applied by an elastic band around the waist.

Circumcised men have lost considerable sensory tissue. Important nerve endings—gone.

"It's cheap and works well enough," says David Steinburg (name disguised) from his home in the Midwest. "While there's still a ways to go, there is no question that the regrowth of some skin has made a real difference in feeling, and I can only imagine what it must be like for those fortunate enough to have avoided circumcision in the first place."

Ron Low of Chicago thought taping lacked something in elegance, so he invented a cone-shaped attachment that pulls naturally after skin is inserted. Obversion, the tendency of skin to roll back, keeps it in place. Low says one can expect to add about one inch per year if the tugger is worn twelve hours a day. His progress with his TLC Tugger is documented on his website [tlctugger.com]. Low says he's sold more than 2,000 with "nothing but positive feedback."

The Joy of Uncircumcising by James Bigelow is the complete guide to restoration techniques.[9]

Whatever the method, the object is to restore enough skin to cover the glans of the relaxed penis, such as happens naturally when the penis is uncircumcised. Complete coverage, which the O'Haras advise, allows the penis to maintain its naturally moist, softly stiff characteristic. (The glans of a circumcised penis is continually exposed, and as a result, can become hardened or keratinized.)

While foreskin restoration can replace this protective covering, merely stretching the skin cannot restore the special orgasmic triggers and glands that were cut and eliminated. Especially the very sensitive frenulum.

The frenulum is the connecting tissue of the foreskin and shaft. Structurally, it is similar to the frenulum that connects the tongue to the base of the mouth. In the same way that the frenulum controls the tongue, researchers believe the penile frenulum controls thrusting. It's on the underside of the shaft, or on top of an erect penis when a man is lying on his back. It, too, is highly enervated, erogenous tissue.

"Often only a remnant of the frenulum is left after circumcision, if it is not also removed," says anti-circumcision crusader Marilyn Milos. "Many circumcised men consider it their 'G-spot,' but only because their 'G-area,' the ridged band and frenular delta, has been removed."[10]

During sex, there is a way to compensate for that loss, Jeff O'Hara found. "The ridged band of the foreskin and the skin of the nipples are comprised of the same specialized nerve tissue called 'rete ridges.' Nipple skin abounds with Meissner's corpuscles (erotically responsive, touch-sensitive nerves), like those found in the foreskin and frenulum.

"When you have your partner twiddle your nipples during intercourse, combined with the increased pleasure experienced after restoration, I reckon that it heightens your sexual feelings to those experienced by the genitally intact man when his penis alone is stimulated during intercourse.... During this activity, the levels of ecstasy are so magnificent, I don't feel cheated in any way, even though I'm missing the nerves of the ridged ban."

"The design of the natural penis indicates that nature intended for pleasure and orgasm to be induced by actions taking place mostly in the upper area of the penis."

Sex as Nature Intended It came about after Kristen O'Hara experienced both natural and circumcised sex and tried to make sense of the difference. While happily married to Jeff, she came to realize that foreskin is what's missing in millions of bedrooms across America—bedrooms where sex is unfulfilling, uncomfortable, and/or avoided.

Her personal experiences[11] and comparisons led to attempts to discover if she was alone in her feelings. She wasn't! Surveys of about 138 women showed that almost all of them prefer natural sex. It was the difference between not being able to get enough and, "There, that'll hold you for a few days." Sitcoms spend a lot of time on male jokes about pursuing sex in the face of expected feminine refusal because it reflects the situation in the real world, she says.

Women in their twenties are often gung ho, regardless; in their thirties, it's okay, she says, but much beyond that age their interest falls off with their lessening vaginal lubrication and the built-up resentment of sex that too often has been uncomfortable and unsatisfying.

Female partners of circumcised men become aroused, crave the sensation of penetration, and enjoy orgasm just as much as partners of intact men. But they express dissatisfaction with the overall experience of sexual relations. Kristen was no different. She loved her husband and they were compatible, but their relationship wasn't good sexually.

"Our love lacked depth," she writes, "the kind of depth that exists when a couple has a deeply satisfying, exquisitely delicious, sensuous, sexual interconnectedness." Because sex with Jeff was annoying, even though desired, Kristen drifted back into her uncircumcised lover's bed.

"During our rendezvous, I couldn't help but notice that his penis felt much more sensuous inside me; it felt infinitely better, deliciously better, indescribably better.

"In characterizing the differences...I would say the circumcised experience is like being repeatedly penetrated in an annoying way, even though simultaneously there is pleasure. And the penis feels too hard, almost foreign-like— you want it, but don't want it, at the same time, driven onward only in hopes of achieving orgasm, the sooner the better. Whereas, with natural, the vagina totally surrenders to the soft sensuousness of lingering ecstasy, as it hungrily caresses and lovingly responds to the erotic movements of the softly-stiff penis, and the penis adores and gently strokes the vagina in return.

"Like two halves of a perfect whole, each organ swoons and sighs to a passionate intermingling...

"With no holding back, you TOTALLY want it, you TOTALLY need it, and you TOTALLY love it."

One explanation: Since the natural penis tends to stay more deeply embedded in the vagina using short strokes, it brings the man's pubic area in frequent contact with the woman's clitoral mound, allowing her clitoris to be pressure-pleasured more often and at a consistent rhythmical rate throughout much of intercourse.

Not only does the circumcised man make longer strokes to stimulate his pleasure areas, he needs to pause, often outside the vagina, to let the nerve endings recharge. The natural man's penis retreats into its foreskin, not having to withdraw from the vagina.

Jeff O'Hara says you can witness the longer strokes and withdrawals in X-rated videos with circumcised men. In fact, he watched a video made of John Bobbitt performing sex. Bobbitt is the man whose wife, Lorena, cut off his penis. Doctors reattached the organ, but Bobbitt lost nerve connections. He performs just like a circumcised man must, O'Hara says: "Pull out, rest, come in fast. Like pile-driving with punishing blows."

Even if the woman can tolerate it, that technique precludes rhythmic build-up for the clitoris.

In her bestselling book, *How to Have an Orgasm...as Often as You Want*, Rachel Swift says a lack of consistent rhythm is one of the chief causes of a woman's failure to climax. "If the pace is broken, so's the ascent to orgasm."

Why do *so many* women fake orgasm? Because *so many* men are circumcised. Women know they're not going to climax the way he's doing it...and they're taking a battering. They might just as well fake it and hope he gets it over with soon. Often the best you can do with circumcised sex is to pleasure the man and woman separately, in succession, rather than simultaneously.

"It was like we were using each other's body to masturbate against," Jeff says of his marital sex before he restored his foreskin, "which is not the same as making love. Lovers totally abandon their individual egos, their individual awareness, and become a union of pleasuring."

Here's a sampling of comments from Kristen O'Hara's survey respondents:

> **My circumcised husband was totally engrossed in satisfying his own sexual needs; therefore, he pounded and banged as if he were having intercourse with a non-feeling person.**

> ~

> **It feels so good to have the feeling of a man's foreskin in my vagina.... [I]t glides easily. Once a natural penis is in your vagina, you wish it could stay forever.**

> ~

> **My natural partner kept more constant pressure on my whole genital area during intercourse. I felt like he was in sync with me.... I had more time to relax, and I would always orgasm before it was over, so afterwards I felt content.**

> ~

> **My sexual experiences with three natural men were extraordinary in the gentleness, sensuality, and mutuality.**

> ~

> **Natural men have a more laid-back approach. They don't seem to feel as rushed or pressed to achieve orgasm. They seem to enjoy the act rather than the resulting orgasm.**

> ~

> **There is definitely more clitoral stimulation with natural.**

> ~

> **Sometimes it's [circumcised sex] too much work for too little reward. When it's over I think to myself, "Thank God he finally came."**

> ~

> **I have noticed that the vagina is much more accepting of the natural penis. Once the head of the natural penis is at the opening of the vagina, it just kind of naturally slides in.**

> ~

> **I've often said to myself after one of these circumcised encounters: I would have been better off masturbating.**

> ~

> **With my natural man, I always glow after intercourse, but with circumcised men, I couldn't wait to get dressed and get away from them. I never glowed.**

> ~

> **The visual effect of seeing an impending erection just starting to peek out of its foreskin is just so much sexier.**

> ~

> **I never made the connection between this feeling of hostility and circumcised sex until now.**

O'Hara's research was first published in the *British Journal of Urology* in 1999. Bestselling author Dr. Christiane Northrup[12] credits the research for helping her fully understand the reasons for the design of the penis and foreskin.

"I always felt that the male foreskin, one of the most richly enervated and hyperelastic pieces of tissue in the male body, is there for a reason," she wrote in an article for her newsletter, *Health Wisdom for Women* (June 2001). "Until recently, I didn't know exactly what that reason was. But now thanks to Kristen O'Hara's well-researched book...I finally understand the reasons for the design of the penis and foreskin and how this design ensures optimal penile function, including the organ's ability to satisfy the female sexually.

"O'Hara makes a compelling argument that circumcised intercourse may frustrate the primordial subconscious that seems to know 'real sex ain't this way.' She also suggested that each circumcised experience has the potential to build-up negative memory imprints so that over time, repeated sexual encounters with the same partner may lead to negative feeling between the two that carry over into everyday life."

As an obstetrician-gynecologist, Northrup said, she performed hundreds of circumcisions. While she stops short of saying she regrets doing them, she does say it's past time to rethink the practice. She reported elsewhere that when she would tell parents at hospital-based childbirth classes that circumcision need not be done, her invitations to such classes were withdrawn.

She quotes obstetrics colleague Dr. George Denniston, co-author of *Doctors Re-Examine Circumcision*: "Circumcision violates the first tenet of medical practice: 'First, do no harm.' According to modern medical ethics, parents do not have the right to consent to a procedure that is not in their son's best interest. The removal of a normal, important part of the male sexual organ is not in their son's best interest."

Jews, Muslims, and a few other groups circumcise as part of their religious practice. But, as a nation, we do not allow parents to impose their religious practices on children to the extent that they do physical harm. Blood transfusions, for instance, are often imposed by court order for children whose parents do not approve for religious reasons. Should genital mutilation[13] be any different?

From a worldwide perspective, the noncircumcised state is the norm for males. Most Europeans and Asians do not circumcise. Wrongful-circumcision attorney David Llewellyn says that he attended a conference in Padua, Italy, in 2004 and told a thirty-five-year-old Italian pediatrician that Americans circumcise about 65% of all boys. "You're kidding!" she said.

Although circumcision rates are dropping in the US, it is estimated that about 60% of newborn males in America are still being cut. If you're an American man between the ages of twenty-five and forty-five, the probability is very high that you were circumcised. Newborn circumcision rates in the US climbed after World War II and peaked at about 80-90% somewhere between 1970 and 1980. If you're older or younger, chances are still good that if you were in an American nursery, you lost your foreskin.

In our cultural acceptance of circumcising males, we keep company with countries like Afghanistan, Algeria, Iran, Iraq, Saudi Arabia, Turkey, Somalia, and the Congo. Some circumcise newborns; most do it at older ages, as a part of religious practice. The United States is the only circumcising country that, generally, has no religious pretense. Circumcisions are usually performed on newborns in hospitals for aesthetic preference, hygienic theory, or for no reason at all. Many parents simply acquiesce to circumcision when the physician offers it, without asking questions. "If it's offered, it must be recommended," seems to be the prevailing view. It's familiar. It's the accepted norm.

Several groups, such as NORM (National Organization of Restoring Men), NOHARMM (National Organization to Halt the Abuse and Routine Mutilation of Males), and NOCIRC, have formed to fight the practice, but it is entrenched. For many it's a matter of "like father, like son." Men who cannot accept that they are less than perfect perpetuate the practice. "Recognizing male circumcision as a mistake reflects on circumcised males."[14] Others, doctors and mothers, may be in denial, as well.

Americans' willingness to conform and disinclination to inquire deeply is another factor. Parents are usually unaware of the extent of the surgery. The amount of skin amputated results in the loss of about one-third or more of the penile shaft skin system. Adult foreskin is about two and a half inches long. It's double layered, so when unfolded, it would be about the size of a 3x5-inch card, enough skin to hold millions of cells and nerves. The removal of the often-described "snip of skin" is considered a major amputaton by some.

It is usually done without anesthesia. Milos, who first witnessed circumcision as a student nurse, went on to make a video of the operation, which she shows to expecting parents. She was told it was too much for parents to see. "Perhaps then," Milos responded, "it's too much for the baby to endure."

"We didn't learn anything about foreskins or circumcision in medical school," says Dr. Paul Fliess.[16] "I watched one, that was it." They were taught that infants don't feel pain, which has been shown to be an absurd notion.

Taylor and colleagues, who discovered the ridged band, have also noted "the current tendency to eliminate the prepuce from anatomy textbooks."

How it became thus is no mystery. Circumcision got its first big jump-start in the US in the late nineteenth century when doctors decided that masturbation was harmful.

A boy with foreskin would have to retract it to urinate, so, they reasoned, he would be more likely to learn to give himself pleasure by self-manipulation. Cutting off the foreskin as a remedy became the rage. In 1888, John Kellogg, of corn-flakes fame, wrote a book blaming masturbation for thirty-one ailments and identified things like shyness and insomnia as symptoms of masturbation.

Soon, circumcision was advocated for infants to prevent, rather than cure, masturbation.

Here are excerpts from medical journals of the late 1800s:

> **There can be no doubt of [masturbation's] injurious effect, and of the proneness to practice it on the part of children with defective brains. Circumcision should always be practiced. It may be necessary to make the genitals so sore by blistering fluids that pain results from attempts to rub the parts.[17]**

~

> **In consequence of circumcision the epithelial covering of the glans becomes dry, hard...the sensibility of the glans is diminished, but not sufficiently to interfere with the copulative function of the organ or to constitute an objection.... It is well authenticated that the foreskin...is a fruitful cause of the habit of masturbation in children.... I conclude that the foreskin is detrimental to health, and that circumcision is a wise measure of hygiene.[18]**

Great Britain joined in the masturbation hysteria, as did Canada, Australia, and New Zealand. Those countries have since rejected arguments for circumcision as fallacious.

Dr. Benjamin Spock advocated circumcision in 1946. He reversed himself in 1976.[19]

The British circumcision rate peaked at more than 30%, then, by the 1950s, fell dramatically. By the time Princess Diana gave birth to Prince William, it was less than 1%. Prince Charles was circumcised, but Diana insisted the young princes be left intact.[20] In her case, the fact that the National Health Service dropped coverage of the procedure probably wasn't a deciding factor. For the majority of Britons, it may have been the biggest one.

By the 1930s, even those who ate corn flakes accepted that masturbation wasn't harmful, but by then circumcision was going strong. Since Jews circumcised for religious reasons, some Jews promoted it for health reasons, too, applying to all, so Jews wouldn't be singled out by the practice. Doctors latched onto the next promulgated theory: Circumcision was more hygienic. After a while, claims were made for its curing or prevention of a host of diseases and disorders, from epilepsy to insomnia. These arguments were debunked one by one, but circumcision still has its proponents. They often tout prevention of penile cancer and cervical cancer as benefits of circumcision. Penile cancer is exceedingly rare, and preventing it is not a reason for depriving millions of their bodily integrity and sexual birthright. Women with uncircumcised partners don't get more cervical cancer. Studies that have shown such supposed links have been seriously flawed.[21]

Recently, AIDS prevention has been suggested as justification for circumcision. This flies in the face of facts. The United States and certain African countries that circumcise also have the highest rates of HIV infection.

Some wonder, might it not all come down to an innate human compulsion to mutilate, especially the sexual organs? Or a drive to control others' sexual behavior? Circumcision is known to harm the bond between mother and son. Does the circumcision-approving parent ever think ahead to the day when the boy is seven or eight and wants to know what was done to him, and why?[22] Does the rise in circumcision in the US correlate with its rise in crime? These questions are being asked.

⌗

It seems that we've gone through a century and a half of searching for justifications for circumcision, seen them debunked, created new ones, and seen those debunked. Now we're waking up to the fact that circumcising has been damaging sexual organs, sexual performance, and sexual relationships. But, in fact, this is something that has been known since antiquity. We just forgot it.

In *Marked in Your Flesh: Circumcision From Ancient Judea to Modern America*, anthropology professor Leonard Glick painstakingly recounts the history of circumcision. It begins

"I have noticed that the vagina is much more accepting of the natural penis."

with Chapter 17 of Genesis. God makes promises to Abraham and puts forth the inexplicable requirement: "Every man child among you shall be circumcised. And ye shall circumcise the flesh of your foreskin; and it shall be a token of the covenant betwixt me and you. And he that is eight days old shall be circumcised among you..."

Why? No one knows. No one single author wrote the Torah. Historically, one function of circumcision, for Jews, was that it identified with whom a Jewess may have sexual intercourse and therefore it served to preserve national identity.[23]

Jews in the Roman Empire knew that others looked down on circumcision. Some did not have their sons circumcised and some tried foreskin-stretching to restore themselves even back then. The ancient Greeks and their Hellenistic successors considered the "ideal" prepuce to be long, tapered, and well proportioned. Removing it was mutilation.[24]

Philo of Alexandria wrote in the first century that circumcision served to excise "pleasures that bewitch the mind." He may have been the first to state that circumcision decreases sexual sensation, Glick suggests.

Later, in the twelfth century, Moses Maimonides, Jewish physician and community leader, wrote, with regard to circumci-

The amount of skin amputated results in the loss of about one-third or more of the penile shaft skin system.

sion: "One of the reasons for it is, in my opinion, the wish to bring about a decrease in sexual intercourse and a weakening of the organ in question.... The fact that circumcision weakens the faculty of sexual excitement and sometimes perhaps diminishes the pleasure in indubitable." He adds:

> The Sages, may their memory be blessed, have explicitly stated: "it is hard for a woman with whom an uncircumcised man has had sexual intercourse to separate from him." In my opinion this is the strongest of the reasons for circumcision....

> [B]ecause his foreskin has been removed from him, and the power of his member has been diminished, he has no strength to lie with many lewd women.

> Women who have had an opportunity to make comparisons, know quite well the difference between circumcised and intact lovers. But it's all for the best, since Jewish men don't waste time and energy trying to satisfy women sexually.

Maimonides understood that the foreskin is a highly sensitive source of sexual pleasure. His words could be slid in between the comments of the women who responded to O'Hara's survey and no one would spot the 800-year gulf between them. Maimonides wrote:

> [W]hen a circumcised man desires the beauty of a woman, and cleaves to his wife, or another woman comely in appearance, he will find himself performing his task quickly, emitting his seed as soon as he inserts his crown.... He has an orgasm first.... She has no pleasure from him...and it would be better for her if he had not known her and not drawn near to her, for he arouses her passion to no avail, and she remains in a state of desire for

> her husband, ashamed and confounded, while the seed is still in her reservoir. She does not have an orgasm once a year....[25]

Even if the various health benefits touted by Schoen were true, and they are hotly debated, medical ethicist Margaret Somerville writes that that wouldn't justify circumcision:

> A common error made by those who want to justify infant male circumcision on the basis of medical benefits is that they believe that as long as some such benefits are present, circumcision can be justified as therapeutic, in the sense of preventive health care. This is not correct. A medical-benefits or "therapeutic" justification requires that overall the medical benefits should outweigh the risks and harms of the procedure required to obtain them, that this procedure is the only reasonable way to obtain these benefits, and that these benefits are necessary to the well-being of the child.

> None of these conditions is fulfilled for routine infant male circumcision. If we view a child's foreskin as having a valid function, we are no more justified in amputating it than any other part of the child's body unless the operation is medically required treatment and the least harmful way to provide that treatment.[27]

Somerville said she once accepted circumcision without a second thought. After studying it, she came to the conclusion that it is "technically criminal assault."

"Once you decide that circumcision is not medically necessary, you take away the therapeutic intent," she says. "Take away therapeutic intent, and circumcision becomes an unjustified wounding."

Dr. Leo Sorger told *ObGYN News* readers that circumcision, "removing normal healthy functioning tissue," violates the United Nations Universal Declaration of Human Rights (Article 5) and the United Nations Convention of the Rights of the Child (Article 13).

Northrup: "I am not Jewish, (or Muslim), but I can assure you that many Jews are rethinking circumcision (I do not have any information about Muslims). As a matter of fact, two of the most well-researched and eloquent books on the harmful nature of circumcision have been written by Jewish men. I urge you to read *Circumcision: The Hidden Trauma* by Ronald Goldman Ph.D. (Vanguard, 1997) and *Circumcision:*

An American Health Fallacy by Edward Wallenstein (Springer Publishing, 1980)."

Restored male David Steinburg is Jewish, and, despite his unhappiness with having been circumcised, he says he's not sure he could resist it for a newborn son in the face of family pressure.

> Many of the rituals of the Jewish community were developed as reminders of "separateness" and don't have any rationale other than ritual—which is fine. I do think it would be healthy—but probably impossible—for society to have something of a discussion about why keeping a foreskin is a good idea. But let's face it—how do you get Americans to talk about sexual pleasure within the context of a newborn? It ties in too many things even open-minded people are squeamish about: Parents don't want to think about their child's sexuality, especially that early on (if ever).

As for Muslims—circumcision is not mentioned in the Koran. According to Islamic websites, "There is no compulsion to circumcision."[28] But Sami Aldeeb found otherwise.

A Muslim lawyer based in Switzerland, Aldeeb would certainly call the circumcision he underwent at age eleven compulsory. Note his discussion of anger, terror, and thoughts of suicide:

> One of the issues rarely discussed in the topic of circumcision is the relation between its damage and the age at which it is done[.] I was circumcised at the age of 11, during the summer break after 5th grade....

> Here a male janitor-nurse pulled open my hospital robe and made a quick mark on my penis. I was then given a shot and carried by that person to the operating table. The last I remember was a nurse arranging "things" on a tray. I never saw the face of the doctor as it took few seconds for me to go under full anesthesia.

> I woke up in a bed with my father beside me, he asked me if I knew what happened, I pulled the blanket because I could feel the dry bandage against my raw glans.... I realized what had happened.... I felt stunned. I could not say a thing. Right then I thought about suicide.

> After I came back home I "surveyed the damage" and counted 10 stitches. My feeling was: now I am just like all of them.

> Years have passed and by the age of 16, I was

> having painful erections....

> At the age of 33, I started to read about the subject on the Internet. I learned about foreskin restoration and tried a technique that worked for me. It was not the aesthetic results that I was looking for, it was the functionality, and that eliminated the premature ejaculation problem I had, just by having some loose skin during erection.

> Physiologically, the experience left me feeling mutilated, for no reason or benefit. It damaged the relation I had with my father, and affected my attitude toward my parents. It also affected my religious beliefs. The effort and pains thinking about the subject, reading literature, and attempting the restoration could have been better spent, if this has not been done.

> A few words about Islamic religion and circumcision. My understanding is that God created the human body in best image; why mutilate it? Islam prohibited practices that cause body harm, like tattoos; and prophet Muhammad himself did not undergo circumcision.[29]

In September 1996 the United States passed a law against female genital mutilation. Opponents of male circumcision are asking for the same. There is some tension with those who crusade against female mutilation, some of them believing that male circumcision is much less harmful and fighting it less urgent. But circumcision opponents say all involuntary genital surgery is mutilation that should be stopped. For now, we can expect that if legal prohibition comes, it will come first in Canada. Canadians are already being warned.

In 1996 the Canadian Medical Association approved a code of ethics that instructs doctors to "refuse to participate in or support practices that violate basic human rights." This suggests, Mark Jenkins writes, "that in the case of circumcision, parental preference should not override the child's physical rights to his body."[30]

The Association for Genital Integrity is in the lengthy process of challenging the ban on female genital mutilation in Canada's Criminal Code as being discriminatory against males, who are not given similar protection.

"Every day in this country a quarter of the boys that are born are having this procedure performed on them without their consent and without any medical need. We don't see why half of our society should be protected by a law and not the other half," said Dr. Arif Bhimji, a Newmarket emergency room physician.

In February 2002 the College of Physicians and Surgeons of Saskatchewan warned physicians against routine circumcision of newborn male infants and essentially told doctors who perform the surgery based solely on parental preference to consult their lawyers![31]

In France, journalist Michel Orcel has pointed out the absurdity of arguing over Muslim head-scarf law when "ritual circumcision is still an elective amputation done on a subject who cannot resist mentally or physically." He says Article 16-3 of the French Civil Code is perfectly clear: "The physical integrity of a person cannot be violated except in cases of medical necessity. The consent of the person must be obtained beforehand except in cases where the person's condition necessitates a therapeutic intervention to which the person is incapable of giving consent..."

In the US, attorney J. Steven Svoboda, a former Human Rights Fellow at Harvard Law School, recently founded Attorneys for the Rights of the Child. "Our position is that circumcision is medical malpractice," he explains. "The medical profession, which has perpetuated this tragic disfigurement of baby boys' genitals, will now be challenged by an organization of legal professionals."

The courts are considering many cases. Samples: On July 22, 1995, a jury in Montgomery, Alabama, found Jackson Hospital and Clinic guilty of negligence in a case where a newborn was mistakenly circumcised against his mother's wishes. The minor plaintiff was awarded $65,000. More recently, a Suffolk County, New York teen won an undisclosed settlement from a hospital and the doctor who circumcised him. He sued because his mother's permission was obtained while she was debilitated by the effects of a Caesarian section and painkillers—a common scenario.

"Never again can someone say that a young man who is dissatisfied with his circumcision as an infant is being frivolous when he objects to his mutilation and brings suit to obtain justice," says Llewellyn, his attorney.

Based in Georgia, Llewellyn's firm specializes in "wrongful circumcision" and has handled about twenty cases, such as where the mother opposes the father's desire to have their son circumcised.

"Doctors need to be sued," he says. "The only thing people seem to understand is lawsuits and money."

He believes it is women who need to take up this issue and defend their sons. "Fathers aren't going to do it because they won't acknowledge the wrong that has been done to them."

And the only way the circumcision rate will be reversed, Kristen O'Hara contends, is to make people aware that women are the primary victims, since they are the ones who enduring discomfort, punishing blows, and lack of orgasm.

"The man suffers too, of course, because when women lose interest in sex, men are deprived. And when it ultimately affects the love bond, and can lead to divorce, it's a tragedy for everyone."

Endnotes

1. A conservative figure, according to restoration activist Ron Low of Chicago. **2.** Taylor, John. The Ridged Band website <research.cirp.org/abstr1.html>. **3.** "The oldest documentary evidence for circumcision comes from Egypt. Tomb artwork from the Sixth Dynasty (2345 - 2181 BC) shows men with circumcised penises.... The examination of Egyptian mummies has found both circumcised and uncircumcised men." "Circumcision," Wikipedia [www.wikipedia.com], accessed 14 June 2005. **4.** Taylor, John, A.P. Lockwood, A.J. Taylor. "The Prepuce: Specialized Mucosa of the Penis and Its Loss to Circumcision." *British Journal of Urology*, Vol. 77 (1996): 291-5. **5.** O'Hara, Kristen and Jeffrey. *Sex As Nature Intended It*. Hudson, Mass.: Turning Point Publications, 2002: 141. **6.** See how the foreskin works in animation: <www.circumstitions.com/Works.html>. **7.** Bullough, Vern L., and Bonnie Bullough, eds. *Human Sexuality: An Encyclopedia*. New York: Garland Pub., 1994: 119-22. **8.** Simple tape—a man stretches his shaft skin then tapes it in place and applies tension with a strap or string; devices such as the TugAhoy <www.TugAhoy.com>; RECAP method <recap_ez@hotmail.com> or <TLCTugger@Juno.com>. For other options, check <www.NORM-socal.org>. **9.** The full title is *The Joy of Uncircumcising!: Exploring History, Myths, Psychology, Restoration, Sexual Pleasure and Human Rights*, 2nd ed. by Jim Bigelow, Ph.D. Hourglass, 1995. **10.** She went on to found NOCIRC, the National Organization of Circumcision Information Resource Centers. **11.** For more details see <www.sexasnatureintendedit.com>. **12.** Northrup is author of *Women's Bodies, Women's Choices* (1998), *The Wisdom of Menopause* (2003), and *Mother-Daughter Wisdom* (2005). **13.** O'Hara and others defend describing male circumcision as genital mutilation. **14.** Goldman, Ron. *Circumcision: The Hidden Trauma—How an American Cultural Practice Affects Infants and Ultimately Us All*. Vanguard Publications, 1997: 73. **15.** For a complete discussion, see Ritter, Thomas J., MD, and George C. Denniston, MD. *Say No to Circumcision!: 40 Compelling Reasons*, second edition. Hourglass Book Publishing, 1996. **16.** Fleiss, with Frederick Hodges, has written "Nontherapeutic Circumcision Should Not Be Performed." *American Medical News*, 38.26 (17 July 1995). **17.** Angel, Money. *Treatment of Disease in Children*. Philadelphia: P. Blakiston. 1887. **18.** Crossland, Jefferson C., MD. "The Hygiene of Circumcision." *New York Medical Journal*, 1891. **19.** Op cit., Coleman: 60. **20.** Op cit., Coleman: 293. **21.** <www.circumstitions.com>. **22.** Coleman discusses the long-term psychological effects of circumcision on children and adults, pp 82-123. **23.** Glick, Leonard B. *Marked in Your Flesh: Circumcision From Ancient Judea to Modern America*. Oxford University Press, 2005: 29. **24.** Ibid: 31. **25.** Ibid: 67. **26.** Schoen's pro-circumcision website is <www.medicirc.org>. **27.** Somerville, Margaret A. *The Ethical Canary: Science, Society and the Human Spirit*. Toronto: Viking/Penguin Canada: 202-19. Also: <www.intact.ca/canary.htm>. **28.** <www.islamonline.net/askaboutislam>. **29.** Aldeeb's homepage: <www.go.to/nonviolence>. **30.** Jenkins, Mark. "Separated at Birth: Did Circumcision Ruin Your Sex Life?" *Men's Health*, July/Aug 1998. **31.** For more legal cases, see <www.circumstitions.com/Law.html>.

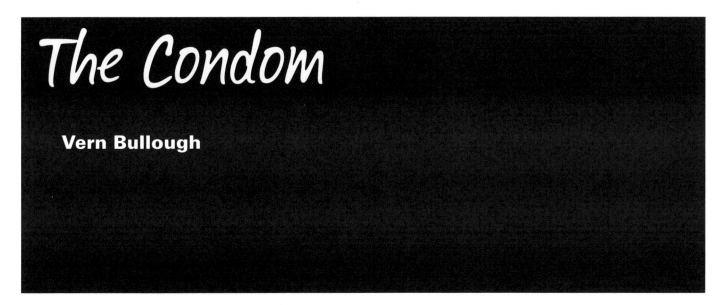

The Condom

Vern Bullough

Technically, the condom is a sheath designed to cover the penis and catch the ejaculate. Condoms are different from penis protectors designed to protect the penis from insect bites or as badges of rank or status, decoration, modesty, or a variety of other purposes. It is, however, possible that the sheath or condom might have evolved from these. The first use of the term in print is by John Wilmot, Earl of Rochester, who in 1665 wrote *A Panegyric Upon the Condom.*

The earliest use of a product to catch the ejaculate is much older. It occurs in a tale told by Antoninus Liberalis, a second-century compiler of Greek mythology who told of the legendary Minos and Pasiphae. According to legend, the semen of King Minos contained serpents and scorpions, and his ejaculate injured all the women who had cohabited with him. To solve the problem, he was advised to slip the bladder of a goat either over his penis or into the vagina of a woman and this would catch all the stored-up serpent-bearing demons when he had sex with her, after which his semen, at least for a brief period, would be normal. In any case, he impregnated Pasiphae successfully, not just once but eight times, resulting in the birth of four sons and four daughters.

As far as I know, there is no other mention of a condom in classical literature. Its mention by Antoninus, however, would indicate that animal bladders or perhaps animal ceca (intestines) were at least occasionally used by either men or women. The difficulty with the use of either is holding it on the penis, or, in case of a vaginal insert, keeping it in place. Ribbons were often put around the top and tied to the body. Another difficulty is that bladders or ceca also deadened the sensitivity so that, if the man used it for contraception rather than for prophylactic reasons, it was more likely to be a tight-fitting cap rather than a full sheath.

The earliest known medical description of a device similar to that used by Minos is by the Italian anatomist Fallopius (1564), but, again, since his mention is rather casual, it gives strength to the idea of a continuing tradition of such devices. He wrote:

> **As often as man has intercourse, he should (if possible) wash the genitals, or wipe them with a cloth; afterward he should use a small linen cloth made to fit the glans, and draw forward the prepuce over the glans; if he can do it so, it is well to moisten it with salve or with a lotion. However, it does not matter; if you fear lest caries [syphilis] be produced in the midst of the canal [vagina], take the sheath of linen cloth and place it in the canal. I tried the experiment on eleven hundred men, and I call immortal God to witness that none of them was infected. [Fallopius, 1564, trans. Himes, 1970]**

At the end of the sixteenth century, the medical writer Hercules Saxonia described a prophylactic sheath made of linen soaked in a solution several times and then put out to dry. From that time on, there are a growing number of references to a penis sheath. Casimir Freschot described one made of an animal bladder that covered the whole length of the penis and was tied on by a ribbon. One physician reported that many a libertine would rather risk getting the "clap" than use such devices.

In the eighteenth century, White Kennet wrote a burlesqued poem about the condom:

> **Happy the Man, who in his Pocket keeps,**
> **Whether with Green or Scarlet Ribband bound**
> **A well made C_____. He, nor dreads the ills**
> **Of shanker or Cordee or Buboes Dire**
> **With C_____ arm'd he wages am 'rous Fight**

Fearless, secure; nor Thought of future Pains
Resembling Pricks of Pin and Needle's Point
E'er checks his Raptures, or disturbs his Joys
[Fryer, 1964, pp. 27-8]

The very crudest of animal condoms were made from unprocessed skins sewn or pasted together to form a sheath. They were both unreliable and unaesthetic. The best condoms from animal ceca were produced by a lengthy and somewhat expensive process that was described in Gray's *Supplement to the Pharmacopoeia*, published in 1828, but the method must have been the same earlier. Gray said the intestines of sheep should be soaked in water for several hours, then turned inside out, macerated again in a weak alkaline solution that was changed every twelve hours, then scraped carefully, leaving only the peritoneal and muscular coats. Next, they were exposed to vapor of burning brimstone and washed in soap and water, after which they were blown up to see if they could hold air. If they passed inspection, they were dried, cut to seven or eight inches, tied or sealed at one end, and bordered at the open end with a ribbon.

Some condoms were made of silk that was cut, sewn, then oiled.

Baudrouches were made the same way but were distinguished from ordinary condoms by undergoing further processing. This entailed drawing them smoothly and carefully onto oiled molds of appropriate size, where they were rubbed with brimstone to make them thinner. Superfine *baudrouches* were scented with essences, stretched on a glass mold, and rubbed with a heavy glass rod to further process them.

There are actually some surviving condoms manufactured between 1790 and 1810, which were found in 1953 preserved in a book in an English country manor.

Probably because prostitutes were often regarded as carriers of disease, many of the surviving references to condoms come from the literature of prostitution. Houses of prostitution are known to have displayed a variety of condoms in the eighteenth century, but they also recommended the use of sponges. Sponges did not protect the customer from disease but did have some contraceptive value, and this might indicate that condoms were sometimes also used as contraceptives, as well as prophylactics.

A good description of condoms appears in the writing of the eighteenth-century Frenchman Jean Astruc, who was determined to prove that syphilis originated in America, not in France:

I heard from the lowest debauchees who chase without restraint after the love of prostitutes, that there are recently employed in England skins made from soft and seamless hides in the shape of a sheath, and called condoms in English, with which those about to have intercourse wrap their penis as in a coat of mail in order to render themselves safe in the dangers of an ever doubtful battle. They claim, I suppose, that thus mailed and with spears sheathed in this way, they can undergo with impunity the chances of promiscuous intercourse. But (in truth) they are greatly mistaken. [Astruc, Book ii, Chap. I, p 2]

Giovanni Giacomo Casanova de Seingalt's (1725-1799) erotic memoirs list 116 lovers by name, although they leave nameless hundreds more women and girls he had sex with, ranging in age from nine to seventy and in occupation and social status from chambermaids to noble women. He reported having intercourse standing, sitting, and lying down in coaches, on boats, in beds, and even in alleys. He also said he knew of and used condoms. Sometimes he called them the "English riding coat," but he also referred to them as "preservative" sheaths and "assurance" caps. Casanova describes an "English overcoat" as being made of "very fine and transparent skin," eight inches long and closed at one end, with a narrow pink ribbon slotted through the "open end" (with which to hold it up or tie it). He apparently used his sheaths not only for prophylactic purposes but to prevent his partners from becoming pregnant. He blew them up like balloons to pretest them. Some were of better quality than others, since he reported that some broke. Some were made of animal ceca, a practice he once mentioned as "suiting" himself up with a piece of dead skin.

It was a common practice to use condoms over and over again, washing them out after each use. The most expensive of condoms were those known as goldbeaters' skins. They got their name from the practice of beating gold into foil or leaf. Such sheaths were carefully processed by beating them until they were elasticized. Madame de Sévigny, writing about contraception in a 1617 letter to her daughter, described such condoms as "armor against enjoyment and a spider web against danger." Some condoms were made of silk that was cut, sewn, then oiled. Condoms made of bladder were advertised in eighteenth-century England. The bladders might well be those of the blowfish common in the Rhine River, which were being described as early as 1788.

Condoms undoubtedly existed in eighteenth-century America, but so far no historical record of them has been uncovered. It is believed that colonists probably fashioned their own condoms for personal use based on English models. It was not until 1844 that one advice book, *The United States Practical Receipt Book; Or, Complete Book of Reference*, gave a detailed description of how to make a condom from the cecum of a sheep. The description was probably based on a standard recipe for homemade condoms mentioned above.

In the first part of the nineteenth century, condoms began to be advertised in some newspapers and other printed material as a preventative against syphilis, and the sellers said they would ship them anywhere in the country. Packages of fish bladder "membraneous envelopes" were sold at $5 a dozen in New York City in 1860. This price would have prevented all but the extremely well-to-do from using such condoms; instead, most used the much cheaper animal ones and washed them repeatedly.

The cost, availability, and material of condoms slowly changed with the vulcanization of rubber by Charles Goodyear and Thomas Hancock in 1843-44. The key development for condoms, however, was the 1853 discovery of liquid latex, which led to the development of thinner and finer condoms. The first latex condom was really a cap designed to cover the glans, not the entire penis. It was described as being made of a "delicate texture" rubber no thicker than the cuticle and shaped and bound at the open end with an India rubber ring. The cap was soon extended to a sheath, and there is a description of a full-length one in 1869 as being effective in preventing conception even though it dulled sensation and irritated the vagina.

These early rubber condoms were molded from sheet crepe and carried a seam along their entire length. Making the latex condoms more effective and useful depended upon further development in rubber technology, and the major innovation was the seamless cement process, so named because the process was similar to that used in producing rubber cement. Natural rubber was ground up, dissolved, then heated with a solvent in which cylindrical glass molds were dipped. As the solvent evaporated, the condom dried. They were then vulcanized by being exposed to sulfur dioxide. These new types of condom were on the market before 1889. The major difficulty was that the finished product had a very short shelf life and had to be used within a comparatively short time of its manufacture. The advantage was that these new condoms were fairly inexpensive and easily disposable. By the 1870s wholesale druggists were selling rubber, skin, and imported condoms at six to sixteen cents each, and in retail outlets or from peddlers they were from $1 to $4 a dozen.

Condoms, as they became more available and trustworthy, were increasingly being used as a means of family planning. Still, only eight of the forty-five women who filled out a sex questionnaire (designed by Clelia Mosher and used over a thirty-year period up to 1920) reported that their husbands had used condoms as part of a means of preventing pregnancy. The ambiguity that some women felt about using condoms was expressed in a letter in 1878 that an Idaho woman, Mary Hallock Foote, wrote to a friend in New York to tell her how she and her husband planned to use a condom to avoid another pregnancy so soon after her current one. She reported that she had learned about condoms from a friend, Mrs. Hague, who told her to have her husband go to a physician and get shields of some kind:

> **They are to be had also at some druggists. It sounds perfectly revolting, but one must face anything rather than the inevitable result of Nature's methods. At all events there is nothing injurious about this. Mrs. Hague is a very fastidious woman and I hardly think she would submit to anything very bad... [Quoted by Brodie, 1994, p 206]**

Availability, however, did not mean widespread usage, and because condoms could not be sold for contraceptive use in many parts of the United States because of state laws copying the federal Comstock Act, they had to be sold as prophylactics. In other countries, however, they were sold as contraceptives as well, and distributed widely, even through dispensing machines. Distribution in the United States was primarily through drugstores and barbershops, but they were also sold by traveling salesmen who visited industrial plants and businesses employing large numbers of men.

By 1890 packages of condoms were available at fifty cents a dozen. The main problem, however, with all contraceptive material in the United States was lack of quality control. There was neither patent nor copyright protection for the manufacturer. None of the major rubber manufacturers, at least as indicated by the archives at the University of Akron (now Kent State University), manufactured them, and this meant that the market was left to a number of smaller companies, some of them with a very tenuous financial base. Eventually, several companies emerged with adequate quality control, including Young's Rubber, Julius Schmid, and Akwell. The entrance of Young's Rubber, founded by Merle Young (a drugstore-products salesman) in the mid-1920s, was particularly important because of his emphasis on quality control. Young's Rubber also began a series of court suits that eventually overturned many of the state laws against condom sales.

In the 1930s, new techniques were developed that enabled rubber plantations to ship concentrated liquid natural rubber latex directly to the manufacturer, and this eliminated the need to grind and dissolve rubber back to a liquid state. Though this proved to be a less costly method of manufacture, the problem of quality control remained. In one of the first American surveys of the efficacy of condoms, that of the National Committee on Maternal Health in 1938, it was found that only about 40% of the rubber condoms sold in the United States were fit for use.

One result of such a finding was a government decision to assign the US Food and Drug Administration control over the quality of condoms sold or shipped in interstate commerce. This marked an abrupt change in federal policy, which went from trying to outlaw contraceptive information, and when this was no longer possible, to ignoring the existence of such things as condoms, and was now recognizing condoms as an important consumer product.

The first governmental effort to look at quality control found that as much as 75% of the condoms on the market had small pinholes caused either by the existence of dust particles in the liquid latex or by improperly vulcanized latex. This situation changed rapidly. By the 1960s, condoms were among the most effective contraceptives on the market and were probably the best prophylactic for use against sexually transmitted diseases. They were simple to use, easy to buy, inexpensive, and did not require a physical examination or a physician's advice. Because they simply served as a container for the semen and did not interfere with any of the bodily processes, they were also harmless.

The use of condoms declined after the 1960s because of the development of oral contraceptives, IUDs, and other forms of contraception, the use of which was controlled by women, but condom use increased in the 1980s with the appearance of acquired immunodeficiency syndrome (AIDS) and the recognition that condoms, used in either vaginal or anal sex, were effective in decreasing the chance of infection. The variety of condoms also increased. Originally, all condoms came in one size, and the assumption of one-size-fits-all was challenged only when the United States began exporting condoms to Asian countries and found that they were too large for many Asian men. Investigation in Thailand, for example, found that the median erect penis length of Thai men was between 126 mm and 150 mm (approximately 5 to 6 inches) whereas that of US men was between 151 mm and 175 mm (approximately 6 to 7 inches). The median erect penis circumference of Thai men was between 101 mm and 112 mm (4 to 4.5 inches), while that of the US measured between 113 and 137 mm (4.5 to 5 inches). This implied that there was also a large variation in the United States, and most large international manufacturers began producing at least two basic sizes, Class I (180 mm in length and 52 mm in width) and Class II (160 mm in length and 49 mm in width). Many manufacturers, fearful of saying

their condoms were smaller than others, advertised them as having a snugger fit. Rubber membranes could also be made thinner, and better testing procedures developed.

As the use of condoms grew, numerous varieties were developed: contoured, textured, ribbed, with a variety of colors and other descriptors such as extra thin, extra strong, or lubricated with spermicides. New designs were developed, as well. The Rumdum Sicher covers both the penis and the testicles and is designed for male-to-male sex. It features a latex band that acts as a "cock ring" to help maintain erection. Manufacturers also began to include better instructions for condom use, and these vary somewhat since those for circumcised men are different than those for uncircumcised ones. Instructions are also given for removal so that sperm do not escape.

Why a condom has been called a condom has been a subject of much debate, with the origin of the word being attributed to several mythical physicians, as well as an actual French village named Condom. The latter seems more a coincidence, although in 1999 this village began to hold an annual condom festival, seeking to attract tourists. If the term was not entirely made up by Lord Rochester, it might have been modified from the Latin *cunnus* (the female genitals) and *dum*, implying an ability to function. There is, however, a continuing and inconclusive debate on the topic.

References

Antoninus Liberalis, "The Fox," Chap. XLI in *Metamorphoses,* edited by Edgar Martin. Leipzig: Teubner, 1896. § Astruc, Jean. *A Treatise of Veneral Disease in Nine Books.* No translator listed. London: W. Innys, et al., 1754, iii, Chap 1, 2. § Brodie, Janet Farrell. *Contraception and Abortion in Nineteenth Century America.* Ithaca, NY: Cornell University Press, 1994. § Bullough, Vern L. "A Brief Note on Rubber Technology and Contraception: The Diaphragm and the Condom." *Technology and Culture,* 22 (Jan 1981): 104-11. § Bullough, Vern L. "Condom." *Encyclopedia of Birth Control.* Edited by Vern L. Bullough. Santa Barbara: ABC Clio, 2000. § Bullough, Vern L., and Bonnie Bullough. *Contraception.* Amherst, NY: Prometheus Books, 1997. § Casanova, Jacques. *The Memoirs of Jacques Casanova de Seingalt.* Translated by Arthur Machen. New York: A.C. Boni, 1932. § Cautley, R.G., G.W. Beebe, and R.I. Dickinson. "Rubber Sheaths as Venereal Disease Prophylactics: The Relation of Quality and Technique to Their Effectiveness." *American Journal of Medical Sciences,* 195 (Feb 1948): 1550-83. § *Consumer Reports,* 54 (Mar 1989): 135-42; 60 (May 1995): 322-4; 61 (Jan 1996): 6-8. § Fallopius, Gabriele. *De morbo Gallico liber absolutismsus.* Pavia: 1564, Chap 89, p 52. § Finch, Bernard Ephraim, and Hugh Green. *Contraception Through the Ages.* Springfield, Il: Charles C. Thomas, 1963. § Foote, Edward Bliss. *Medical Common Sense.* New York: n.p. 1862. § Fryer, Peter. *The Birth Controllers.* London: Secker and Warburg, 1964. § Grady, W.R., et al., *Contraceptive Failure and Continuation Among Married Women in the United States, 1970-1976. Working Paper No. 6.* Hyattsville, MD: National Center of Health Statistics, 1981. § Gray, S.F.A. *Supplement to the Pharmacopoeia.* 4th ed., London: n.p., 1928. § Himes, Norman. *Medical History of Contraception.* New York: Schocken Books, 1970. § Kestleman, P., and J. Trussel. "Efficacy of the Simultaneous Use of Condoms and Spermicides." *Family Planning Perspectives* 23.5 (1991): 226-7, 232. § Redford, Myron H., Gordon W. Duncan, and Dennis J. Prager. *The Condom: Increasing Utilization in the United States.* San Francisco: San Francisco Press, 1974. § "Update on Condoms – Products, Protection, Promotion." *Population Reports,* ser H., no. 6 (Sep-Oct 1982), vol. 10, no. 5. § W.A. Week and Company. *Illustrated Year Book.* Chicago: n.p., 1872.

Hooray for Sodomy

Is the Rectum an Easter Basket?

Simon Sheppard

Easter, 2005

I've just finished fucking this guy, a tall, odd-but-handsome-looking fellow whose family, he's told me, is Irish Catholic, a nice touch for the holiday. He's proven to be a great lay, with a passionate attitude and an ass that fairly sits up and begs for more. It's the second day in a row he's come over to have sex, and he once again put his legs in the air while I slid my hard-on into his lubed-up ass and cheerfully obeyed his exhortation: "Plow me hard with that beautiful dick." Absolutely, Patrick. Sure thing. Happy Easter, dude.

There's a passage by the late French queer theorist Guy Hocquenghem that I love, even if I'm not quite sure just what it means. It's from a book titled *Homosexual Desire*, published way back in 1972:

> **If the homosexual image contains a complex knot of dread and desire, if the homosexual fantasy is more obscene than any other and at the same time more exciting, if it is impossible to appear anywhere as a self-confessed homosexual without upsetting families...then the reason must be that for us twentieth-century westerners there is a close connection between desire and homosexuality. Homosexuality expresses something— some aspect of desire—which appears nowhere else, and that something is not merely the accomplishment of the sexual act with a person of the same sex.**

Oh-KAY, Monsieur Guy!

I've slogged my way through a bit of Foucault and stuff, but let's face it—unless you're shooting for academic tenure, it's hardly the kind of thing you read in an odd moment on the toilet. But as I understand it, the gist of Hocquenghem's thesis is that—well, that fucking butt has nothing productive about it, that's it's just about pleasure, pure and simple. No wonder right-wingers hate the idea of queer sex. It's so...noncapitalist.

And then there's the "appears nowhere else" thing. Don't we all want to believe we're, as Radiohead elegantly put it, "so fucking special?" So if a guy can become as ineffably ineffable as Cher simply by taking cock up his butt...well, why the hell not?

Looking down at Patrick, at his big, lean body, his hard cock leaking precum on his belly, making him moan with stroke after stroke, then leaning over to kiss him while my condomized cock slides in and out of his yielding hole—it was all more than pornographic. It was both friendly and predatory, animal and human. Holy and profane. It was...um...hot.

No wonder right-wingers hate the idea of queer sex. It's so...noncapitalist.

I've been passing myself off as a sex advisor for quite a while now, and I've always maintained that anal sex is strictly optional for queer men, just one carnal choice among many. Which is to say: Committing sodomy is not required to be a sodomite. (And yes, I know that some benighted souls define even a quick blowjob as "sodomy," but fuck 'em.) Lately, though, I've been wondering if perhaps that approach isn't just a tad too liberal, if the essence of male queerness is not in fact somehow fully dependent on getting (or giving) it up the ass. Certainly it's a familiar whine of homophobes: "That's an exit, not an entrance, you stupid fag."

Those same homo-haters may in fact jack off to pictures of women getting it on with each other, but lesbians don't fuck each other up the butts. (Or, if they do, at least they sensibly use dildos.) Queer men, on the other hand, insist on shoving our very own flesh up each other's poop chutes, and that squicks numerous straight men—the ones who aren't doing their girlfriends up the ass, anyhow. (I have it on good authority that some straight boys, as part of their countless appropriations of gay male culture, are getting fucked by women wearing strap-ons...so maybe it is a small world after all. Still, I think that most of us would agree that when it comes to buttfucking in theory and practice, homos hold most of the important patents. How many women, for instance, do you think have fisted their husbands? Not nearly enough, I'll venture.)

Queer essentialist Leo Bersani, in the title of a famous essay, asked: "Is the rectum a grave?" Well, unlike your basic, garden-variety vagina, the nether rosebud is more likely to issue feces than rugrats. And certainly, the advent of HIV has made the gentle art of sodomy seem even more fraught, more freighted with fateful whatever. But a *grave*? Isn't that a bit extreme?

If the universe has an endpoint, the pious Christian would rather it not be located just slightly above the perineum.

Perhaps the basic issue, the *leitmotiv* as 'twere, is mortality. You know: death. Entropy. Dissolution of all that is, including our precious egos. To put this as inelegantly as possible, yesterday's food is today's shit. We're not only *part* of the food chain, we *are* the food chain, in miniature. Every dump we take is a *memento mori*. Nothing is forever. Everything passes. And is flushed.

This is distressing to some folks. Not just on a visceral, "Phew! That stinks!" level. On an existential level. On an "I can't stand the thought that someday soon, I'll be no more" level. You know.

⊗⊗

After I fuck Patrick and see him out the door, I microwave a cup of leftover coffee and sit down to read the Sunday newspaper. Seeing as how it's Easter, there's an investigative arti-

cle on the Resurrection, real hard-news stuff. And one young born-again fellow is quoted as saying, "If there weren't eternal life through belief in Jesus, then it would make no sense to be a Christian." Well, say what you will about God's love, about the pleasures of doing good and all that swell stuff, let's face it—eternal life is clearly Christianity's Big Gimmick, the free toaster when you open a new account. Traditionally, Jews haven't focused on the afterlife: You did the right thing because G-d told you to, and that was that. After all, wasn't it those rotten ol' pharaohs who were always fretting about what would happen to them after they died?

Then the Christians came along and started offering Heaven as the carrot and Hell as the stick. Sure, the Egyptians had already come up with the dead-and-resurrected-god shtick. Lots of other religions had, too. But Christianity doesn't require mummy wrappings and gilded tomb *tchotchkes* to assure immortality. You just have to do good. Or, if you're part of the salvation-by-faith crowd, even that's not a prereq. You just have to say the magic words, and hey, presto, your self will never, ever die.

Mid-April

A new Pope has just been elected; a job promotion for the erstwhile Cardinal Ratzinger, the ex-Hitler Youth Inquisitor who's stated that he and his god think what I do is an "evil... disorder." Yet another reason to wonder why an organization of supposedly celibate men—albeit one riddled with child molesters—should be allowed to pontificate on hot sex between consenting adults. And yet another reason to prefer the Dalai Lama.

The same day, I go over to visit a chunky Latino boy, figuring I'm going to be the Daddy top. But Junior has other ideas. Soon enough, I'm flat on my back while the boy slides his smallish, delightfully uncut, and very hard dick into me. Since I'm in the middle of writing this extended essay on buttfucking, I try to maintain a certain reportorial objectivity. Nope, can't do it. I don't get fucked all that often, and *mi hijo* knows what he's doing; whatever he lacks in genital heft, he more than makes up for in brutal enthusiasm. He pounds into me, whispering sweet nothings like, "Does Dad like having his boy's cock up his ass?" Well, yes, as a matter of fact, I do. And when Ernesto comes into his condom while I shoot messily onto my belly, I think "Hey, Pope Benedict the Whatever, that one was for you."

Well, actually I didn't think that, not then, but I wish I had.

I know, I know. Childish anti-authoritarianism, right? I should really grow up. That's a way the Freudians have put queers down, actually: Since the only "fully mature" manifestation of sexuality is vaginal fucking, queer men are fixated at the oral or anal stage of development. How immature. *Grow up, you fags!* (Of course, believing in a fatherly sky god who'll reward or punish his children has a certain infantilism to it, too, but let's let that pass for now, shall we?)

Let's get back to buttholes.

There's something Hindu—Shivaite—about the cycle of nutrition and excretion, as though we're just meat-tubes through which flow eternal patterns of destruction and rebirth. Christianity, on the other hand, is all about The End Of Time, and if the universe has an endpoint, the pious Christian would rather it not be located just slightly above the perineum. If, after all, Mr. Priest is feeding us the body of Christ, wouldn't we rather not think what happens to the swallowed Host once it makes it to the colon?

Let's face facts: Transubstantiation ends up, as does so much else, in the toilet. Unlike some other worldviews, Christianity is kind of hinky about the body, with its pleasures and limitations. Blame the Gnostics, maybe, but the corruption of the body is something to be sidestepped on the way to the Pearly Gates, not something to be accepted and dealt with. So, as stupid as it may have seemed to me, maybe that born-again who was quoted in the paper was right. Maybe the irreducible essence of Christianity is in fact the denial of mortality. Stack that on top of the Levitical obsession with cleanliness (Moses should have met my mother), and you know what that means. No shit. And no shitholes.

Late April

Daniel. Daniel is a college kid, and he'd never had sex with a guy before he met me. He's sweet, slightly geeky, and utterly delightful. He also, not so incidentally, has a marvelous asshole. When I first fingered it, it responded by inviting me in, rare for a guy who's never been fucked. (Though Daniel had, he'd told me, played with dildos a few times.) The third time we met, I got a couple of fingers inside him.

The fourth time he asks me to fuck him.

"You've never been fucked before?"

"Nope. Would you tell me what to do?"

It's a simple, sincere question. It's a breathtaking moment.

I suggest he straddle me and lower himself down on my hard-on, a position preferred by many first-timers, since they can retain control. But Daniel wants to get on his back, me on top, and I'd be a fool to refuse him. I go in slowly, figur-

ing he has a hole that will open up for me with a bit of penile persuasion.

I'm right.

Daniel gets a beatific look on his young face as I plumb his guts.

"Fuck," he says, "that feels good."

"To me, too." I'm inside him. A part of me is inside him, inside the ass of this formerly ostensibly-het kid who trusts me enough to let me fuck him. As nice as it's been to suck his cock, to eat his ass, to fingerfuck him, this is something else. This is rhapsodic. This is fucking great.

"So you're always a top?" he asks. I have no problem making small talk with Daniel while my cock's in his ass; I'm just wondering whether he's obliquely suggesting he dick me with his thick meat, a slightly daunting idea.

"Well, mostly. Why, you want to fuck me?"

"No, nothing like that. Guess I'm just a bottom."

"Well, most guys are."

"Really?" Daniel is endlessly curious about queer folkways, it seems.

"Yeah."

"Hey, can we try it doggy-style?"

After we've both come—Daniel while I was fucking him, me while he was sucking me off—we lie around drinking Dr. Pepper and talking.

No wonder I've woken up with a yen to eat ass.

"Anal sex is really cool," he says.

It's hard to argue with that. I don't even try.

"I mean, there's so much interesting about it, huh?" Daniel is a linguistics major.

I tell him there had better be a lot, since I'm just partway through writing a major essay on buttfucking.

I start gassing on about Christianity and transgression and all that stuff. But meanwhile I'm thinking that really what's most interesting to me about fucking Daniel is how thoroughly fine it is. It's not that blowing him, rimming him, and fucking his face haven't been fun. But I'm wondering if maybe I was wrong all along. Perhaps, in the immortal words of a Craigslist ad, "If it isn't fucking, it isn't sex."

Later, after Daniel leaves, I have third thoughts about the indispensability of sodomy. No, fucking isn't the be-all and end-all of male/male sex. Still, when my cock went up Daniel's sweet ass, it was as if some final barrier was crossed, some Rubicon of the rump. So I'm gratified when the next day I get email from him that reads, "I can't believe how great it was to get fucked by you. I really wanna do it again."

Gratified, because the feeling is mutual.

→

Many heterosexuals, whatever faiths they may or may not follow, have a good deal invested in passing on their DNA through breeding. Gay men, meanwhile, are more or less un-interested in the life-generating pussy. No offense, ladies, but we'd rather deal with ass. For some odd reason, this anal ob-session seems to get puritans' (and not just of the Christian variety) noses out of joint.

When the fire-and-brimstone fulminators talk about "the gay deathstyle," just what's happening there? Sure, there are health issues to think about. But since some of those very same homophobes are 300-pound cigarette-smokers head-ed to McDonald's in their pollutant-spewing SUVs, the health concerns seem iffy. It seems more likely that by marrying, breeding, and raising kids, Mr. Het may well feel he is, per-haps grimly, doing his duty, keeping the ol' human race afloat. A queer guy, though, can say, like some buggering Bartleby the Scrivener, "I'd prefer not to," and stick his dickie up a butthole instead. The sheer, brazen, nonreproductive effron-tery!

Blowjobs, no matter how nonreproductive, are a different

When my cock went up Daniel's sweet ass, it was as if some final barrier was crossed, some Rubicon of the rump.

matter. For one thing, there's hardly a straight guy alive who doesn't like getting sucked off, and not a few avail themselves of the oral services of expert queers, in online-arranged dates or brief encounters down at the rest stop on the interstate. Even when it comes to ass, a not inconsiderable number of het boys have persuaded their girlfriends or wives to let them inside their tight, wet rears. But only a select minority of non-queer men—the few, the proud, the buggerees—ever deign to let down their armor and throw their legs in the air.

Early May
Spring has come. I'm still seeing Daniel every once in a while. Meantime, out in the world beyond the bedroom door, there's a Pope who hates fags (though I'm sure he would,

full of Christian charity, claim otherwise), a US President who thinks Jesus talks to him (no doubt denouncing queer sex when he does), and a California governor who denounces "girlie men." No wonder I get out of sorts.

No wonder I've woken up with a yen to eat ass.

I've come to realize that, in fact, I'd often rather stick my tongue up a hole than plunge my dick in there. I'm not sure where that comes from, but I know when I lick a guy's hole, it's a powerful moment for me. Ostensibly, it's a very bot-tom-y thing to do, I guess, but I've hardly ever met a bottom guy who didn't like getting his hiney licked. It feels great, of course, and often loosens a pucker for boning. To me as rim-mer, it's a bit of a wallow, a radical commitment to the food chain, a violation on both our parts. And, given the potential health risks, eating ass is a tempting of fate; I'll readily con-cede that.

It's as close as I get to taking Communion.

I've heard that novice Tibetan Buddhist monks go through an initiation called "sleeping with corpses," which is pretty much what it sounds like. It is, I'm supposing, a way to ac-cept the transitory nature of all things, to learn the lesson that we're all going to die. Even that monk over there in his saffron robes is going to croak. Even, dear and gentle reader, you.

Buddhists, of course, believe that until we learn to behave ourselves, we're doomed to countless rebirths. Christians believe that unless we learn to behave ourselves, we're doomed to die. Whichever. Whatever. I'm pretty damn sure I'm doomed to something or other. Be that as it may, I truly, madly, deeply love eating ass; it's my very own version of sleeping with corpses, I guess. Only it has to do with "stiff" in quite another sense of the word.

Madonna, profound thing that she is, once pointed out that life is a mystery. Well, sexual attraction is a mystery, too. Maybe even a bigger one. And each of those beautiful men out there has an asshole, a portal into his guts. Hawkers of hetero hegemony will tell you that when it comes to sex, the anus is just a poor substitute, a second-rate vagina. But what if it's precisely the other way around? What if the very best sex is supposed to be nonpro-ductive, dangerous, messy, queer? What if cunt is just a poor substitute for asshole?

Well, I'm just asking…

Mid-May
I'm in luck. Juan is free to stop by.

Juan is a guy in his late twenties. We met, as I often meet play partners, over the Internet. The first time he showed up at my door, I was more than a little dazzled by his good looks, trimly buffed body, and stunning smile. And by how much he liked to get fucked.

Though he's a busy guy, today he's made some time to come over after work.

"Hi, *papi*," he says when he walks in. His smile's even more amazing than I remember. "It's good to see you."

It's good to see him, too. It's good to look down and see him sucking my cock. It's good to pry apart his asscheeks and taste his hole. (And Juan has a very, very pretty hole. Remember, I'm a connoisseur.)

———3

I remember the first time I fucked ass. It was with my first boyfriend, my first, tritely tragic love. I'd read an erotic novel, a rather good one as it happened, that explained how anal sex was the ultimate joining, a momentous pledging of devotion.

So when I tried to jam my dick into Jim's unready ass, when things collapsed into tears, neuroses, apologies, it all seemed so damn fraught. We broke up soon after, him leaving me to get married; I'm assuming his wife never did him with a dildo. But who knows?

I do not, oddly, recall the first time I got fucked. I do remember this cute, curly-haired insurance salesman who used to come over to my place in the Haight, many years ago, and pound my ass till I was ready to beg him to stop (though I'm hoping I never actually begged him).

Back then, I used to think I was doing a top a Real Big Favor if I let him use my ass. What can I say? I was young and foolish. I think I've learned a lot about sex since then. Buttfucking in theory and practice.

✕✕

And, most of all, it's good to have my "son" Juan ride my dick. I do enjoy being on top, but as I suggested to Daniel, I also love to lie back and feel a guy ease down on my hard-on, and that's just what Juan does. I look up into his dark eyes as I feel his sphincter relax, his delectable ass open up for me.

"Ay, *papi*," he gasps. "It's so big." (I'm not boasting here, only reporting.)

We shift positions so I'm hitting his prostate, over and over and over again.

And it's Easter all over again.

♡♡

So *is* the rectum a grave?

Well, yes. Insofar as the body itself is a grave. Insofar as all our pleasures are mortal. Insofar as the corpses we sleep

If the ass is a tomb, it's like the one Jesus allegedly was left in.

with are, ultimately, ourselves. And, yes, insofar, as the Buddha said, as our pleasures are what bind us to these pieces of walking meat we call "I."

But, at the risk of, oh, a thousand more incarnations or so, I find myself unable to stay away from the amazing beauty, the life force, of a good fuck. Hell, I'm not even trying very hard.

Because if the ass *is* a tomb, it's like the one Jesus allegedly was left in: It may seem like a dead end, but it's a portal to transcendence, too. And if that transcendence is fleeting, equivocal, even stupid, well....

Nothing says "trapped in a body" quite like anal sex does. And nothing else better says, "What the hell?"

The transformational powers of anal sex are immense. What had been a functional aperture becomes a site of pleasure, replete with multiple meanings. It's positively alchemical. Dross into gold. Asshole into pussy. Shit into glory. Magic, pure magic. And beauty. Beauty, beauty, beauty.

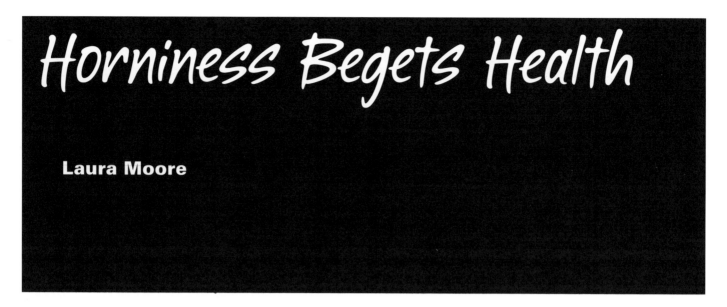

Horniness Begets Health

Laura Moore

Editor's Note: Sex radicals Susie Bright, Annie Sprinkle, Marcy Sheiner, and Bob Flanagan, among others, have written about using orgasms and/or sex to quell pain and for other health reasons. With her book Sex Heals, *Laura "The Healthy, Sexy Mom" Moore joins their ranks, revealing her experiences and explaining the science behind the humping-healing connection. Chapter three, below, discusses some of this. Several of the points are expanded in other portions of her book, which is available through <www.thehealthysexymom.com>.*

"When I get that feeling, I need sexual healing."
—Marvin Gaye, "Sexual Healing"

Have you ever stopped to wonder why our sex drive is so strong? We don't want sex just when it's time to continue the species. We want it all the time. We think about it every day. We are bombarded with advertisements that use sex as a selling point (and they usually work!), and the funniest jokes seem to be related to sex...or the lack thereof.

Could there be an underlying biological motivating factor, other than procreation, involved with our sexuality? Does our innate horniness have beneficial effects besides mere pleasure? Certain scientists believe so, and I will bet my life on it. Being sexually driven and satisfied helps to keep our hormones balanced so that our bodies can be as robust as possible.

Certain hormones, such as prolactin, growth hormone, and oxytocin, help to keep our immune systems strong. These same hormones (along with many others) are released during orgasm. Our immune systems are responsible for fighting off microorganisms and toxins that make us sick and cause allergic reactions. When we have stronger immune systems, our bodies are better able to combat these substances. Our sex drive is a built-in immune booster.

Let's take John L. as an example of how much influence sex can have over our health. John had been married for over fifteen years and was always the picture of health. When he got divorced, however, his health rapidly declined. His doctor was puzzled because his eating and exercise habits remained constant. His doctor simply diagnosed him with depression and gave him a prescription for the antidepressant Zoloft. Before filling the prescription, though, John came to me to ask for my insight. After a series of questions regarding his personal life, I noticed that the only thing missing from John's life was a lover. I asked if he had had sex since his divorce, and he was flabbergasted. "Dear God, no! That would be immoral!"

"Well, how do you feel about masturbation?" I quickly replied. Luckily for John, he didn't consider jerking off a one-way ticket to hell, so after a month's worth of solo sex, his immune system seemed as strong as ever...and he never did fill that Zoloft script. Which, by the way, would have probably suppressed his immune system even more because antidepressants put big dampers on libido.

Here's an even better example of sexual healing: Not too long ago I was attacked by a very nasty stomach virus. I couldn't keep anything down, my head throbbed, and I was terribly weak and nauseated. One of my editors called during this plague and told me he needed an article by the next day. Yikes! I sat with pen in hand for fifteen minutes—nearly in tears—thinking, "There's no way I can write anything feeling this horrible."

Then, eureka! The sexual healing goddess awoke within me, and I knew what had to be done. I went straight to my bedroom, pulled out my most trustworthy vibrator, and got busy. As soon as my mechanical love tool touched my clit, all discomfort and pain melted away. I made sure to complete the sexual therapy with an orgasm (well, actually it was two orgasms!) to ensure a complete healing. Afterwards, I worked on my article for four hours, then had dinner with friends that night. Bye-bye, virus!

Sex Is a Healer

How can sex be such a healer? Low-to-moderate intensity exercise, such as what we get when we have sexual intercourse, is one explanation for an improved immune system. It has been proven that endurance exercise triggers neutrophil (the powerhouses of our immune system) activation and also helps them to do a better job protecting our bodies.

David Nieman, D.H.Sc., chair of the Department of Health Science at Loma Linda University in Southern California, assigned fifty non-exercising women to one of two groups. Half continued their sedentary ways, while the other half took brisk walks for forty-five minutes a day. (By the way, brisk walking burns approximately four calories per minute, and sex with an active partner burns approximately 4.5 calories per minute.) After fifteen weeks, the exercisers reported only half as many days with cold symptoms.

Another reason sex helps with immunity is because of the hormone oxytocin, utilized to help process white blood cells that work to engulf foreign particles (such as bacteria, viruses, allergens, and carcinogens) that invade our bodies. Normal levels of oxytocin help stimulate these cells to work harder. For example, it is a known fact that women who breastfeed their young have a much lower incidence of breast cancer. The stimulation of the nipple and the cuddling with the infant produce high levels of protective oxytocin. As we now know, we can prompt our bodies to produce more oxytocin by having frequent orgasms and even by having loving or lustful thoughts. And if you're lucky enough to have a lover who is lactating, drinking her milk will improve your immune system and help you build more lean muscle mass because of the high level of immune-boosting substances and growth hormone.

Frequent Sex = Stronger Immune System

According to a study conducted by Carl J. Charnetski, professor of psychology, and Francis X. Brennan, Jr., assistant professor of psychology, both at Wilkes University in Wilkes-Barre, Pennsylvania, it seems that persons who engage in frequent sexual activity (once or twice per week) have substantially higher levels of the antibody immunoglobulin A (IgA) than those individuals who have sex less than once per week or who have no sexual activity. IgA, which is found in all mucosal linings of the body and in the blood, is the most prevalent of the five major antibodies that work as part of the body's defense mechanism against disease. The general function of one's immune system can be inferred by measuring IgA levels.

In the study, IgA was measured in saliva samples obtained from a group of male and female undergraduate students. The researchers asked those students about their sexual encounters that included some sort of genital contact with a partner, length of their relationships, and their satisfaction with their sexual relationships.

The collected data revealed four distinct classifications of sexual frequency: no sexual activity, infrequent sexual activity (less than one occurrence per week), frequent sexual activity (one or two occurrences per week), and very frequent sexual activity (three or more occurrences per week). The researchers found that the concentrations of IgA were approximately one-third higher in the frequent group as compared to all other categories, including the very frequent group.

So, according to this study, we shouldn't get greedy when it comes to planning our coital calendars. This particular study

Being sexually driven and satisfied helps to keep our hormones balanced so that our bodies can be as robust as possible.

shows that sexual activity (with genital contact with a partner) once or twice per week appears to be the optimum frequency in order to have a stronger immune system. Personally, I think I do better healthwise with a slightly higher quota of orgasms per week. They didn't mention the positive effects of masturbation in this study, but we'll get around to that!

An Orgasm a Day Keeps the Doctor Away

Twice a week doesn't seem like enough sex for you, either? Here's a study that will impress the pants or panties off of you. Scientists at the Department of Social Medicine, University of Bristol, performed a study on the relation between frequency of orgasm and mortality. They studied 918 men aged forty-five to forty-nine and followed up on the study until all of the men had died. The results showed that the mortality risk was 50% lower in the group of men who had high orgasmic frequency than in the group with low orgasmic frequency. In other words, the more orgasms, the lower the mortality; the fewer orgasms, the higher the mortality.

At the point when the group's number of orgasms equaled 100 per year (twice a week), the death rate was significantly lower (68% less mortality) than that of the lowest frequency group (less than one month). (How did those guys manage with just one nut a month?!) The scientists concluded that sexual activity seems to have a protective effect on men's health.

Even better news for you sex junkies is that this study provides strong evidence that there is a "dose-response" relation with sex. This means that the improved mortality benefits from orgasm frequency continue all the way up to daily "doses" (one orgasm per day, or 365 per year) and possibly beyond! This association for lower mortality in high-frequency orgasm groups was most pronounced in those men with coronary disease. Makes you wonder why we sometimes hear of men kicking the bucket during sex, doesn't it?

A follow-up study performed with women proved that sex is just as important in extending the life span of the fairer sex. There was a minor difference, however. The scientists concluded from the results that for men the *quantity* of sexual activity is paramount (more sex, less death), while for women *quality* is more important (more sexually-related pleasure, less death). Must be a Mars and Venus kind of thing.

There was also a case-controlled study of middle-aged women who expressed dissatisfaction with the quality of

I even had orgasms when I had to stay in the hospital hooked up to IVs and after a spinal tap!

their sex lives—primarily because of premature ejaculation or impotence of their partners—in which researchers found an increased risk of acute myocardial infarction (heart malfunction). So, guys, if you want to keep your women healthy and happy, work on ways to transport them to their particular sexual nirvana. Ladies, if you're concerned about your men's health, just keep 'em coming!

Sex and the West Nile Virus

My book *Sex Heals* was delayed in its initial publication because I was struck ill with the potentially fatal West Nile Virus, transmitted to me by one of the gargantuan mosquitoes that dominate the southern US. That nasty microorganism wiped out over a month of my life, but in retrospect I'm actually grateful for the opportunity it gave me to put my sexual healing theory to the ultimate test.

The symptoms incurred from the West Nile Virus included severe headaches (my brain was swollen from encephalitis), high fever, nausea, muscle weakness, vertigo, and general malaise. Admittedly, for the first few days of my illness, I didn't feel like doing anything except trying to sleep away the

pain.

When I partially came back to my senses, I put my best masturbatory talents to work and began to feel just a bit better. Immediately after my orgasms, I experienced the greatest relief from the pain and discomfort…but it was always short-lived. That vexatious pathogen called for intense orgasmic therapy, so some nights I brought myself to my sexual zenith up to four times straight in a row. I even had orgasms when I had to stay in the hospital hooked up to IVs and after a spinal tap! It was exhausting, but aside from the instantaneous gratification, I could actually feel the healing hormones gushing through my blood vessels and purging my diseased body of toxins. After each orgasm, I lay on my soaked bed linens, taking deep, replenishing breaths and welcoming the sexual healing.

Many people have died or suffered some type of permanent damage from the outbreak of West Nile Virus. I believe that my overall good health and my extremely healthy libido saved my life. Take care of yourself, too, by enjoying more orgasms. And watch out for them skeeters!

The Real Fountain of Youth

One of the reasons sex plays such a vital role in longevity is that it helps increase our levels of growth hormone. Growth hormone is responsible for helping our bodies rejuvenate. Some eccentric millionaires take injections of synthetic growth hormone in the hopes of staying young forever. It works to a certain extent, but all of us will age eventually. To avoid the side effects of the synthetic growth hormone, we can engage in frequent sex to increase our natural levels of the substance that Ponce de Leon would have given his left nut for.

Increasing your deep sleep will also pump up your growth hormone levels, and sex is just the ticket for getting some quality Zs. Don't you find you sleep like a baby after bumping nasties for an hour or two? Researchers at the University of Chicago found that the quality of sleep decreases with age, along with the body's production of growth hormone. As the subjects' deep sleep was increased, so were the levels of growth hormone.

Studies show that as levels of oxytocin rise in the brain, subjects are induced to go into a deep sleep. You know that orgasms increase your oxytocin levels, so if your lover ever complains about you drifting off to dreamland immediately after sex, just plead, "Oxytocin overload, babe." She or he should take it as a compliment. But please be sure you reciprocate that gushing of the love hormone before you knock on out.

The most intriguing aspect of sex and longevity deals with the hormone prolactin, practically the only hormone that increases with age. We know that prolactin levels increase after orgasm, but we have also seen that more sex equals longer life. This leads me to hypothesize that when we increase our levels of prolactin via orgasms, it is as if we are taking in exogenous (outside source) prolactin.

When the body detects an overabundance of a particular hormone in our system, it will automatically shut down its own production of that hormone. This is why so many bodybuilders who take huge amounts of exogenous testosterone have nuts that look like raisins. Their testicles figure, "Heck, we don't have to work any more. This guy's getting all the testosterone he needs from his pills and injections." This is why I think increased levels of prolactin from an active sex life protect our bodies from the aging effects prolactin normally produces. Sexually active people get surges of prolactin so constantly that their bodies slow down the regular production of prolactin. I haven't seen this theory in any medical research. This is just my scientifically creative mind at work.

Sex Heals Pain

Dr. Jorge Flechas, a family practitioner in North Carolina, specializes in patients who suffer from fibromyalgia and chronic fatigue syndrome. He has developed a new protocol for the treatment of these illnesses using oxytocin, DHEA, and other natural nutrients. (Just before orgasm and ejaculation, oxytocin and DHEA levels spike to levels three to five times higher than normal.) Dr. Flechas theorizes that an empty receptor for oxytocin can potentially cause pain. Administering oxytocin causes the empty oxytocin receptor sites to become full, thereby diminishing or completely obliterating pain. Oxytocin has been given to humans to kill cancer pain, ovarian pain, lower-back pain, and bowel pain from irritable bowel syndrome. Isn't it wonderful to know that we can produce our own endless supply of oxytocin just by enjoying a healthy sex life? How much simpler could it get?

Sex can also help in the management of "arthritic pain, whiplash pain, and headache pain," according to Dr. Beverly Whipple, president of the American Association of Sex Educators, Counselors, and Therapists. Hormones released during sexual excitement and orgasm can elevate pain thresholds. Also, by going through the different movements of the sex acts, one can put the joints through their full range of motion (hopefully), thereby pumping lubricating fluids through the joints, which helps keep them pain-free. Sex (and sexercise) also releases endorphins, the body's own pain-relieving chemicals.

One of my radio listeners (who asked to remain anonymous)

emailed me with this to say: "I would love to get an autographed first edition of your book, *Sex Heals*. And as an aside, the title is great! I have two arthritic knees and a bad back due to a bicycle accident, and there is a certain act my wife refers to as 'The Treatment' because for about two hours later, I feel NO pain."

Keeping oneself happy with an active sex life can definitely keep back pain at bay. Dr. Eugene Carragee, associate professor of functional restoration at the Stanford University Medical Center, is the lead author of a study published in the medical journal *Spine*. Dr. Carragee and his team compared the results of MRI and vertebral disc tear tests of patients who had known risk factors for disc degeneration. Disc tears have traditionally been thought to directly cause lower back pain, but the researchers were surprised to find that patients with disc problems were only slightly more likely to have back pain than those without any disk degeneration. Furthermore, 25% of those who did have disc problems had no lower back pain at all.

This prompted the researchers to perform psychological tests on these patients, which showed that back pain is strongly associated with the patient's state of mind. It seems that depression and poor coping skills are often a better predictor of back pain than disc damage. The researchers emphasized that treating a patient for emotional and perceptual concerns may be more beneficial in reducing lower back pain than the more conventional invasive, costly, and oftentimes unsuccessful back surgery option. Can you think of something that would keep you from being depressed? A healthy, active sex life is the first thing that pops into my mind!

Michael Teague, a recreational hockey player, claimed that just cuddling with his special someone eased the intense pain in the knee he twisted during practice. This is because his body kicked into overdrive pumping out the cuddle-chemical oxytocin once he felt the softness of her skin, tasted the warm wetness of her breath, and smelled her candied scent.

No More "I've Got a Headache" Excuses!

Sex releases tensions that restrict blood vessels in the brain, which is the cause of many headaches. Mary Everett, a school teacher, credits having sex on a regular basis (twice a week) for keeping her migraines at bay. She claims, "I have suffered from severe migraine headaches since I was a teenager. The only thing that would help was a prescription narcotic. Ever since I started my 'sex therapy,' I have been pain-free. If my husband isn't available to help me out, I just masturbate when I notice the first twinge of pain. After the first orgasm the migraine goes completely away. I am a firm believer that sex really does heal!"

This testimony should give hope to those lovers whose romantic advances are constantly thwarted because of the dreaded statement, "Not tonight, dear. I have a headache." The next time you hear that lame excuse, simply say, "Darling, I've got just the thing for you!"

Sex Heals Vision Problems

Reduced levels of oxytocin can cause pain so severe in the posterior eye that only narcotics provide effective pain relief. A decrease in oxytocin levels can also cause problems with intermittent blurring of vision. But when synthetic oxytocin is given to patients suffering from this malady, their vision is sharpened. Since oxytocin is released during orgasm, this certainly doesn't lend any credence to the old wives' tale, "Don't play with yourself or you'll go blind." And you won't have to start shaving your palms, either!

Sex and Diabetes

Many diabetics suffer from some type of sexual dysfunction such as fatigue, vaginitis, decreased sex drive, decreased vaginal lubrication, longer period of time to reach orgasm, impotence, or frigidity. The ironic thing is that sex can actually help keep insulin levels in check and improve these conditions, along with many others associated with diabetes.

"Excuse me, honey, could you jack off on this annoying rash, please?"

Forgive me if I get on my soap box for a few paragraphs…. Did you know that in the past decade there has been a 70% increase in the occurrence of type II diabetes? Probably not. Diabetes is a silent killer, and unfortunately most people just seem to accept it because they think there is little they can do about it. Type II diabetes occurs later in life because the person ate too many starchy carbohydrates and sugars, which made their insulin levels rise too high and too quickly, eventually causing their bodies to become insensitive to insulin. Type I diabetics have a genetic factor causing them not to produce enough insulin. Insulin is one of the most important hormones in our bodies because it transports blood sugar to cells to be used for energy.

Aside from how we poison our bodies with sugar, the point I'd like to make is that as long as diabetes is on the rise, for our health's sake there should be a rise in sexual behavior, too. A study by the US Department of Agriculture showed that as oxytocin levels decrease, so does one's sensitivity to insulin. Inversely, as our oxytocin increases, our bodies become more sensitive to insulin.

An extra bonus from having sex if you're a diabetic is the surge of prolactin you get from orgasm. We've shown that prolactin is a stimulating factor for the immune system, but it is especially helpful in reducing elevations in blood glucose (sugar) levels in persons with type I diabetes, according to studies performed by the Department of Medical Cell Biology, Uppsala University in Sweden.

Now, class, what's the best way to naturally increase your oxytocin and prolactin levels? Anyone? Yes! Have orgasms… and lots of them. Well, at least two or three a week.

Sex is also a great way to reduce your risk of diabetes because of the exercise it provides. JoAnne Manson, MD, assistant professor of medicine at Harvard, analyzed health and exercise data from the ongoing Nurses Health Study and found that exercises, such as mattress surfing, performed just one day a week can significantly reduce the risk of diabetes. Glenn Gaesser, PhD, an associate professor of exercise physiology at the University of Virginia in Charlottesville, found that even a leisurely lap or two around the typical mall significantly decreases insulin resistance. He further stated that a few modest walks a week can reduce insulin needs, possibly allowing people with type II diabetes who take insulin to get off it altogether.

Don't you think you could work up just as much of a sweat doing the horizontal bop as you could walking around the block? And most people aren't rewarded with rushes of orgasmic pleasure (not to mention the extra health benefits orgasms give us) while strolling around the block.

Sexy Smile

Someone sent me an email that listed the top ten reasons to make love. One of them was that kissing increases your saliva content and therefore cuts down on cavities and plaque build-up. The list didn't mention anything about cunnilingus or fellatio, but I can't think of many other acts that make us salivate more. Can you?

In addition, vaginal fluid has immune-enhancing properties, and semen contains muscle-building protein and energy-giving fructose. Of course, you would have to drink at least a gallon of semen to receive optimal benefits. Baby steps, baby steps….

Sexy Skin

Hopefully, you put enough energy into your lovemaking sessions to work up a good sweat. Sweating helps to cleanse your pores and make your skin glow. The hormone estrogen is also increased in men and women during sex, which helps to keep skin smooth…and gives women their sweet scent. If you want a clearer complexion, do not neglect your sex life.

Are you familiar with that warm, rosy flush you get all over your skin after you orgasm? This sex flush occurs because of an increase in blood flow throughout your skin, which brings vital nutrients that nourish and rejuvenate our external covering. If you have problems with acne or dermatitis, try having more orgasms than normal and watch those pimples or rashes fade away. An active sex life also cuts down on stress levels that can cause skin outbreaks. And if you were to put a dab or two of certain bodily fluids on bug bites, minor scrapes and bruises, rashes, or pimples, you would be amazed at how quickly those problems heal.

Medicine Chest
Breast milk is one such secretion that performs miracles on skin problems, and, as mentioned earlier, if you drink it, your immune system gets an incredible boost. Mother's milk contains immunoglobulins and other substances that have wondrous healing properties, whether applied topically or taken orally.

When I was lactating (which was for six years straight), any time someone close to me had a cut, burn, bruise, bug bite, pimple, etc., I expressed a bit of my milk to apply to it. Within seconds the pain went away. Breast milk also cuts in half the healing time of minor boo-boos. And when someone has a cold or flu, a cup of breast milk can be better than chicken soup. God has given women their very own "medicine chest."

"Breast Milk: It does a body good!"

Love-Juice Ointment
Understandably, women don't lactate all the time, so breast milk can be a little hard to come by, unless you run across someone selling it on some obscure website. This led me to experiment with another fluid, which also contains many healing substances, that most women can manufacture in their bodies. Mm-hm. Vaginal fluid.

The immunity of the female reproductive tract is influenced by immunoglobulins, cytokines, and hormones. Vaginal fluid is rich in these healthy essences. I bet you're dying to know how I tested it, huh? Well, as I mentioned earlier, down in the Deep South where I was raised, we have mosquitoes that have been known to carry away small children. One of these little suckers bit me while I was in bed one night, and it itched horribly! Since my youngest son had pretty much drained all

of my breast milk for the night, and I was too tired to get up for a salve, I decided to get my finger wet by sliding it inside my vagina, then I saturated that bulging, stinging irritation. Instantly, the itching and burning ceased, and I fell peacefully back to sleep, right after making a mental note to add that juicy bit of information to this book.

The only real experience I've had with the healing benefits of semen on my skin is that I notice when my lover ejaculates on my tummy, back, face, or other parts of my body, I feel silky smooth for the next few hours after I clean up. And when I swallow his ejaculate, I feel energized.

According to a recent study by scientists at the State University of New York, it appears that the mood-enhancing hormones in semen—namely testosterone—are absorbed through the vagina and by swallowing semen. I haven't had an opportunity to experiment with semen on any boo-boos yet, however. "Excuse me, honey, could you jack off on this annoying rash, please?" If any of you do, please contact me with the results <www.thehealthysexymom.com>.

Sex Heals Incontinence
Speaking of bodily fluids.... Incontinence (losing voluntary control over urinating) occurs when the weight of the bladder, unable to be properly supported by damaged PC mus-

Hormones released during sexual excitement and orgasm can elevate pain thresholds.

cles (the muscles that you press down on to stop the flow of urine) causes it to sag. This changes the angle of the bladder, the bladder neck, and the urethra (the canal through which urine flows out of the body), and weakens the bladder neck seal. Wetting oneself unintentionally can then occur under the stress of exercising, sneezing, coughing, lifting, etc. or under the urge of a filling bladder. By engaging in regular sexual activity and having orgasms, the muscles that support the bladder are given a great workout and thereby strengthened and toned.

Sex improves our immune system. Sex helps us live longer. Sex relieves pain. Sex can improve vision and skin. Sex can reduce our risk for diabetes, as well as improve conditions in people who already suffer from the disorder. To screw or not to screw? You decide.

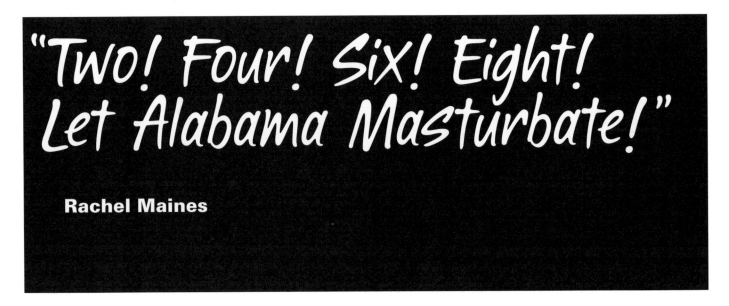

"Two! Four! Six! Eight! Let Alabama Masturbate!"

Rachel Maines

When my book *The Technology of Orgasm: "Hysteria," the Vibrator, and Women's Sexual Satisfaction* was first published by Johns Hopkins University Press in 1999, I received a call from a Swiss manufacturer of upscale vibrators. He was in the United States trying to buy advertising for his company's device and had targeted slick, upmarket women's magazines like *Vogue* and *Glamour*, which were publishing ads for Viagra. None would accept his company's advertising. Baffled and frustrated, he asked why and was told, "Viagra is for men having sex with women. Vibrators are for women having sex by themselves, and we can't endorse that." Looks as if the double standard is alive and well, raising both its ugly heads in American advertising, as well as American law.

According to the FBI's Uniform Crime Report, more than 16,000 murders were committed in the United States in 2003, along with more than 93,000 rapes and 413,000 rob-

Southern legislatures acted against the dire threat represented by women discovering that vibrators produce their orgasms much more reliably than penises do.

beries. In Alabama, Texas, Georgia, and Kansas, law enforcement extends beyond these obvious threats to what some legislators apparently believe is a more subtle and insidious threat to American morals: the sale of vibrators and dildos.

Until the arrest of Passion Party's Joanne Webb in Burleson, Texas, in 2003, which generated a veritable storm of media hilarity and bad jokes, few Americans were even aware that the sale of vibrators and the possession of more than five (count 'em!) is against the law in some states. Those who did know

usually assumed that the laws against them were decrepit survivors of the Comstock era. Some of them are—Massachusetts still has such a law on its books, dating from 1879, in the same section of code that prohibits the dispensing of contraceptives, both judiciously and judicially ignored since *Griswold v. Connecticut* (1965). The anti-obscenity laws of Texas, Alabama, and Georgia, however, don't even have the excuse of antiquity to explain their existence, let alone their enforcement.

South Dakota has the dubious distinction of having led this modern wave of sex-negative legislation in 1968 by including vague warnings in its anti-obscenity act, SD Code § 22-24-27, regarding unspecified "equipment, machines or materials" that might appeal "to the prurient." That same year, Kansas drafted legislation, KS § 21-4301, which in its present (amended) form prohibits the sale of "a dildo or artificial vagina, designed or marketed as useful primarily for the stimulation of human genital organs, except such devices disseminated or promoted for the purpose of medical or psychological therapy." This statute was successfully challenged in 1990 and has not been officially enforced since, although a citizens' group in Abilene recently convened its own grand jury and indicted a local sex-toy store owner.

Texas' and Georgia's statutes date from the mid-1970s, apparently a response both to technological change in the sex-toy industry that made possible more lurid anatomical representation, and, more ominously, to the then-new association of vibrators with feminism. Betty Dodson had begun her campaign of teaching us to reclaim female sexuality from the tired old "all she needs is a good fuck" model, and Dell Williams had recently launched the world's first feminist sex-toy store in New York City, Eve's Garden. Southern legislatures acted against the dire threat represented by women discovering that vibrators produce their orgasms much more reliably than penises do. Apparently they'd all heard the old joke that goes: "When did God make men? When she found out vibrators couldn't dance."

Although one would intuitively suppose that legislatures had better things to do, other states with apparently similar fears followed suit: Colorado's Rev. Stat. § 18-7-1-101, 102 to the same effect was passed in 1981 and overturned in 1985. Georgia passed § 16-12-80 (c) on this question in 1975. The Texas statute, § 43.21, revised in 1977, was the model for some of the later laws, including Alabama's 1998 Anti-Obscenity Act. These statutes prohibit the sale of "a device designed and marketed as useful primarily for stimulation of the human genital organs," making it an offense to possess "six or more obscene devices or identical or similar obscene articles," because such possession indicates intent to sell. Nebraska legislated in 1977 against any "article, or device having the appearance of either male or female genitals" (Nebraska Code § 28-808), clearly reacting to the appearance rather than the function of sexual devices.

In 1983, two more states weighed in, Indiana with a statute (IC § 35-49-1-3) as vague as South Dakota's and probably copied from it, and Mississippi with what was already becoming the standard wording for this new type of legislation, prohibiting the sale of any "device designed or marketed as useful primarily for the stimulation of the human genital organs" (Mississippi Code § 97-29-105). In these legislative novelties, appearance, packaging, and marketing rather than functionality seem to be the decisive factors in whether or not a device is "obscene." So you can sell whatever you please, as long as you're sufficiently hypocritical about what the device is good for.

The American Civil Liberties Union challenged the Alabama act of 1998 almost as soon as the ink was dry, and it was twice upheld in the (Federal) District Court for the Northern District of Alabama. In 2003 Alabama's law was upheld as absurd but constitutional by the Eleventh Circuit Court of Appeals, the same Atlanta body that ruled in George W. Bush's favor in the 2000 election. The laws remain on the books, and the threat of enforcement remains, as well. Georgia's law was challenged a few years ago by a sex-toy store and was upheld.

Despite the best efforts of Eve Ensler of *Vagina Monologues* fame, Joanne Webb of Burleson, Texas, and an article by Jennifer Senior in the *New York Times Magazine* of July 4, 2004 (Independence Day!), reactions from the feminist community since 1998 have been muted. Some of us have trouble believing that anything as ludicrous as this could possibly be going on in a modern industrial democracy. Others assume that women in the sex-toy-prohibition states can still buy their favorite gadgets legally over the Internet, which unfortunately isn't the case. The seller is still technically violating the law by completing the sale within the state, although so far there have been no indictments of out-of-state sellers.

Thousands are dying in Iraq, global warming is a fact, certifiable wackos roam the streets with dangerous firearms, and

These statutes prohibit the sale of "a device designed and marketed as useful primarily for stimulation of the human genital organs."

what do Southern legislatures and law enforcement agencies worry about? Women having more fun by themselves than they might be having with men. With fun-loving guys like them in charge, maybe they *ought* to worry. Hell, they probably can't dance, either.

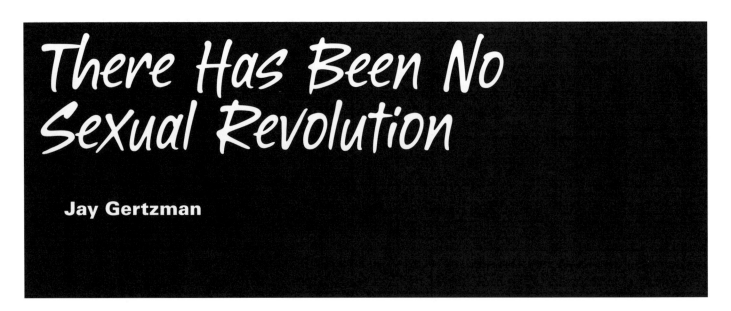

There Has Been No Sexual Revolution

Jay Gertzman

"American reality . . . stupefies, it sickens, it infuriates, and finally it is a kind of embarrassment to one's meager imagination."

–Philip Roth, 1962

A glimpse of one hot babe's nipple excited a load of hard-ons—many of the figurative kind—during 2004's Super Bowl half-time show. Those made rigid with moral indignation included the FCC, Bill O'Reilly, Laura Bush, the Parents TV Council, and Concerned Women of America. Clear-eyed columnist Frank Rich saw that Janet Jackson and Justin Timberlake's presentation was as a whole a seduction dance, previewed

I am convinced that the very same attitudes and procedures apply now as did a century ago regarding the red flags, or taboo signals, that sexual explicitness raises.

(presumably sans nipple) by CBS and approved as sanitized, rocking fun that would hold audience attention through the next $80,000-a-second commercial.[1]

The next pigskin season was half over when another hottie visited a team locker room; a star receiver's eyes widen as she drops her towel and jumps into his arms. The ball player, not the audience, sees the goods; no way he's going back on the field. It's a *Monday Night Football* lead-in. ABC's ratings for the games were down; the controversy could not but help. More hands wrung in dismay—kids are still up. Parents hate to let them see hot sex. Adults' own ambivalence when exposed to it, a mixture of prurience and moral chagrin, makes it hard to talk about indecency with their children. The towel-off gives commentators on the corporate sports network a debate topic, a laugh, and a platform spanning several commercials. And the actress' show, *Desperate Housewives*, gets a ratings goose, even if ABC does not. So does a CBS outlet in Cleveland. That same night, a local "news journalist" takes off her clothes to join other volunteers for an (ephemeral) installation of street art. Among those outraged was the artist—at the exploitation of his art form. In mainstream American TV, prurient escapism is a staple even of local "news" broadcasts.[2] After all, they have to compete with *Entertainment Tonight*.

January 2005: Outgoing FCC commissioner Michael Powell fails to get a conviction in the case of an Internet distributor of videos dedicated to storylines of extreme abuse, including rape, of women. *Nightline* has three obviously biased principals as talking heads: an outraged feminist, a Justice Department official, and the gonzo pornographer who owns Extreme Associates (his wife is one of the performers). Ted Koppel, who is leaving ABC, is not hosting. No First Amendment lawyer appears. The program is titled "Privacy vs. Morality," although public morality can hardly be affected by what all but a few will not pay to download. The question of harm is begged, and the distinction between narrowcasting and broadcasting is not mentioned. Nor is the distinction between how a few psychopaths and the vast majority of people react to what they choose to see and hear. There is no study that shows a correlation between a sane person's private fantasies and his actions, but the last word is granted to the Bush administration official, who vows a full attack on all kinds of obscenity. He reiterates the 1986 Meese Commission's conclusion that all sexually explicit representations are harmful, in an escalating scale from pin-ups to *Playboy* to hardcore videos.

George W. Bush's chief political advisor, Karl Rove (whom

his boss has endearingly, and coarsely, dubbed "Turd Blossom"), opines that a desire to fight immoral TV and films was the reason Bush won re-election. "I think it's people who are concerned about the coarseness of our culture, about what they see on the television sets, what they see in the movies." *Desperate Housewives'* popularity in the Bush-friendly states aside,[3] this has to be the last word. Rove engineered the defamation of three military heroes as variously mentally unbalanced (John McCain), unpatriotic (Max Cleland), or dishonest (John Kerry).[4] Each was running against either a prominent Republican or Bush himself, whose tour of duty was in a National Guard office. In any discussion of hypocrisy, and of the way well-spun, sickening fantasies about political opponents fuck with the facts on the ground, Rove on indecency is an obscenity no one can beat.

Having studied the publication, distribution, and prosecution of pornography in America in the twentieth century, I am convinced that the very same attitudes and procedures apply now as did a century ago regarding the red flags, or taboo signals, that sexual explicitness raises. Regardless of the groundbreaking changes in obscenity law, there has never been a sexual revolution in America. A New Deal, yes. Progress toward social equality, fine. In Bushworld, these are endangered, while under its watch the following revolutionary developments have progressed: destruction of safety nets protecting citizens from loss of job and Social Security benefits, faith-based initiatives that would put institutions with a specific religious *raison d'être* in charge of medical and educational public services, militarized police forces, cynicism about how America has controlled other nations' destinies, and the capitulation of professional journalists to the demands of their employers' PR offices.

This President has also embraced ideas geared at initiatives regarding faith-based and, thus, abstinence-only programs here and abroad. He is "pro-life," anti-abortion, anti-gay marriage, anti-adult entertainment. As Attorney General, John Ashcroft attempted to block any website adjudged indecent in order to protect young people, even if it meant ignoring principles established half a century ago stating that adults cannot be prevented from accessing what might unbalance the most impressionable members of a community. Yet Bushworld's agendas concerning the morality of what people can do or vicariously experience sexually cannot be called radical. As I hope this essay shows, there has never been a revolution in the prurient ambiguities and anxieties that sex stimulates in the American consciousness. The prurience leads to censorship or five-second delays in transmission or decency codes. Any such actions just shift the temporary onus from one bookseller, one company or medium to another, and make it

harder to determine the hidden source of the sexually explicit entertainment. The result is better and better for business.

I

The present generation has witnessed the tolerance of sexual subcultures as legitimate consumer groups, legalized abortion, a narrower range of obscenity prosecutions, and different erotica-distribution methods. Once-taboo "perversions" are now the subject of titillation on sitcoms. Also as part of the mainstreaming of porno into popular culture, fetish costuming and accessorizing have taken their roles in the drama of high fashion. One socioeconomist opines that the bear market is an explanation for the mainstreaming phenomenon, which has produced lucrative gentlemen's clubs, ladies' nights at the Penthouse Boutique, autobiographies of porn stars, and Fortune 500 adult-entertainment corporations.[5]

But mainstreaming means that what made individual pornographers wealthy fifty years ago makes a fortune for corporate sponsors now. Anyone who thinks that 1950s erotica customers couldn't have imagined what is available today was never below the counter in a Times Square adult bookstore. Those cheaply produced booklets, photo sets, and films allowed a few porn kings to buy homes in exclusive New York and Connecticut suburbs. Distributors themselves have

There has never been a revolution in the prurient ambiguities and anxieties that sex stimulates in the American consciousness.

morphed from Jewish middlemen to Mafia lieutenants to upper-middle-class Internet providers with college degrees.

There are no more Societies for the Suppression of Vice or citizens privately deputized to spy and inform on publishers and booksellers of erotica, but associations dedicated to protecting the "traditional" (i.e., now nearly obsolete) family unit, federal obscenity task forces, and anti-indecency clauses in NEA grants have taken up the slack. Bush's Secretary of Education Margaret Spellings began her reign by attacking a PBS children's TV show that, in just one episode, portrayed gay moms as ordinary folk one's kids might enjoy meeting. Faced with a loss of funding, the network voluntarily pulled the episode. It couldn't afford to dissent from a "healthy marriage initiative" which a godly administration has managed to fund with taxpayer's money.[6]

We are still making the same fantastic distinctions between acceptable mass entertainment and obscenity as we did when pin-ups on magazines were red-blooded fun but the same newsstand publications showing cover girls brandishing whips or wearing spiked collars were confiscated as degenerate. Janet Jackson's exposed nipple: an outrage. The Super Bowl's beer commercials featuring (as Frank Rich observes) "a crotch-biting dog, a flatulent horse and a potty-mouthed child": that's entertainment. In the late 1990s, with the Giuliani administration tearing down the Times Square porn shops, a giant Calvin Klein poster towered over 42nd Street featured teenage rapper Marky Mark in form-fitting Calvin Klein jeans and little else. Rebecca Robinson of the Times Square Business Improvement District had to wonder "how far we'd actually come."[7]

That question could have been asked about the mayoral strategies that led to the eradication of the Times Square porn stores themselves. Over sixty-five years ago, in 1937, Mayor LaGuardia earned himself quite another epithet than Little Flower among New York's young men by initiating the process, completed in 1942, of closing down burlesque. As in Giuliani's time, it was not obscenity legislation but zoning that stamped out the offending blight (42nd Street was a dangerous place to be by the mid-1980s, although not because of the porn-strip-peep palaces, but due to Mob involvement in drugs and prostitution, to which the porn stores were ancillary). During the Depression, Times Square had lost its elite theaters and speakeasies, and had become increasingly a

The remedy was a draconian exercise in self-censorship, the Comic Book Code.

cornucopia of mass entertainment, or honky tonk. As tabloid editorials verbally strafed the Minsky-owned burlesque theaters as "plague centers," LaGuardia attacked especially the Minsky chain as places of "incorporated filth," and opined, without supporting evidence, that the striptease had incited the recent sex crimes that the New York dailies ballyhooed.[8]

Mayors Wagner, Lindsay, Beame, and Koch, as well as Giuliani, later similarly described the Mobbed-up, increasingly sleazy sex carnival that Times Square was becoming. Garish, erotically-focused signage, all-night sex emporia, streetwalkers, pavements littered with flyers for peep shows and massage parlors, shouted insults, and bottle gangs were part of this late-twentieth-century vice center. But both LaGuardia and Giuliani knew that First Amendment cases were hard to win, especially with brilliant lawyers such as Morris Ernst in the 1930s and Herald Price Fahringer in the 1990s declaring that there were specific criteria separating the sexually explicit from the legally obscene.

After winning the obscenity conviction of a single burlesque show, LaGuardia's License Commissioner resorted to his power to refuse to renew the permits of any burlesque the-

ater. The Commissioner based his decision on two separate observations, shared by area businessmen. He said that the burlesque, from lobby card and marquee to runway and stage, had encouraged rowdiness, was "completely sex-centered," and was "poisoning" the district's social life. He also pointed out—and this was why he used his licensing power—that their youthful and working-class clientele, gaudy billboards, and flannel-mouthed barkers had brought down property values in the area.[9] It was the 42nd Street Property Owners and Merchants Association, complaining since 1919 of the decline of respectable businesses on the street, that alerted the local anti-vice organizations to the problem in the first place.

In the 1990s, after the Times Square Business Improvement District (BID) interpreted a neighborhood survey as revealing the negative "secondary effects" of the porn shops on other businesses, similar zoning regulations went into effect. The BID surveyed owners of "major chain" and "well known" restaurants, apartment houses, and hotels; real estate brokers; church and community groups; and public-school principals.[10] There was general agreement among those interviewed that the sex businesses brought down property values, discounted tourism, and increased crime. The sample used was criticized, and statistics regarding these effects were disputed as inconclusive.[11] Bottom line: The Disney organization demanded that before they would invest in 42nd Street's redevelopment, the Deuce's sex businesses had to go.[12] Property values and city revenues certainly did soar with the clearing of the redevelopment area and Disney's purchase of the New Amsterdam Theater.

In both cases, the losers were the *hoi polloi*. In the 1930s, they filled the grinder movie houses, taxi dancehalls, shooting galleries, juice stands, carny flea circuses, and cafeterias. The gay population in the nearby residential hotels enjoyed the same attractions and had its own hangouts, as well.[13] In the 1970s and 1980s legions of underclass and middle-class adolescent males and adults wanted the peep booths, porn theaters where whatever kind of alternate sexuality was tolerated, and non-sex outlets such as the delis, cut-rate drug, electronic, and clothing stores, army-navy outlets, and novelty shops.[14] Moreover, it is doubtful that owners of these latter business really would object to neighboring sex emporia, since they served many of their patrons. People who need inexpensive goods and services, who in the 1930s could not afford call girls, night clubs, or under-the-counter photos and books, and who in 1995 could not afford Internet porn, phone sex, or gentlemen's clubs, needed to venture to the peep booths and browse magazines, photo sets, and used videos.

The essential fact was and is that commercialized sex, partly because it is widely affordable, is incompatible with the status with which an elite must identify itself. Therefore, the latter will remove it from an urban neighborhood in which it plans to invest its power. Ironically, that same elite includes the entertainment, clothing, and publishing empires that exploit prurience to contribute to our most powerful economic institutions and political officeholders. Thus the Marky/Calvin Klein billboard, as well as the Janet Jackson Super Bowl show and the revenue Fox and other media giants garner from cable and hotel-room porno.[15]

Also ironically, in the case of Times Square, its re-creation as a city center with corporate towers and chain restaurants and upscale stores meant the renewal of creative vitality in architecture, theater, and music. Even a progressive social observer like Frank Rich acknowledged this.[16] The Business Improvement District was fortunate to have talented administrators such as William Daly, Gretchen Dykstra, and the aforementioned Rebecca Robinson. New Yorkers have learned never to underestimate the dynamic duo of Rudy G. and Micky M.

II

How far have we come? Rich's essay on the 2004 Super Bowl is a reality check to those who feel "the censorship is over." He finds an antecedent to the "healthy family initiative" in the mid-1950s agitation over comic books that—energized by a congressional committee and an influential study of mass culture called *Seduction of the Innocent* which helped develop its agenda—asserted that rape, gang violence, and latent homosexuality were generated by depictions of bloodthirsty gangsters and their busty molls in crime comics.[17] Their opportunistic publishers, it was widely believed, had the morality of gutter rats.

Apparently, the remedy for troubled youth fascinated by sex and violence did not require that parents, teachers, and religious advisors reassess why they were being ignored, or that they consider how popular entertainment reflected what young people learned about power and violence from looking around them as the Korean War ended. People were being dismissed from their jobs through blacklisting; alcoholism and divorce were increasing; school students were taught how to "duck and cover" in case of atomic attack; and hydrogen bombs were being tested in the Western deserts. Politicians, clergy, teachers, and businessmen too seldom discussed core reasons for such events or their effects on young people's attitudes. Instead, parents were advised to be more insistent in teaching right from wrong, to go to church more often, and to condone more censoring of what did not accord with their tastes and values since, as J. Edgar Hoover preached, obscenity and indecency might be "pinko"-inspired.[18] The coarse-

ness of our culture, then as now, might be the enemy within. Coarseness in this context means indecency and obscenity. The qualifying adjective was, and is, *insidious*. *Coarse*, or the earlier words *dirty*, *lewd*, *smutty*, and *filthy*, refer to the pariah middlemen, those "polluters of our culture," who distribute it. Behind them were thought to be the malcontents, anarchists, communists, or America-haters.

The investigation of crime comics was typical, as was the response by the publishers.[19] That response was not to deplore the snarl words authorities used or the humiliation suffered by subpoenaed publishers. Rather, the industry addressed the fact that the criticism could not be good for business. The remedy was a draconian exercise in self-censorship, the Comic Book Code. It outlawed nudity, any form of indecent words or phrases "which have acquired undesirable meanings," stories involving "illicit sex" and "sexual abnormalities," and female costuming that "exaggerat[es] any physical qualities" or is not "reasonably acceptable to society." In addition, "respect for parents, the moral code, and for honorable behavior shall be fostered." Profanity, obscenity, smut, and vulgarity were forbidden. Finally, "policemen, judges, government officials, and respected institutions shall never be presented in such a way as to create disrespect for established authority."

One comic book that couldn't pass muster with the enforcement agency, the Comic Code Authority, was the fledgling *Mad*, since it dedicated each issue to satirizing injustice. Therefore, it could not be handled by the industry's distributors. The solution was for it to avoid the standards for publications aimed at a readership under age fifteen by becoming a magazine.[20] Apparently publishers of comic books did not share *Mad*'s desire to teach or inform, if it got them bad press and parental disapproval. They might, if they wished, show that they could enlighten readers by pointing to the "Classics Illustrated" series. However, that publisher took advantage of the fascination with the dark and violent side of human nature by putting out another edition of Mary Shelley's *Frankenstein*. Equally hard to defend, and good for business, was the program of Dell comics. Exempted from the Code because they published the Walt Disney line, Dell took advantage by doing horror comics, including *Tales From the Tomb* in 1962.[21] Avidity for profit trumped all other goals.

For several years, Wal-Mart, K-Mart, and Blockbuster have been no less vigilant than the Kefauver Committee and its supporters. Rock and rap musicians can't afford not to comply with the decency standards of the giant store chains, so they have albums specially edited for these outlets. The revised lyrics and album covers exclude the erotic and scatological words and images in packages distributed elsewhere. This means that their fans in many rural areas of the country

THERE HAS BEEN NO SEXUAL REVOLUTION   *311*

have no choice regarding the music and lyrics they purchase. Wal-Mart and K-Mart assert that the surveys they rely on for verification show customers approve of the practice (how were those questions phrased?). Therefore, they deny that the revisions of the music are prior restraint. It takes open-mindedness to listen dispassionately to many rap and rock lyrics glorifying fighting and gang solidarity, as well as contempt for "bitches," white people, teachers, and police. But at least part of the defiance serves as a wake-up call about the astonishing inequalities between classes and races in America and the results of those inequalities. It's foolish to ignore the messages and silence the messenger.

It is as regressive now as it was half a century ago to insure that teenagers never criticize what teachers, policemen, judges, clergy, or other "established authorities" tell them about sex and violence. If it was disingenuous to impose censorship then by calling it a code of decency, it is even more so to use current economic jargon to redefine it as "target marketing."[22] All it is, is good business and the tyranny of the majority, as was the Code for the comic-book industry. In a country which prides itself on raising young people to understand all sides of an issue and to make independent choices, the behavior of the chain stores, as that of the comic-book industry, is coarse and vulgar.

The 1990s brought to the Western world designer clothing, Hollywood's NC-17 films, day spas for men, gentlemen's clubs, and erotic experiences via telephone, hotel-room cable TV, and the Internet. The general population's increasing exposure to sex has been good for the entertainment business. In the liberal 1960s, when the so-called sexual revolution was jump-started, sex was equally good for the publishing business. The best evidence is Ralph Ginzburg's performance, in an inappropriately colorful blazer and straw hat, before the Supreme Court, which helped get him a jail sentence in 1963. He was brashly proud of appealing to prurience in his advertisements, inflicting a reality check on the Supremes that made them judge the man, not the material.[23] Ginzburg's point was that differences between Grove Press' scholarly editions of *Tropic of Cancer* and *Lady Chatterley's Lover* and his *Eros* magazine's erotica were only a matter of the cosmetics of packaging and blurbs. For most purchasers, furtive curiosity is a prime impulse. Therefore, Grove benefited less from the Brennan Court's rulings than did TV, movies, magazines, and mass-market paperbacks. Ginzburg implied that the Court, however idealistic, was being neither logical nor realistic about the underlying reason—the health of the economy—for its de-censorship rulings. Who could blame them, since they were not at all venal and Ginzburg clearly was a pitch man?

In the mid-twentieth century, and equally today, many people handled the sex side of their lives in such a way as to en-courage self-respect and a path to honest affection. When that happens, the symbiosis between erotica distributors and authorities who reinforce their power by identifying illicit sex with degeneracy has truly been subverted. With successful advocacy of the rights of sexual minorities, and the frank expression of their desires and sex practices, the subject of sexual expression has been taken from the closet and asserted—by a much criticized minority—as legitimate and necessary. Yet, next to terrorism, and with an equally feverous distinction between us and them, "sexual permissiveness" is the easiest straw man to rage against. Karl Rove's "moral values" shtick, his focus on the culture war as opposed to the horrible facts of the unilaterally-waged Operation Iraqi Freedom, was a factor in the 2004 election.

Comforting belief systems shared by trusted friends and co-workers are much easier to ratify than unsuccessful wars started for discredited reasons. The indignation generated by Republican spin artists hungry for the votes and money of Christian fundamentalists has resonance in the hearts and minds of Americans trained to see survival as a battle between us and them. Gay marriage, abortion rights, and high-school sex-education courses seem more personal to many Americans than the daily horrors characterizing the Bushite occupation of Iraq. Moral crusades are always political, none more intensely so than those which occur in times already scarred by national emergencies. So how far have we come since J. Edgar Hoover explained that the Reds were planting pornography in order to demoralize our people and debauch their children?

III

The eagerness of journalists to cover prurient-interest stories, be they about erotic images of children or salacious advertisements, is as regular as cable TV tabloid news. Spokespeople for sexual decency, whether clergymen, public officeholders, or police officials, are—as they have been for a century—entrepreneurs, identifying themselves with their cause and its righteousness. Erotica distributors do much the same thing. Whenever it is to their advantage, they say they are furthering First Amendment and privacy issues, but they are making a living as middlemen, doing the unpleasant job of providing taboo material. And how well they have learned the variety of stories and pictures that would do that! *Desperate Housewives* and Extreme Associates are examples. So were the 1950s sex pulps, 1960s sexploitation movies, and pioneering porno-chic films like *Deep Throat* and *Behind the Green Door*. Erotica exploits fantasies with which customers are enthralled, however ambivalent about what they see. Its distributors' best friend has always been the opportunistic moralist who allies with political authority to deplore sexually explicit texts and images.

In both the 1950s and today, moral crusaders think they defend an otherwise virile, clean-minded nation against an alien infection which coarsens and debilitates by unleashing "the virulence of sex." In the 1920s, that phrase was a shibboleth of the New York Society for the Suppression of Vice. It remains to be seen whether Michael Powell's successor at the FCC, Kevin J. Martin, will resurrect it. Maybe he'll prefer the connotations of "coarseness." He undoubtedly will not allude to two examples of sanctioned sexual humiliations: those routinely inflicted on fraternity pledges and on Guantanamo and Baghdad prisoners of Operation Iraqi Freedom and the "War on Terror."

There are other possible, but highly improbable, targets. Frank Rich offers wonderfully infuriating examples of how sex's most successful purveyors make financial and moral capital simultaneously. At the same time as Fox "News" plumps for decency, its sports division replays the one titillating ad in the 2005 Super Bowl broadcast, as well as gyrating *Playboy* bunnies, on its "Funhouse Fox of the Week" website. Adelphia Communications, ardent supporter of homophobic, pro-life Senator Rick Santorum, offers XXX cable porn, as does Comcast, prime contributor to George W. Bush.[24] As of March 2005, five of the Senate's most indignant critics of "the coarseness of our culture" had accepted campaign contributions from the Marriott and Holiday Inn hotel chains, which realize enormous profits from hardcore movies offered in their rooms.[25] Contributions from Comcast, Time Warner Cable, Charter Communications, Cablevision, EchoStar (parent company of the DISH Network), and DIRECTV, all of which draw enormous profits from adult programming, regularly are gratefully accepted by members of Congress.

This kind of hypocrisy is common because of the prurient curiosity with which sex, the ultimate and universal form of human intimacy, is bonded. As long as this is so, sex will be integral with money and power in America. If "sex is like money" is a stupefyingly twisted maxim, money does flow from the deep mine of profit yielded from the bonding of sex with prurience. Just follow the career of any twentieth-century bookseller who supplemented general literature and magazines with erotica and thenceforward flourished: Eddie Mishkin, Irving Klaw, and Bob Brown (New York), James Delacey (Boston), Horace Townsend (Philadelphia), Lou Saxton (Pittsburgh), Reuben Sturman (Cleveland), Mike Thevis (Atlanta), Harry Schwartz (Milwaukee), Stanley Rose (Los Angeles), N. M. Gordon (Hollywood).

Almost any event in which the subject becomes notorious

conceals a kaleidoscope of motives. Those ran close to the surface in the Clinton impeachment scandal, in which the President was shamed with oral sex, former judge Kenneth Starr's report became a pornographic milestone, William Bennett despaired that Americans could not share his moral indignation, and the sanctimonious Newt Gingrich's and Henry Hyde's affairs were exposed by Larry Flynt.[26]

For perspective, let's take a look at a major celebrity event of 1953: the headline-grabbing vice trial of one Mickey Jelke, a wealthy young playboy who, awaiting his large inheritance to come due, had been for several months pimping café-society showgirls. No one revealed the concealed motives governing the way Jelke's trial was conducted, but at least some of them can be surmised. The presiding judge refused to allow the press to cover testimony of the District Attorney's glamorous star witness. He said that the sexually explicit details would debauch the impressionable young people of Manhattan. Regardless of First Amendment principles, it was wrong, he opined, to allow sensational tabloid coverage of "proceed-

As of March 2005, five of the Senate's most indignant critics of "the coarseness of our culture" had accepted campaign contributions from the Marriott and Holiday Inn hotel chains, which realize enormous profits from hardcore movies offered in their rooms.

ings...permeated with crimes and acts of a salacious or sexual nature." The ruling was patently absurd, given what was available in theaters, on newsstands, and on TV screens. It earned Judge Valente shouts of derision from the New York dailies. With it, however, several famous actors and performers on both coasts (Mickey Rooney, Bob Hope, George Raft, Joey Adams, and Martha Ray were some of those who might have been involved), and especially their agents (whose way of doing business was a template for the accused), breathed easier, as did the owners of midtown nightclubs and Hollywood studios.[27]

Protecting Jelke's more seasoned associates in "vice" was especially incongruous in light of the presiding judge's decision that the convicted Jelke couldn't be released on bail pending his sentencing. His Honor singled out the hapless playboy as in need of an immediate start on rehabilitation, for he had been "flagrantly oblivious to the barest standards of decency in his personal relationships." Apparently, the distinction between Jelke and the more veteran and well-connected members of the café-society crowd was the flagrancy angle, although any such statement would have made Valente hit the ceiling in a hopping, howling fit.

Jelke and a confederate went to prison, an already declining café society lost more glitter, and neither the stars, their agents, nor their studios were subject to public scrutiny. Nor, save one dress manufacturer with a salacious and kinky photo collection, were the Garment District executives and their clients. The latter routinely asked their hosts to set them up with "dates" and therefore comprised most of the high-rolling johns. The manufacturer with the collection (a former husband of famous designer Ceil Chapman) spent a night in jail but apparently was never brought to trial.

Today, as in the twentieth century, politicians, lawyers, and opinion-shapers use scapegoats, snarl words, and automatic responses to get citizens to conceive of coarseness (indecency and obscenity) as a social evil that true leaders can eliminate, if not impeded by smutmongers who will do anything for a buck. No one wants to admit that the sin is in his own mind and heart. Our leaders tell us whom to punish. But as far as the porn profits of Fox, Comcast, ESPN, ABC, CBS, Adelphia, and other corporations are concerned, they and the executives who conceived the relevant deals are almost invisible. Fifty years ago, so were the Garment Center executives, their clients, and the Hollywood agents and actors who disappeared in the not-so-deep background of the Jelke case. For a century now, the same can be said of real estate agents,

As long as we equate sex with dirt, weakness, and guilt, a powerful weapon exists for demagogues.

police officials, district attorneys, elected officials, major movie studios, and TV networks, not to mention their banks and investment counselors. Many resourceful professionals in these fields either took "clean graft," turned enormous profits, or won municipal, state, and national elections by offering simplistic and indignant attacks on the easily exposed, publicly vulnerable, street-level corruptors of youth. Ah, the power of sex...and money. The more things change....

One final word. Political discourse about sex need not be a matter of us versus them, purity versus degeneration. It need not be restrained by intractable dogma. Predictably, that is what has been happening. An example is the case of the emergency "morning after pill," which FDA analysts approved for use in 1999. The FDA Commissioner said in 2003 that he would soon release the product. But it has not happened as of April 2005; therefore, Democrats are holding up approval of President Bush's choice for a new FDA head. Conservatives have condemned this pill as "always producing abortion" and, thus, murder. They've also asserted, much as the

1920s anti-vice societies said of teaching poor women about contraception, that it would cause irresponsible behavior.[28]

But on other sex-specific issues there has been a more hopeful and democratic response. FCC Chairman Martin has declared, in response to parental concern about sexual content on cable TV, that he prefers not to use legal measures to restrain it.[29] Even Senator Joseph Lieberman is capable of tolerance, although his history would dictate otherwise. This is the Democrat who rose on the Senate floor during the Lewinsky scandal to reinforce the impression that Clinton's sexual behavior was grounds for impeachment. He joined C. Delores Tucker and William Bennett in warning parents against letting teenagers hear and thus think about what rappers such as Snoop Doggy Dogg say in their "obscene music." Lieberman, Tucker, and Bennett, along with Bob Dole, shamed Time Warner into selling its shares in the record company that was distributing the gangsta rappers and thus "marketing...evil."[30] But even Lieberman has recently acknowledged that more studies are needed to ascertain if listening to violent songs actually causes criminal behavior.[31]

Perhaps we can even be sensible enough to give young people credit for being able to distinguish fantasy and reality. (In fact, despite the increasingly more explicit music and prime-time TV shows, teenage pregnancy, abortion, and intercourse are down by as much as a third in the last decade.[32]) Half a century ago, Senator Kefauver himself baulked at declaring that comic books were the sole source of juvenile rape, sadism, and gang warfare, although the author of *Seduction of the Innocent* had convinced many Americans that this was true. When Catherine MacKinnon and Andrea Dworkin got an ordinance passed in Minneapolis in 1984 equating pornography with whatever might harm women, the mayor understood that it ignored any objective definition of harm, that it made hash of the Bill of Rights, and would have been a nightmare to try to enforce. He knew it would never stand the test of court challenge and vetoed it.[33]

Not every issue involving personal behavior need be determined by political interests in order to build constituent support or by powerful business interests in order to make their customers feel they can respect and trust the people from whom they purchase goods and services. Or does it, in today's atmosphere? There's a big payoff for expurgating popular songs before young people can access them. It's equally lucrative to get urban renewal projects approved by removing sex shops as blight without proving that, although they are in commercial neighborhoods, they actually hurt, or are a problem for, the shops surrounding them. There are obviously disingenuous reasons for crafting ordinances dealing with public morality so that they interdict premarital sex and gay marriage as subverting the American way of life. Why are requests to put on sale safe medication to prevent conception stonewalled? It's hard to separate sincere conviction about when life begins from the fact that Christian fundamentalists are a powerful voting block.

As long as we equate sex with dirt, weakness, and guilt, a powerful weapon exists for demagogues who not only flatter supporters that they are disciplining their own erotic instincts correctly, but also advertise the values they profess as essential to living a good life. Political "architects" will exploit these identity politics to make life a contest between us and them, between "people of faith" (who don't have to reveal their own sexual desires) and "liberals" or "atheists," whose coarseness needs to be investigated and restrained. Phyllis Schlafly has said that the chief problem for the country today is whether "we as a people acknowledge that God exists."[34] Those who do not are pro-abortion, like the state and federal "secularist" judges who "hate religion" and the Healthy Marriage initiative. Equally degenerate, according to this kind of discourse, are the liberal Democrats who want to keep them on the bench so they can keep abortion legal, prevent the "Intelligent Design" doctrine from being taught, and help pornographers keep the Internet unsafe for children to access. Us vs. them. Similarly, patriotism is equated with fighting terrorists, and wars of choice with removing tyrants. It's infuriating, but hey, it's worked so far.

Endnotes

1. Rich, Frank. "My Hero Janet Jackson." *New York Times*, 15 Feb 2004: Arts Section. **2.** Carr, David. "When a TV Talking Head Becomes a Talking Body." *New York Times*, 25 Nov 2004: E1, E5. **3.** Tucker, Cynthia. "Now on FOX: Immoral Values." *Atlanta Journal-Constitution*, 2 Jan 2005. **4.** Davis, Richard H. [McCain's campaign manager in 2000]. "The Anatomy of a Smear Campaign." *Boston Globe*, 21 Mar 2004; Kerry-Edwards 2004. "Bush Waged Nasty Smear Campaign Against McCain in 2000." Press release, 21 Aug 2004; McGrory, Mary. "Dirty Bomb Politics." *Washington Post*, 20 Jun 2003: A23; Moore, James. "Smear Artist." Salon.com, 28 Aug 2004; Moore, James, *et al.* Bush's Brain. John Wiley & Sons, 2003; Siddall, Eric. "How Karl Rove Uses Vietnam Against Kerry." The Simon [www.thesimon.com], 2 Aug 2004. **5.** Folsom, Robert. "Porn and the Bear Market." Bearmarketcentral.com, 27 Sep 2004. **6.** Rich, Frank. "The Year of Living Indecently." *New York Times*, 6 Feb 2005: sec 2, pp 1, 7; Chasnoff, Debra. "Bluster over TV's 'Buster' Only Splits Us Further Apart," *Houston Chronicle*, 4 Feb 2005. **7.** Eliot, Marc. *Down 42nd Street: Sex, Money, Culture and Politics at the Center of the World.* Warner Books, 2001: 254. **8.** Alexander, H.M. *Strip Tease: The Vanished Art of Burlesque.* Knight, 1938: 113; Senelick, Laurence. "Private Parts in Public Places." In William R. Taylor, ed. *Inventing Times Square.* Russell Sage Foundation Publications, 1991: 335; Shteir, Rachel. *Striptease: The Untold History of the Girlie Show.* Oxford University Press, 2004: 92-93,170-76. **9.** "*People v. Moss* – Undecided," p. 7, File no. 391, Morris Ernst Papers, Humanities Research Center, University of Texas at Austin; *op cit.*, Senelick: 337; Friedman, Andrea. *Prurient Interests: Gender, Democracy, and Obscenity in New York City, 1909-1945.* Columbia University Press, 2000: 83-90. **10.** "Report on the Secondary Effects of the Adult Use Establishments in the Times Square Area," Times Square BID, 1994: 12-4, 37-9. **11.** For the responses of lawyers for the sex shops who appealed the zoning regulations on First Amendment grounds, see Traub, James. *The Devil's Playground: A Century of Pleasure and Profit in Times Square.* Random House, 2004: 194; "Lawyer for Sex Shops Predicts Failure of Mayor's Crackdown," *New York Times*, 27 Mar 2001: 97; "Court KO's Closing of XXX Shop," New York *Daily News*, 21 Dec 1999: 6. For a discussion of the complex racial and ethnic groups making up the "community" of late-twentieth-century Times Square, see Kornblum, William, and Terry Williams. "Methodological Notes for a Times Square Field Station," in Robert McNamara, ed. *Sex, Scams, and Street Life: The Sociology of New York City's Times Square.* Prager, 1995. Volume I of the New York State Urban Development Corporation's "42nd Street Development Project: Final Environment Impact Statement," Aug 1984, Section 10 contains a large selection of pro and con comments to the 1984 Project by academics, city planners, representatives of neighborhood associations, and spokespeople for concerned businesses. **12.** *Op cit.*, Eliot: 245-7; Sagalyn, Lynne B. *Times Square Roulette: Remaking the City Icon.* MIT Press, 2001: 346-9. **13.** Gilfoyle, Timothy. "Policing of Sexuality." In William R. Taylor, ed., *Times Square: Commerce and Culture at the Center of the World.* Johns Hopkins University Press, 1996: 317-28. **14.** The best book on what was lost—and why—by Disneyfication is by a frequent customer of the movie theaters of the old Deuce: Delany, Samuel. *Times Square Red; Times Square Blue.* New York University Press, 1999. **15.** More accurately, the entertainer formerly known as Marky Mark, now the fine actor Mark Wahlberg. **16.** *Op cit.*, Sagalin: 343-4. **17.** *Op cit.*, Rich, "Year": 7. For *Seduction of the Innocent* and the public response to it, see Gilbert, James. *A Cycle of Outrage: America's Reaction to the Juvenile Delinquent in the 1950s.* Oxford University Press, 1986: 91-108. **18.** *Report of the New York State Joint Legislative Committee to Study the Publication of Comics.* Williams Press, 1955: 22. **19.** US Senate, Committee on the Judiciary, Subcommittee to Investigate Juvenile Delinquency. *Hearings on Juvenile Delinquency (Comic Books),* 83rd Cong., 2nd Sess., S. Res. 190 (Washington, DC: GPO, 1954). See Gilbert: 143-61. **20.** Sabin, Roger. *Adult Comics: An Introduction.* London: Routledge, 1993: 157-70, 251-4. **21.** *Ibid.*: 166. **22.** Rolfe, Dick, "Wal-Mart Sells 'Sanitized' Music, Film-Censorship or Customer Service." The Dove Foundation, Dec 1996; Hoffman, Hank. "Wal-Mart Blues." *Sonoma County Independent*, 9 Jan 1997. **23.** de Grazia, Edward. *Girls Lean Back Everywhere: The Law of Obscenity and the Assault on Genius.* Vintage, 1993: 502-12. **24.** Rich, Frank. "Hollywood Bets on Chris Rock's 'Indecency,'" *New York Times*, 27 Feb 2005. **25.** The Senators are Sam Brownback (R-KS), Joe Lieberman (D-CT), and John McCain (R-AZ); the Representatives are Tom Delay (R-TX) and Fred Upton (R-MI). See Citizens for Responsibility and Ethics in Washington. "Addicted to Porn: Members of Congress Accept Contributions from Porn Purveyors." www.citizensforethics.org, 10 Mar 2005. **26.** In *The Flynt Report*, 4.1 (1999). **27.** The Archives of the City of New York District Attorney's records have a large file on the case: ACCN#93-39, shelf collection 130218. There were numerous newspaper and magazine articles on the case. Some relevant ones are "Decision Reserved on Jelke Press Ban." *New York Times*, 20 Feb 1953: 14; "Bail Denied Jailed Jelke." *New York Times*, 3 Mar 1953: 22; "Jelke Gets 3-6 Years on Vice Conviction." *New York Times*, 28 March 1953: 1, 243. Jelke was Minot Jelke, heir to a family oleomargarine fortune, but not old enough to receive money from it when he was involved in the pimping. The chief witness, Pat Ward, subsequently attempted a career in show business but failed. The other agent to be convicted, and sentenced to one year in prison, was Ray Daviani. No callgirls were sentenced. **28.** Paynter, Susan. "We've Waited Long Enough for the 'Morning after Pill'," *Seattle Post-Intelligencer*, 13 Apr 2005; Schultz, Connie. "Hard to Swallow Objections to Pill," *Cleveland Plain Dealer*, 18 Dec 2003. **29.** Ahrens, Frank. "FCC Head Downplays Regulation," *Washington Post*, 6 Apr 2005. **30.** "Know Your Enemies," Mass Mic: Preserving Free Expression in Music [www.mass-mic.com]. **31.** "Prepared Statement of Senator Joe Lieberman Media Research Forum...." Digital Kids [www.digital-kids.net]. **32.** Brooks, David. "Public Hedonism and Private Restraint." *New York Times*, 17 Apr 2005: 14 (Op-Ed section). **33.** *Op cit.*, de Grazia: 612-6. **34.** Ridgeway, James, "Mondo Washington: Stalin to the Rescue." *Village Voice*, 13-19 April 2005: 24; Milbank, Dana. "And the Verdict on Justice Kennedy Is: Guilty." *Washington Post*, 9 Apr 2005: A3.

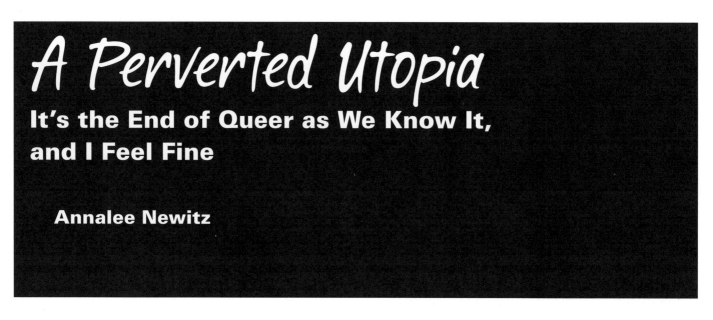

A Perverted Utopia

It's the End of Queer as We Know It, and I Feel Fine

Annalee Newitz

I always knew I was a queer, ever since I got a thrill out of chasing the boys at lunchtime in elementary school. I would run as fast as I could after those preadolescent objects of my desire, grab them in the fists of my seven-year-old grip, and kiss them hard, on the lips or the shoulder or anywhere. It didn't matter. I just wanted to give in to the delirious, seductively violent wrath of a feeling I couldn't quite define.

During those same so-called innocent years, I began playing horsey games with a group of wild, outcast girls. We would wind jump ropes—the bridles, we called them—around one another's bodies and lead each other around, occasionally using an extra jump rope as a whip. After all, horses are supposed to be whipped, right? I had no other choice if I was

I was coming out as bisexual, kinky, and radically, massively genderfucked. I didn't even have words for the thing I would be when I came out.

going to play the game in a fashion true to my beloved *Black Stallion* novels.

I had no choice, in my teens, but to follow my proto-pervert desires into situations far weirder than those I heard described by my peers in the local Orange County gay and lesbian center's youth group. I wasn't just dealing with coming out as a lesbian, which would have been blissfully simple, although no doubt just as painful. Instead, I was coming out as bisexual, kinky, and radically, massively genderfucked. I didn't even have words for the thing I would be when I came out.

But I had actions. I wore men's clothing. I initiated threesomes with my gay male friends so I could watch them fuck.

I begged my girlfriends to have sex with me. I begged my boyfriends to let me take them by force. I refused to be monogamous. Even to my homosexual friends, I seemed like a sexual deviant.

But I knew, somehow, that I was a damn fine queer, and I dreamed about coming to San Francisco, where I imagined that my confusion would give way to coherence. I didn't make it to the city of my dreams for almost a decade, however, and spent the intervening years languishing in East Bay queer circles, where gay men dominated the scene, lesbians had their own separate spaces, and bisexuals and transgendered people showed up at events once in a while only to find themselves part of such a small minority that they never came back. A gay male friend I had at that time tried to explain my sexuality and finally said helplessly, "Well, you're the kind of woman who gay men have sex with."

It was all too much, and I fled to San Francisco in 1997, hoping to find what seemed at the time like science fiction: a radically queer community of bisexual, transgendered, kinky sex freaks who would do anything that moved (as long as they found it attractive, of course). And I found it, buried in the hidden cracks of the "legitimate" queer community, which seemed to be all about legalized marriage and adopting kids and earning enough money to keep up with the dot-commers next door.

Members of the group I found sometimes call themselves the "sex community," a relatively unused term that seems to designate all the unassimilated sexual minorities whose lives don't inspire HBO specials, national sex-advice columns, or life-affirming novels. And yet nearly everyone in the sex community could also be called "queer," an outlaw word that designates a whole range of people who can't be divided up into the rigid binaries of homo/het or male/female. We are the transgendered, the bisexual, the kinky, the nonmonogamous, and the sexually undefined. We are the people whose sexual desires and gender identities make us outcasts, even in a queer community whose founding principle was sexual freedom at any cost.

Bill Brent, publisher of Black Books Press and radical sex magazine *Black Sheets,* remembers that the gay community of the 1970s was more like what the sex community is now. "I think that a lot of things shifted in the gay community when it became more aggressively political around 1978. It was necessary, but there was a sacrifice in terms of a certain *laissez-faire* attitude about an individual's right to invent their own sexuality."

As the gay community slowly emerged from the underground, its values shifted. Rather than being a radical experiment, gay life was codified and defined. The "Castro clone" emerged, a reminder that what it meant to be and act gay was no longer up for grabs. There is a well-defined gay type: clean, professional, white, mono-gendered, and unambiguously attracted only to the same sex. Queer-friendly books, movies, and TV shows offer us images of homosexuals who are fundamentally nice boys and girls with the same values as your typical middle-class suburban family. None of these happy homos are fistfucking at naughty clubs or enjoying more than one lover or changing their sex.

The more inclusive term *queer* became popular in the 1990s as a way to combat the cloneish aspects of the gay community. But when the Pride parade rolls around, for example, it's clear that the queer community is largely dominated by homosexuals, and the rest of us are relegated to some sort of "queer runoff" status or worse.

Brent, a longtime participant in what he calls "mixed-gender sex spaces," says, "Most of my sexual activity is with men, but I get tired of gay men who act like my playing with women is some kind of aberration. To them, we're exotic, just as gays and lesbians seem exotic to a lot of straights. And this can be a little frustrating when you're trying to deal with a lot of the same issues, like social acceptance, health care, and individual sexual freedom."

Ironically, the mainstream queer community has created its own seething, semi-invisible underground of individuals whose sexual choices don't register on gaydar. I would argue that just as we look to the cultural underground for the future of art and entertainment, we must look to the sexual underground for the future of queer. Just because Ellen DeGeneres can display her well-aerobicized girlfriend on TV and Dan Sav-

age can adopt a kid doesn't mean the revolution is over. It's just gotten started.

Carol Queen, a bisexual pioneer, writer, and much-loved organizer in the sex community, suggests that gender identity is one of the new frontiers in queerness. She explains that one of the things that makes people identify as queer these days—even if they aren't a card-carrying homo—is "a gender-role critique, particularly in sexual relationships." Even heterosexuals are attracted to this aspect of queer, she says. "Plenty of hets aren't crazy about gender roles. That's the first thing people turn to queers for—a living, breathing, loving critique of the pink/blue dichotomy."

Transgender politics, displayed forcefully in 1999's hit indie film *Boys Don't Cry*, are just the tip of the iceberg. As more female-to-male (FTM) transsexuals become visible and male-to-female surgeries improve dramatically, new permutations of transgenderism have surfaced. San Francisco's Cheryl Chase heads the Intersexual Society of North America [www.isna.org], an activist organization for intersexuals (people born with physical characteristics of both sexes). And activists like Matt Rice and Patrick Califia—both FTM—are making it obvious that being a transsexual isn't about using hormones and/or surgeries to "go straight."

Ironically, the mainstream queer community has created its own seething, semi-invisible underground of individuals whose sexual choices don't register on gaydar.

Rice says that people's reactions to his identity have changed a lot over the past ten or more years. "When I started working at [San Francisco gay bar] the Lone Star, and I said I was transsexual, men would assume I meant I was MTF [male to female]. They had no idea that FTM existed, and they would say, 'Aw, don't wear dresses—you're such a cute boy!' Now when I tell them, they say, 'So what?'" Rice explains that he's had to educate men in the queer community in order to be accepted, but that acceptance was generally given willingly. "It does take the support of a community to make that kind of change," he says. "And what I didn't expect was that my friends ended up being gender activists too. They stuck up for me when people talked behind my back."

And of course, FTM and MTF aren't the end of the story, either. Plenty of transgendered people in the queer underground aren't in any hurry to pick male or female. They might take hormones but not get surgery. Or they might crossdress without having any plans to ever change their biological sex. And when sexuality gets thrown into this genderfucked mix, all kinds of permutations result. Is a crossdressed boy who has sex with a girl having homosexual or heterosexual sex? What if the individual in question has taken hormones and has breasts but also a penis? What kind of sexual orientation is that for the people involved?

Laughing, Rice says, "It's not the 1970s—it's not the Stone Age—and it's okay to be queer and transsexual." His joke cuts to the heart of what's happening in the queer community right now. Things have gone so far beyond the 1970s post-Stonewall days that it's high time we acknowledge it.

Queen notes that sometimes queers are far more sexually conservative than most people assume they are. "There is still a fair amount of controversy about sexuality which isn't specifically genitally focused," she says. She's referring not just to bisexuality, an orientation that is less about a specific type of genitals than about a specific sort of person, but also to kinky sex, which might be focused on leather, latex, feet, piss, bondage, or any number of other things that have nothing to do with the genitals of your object of desire. For homosexuals, whose sexuality is genitally focused (they want partners with only one sort of genitalia), queer sexuality that goes beyond genital preference can be upsetting and challenging.

But, as Queen points out, "If being radical outsiders is part of our queer history, then other radical outsiders who challenge the same things we challenge must be in the club part of the time."

The queer community needs to continue the social critique that got started several decades ago in a small New York gay bar that was busted by the cops. While some queers are happy to settle into marriage and family life, many of us can never do that. We cannot assimilate. And when homosexuals react in horror to bisexual kisses and kinky, nonmonogamous sex and transgendered bodies, it's as if we've come in to pervert

Is a crossdressed boy who has sex with a girl having homosexual or heterosexual sex?

their perfect gay utopia.

So at the edges of acceptability, in hidden places, we're building our own perverted utopia, and our strange new sexualities and genders lurk in your future. Join us. We're inventing ourselves right now.

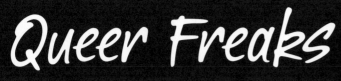

Queer Freaks

Why Legalized Sodomy Is Just Political Foreplay

Patrick Califia

In June 2003, when the Supreme Court decided, in *Lawrence v. Texas*, to decriminalize sex acts that people have been doing ever since they had genitals and other orifices, I was as happy as any other AmeriKKKan queer. San Francisco's gay pride parade followed soon after, and the city was full of delirious fags and dykes, bisexual (speak it under your breath) men and women, and even those do-they-have-to-be-so-obvious transgendered *people* ("Well, you can't call them men or women, can you?" say the gym-toned gay Democrats and the lesbian soccer moms), celebrating the good sense of our highest court. All of them far too stoned to follow such a long sentence. Like Nancy Reagan, I just get high on life. Maybe I'll be named the next Drug Czar. Anything's possible now that I'm no longer a sex offender.

Frankly, I didn't think I would live long enough to see this much sexual sanity in the United States of Gunpowder and the Indian reservations it made possible. Especially not under the reign of failed energy magnate George W. Bush. Maybe the Supremes felt that they owed us something for letting Bush steal the election? My dance of gratitude falters, because I very much fucking doubt it. While the rest of you laugh at Dubya for not being able to find weapons of mass destruction in Iraq, I will fortify myself with a Frappuccino from the Sodomites' Starbucks at 18th and Castro, and hope this should-be-bankrupt dude-ranch cowboy will have an equally difficult time finding our very own WMD. How do you say "Put down the red telephone" in Korean?

Bitter, table for one! Or two, since you're here now. Stick around, I've already ordered for both of us. Service is slow, which is odd when you think about how many self-proclaimed bottoms there are in this town, so let me throw out a few conversation stoppers while we're all chipper enough to deserve a chewing out.

I'm a queer freak. I'm a promiscuous, bisexual, female-to-male transsexual, and a sadomasochist. Do you mind if I grope your ass, lick your ear, and whisper, "Since my dick isn't long enough to go up somebody's ass, is it at all helpful to me to know assfucking is now as legal as taking fertility drugs to conceive a litter of Southern Baptists?" Here's my next question. If you've been accused of witchcraft by your Puritan neighbors, and they hang you, does it really matter a lot if one of them doesn't watch so he can take a discreet leak on your pansies? Is that a breath of fresh air? Is that freedom? No, of course not, and I don't feel particularly free if I'm told that there's nothing illegal about my sex life yet I'm still not allowed to get married, serve in the military, or partake of other dubious heterosexual privileges. We aren't even at the point of being "separate but equal."

Frankly, I didn't think I would live long enough to see this much sexual sanity in the United States of Gunpowder and the Indian reservations it made possible.

Despite a long overdue Supreme Court verdict in favor of sexual privacy, the public policy in America and other Western countries remains hostile toward gay, bisexual, and transgendered people and folks of any sexual orientation who pursue consensual but nonstandard forms of pleasure and intimacy. Like outsiders in a Puritan village, we are still vulnerable to prosecution and persecution. One of the problems with assimilationist politics is its short-sighted view of what should be on the queer political agenda. The most privileged among us—gay men and lesbians with good educations and upper-class backgrounds or middle-class jobs—are easily placated. Assimilationist gay activists think in terms of seeking equality. But what does equality mean in a society that is designed to maintain wide gaps between classes, genders, sexual orientations, and races? Trying to reform the systems that punish people for wanting the wrong kind of sex or people whose gender expression deviates from the norm is like putting rotten meat back into the freezer, then defrosting it and assuming it will now be fit to eat. I want fresh meat, and so should you.

Not ready to be a queer revolutionary? Go on your merry way, then. All the more high dudgeon for me to consume on my lonesome. Oh, dammit, I told the waiter to bring the irony on the side, not ladled all over it like gravy. Yuck. Dear me, now the manager's headed this way, and he says, "Do we have a problem here?"

There are still far too many deviants who can't see beyond the edges of their own oppression, to see where all the freaks are connected in a crazy quilt of sexual repression and misrepresentation.

The problem is that I don't even know how to start telling you what the problem is. The repression of sexuality in this country goes far beyond the homophobic stigma placed on butt piracy, muffdiving, and cocksmoking. There's a connection between that taboo and the fear of nudity, the prohibition against talking honestly with children and teenagers about their bodies, the chipping away at abortion rights, and a multitude of other expressions of sexual shame and fear of diversity. That sexual repression is held in place by a multitude of misogynist attacks on the equality, self-esteem, and safety of women. There are related, complex, rigid, and punitive standards for the expression of masculinity and femininity. Racism and class oppression are intertwined through all of these institutionalized forms of discrimination and cruelty. A movement focused on gay rights—or feminism or transgendered rights or sexual liberation—has far too narrow a scope to elucidate these links or form alliances based upon resisting social control.

It's a big, big problem. It's bigger than the one that got away. Even bigger than the one you had last night at Blow Buddies. We're a society in need of a revolution, but the left has been terrorized into silence on that topic. You don't need a Weatherman to know that there aren't any more Weathermen. The hard rain Bob Dylan sang about did indeed come, but it fell only on the people who could not take shelter in the Estab-

lishment. And now, forty years after the war in Vietnam, the United States is once more embroiled in an illegal war on foreign soil. The only people who believe in armed uprisings are the pale-faced crazies who want to kill all of the fags, Jews, and...oh, you know the whole sick, sad list of hatreds. There are days when I almost wish they would reinstate the draft, because it will take something like that to make Americans desperate enough to learn something about radical politics and stop watching television long enough to fight back.

But this is just about sex. Sex and gender. Two things that have nothing to do with war. And if you believe that, you deserve to be an Army reservist who is getting called back to Iraq even though he's already served a tour of duty there, big boy. Uncle Sam is dressed up as Mae West, but he doesn't need to ask if you're just glad to see him, because he put that pistol in your pocket. Shoved it in there like a prison convict named Killer puts it to a check-kiting, bubble-butted newbie. You don't want to be a victim doing time in a military stockade, so you're going to pick up your weapon and drill somebody else. Flies trapped in amber have more free agency.

§§

But let's get back to our more appetizing main course of Vaseline and fudge-packing.

The problem is that even though they've decriminalized sodomy in Canada and authorized monogamous gay marriage in Ontario, Canadian customs agents still seize books that depict anal sex or images of bondage, fisting, or any sort of sexual fun between two men or two women. There's almost no pornography depicting the bodies and desires of differently-gendered people like me, so they don't even need to confiscate it to make my sex life invisible.

At the same time as the Supremes have given their blessing to oral sex and anal sex and other alternatives to breeder screwing in the dead-bug position, the Department of Justice has declared a new war on "obscenity" in this country. You can have queer sex (in private, with one other person over the age of eighteen), but you'd better not photograph or videotape it and sell those representations to other happy practitioners of buggery. If sodomy is not a crime, just like eating or sewing, making art about it should be as innocuous as a photograph that accompanies a recipe or a television show about quilting.

Our elected representatives continue to angle for ways to get depictions of sex off the Internet, and that includes information about birth control, abortion, and how to have sex without getting infected with HIV, hepatitis, or other STDs. Agencies that do HIV-prevention work are being accused of circulating material that advocates queer sex and are being harassed with federal audits. Why is a pamphlet about how to put a condom on a hard cock more obscene than a teenage girl with an unwanted pregnancy or an adolescent boy who just learned he's HIV-positive? A teacher who hands out lube and condoms would lose his job, but a teacher who tells his students that condoms don't protect you against HIV will not be prosecuted for murder.

Meanwhile, in the Gay Pride Mecca of San Francisco, 85% of the gay men I know have to snort, smoke, or inject crystal before they can get their freak on. We're all very happy after we've taken our party favors, but if we were happy in the first place, would we really be making sure we didn't leave home without a bump and a straw? Is the music so loud because we don't really want to talk to each other or because we can't stand the voices in our own heads? All of us grew up being spit on, hit, and kicked around for being sissies, but as adults, the only guys we want are the ones who hold up the most brittle façade of muscular virility. If the only thing that matters is how good you look and how butch the people you're having sex with look, all you've got is a room full of pretty but very depressed men. Trying to get rid of internalized homophobia when there's so much hostility all around us is like, shudder, washing your hair in dirty water. But, hey, it's our fault that syphilis rates are rising, because fags are self-indulgent and irresponsible. Go to it—it's legal!

♛♛

We have more codified gay rights than we did when I went to my first gay bar in 1971 and saw cops take a payoff right over the counter. But there are still too many straight people who hate us. There are still far too many deviants who can't see beyond the edges of their own oppression, to see where all the freaks are connected in a crazy quilt of sexual repression and misrepresentation. A few examples follow that tirade.

The Human Rights Campaign still won't advocate writing transgendered people into the Employment Non-Discrimination Act (ENDA), a proposed federal anti-discrimination law, and when gay civil-rights laws are being debated at the local level, more often than not the lesbian and gay activists who are pushing for those laws actively resist extending that umbrella of protection to transpeople. These are the same kind of people who would have pushed other Jews out of line to make sure they got one of Raoul Wallenberg's fake German passports out of the Third Reich. Let's keep on making sure there's never enough to go around, shall we? The surest sign of being a shit is the drive to make other people live in it. Ah, the sweet smell of capitalism, the rim seat of economic systems.

Sodomy is legal, but what if you want to wear a latex strait-jacket and whimper, "Oh, sir, please flood my pig pussy with your dirty spunk," while a hard dick is pressed against your bruised and greedy butt? Leatherpeople have been deplored and harassed in every single gay rights march we've had in Washington, DC. And I'm not fingering Fred Phelps or the Sons of Saint Patty here. (Eeew. Gotta wipe that off my imaginary digit.) Mainstream lesbians and gay men apparently think that those of us who are drag queens or wielders of bullwhips enjoy being turned into the home-movie stars of homophobic Christian propaganda. In fact, it's a problem for us, too. We don't want to do anything to set gay liberation back, but we also want a chance to publicly celebrate who we are. We've already been shoved into the closet as far as we can go without getting turned into pathologized mashed potatoes. Unlike same-sexers, "sexual sadists" and "sexual masochists" are still in the damned DSM-IV-TR, tagged along with trannies as a mental disorder.

The cross-waving addicts of flaming holy writ are not after just you, bubba, with your domestic partner and Jack Russell terrier. The religious right has targeted leather conferences, fetish parties, and S/M clubs all over the country in a well-organized campaign to prevent us from meeting or playing in public. Just as bars were once threatened with losing their liquor licenses if they allowed homosexuals to congregate on their premises, hotels and other establishments are turning us away because the vice squad has had a little talk with

The repression of sexuality in this country goes far beyond the homophobic stigma placed on butt piracy, muffdiving, and cocksmoking.

them. Kinky people come to these events and clubs in part because it's often not safe for us to have the kind of sex we want to have in our own homes or apartments. We don't usually meet compatible tricks at the laundromat, PTA, or down the hall in our offices.

People in the leather-S/M-D/S-fetish community lose our jobs, have our children taken away from us, get thrown out of housing, are made to leave job training or school, get beaten up or killed, and have to cope with the stress of being stereotyped and hated. We are depressed and angry. We are isolated and self-destructive. And that's just the BDSM activists I'm talking about. When will there be some kind of legal protection for us? Can we join gay men and lesbians in doing sensitivity training for the police so they'll stop trying to close down our bars and will listen to us when we get assaulted or blackmailed? You honestly don't have to worry about sadomasochists running amok and flogging people at random; there are so many people out there who need to be spanked that just thinking about it has confined me to my bed with a restorative cup of cocoa and a double dose of Wellbutrin.

In the wake of the 9/11 attack and passage of the USA Patriot Act, our elected representatives handed the Justice Department sweeping new powers of censorship surveillance and the ability to effectively repeal *habeas corpus*. Your government wants to know what you check out at the library and where you go on the Web. The Feds want to know where your charitable contributions go, which foreign languages you speak, how you worship, and where you go if you leave the country. You'll probably never know you've had your pockets and your credit report turned inside out by the Powers That Be, because it's illegal for anyone who rats you out to tell you Uncle Sam is looking over your shoulder at ads for piercing jewelry, VCR head cleaner, and used jock straps. Have you seen any coverage of the Patriot Act in your local homo bar rag, perhaps between the ads for gay dentists and lesbian realtors and the outcall masseurs?

In guidelines issued by the Justice Department, transgendered people have been singled out for special scrutiny under the guise of rooting out terrorism. Our ability to change our legal documents, work, or travel freely was curtailed by an Attorney General who seemed to think he was the progeny of Senator Joe McCarthy and J. Edgar Hoover. Talk about unsafe

If you hate taking off your shoes at the airport, think about what they're going to want *me* to take off. I can't pay my rent, much less buy a penis.

sex. Throw a blanket over that image, will ya? Is there a doctor in the house who can perform an emergency vasectomy? Don't forget to ask which one of them plays the woman.

This is my life. I have a full beard and a driver's license that says I'm a girl. I can't change it because the Department of Motor Vehicles wants an affidavit that says I've had genital surgery. Even if I had health insurance, it wouldn't cover that procedure. So if I want to travel, I have to do it with a passport that doesn't match my gender. If you hate taking off your shoes at the airport, think about what they're going to want *me* to take off. I can't pay my rent, much less buy a penis. I don't even think I could afford an hour with somebody else's penis.

I fuck anyway, of course—I enjoyed witnessing and executing penetration long before I became a testosterone-based lifeform. But the dildo in my strap-on harness is illegal in several states. Right-wing think tanks have written model obscen-

ity legislation that includes banning sex toys along with titty mags and boy-boy X-rated videos. If I try to sneak my dick into my native state of Texas, perhaps when I'm over there petitioning a court to revise my birth certificate, I'll have to tell the nice rent-a-cop at the airport that it's a dog retrieval dummy. But I won't be making that trip any time soon because, guess what, no frankendick, no piece of paper that says you're a guy. It's wonderful, being pre-op. All of a sudden, nobody wants me to use their bathroom. Better start walkin' like a camel, because I'm going to have to hold it forever.

The sad thing is that oblivious straight people usually treat me better than gay men or lesbians. The fags are afraid I've got cunt cooties, and lesbians have never been nice to "dykes who just gave up when it got too hard to be a butch woman so they traded it all in for male privilege." Yeah, I've got so much male privilege that I am constantly sick to my stomach for fear I'll say the wrong thing, be seen reading the wrong book or talking to the wrong person, and be read as a tranny and stomped. My male privilege only lasts as long as nobody knows. Kind of like when everybody is nice to you at work until you bring your same-sex lover to the company picnic. No more heterosexual privilege for you.

Now that sodomy is legal, the part of my sex life that I refer to as "foreplay" is no longer a criminal act. Until the handcuffs come out. Then it might be assault, even if the person in the handcuffs is dribbling quarter-cups of precum and consent. Sodomy is legal in England, too, but after a 1987 investigation of a circle of friends who played in one another's homes and videotaped some of their parties, British courts sent three gay men to prison for participating in S/M activities with one another. The Operation Spanner case included about a dozen defendants, and the bottoms were convicted of assaulting *themselves*. And you thought it was hard for Scott O'Hara to suck his own dick! In the last few years, people in New England and San Diego have been arrested at play parties and charged with public indecency, assault, possession of weapons, and other rot. So why do it? Especially, why do it someplace other than my bedroom?

I won't deny that I'm an exhibitionist who enjoys casual sex and mayhem with strangers. But I also want to participate in the public life of a community. If I stay home and watch television or go to the supermarket, I'm not going to see any people who are like me. S/M play parties are not just opportunities to do elaborate scenes on equipment that won't fit in a studio apartment. They also offer a chance to see old friends, make new ones, teach someone how to play safely, learn a new bondage trick, eat potato chips, show off a new outfit, show off a new relationship, ease loneliness, and bolster our ego strength and survival skills. Where else am I going to find people who will think I am just dandy because I can cane someone for an hour without making them bleed? Assimilate that.

××

When the term *queer* first came along, it was such a relief to be able to embrace a label that encompassed so much of my experience and identity. But normalization is as relentless as a marching troop of army ants. *Queer* is on the verge of becoming nothing but a synonym for *gay*. Just the way *bisexual* has come to mean *gay*, under the rubric of being inclusive. After decades of active attempts to purge bisexual women, a few lesbian groups now supposedly include bisexual women, but if these women talk about their male lovers, the atmosphere in the room is damn chilly. AIDS-service organizations pull the same lame maneuver. "Please come to our inclusive safer-sex workshop for gay/bisexual men, where we will only talk about your MALE sex partners." You can't expect Kinsey-6 men to stay in the same room with the word *vagina*. There's not enough Viagra in the world to erase that trauma.

And what about those diversity-loving political leaders who blithely refer to transgenderism as a sexual orientation? Hello, not all transgendered people are gay, and the norms for gender identity are not enforced the same way that norms for sexual conduct are regulated.

"Gay Liberation" never included sadomasochism. Never saw any potential for pride or dignity in the eroticism of physical restraint and the judicious application of intense physical sensations. Doesn't believe in the spiritual surcease of being forced to slow down, go within, escape the confines of the flesh, and fly up to a blissful realm of communion with the divine. Never saw any value in the establishment of a fantasy realm in which people actually get to decide what they will experience, and can let go and trust that their limits will be respected and everything that happens is done for their benefit. It's too big a reminder of what we don't have in real life—justice, consent, loving kindness, acceptance, pleasure, attention.

Living in a human body subjects us to unregulated and un-

fair pain and suffering. And we all cooperate in a system that multiplies that agony. Even when we gratify our basic needs by eating or sleeping in a warm bed, we enjoy those privileges on the backs of people who are hungry and sleeping on cold, dirty streets. At least my slaves can take off their collars when we're done playing.

I don't want to give up the term *queer* because it still bugs people like the middle-class gay homeowners in the Castro who have halted plans to open a shelter for homeless queer youth in their beautiful neighborhood. I use it because every time I say it, I get an unpleasant jolt of memories of being called vile names or bashed, and I guess I hope that if I say it with enough aplomb and nonchalance, those memories will lose their power to subdue and terrorize me. The jaws of assimilation have closed around the word *queer*, but they haven't managed to crush it into dust just yet.

I think the term *freak* has to be reclaimed, as well. A freak is somebody who is unusual, stared at, upsetting, revealing

Why is a pamphlet about how to put a condom on a hard cock more obscene than a teenage girl with an unwanted pregnancy or an adolescent boy who just learned he's HIV-positive?

by their difference what is wrong with the status quo. When a freak appears, the world is instantly divided into gawkers and the unique, solitary individual who has given them pause. There are those who cannot hide their shameful or alarming attributes, and those otherwise apparently normal people who love them. The cloak of the exile falls upon them, too, because their eyes and hearts have persuaded them to be loyal to people who are shunned. Freaks are entertainers, jesters, satirists, artists, beautiful in a way that few can endure or savor, intelligent in a way that makes others angry.

If you don't want to be a gawker and a rube, you gotta join the circus. Goddess knows I wish I could run away to one.

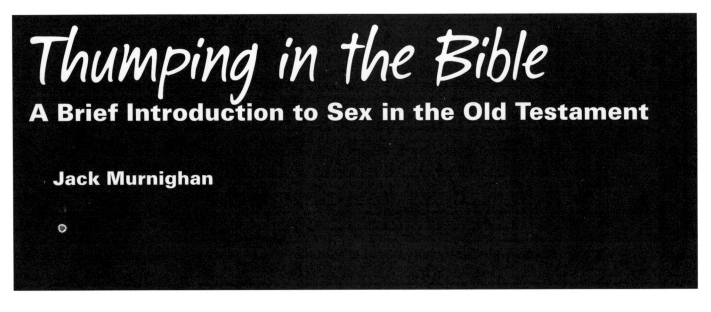

Thumping in the Bible

A Brief Introduction to Sex in the Old Testament

Jack Murnighan

I think it was Umberto Eco who said that he dreaded reading the Bible as a teenager until he discovered how much sex was in it. He has a point: Not too far into Genesis (2), God says, "It is not good for a man to be alone" (a belief I've long subscribed to), and first he makes the animals, then Eve. I'd rather not comment on the order of these events—the implications are clear to those who want them to be clear—I'd rather point out that Adam gets a partner in Eden faster than most of us would in a sex addicts' convention.

And such is the nature of the Bible as a whole: Couplings are common, incest omnipresent, and innuendo aplenty. The

So much happens so fast in the Bible that reading it for naughty bits is like trying to distinguish body parts in scrambled adult channels on TV.

Good Book does not lack for good parts, especially the Old Testament; you just have to sift through endless lists of progeny and litanies of the scourges inflicted on the Israelites to get to them.

Take the story of Abraham and Sarah (originally Abram and Sarai), the second example of sex in Genesis. In the course of a few chapters, Sarah, while pretending to be Abram's sister to protect him, gets abducted into the Pharaoh's harem (bad Pharaoh, bad Pharaoh), proves herself to Abraham's half-sister, gets released, then gets taken into Abimelech's harem (who is warned by God not to go near her), gets released, convinces Abraham to have a baby (Ishmael) with the maid Hagar, and eventually has a baby (Isaac) with him herself. So much happens so fast in the Bible that reading it for naughty bits is like trying to distinguish body parts in scrambled adult

channels on TV. If your attention wavers for even an instant, you risk missing the enchilada.

Amid all the wham-bam sex tales in the early books of the Old Testament, the most interesting involve Lot and his daughters. Lot, you'll remember, was the one man in Sodom that the LORD decided to save from the fire and brimstone. So he sends two angels to Lot's house to warn him of the destruction and give him instructions for getting himself and his family out of Dodge.

Now, the inhabitants of Sodom were not called Sodomites for nothing, so when they see the two male angels—certified hotties—going into Lot's house, they want a piece of the action. "Both old and young, all the people from every quarter" circle around Lot's house, banging on his door, calling, "Where are the men which came in to thee this night? Bring them to us that we may know them." Among the fabulous euphemisms for sex in the King James translation, "to know" is one of my favorites. I envision a mob of sex fiends hemmed in around Enrique Inglesias, screaming, "We want to know you; we just want to know you." You get the point.

Lot realizes he has a difficult situation on his hands. So he goes out to the throng, locking the door behind him, and says:

> **I pray you, brethren, do not so wickedly. Behold now, I have two daughters which have not known man; let me, I pray you, bring them out unto you, and do ye to them as is good in your eyes: only unto these men do nothing; for therefore came they under the shadow of my roof.**

Here is a good example of what can transpire in the course of a few biblical words. You scan the line, scan it again, and say to yourself: In place of the angels, did Lot just offer the crowd his virgin daughters to do with what they will? I mean, being a good host is nice and all, but that seems a bit extreme. The mind reels—not unproductively—at what would befall the innocents if they were cast to the awaiting wolves.

Thankfully, the angels intervene. They pull Lot back into the house and blind the Sodomites pressing against the door. Then they facilitate Lot's exit, with wife and daughters in tow, but, in their flight across the plain, Lot's wife makes the mortal mistake of looking back (like many of us toward old relationships) and is turned into a pillar of salt.

Yet the saga of Lot and his daughters is not over. Having fled to the town of Zoar, he eventually becomes afraid and moves himself and his daughters to the mountains. Apparently it was a little underpopulated up there, and his daughters begin to despair of ever getting nookie. The older says to the younger, "Our father is old, and there is not a man in the earth to come in unto us after the manner of all the earth. Come, let us make our father drink wine, and we will lie with him, that we may preserve the seed of the father."

Ah, the old *Get Dad Drunk and Have Him Impregnate Us* trick—pretty sneaky, Sis! So on consecutive nights the daughters get Lot schnookered and go lie with him (again, a nice euphemism, though not as good as "come in unto"). Lot, the sod, doesn't seem to notice either time. Eventually each of his daughters gives birth to a son.

Now, mind you, all this has happened in the first 20 pages of the Bible (at least in my edition). This is some kind of book. By comparison, the first 20 pages of a *Best American Erotica* contain nowhere near as much sex and a fraction of the scandal. True, conventional erotica tends to have more adjective-heavy descriptions of sex than one finds in the Holy Book (the Song of Solomon is the exception, as we will see), but for sheer quantity of nudge nudge, the Bible is up there.

By and large, the Old Testament is a very weird document, full of bizarre and rather unsavory tidbits that the New Testament tried to smooth over. Even God himself had to be rendered kinder and gentler the second time around, for in the Hebrew books he was forever casting plagues and famines down on the people and insisting on himself as a "consuming fire" and a "jealous God." In Isaiah 3, for example, the "haughty" daughters of Zion, with their "wanton eyes, walking and mincing as they go and making a tinkling with their feet," will be smote down by the LORD, and he will discover

their "secret parts." Ooh. Best take off those bangles before it's too late.

But my favorite Old Testament oddity occurs in Deuteronomy 23, where, in a list of all those who will not be making it to Heaven, it is written: "He that is wounded in the stones, or hath his privy member cut off, shall not enter into the congregation of the Lord." Rum thing: not only do you have to go through this life without the priviest of privies, but the gates of Paradise are closed to you, to boot (and the fact that you can sing a decent falsetto is pretty minor recompense). Yet the intrigue of this passage doesn't end there: Why, in fact, are the memberless or the crushed-testicled not welcome in the New Jerusalem? Interesting question. There are numerous medieval theological debates about whether angels eat and drink, piss and shit (and where it would go if they do), but I've never heard anyone ask if they screw. Yet here, perhaps,

Why, in fact, are the memberless or the crushed-testicled not welcome in the New Jerusalem?

is evidence that the celestial nightclub serves up more than just juice and cookies.

Perhaps this is not the venue to reinscribe us in thirteenth-century scholastic arguments, but the point is still intriguing: If it was just sex the elect were after, the penis would be enough. But if the balls are also necessary, this suggests a certain import to the male ejaculate as well. To my mind, this complicates Aquinas' notion that the postprandial material discharge of angels is only a vapor (but not a flatulence, mind you); for even if we agree that angel excretion is but gas, what are we to do with angel jizz? Aquinas would probably have described it as some kind of noumenal hand lotion.

✕✕

Even in the briefest introductions to sex in the Old Testament, no account can ignore one of the most erotic, exquisite texts not just in the Bible, but in the whole history of Western literature: the Song of Solomon. In all the reams of Biblical interpretation, this is the text that has received the most treatment. The reasons are twofold: The Song of Solomon is sufficiently explicit to be embarrassing to the anti-sensuality of the later Christian church, and thus required extensive backpedaling. This is the obvious, confessed reason so many monks spilled their ink on its pages. The other, only slightly less obvious, is that it is very fun to read and decidedly arousing, especially if the only other thing you're reading is Samuel and Jeremiah's accounts of the punishments visited upon the wicked.

In effect, the Song of Solomon is generally agreed to be a dialogue between two lovers (although I, for one, detect more than two total speakers, but that truly is a debate outside our scope), one called Solomon (not necessarily the famous King who appears elsewhere in the Old Testament), the other his unnamed lover, who, by some accounts, may have written the piece. Orthodox Christian interpretations attempt to downplay the hot and heavy eroticism in the Song by saying that the female lover is the Church, Solomon is Christ, and their love is the spiritual union of the material Christian apparatus with the higher spiritual forces.

Yeah, right. The Song begins: "The song of songs, which is Solomon's. Let him kiss me with the kisses of his mouth: for thy love is better than wine." If the point here was supposed to be that the Church wants to merge itself with the love of Christ the Savior, there would have been considerably less distracting ways of saying it. No—the Song of Solomon is a

"Blow on my garden, that the spices thereof may flow out."

love poem, and the love is a very corporeal one. That it made it into the foundational book of Christianity is a mystery beyond my comprehension. But, like the Psalms, here is a part of the Bible that can be read purely for the love of its poetry.

There is no need for an exegesis of all the evocative imagery in the Song; most of it speaks for itself. There are, however, a few highlights, such as when the lover says that her beloved "feeds among the lilies" and that her hands, when she rises up to him, "dropped with myrrh." And Solomon, meanwhile, says to her, "Thy lips, O my spouse, drop as honeycomb: honey and milk are under thy tongue." And she back to him: "Blow on my garden, that the spices thereof may flow out. Let my beloved come into his garden, and eat the pleasant fruits." Heart be stilled!

Even amid the glories of these and similar passages, the author of the Song does strike an odd chord or two. Such compliments as "thy neck is like the tower David builded for an armory" or "thy hair is as a flock of goats, that appear from mount Gilead" have perhaps lost some of their charm in the last few thousand years (a modern adaptation might be: thy hair is like Cornell freshmen plunging into the gorges of Ithaca). Furthermore, the line that precedes the one about the myrrh-drenched hands always struck me as a bit overdone: "My beloved put in his hand by the hole of the door, and my bowels were moved for him." Yes, well, I'm all for psychosomatic response, but that's a bit much.

Fan though I am, I hadn't read much of the Bible until I went to graduate school and, on a rather prolonged lark, decided to become a medievalist. As a result, I found myself a late twenty-something pagan having to read the whole of the Good Book. I did it straight through—not quickly, mind you, but steadily. What I discovered between the now worn-off covers of my Red Letter edition corresponded so minimally to what I had anticipated, I wondered if I had the right religion. The sex and sexual oddities were only some of the Bible's unforeseen pleasures (others include the almost James Bond–like coolness of Christ, the beauty of Paul's prose, the phenomenal stories of Job and Ruth, the bombast of Ezekiel, etc.).

Having now read the entire Bible, multiple times over, I am still a pagan, but I'm all for placing copies in every hotel room. It's the most influential book in Western culture, and it's a lot better than dial-up porn.

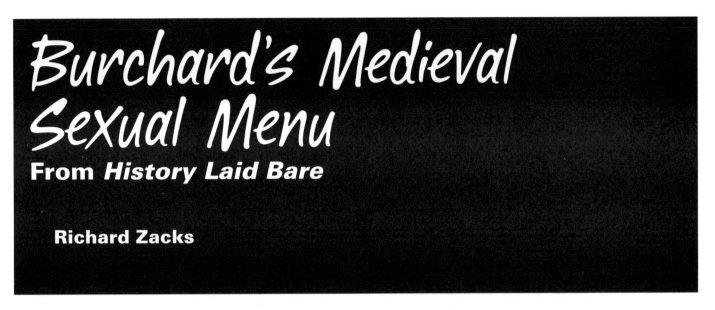

Burchard's Medieval Sexual Menu
From *History Laid Bare*

Richard Zacks

The following is unquestionably the longest and kinkiest list of medieval sexual practices still in existence, and much of it has never before been translated into English from the original Latin.

In 1012, a German bishop with the unlikely name of Burchard of Worms wrote his Penitential. Most of Burchard's twenty-volume tome covers the usual lying, cheating, stealing, and so on. But in volume nineteen, chapter five, he runs down an astoundingly varied menu of 194 different sexual sins. Burchard combines Teutonic thoroughness with a vivid imagination:

Questions for Men
Nuns

Have you committed fornication with a nun, that is to say, a bride of Christ? If you have done this, you shall do penance for forty days on bread and water, which they call a "carina," and [*repeat it*] for the next seven years; and as long as you live, you shall observe all six holy days on bread and water.

"Retro, Canino"

Have you had sex with your wife or with another woman from behind, doggy style? [*Latin: "retro canino"*] If you have done this, you shall do penance for ten days on bread and water.

Sunday

Have you had sex with your wife on a Sunday? You shall do penance for four days on bread and water.

Sister-in-Law

If in your wife's absence, without your or your wife's knowledge, your wife's sister entered your bed and you thought that she was your wife and you had sex with her, if you have done this, then if you complete the penance, you can keep your lawful wife, but the adulterous sister must suffer the appropriate punishment and be deprived of a husband for all time.

Stepdaughter

Have you fornicated with your stepdaughter? If you have done this, you shall have neither mother nor daughter, nor shall you take a wife, nor shall she take a husband, but you shall do penance until death. But your wife, if she only learnt afterwards that you committed adultery with her daughter, shall not sleep with you but marry again in the LORD if she wishes.

Son's Fiancée

Have you fornicated with your son's fiancée, and afterwards, your son took her to wife? If you have done this, because you concealed the crime from your son, you shall do penance until death and remain without hope of marriage. But your son, because he was ignorant of your sin, if he wishes, may take another wife.

Have you had sex with your wife or with another woman from behind, doggy style?

Mother

Have you fornicated with your mother? If you have done this, you shall do penance for fifteen years on the legitimate holy days, and one of these [*years*] on bread and water, and you shall remain without hope of marriage, and you shall never be without penitence. But your mother, if she was not consenting, shall do penance according to the decision of the priest; and if she cannot live chastely may marry in the LORD.

Sodomy

Have you fornicated as the Sodomites did, such that you inserted your penis into the rear of a man and into his posterior, and thus had intercourse with him in the Sodomite manner? If you had a wife and did this only once or twice, you should do penance for ten years on the legitimate holy days, and for one of these on bread and water. If you did this as a manner of habit, then you should do penance for twelve years on the legitimate holy days. If you committed this sin with your brother, you should do penance for fifteen years on the legitimate holy days.

Interfemoral

Have you fornicated with a man, as some are accustomed to do, between the thighs, that is to say, you inserted your member between the thighs of another and by thus moving it about ejaculated semen? If you did this, you shall do penance for forty days on bread and water.

Homosexual Mutual Masturbation

Have you fornicated, as some are accustomed to do, such that you took another's penis in your hand, while he took yours in his and thus in turn you moved each other's penises in your hands with the result that by this enjoyment you ejaculated semen? If you have done this, you shall do penance for thirty days on bread and water.

Have you fornicated with a man, as some are accustomed to do, between the thighs?

Masturbation

Have you fornicated with yourself alone, as some are accustomed to do, that is to say, you yourself took your penis in your hands and thus held your foreskin and moved it with your own hand so that by this enjoyment you ejaculated semen? If you have done this, you shall do penance for twenty days on bread and water.

Masturbation With Sex Aid

Have you fornicated, as some are accustomed to do, such that you inserted your penis into a hollowed-out piece of wood or some such device, so that by this movement and enjoyment you ejaculated semen? If you have done this, you shall do penance for twenty days on bread and water.

Kiss

Have you kissed some woman due to foul desire and thus polluted yourself? If you have done this, you shall do penance for three days on bread and water. But if this happened in a church, you shall do penance for twenty days on bread and water.

Bestiality

Have you fornicated against Nature, that is, you have had intercourse with animals, that is, with a horse or a cow or a donkey or with some other animal? If you did this only once or twice, and if you had no wife, so that you could to relieve your lust, you must do penance for forty days on bread and water, which is called a "carina," as well as [repeating it] for the seven following years, and never be without penitence. If, however, you had a wife, you must do penance for ten years on legitimate holy days; and if you were in the habit of this crime, you must do penance for fifteen years on the legitimate holy days. If, however, this occurred during your childhood, you must do penance on bread and water for 100 days.

Questions for Women
Lesbians With Sex Aids

Have you done what certain women are accustomed to do, that is, to make some sort of device or implement in the shape of the male member, of a size to match your desire, and you have fastened it to the area of your genitals or those of another with some form of fastenings and you have fornicated with other women or others have done with a similar instrument or another sort with you? If you have done this, you shall do penance for five years on legitimate holy days.

Female Masturbation With Sex Aid

Have you done what certain women are accustomed to do, that is, you have fornicated with yourself with the aforementioned device or some other device? If you have done this, you shall do penance for one year on legitimate holy days.

Mother With Son

Have you done what certain women are accustomed to do, that is, have you fornicated with your young son, that is to say, placed your son above your "indecency" and thus imitated fornication? If you have done this, you must do penance for two years on legitimate holy days.

Bestiality

Have you done what certain women are accustomed to do, that is, you have lain with an animal and incited that animal to coitus by whatever ability you possess so that it will thus have intercourse with you? If you have done this, you shall do penance for one "carina," along with [each of] the seven following years, and you shall never be without penitence.

Aphrodisiacs and Superstitious Practices
Semen Swallowing

Have you tasted your husband's semen in the hope that because of your diabolical deed he might burn the more with love for you? If you have done this, you should do penance for seven years on the legitimate holy days.

Live Fish and Childbirth

Have you done what certain women are accustomed to do? They take a live fish and place it in their afterbirth and hold it there until it dies, and then after boiling and roasting it, they give it to their husbands to eat in the hope that they will burn all the more with love for them. If you have done this, you shall do penance for two years on the legitimate holy days.

Bread and Buttocks

Have you done what certain women are accustomed to do? They prostrate themselves face-down and uncover their buttocks, then they order that bread be prepared on their naked buttocks; when its baked, they give it to their husbands to eat so they will burn more for love of them. If you have done this, you shall do penance for two years on legitimate holy days.

Menstrual Blood

Have you done what certain women are accustomed to do? They take their menstrual blood and mix it into food or drink and give it to their husbands to eat or drink so that they might be more attentive to them. If you have done this, you shall do penance for five years on legitimate holy days.

Selective Impotency Spell

Have you done what some adulterous women are accustomed to do? When they first find out that their lovers want to take legitimate wives, they then by some trick of magic extinguish the man's lust, so that they are impotent and cannot consummate their marriage with their legitimate wives. If you have done this or taught others to do this, you should do penance for forty days on bread and water.

Aphrodisiac Loaf?

Have you done what certain women are accustomed to do? They take off their clothes and smear honey all over their naked body and then lay down their honey-drenched body onto some wheat scattered upon a linen on the ground; they then roll around a lot this way and that, and then carefully collect all the grains of wheat which stick to their wet body, and place them in a mill and make the mill go backwards against the sun

They prostrate themselves face-down and uncover their buttocks, then they order that bread be prepared on their naked buttocks.

and grind it to flour; and they make bread from the flour and then give it to their husbands to eat that they may become feeble and waste away. If you have done this, you shall do penance for forty days on bread and water.

—BURCHARD OF WORMS

Over the years, the nature of penance changed away from being exclusively prayer and fasting. Many of Europe's glorious medieval cathedrals were built by peasants sweating off their sins through public works. And for the rich, gaining absolution became easier. By the mid-1200s, churchmen with the pope's blessing were selling "indulgences." A sinner with a bankroll could try out a smorgasbord of Burchard's sins and, if caught, simply buy forgiveness and another shot at heaven.

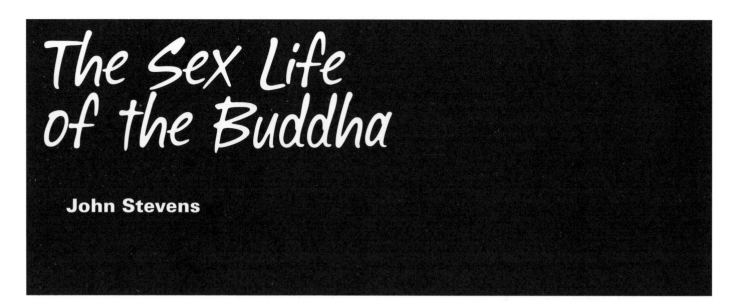

The Sex Life of the Buddha

John Stevens

The Buddhist experience relies on higher truths, and it does not really matter, ultimately, whether or not there was an historical Buddha; however, the traditions and legends that surround the life and teaching of Gotama, the Awakened One, born in what is now Nepal sometime around 500 BCE, are based on perceptions that shape the Buddhist vision of the universe.

Even texts compiled by puritan Buddhists contain a wealth of information on his birth, early manhood, and sexual experiences, and it is not difficult to flesh out the romantic legend of Gotama in loving detail.[1]

Her eyes were clear as a blue lotus leaf and her lips red as a rose.

The requisites for being the mother of a Buddha, for instance, are clearly delineated: She must be beautiful in facial appearance, figure, limb, and bearing; virtuous, of pleasant disposition, polite, patient, modest, chaste, obedient, reflective, and religious-minded; gracious and not facetious or quarrelsome; skilled at feminine pursuits; pure in body, mind, and speech; free of evil thoughts, anger, hatred, and the "faults of ordinary women."[2]

Queen Māyā met all these requirements and was a stunning beauty as well: Dark, perfumed curls surrounded her unblemished, perfectly proportioned face; her eyes were clear as a blue lotus leaf and her lips red as a rose; her teeth shone as brightly as the stars in the sky, her breath was as fragrant as incense, and her voice as soft as a dove's; her body was smooth, firm, and lusciously shaped. Queen Māyā was, in short, ravishing to the eye and heart, "radiant, alluring, and gleaming with a sheen of gold," so comely that even the gods envied her. In fact, she was called Māyādevi, "Goddess of Illusion," because

her body was too beautiful to be believed.[3] Her husband, King Śuddhodana, was the ideal mate, supremely handsome, with a powerful, well-formed body, and neither too young nor too old.

Although the mother of a Buddha need not be a virgin, she must not have borne a child, and once the would-be Buddha enters her womb, she naturally becomes devoid of all lustful thoughts and emotions.

That is why, it is said, when Queen Māyā realized she had conceived "spiritually"—tradition states that the Buddha-to-be descended into her womb as she slept—she asked her husband to allow her to take a vow of celibacy (along with vows not to kill, lie, steal, cheat, slander, engage in worldly talk, or be covetous, angry, or foolish). The king readily agreed and, we are told, thereafter regarded her as he would his mother or sister.

Exactly ten (lunar) months later, Māyā gave birth to a child unsullied by blood, mucus, or other discharge. The newborn was perfectly formed and was able to speak and walk, startling everyone present by immediately taking seven steps and declaring himself "the Honored One of Heaven and Earth." He received a natal bath from two water dragons, and flowers poured down from the sky. Seven days later Queen Māyā suddenly died,[4] and the infant was adopted by Mahāprajāpatî, his mother's sister and his father's second wife.

Not long after Gotama's birth, a soothsayer named Asita visited the palace to examine the unusual child. "This boy is destined to become a great leader," the sage declared solemnly. "If he remains in the palace he will become a universal monarch, but if he enters the religious life he will become an enlightened being, a teacher of men and gods."

The king, determined to make the first prediction of Asita come true, lavished care and attention on his son. He was raised by a host of doting wet nurses and nannies, and when he grew older, nothing was denied him. Gotama used only the sweetest-smelling incense and wore the finest, most costly cloth; day and night a canopy shielded him from heat, cold, wind, and dust; he had three magnificent residences, one each for summer, winter, and the rainy season; the choicest delicacies graced his table; he was serenaded from morning to night by court musicians; and servants were always on hand to cater to his every need.

Gotama grew into an extraordinarily handsome prince with all the marks of a world conqueror:[5] He was well built and agile, with cool, smooth skin; he had golden hair (in some accounts), intense black (or dark blue) eyes, perfectly symmetrical features, a lustrous complexion, and a voice of the purest tones. His well-formed sex organs were "enclosed in a sheath," so that they were hidden from view even when he was naked. (That unusual characteristic explains why most statues of Gotama do not show even a hint of his private parts.)[6]

In order to further bind the prince to worldly life, the king decided to find him a chief consort and devised the following plan to secure the best bride for the finicky Gotama: "I'll have heaps of jewelry made for the prince to distribute as gifts to all the eligible maidens of the land and instruct my aides to carefully observe which of the girls catches the eye of my son."[7]

On the appointed day, however, the girls gathered at the palace merely swooned in the presence of the dashing prince, and Gotama did not appear to be interested in any of them. Suddenly, though, at the very end of the reception, a stunning beauty appeared with a huge entourage in tow. The lovely maiden walked up to the prince without hesitation, looked him directly in the eyes, and asked for her present.

"I am sorry," the prince said as he gazed back, "the jewelry is all gone. You should have come sooner."

"Why didn't you save something for me?" she asked in a hurt voice.

"Here, you can have my ring. Or how about my necklace?"

"No, thank you," said the girl petulantly, and she turned away as Gotama watched in rapt attention. (In another version, the girl took the necklace but added with a coy smile, "Is this all I am worth?")[8]

A full report of the encounter between Gotama and the girl, whose name was Yaśodharā (or Gopā in some accounts), was

given to the king. When he was told how their eyes met and of Gotama's obvious fascination with the elegant maiden, the king immediately sent a messenger to Yaśodharā's father to ask for her hand on behalf of the prince. To his chagrin, the king was rebuffed: "I will consent to give my beloved daughter only to the young man who can prove he is superior to all the others."

An assembly of all the young men in the kingdom was quickly arranged, and Gotama squared off against the others in contests of writing, arithmetic, archery, swordsmanship, horse-riding, and boxing. Gotama emerged victorious in all the events and claimed his willing prize. They were married in a magnificent ceremony, and court poets sang that the fair Yaśodharā afforded the prince every sort of pleasure as they spent themselves in nuptial bliss—a delightful union of the choicest butter and the finest ghee.[9]

His well-formed sex organs were "enclosed in a sheath," so that they were hidden from view even when he was naked.

Yaśodharā was an independent sort, refusing to don a veil in the presence of her in-laws, the king and queen, and, more scandalously, in front of the other men of the household. When criticized for such behavior, Yaśodharā replied, "A noble woman, one who guards the mind and controls the senses, will be properly veiled even if she happens to be naked—one cannot cover up sins with a pile of robes and a veil."[10]

As was the custom in those times, Gotama apparently had several other official wives[11]—one for each of his palaces?—and his courtship with the one known as Gotamī is also classic romance.[12]

The beauty Gotamī was desired by hundreds of suitors, but the girl, just as independent as Yaśodharā, steadfastly rejected all offers of an arranged match, even with the king's son, and insisted on making her own choice. "Let it be known that in one week I will select a husband. Have all the eligible men gather in the palace."

On the morning of the seventh day, Gotamī bathed in scented oil, decorated herself with the prettiest of flowers, put on her finest jewelry and robes, and made her way to the palace with her mother and several other attendants along to act as advisors. Surveying the crowd of dandies dressed to the teeth in fabulous garments and elaborate coiffures, weighted down with jewelry and reeking of perfume, Gotamī exclaimed with disgust, "These fops all look like women! They are more dressed up than I am!"

"Isn't there anyone here who catches your fancy?" her mother asked.

"Yes. One, and only one. That prince over there in the simple robe and radiant smile. At last, a real man."

In one text the girl is named Splendor of Delight, and she calls out to the prince:

When I saw you, young man, excellent
In form and strength, endowed with virtue,
All my senses were delighted,
And immense joy arose in me.
Your complexion is like a pure shining jewel,
Your hair is black and curly,
You have a fine brow and nose;

Your tongue is long and broad, Coppery red, soft, shining like a jewel

I offer myself to you.
You have excellent features.
Resplendent, you are like a mountain of gold.
In your presence I do not shine;
I am like a pile of charcoal.
Your eyes are large and dark,
Your jaw is like a lion's, your face like the full moon.
The fine sound of your voice is irresistible;
Please take me in.
Your tongue is long and broad,
Coppery red, soft, shining like a jewel;
With your superb, clear voice
You delight people when you speak.
Your teeth are even, shining white,
Clean and well-spaced;
When you show them as you smile,
You delight people, O hero.

Then the girl's mother, the supreme courtesan called Beautiful, extols her daughter's charms to the prince:

With dark hair, lotus-blue eyes,
A clear voice, and golden complexion,
Finely clad in garlands, she emerged
From the lotus, resplendent as pure light.
Her limbs are bright, her body evenly balanced;
Her limbs are complete, her body well-proportioned;
She shines like a golden statue adorned with jewels
Illuminating all directions.
The finest fragrance of sandalwood wafts from her body,
Filling the air around her;
As she speaks, with celestial sweetness,
A scent like a blue lotus comes from her mouth.
Whenever she smiles,
Heavenly music plays;
This treasure of a woman should not be abandoned
To control of the vulgar.

She is not short or too tall,
Not stout or too thin;
She is slender at the waist, full-breasted,
Suitable for you with an impeccable body.[13]

A splendid ceremony was performed, and the couple retired to the palace to partake of the joys of wedded life.

Since the king's ministers suggested that the prince be enticed with all the pleasures of love in order to keep him addicted to the palace, in addition to his wives Gotama was waited on by an army of the most beautiful, accomplished, and adoring women in the kingdom, all vying to provide him the utmost in attention, service, amusement, and comfort.

It is possible to conjure up an idea of what these pleasure girls looked like from ancient Indian texts on love and classical Hindu and Buddhist iconography—indeed, Buddhist iconography is distinguished by its lavish use of the female form in all its sensuous glory.[14]

A pleasure girl of the Buddha's time was typically dressed in a red and gold girdle, with bracelets around her wrists and ankles. Her long, jet-black hair was adorned with flowers and ornaments. She possessed a face as lovely as the full moon, with doe eyes, a delicate nose, and red lips set off against a golden complexion. Naked above the waist, she wore necklaces and strings of pearls to grace her swelling, close-set breasts, which were shaped like golden cups, black-nippled, and rubbed with sandalwood oil. Her skin was as soft as rose petals; her navel was deep, her belly rounded with soft folds of skin, her hips ample, her buttocks high and firm, and her thighs like the stem of the banana tree. Her *yoni* (vulva) resembled a lotus bud and had the fragrance of a newly burst lily or fresh honey. She had a voice a cuckoo would envy, and she moved like a swan. The girl was well-versed in the arts of speaking, singing, dancing, and playing musical instruments; she was a teller of erotic tales, a weaver of spells, a creator of aphrodisiacs and potent perfumes.

Supremely skilled in the practice of love, having been taught by the sages of divine love, she was expert in imparting bliss to her partner; she was a sexual gymnast of the highest order. The girl was a master of the various types of kisses—moderate, contracted, pressed, soft, clasping, throbbing, the "war of tongues," the "secret of the upper lip"—and all other forms of oral love: side-biting, outside pressure, inside pressure, "kissing the stalk," "sucking a mango," "swallowing up." She was talented in every sort of embrace, familiar with the most effective love bites and scratches, and well-schooled in the techniques of physical union—widely open, yawning, clasping, twining, feet in the air, one leg up, inverted, reversed, supported, suspended, rising, all-encompassing, "packed," and the other specialties: "wheel of love," "opening and blossoming," "the bow," "splitting a bamboo," "fixing a nail," "pair of tongs," "spinning top," "the swing," and the postures of the crab, the tortoise, the crow, the monkey, the cow, the mare, the bird, the jumping tiger, the union of cats, the pressing of an elephant, the rutting of the boar, the bee buzzing over the honey, and (with another girl) the union of three. The girls also teamed up to perform the *yogini chakra* with the prince, a rite in which he made love simultaneously with three, five, seven, or nine partners.[15]

The king had a special "chamber of love" constructed for Gotama, decorated with erotic art and illumined with subdued light "like that of the hazy autumn sun."[16] Captivated by sexual extravagance, the prince spent his days and nights in continual dalliance, experiencing every imaginable sensual delight of heterosexual intercourse with the indefatigable beauties of his vast harem and, when he tired of them, with the professional goddesses of love in neighboring pleasure groves.[17] Gotama's life consisted largely of opening women's skirts, unfastening their girdles, pressing their swelling breasts, caressing their secret parts, and devouring them with love.[18] So intense was Gotama's lust that even the miracles attributed to him had to do with sex: Once in hot pursuit of one of his maidens, Gotama inadvertently stepped off the roof of the palace and found himself suspended in midair.[19]

Gotama's life revolved around the five elements of physical delight beautiful women, excellent music, pleasing scents, fine food, and the best in raiment—corresponding to the senses of sight, hearing, smell, taste, and touch.

Yet despite his incomparable comfort, the prince was not at ease. His father made every effort to shield the prince from anything remotely unpleasant or upsetting by imprisoning him in a fantasy land, but Gotama was sorely troubled by his rare glimpses of the real world. Once, as a boy, he was taken to a plowing festival that marked the beginning of the planting season. Instead of enjoying the festivities, Gotama was appalled at the sight of sweat pouring off the men and oxen as they scarred the earth with their plows. Blood dripped from the bridles of the struggling oxen as man and beast strained and suffered in the scorching sun. Flocks of birds swooped down to feast on the hapless insects unearthed by the plow, and hawks, in turn, preyed upon the smaller sparrows and swallows. Filled with pity at the plight of all these creatures, the prince said to his father, "I need to be alone," and he went to sit beneath a tree to contemplate the meaning of it all.

Years later, Gotama received several more rude shocks. Despite the king's command to clear the streets of all refuse, material and human, when the prince was on an outing, Gotama

was eventually confronted with the three ugliest facts of life. First, he encountered a decrepit old man, bald, toothless, bent with age, racked by a rasping cough, staggering along on crutches; next, he saw a diseased person with a swollen belly and crooked limbs, pale and miserable, covered with filth and flies and gasping for breath; then he witnessed a shroud-covered corpse being carried through the streets, the dead man's relatives following behind, wailing terribly and beating their breasts. When he asked his attendant the significance of each incident he was told, "All human beings face the same fate."

After each of these frightful experiences Gotama tried to further abandon himself to the world of the senses, but to no avail—he became increasingly self-absorbed and withdrawn. On another trip outside, Gotama caught a glimpse of a serene mendicant monk; the homeless sage seemed to be at peace with himself and with the world. Gotama was neither, and he cut short his trip in disgust with himself and returned to

The girls also teamed up to perform the *yogini chakra* with the prince, a rite in which he made love simultaneously with three, five, seven, or nine partners.

the palace. On the way back, one of the young women who thronged to the balconies for a glimpse of the dashing prince as he drove by saw him and sang out his praises: "Blessed indeed is the mother, blessed indeed is the father, blessed indeed is the wife of such a glorious Lord!"

Upon hearing that, Gotama realized that he would only truly be blessed when he solved the riddle of life. In appreciation for the girl's prompting, Gotama sent her a pearl necklace (which she mistakenly took as a declaration of his love for her). Thereafter, he longed to break free from the confines of his pleasure palace and seek the truth before his mind was hopelessly clouded and his spirit totally debauched.

The king and Gotama's stepmother sensed the prince's growing dissatisfaction with his life; Mahāprajāpatî ordered the concubines to envelop the prince in "a cage of gold," taking care never to staunch the flow of narcotic wine or erotic entertainment.[20] In desperation, the king invited all the damsels in the realm to sport with the prince in a pleasure garden. The girls—intoxicated by wine, redolent of sweet perfume, and overcome with desire—rubbed against the prince with their fragrant breasts, and wrapped their legs around him. They slipped out of their robes and made every sort of tantalizing proposal, all to no avail.[21] Gotama's heart was elsewhere. "How can there be mirth and laughter," he sighed, "with so much suffering present in the world?"[22]

Gotama's closest friends were sent by the king to remind the prince of his duties toward the country and the women who lived only to love him. "How can you be unhappy with all this when you are so young and full of life? Follow tradition, and abandon the world when you are an old man."

Gotama's chief consort Yaśodharā had a nightmare about his leaving her and their newborn son. She was the only one who still had a hold on Gotama, and it is recorded that he consoled her gently and spent that night in loving embrace with her.[23]

Still, Gotama was in torment. When his anguished father asked, "What is the matter? Name your heart's desire and it will be yours," Gotama replied, "Promise me that I will always be youthful; that I will never be sick; and that I will never die. Promise that I will not lose you, nor the girls in my harem, nor my kinfolk. Promise me that this kingdom will never crumble or be plagued by evil." Those were wishes that even the greatest king could not grant. Palace life began to suffocate the prince.

Some were naked, contorted into unseemly positions with legs and arms askew.

Gotama's gloom spread over the kingdom. Birds stopped singing; flowers ceased to bloom; lakes and rivers dried up; crops withered; musical instruments shattered; and people became fitful.[24]

One night, following what was evidently a frenzied orgy, Gotama awoke from a troubled sleep and took a hard look at the harem women surrounding him in the love chamber. Lying about in torn clothing and disheveled hair, with their ornaments, tiaras, and musical instruments strewn about, the girls were far from a pretty sight. Some were naked, contorted into unseemly positions with legs and arms askew; others were snoring loudly with their mouths agape, mumbling to themselves in their sleep, or drooling in a drunken stupor. In the lurid light of the oil lamps, the girls had lost all their allure—for the first time Gotama noticed the blemishes and flaws of each girl. Revolted by such meaningless excess, he felt as if he had come to in a cemetery full of the living dead.[25]

Gotama sighed wearily:

This world is full of deception and falsehood
and nothing is more deceiving than a woman's appearance;
Attracted to fine clothes and trinkets,
Foolish men become mad with desire,
But when one realizes that a woman's charms are mere illusion,
He will no longer be deceived.

This is the way to liberation and purity of body and mind.[26]

The repugnance Gotama now felt toward his life of frivolity and hedonism in the palace galvanized the prince, and he resolved to flee "this swampland of sex"[27] that very night to seek a path of deliverance.

Before fleeing the place, though, as legend maintains, Gotama had a last look around his domain and went to Yaśodharā's chambers to gaze upon his wife and son. The infant was sleeping peacefully next to his mother's breast, and Gotama moved to embrace him.

"No, I cannot," the prince whispered, restraining himself. "If I lift the queen's arm I will disturb her and waken them both. When I attain the truth I will be back to see them."[28]

So saying, Gotama summoned his faithful servant, the groom Chandaka, and called for his horse. Chandaka made a final appeal against Gotama's act. Among many other objections, Chandaka protested, "If you remain here and become, according to the prediction, a universal monarch, you could establish a kingdom of peace and plenty and create tremendous good."

But Gotama replied, "Even if I became ruler of the world and were able to provide my subjects with every physical need, they would still suffer from sickness, old age, and death. If I attain enlightenment, I can cure the spiritual anguish of all beings."

Gotama resolutely went forth from the palace into the gloom to seek enlightenment. The next morning he exchanged his silk robes for the tattered rags of a woodsman and shaved off his luxurious curls with his sword, symbolizing his renunciation of sex. (Long hair was believed to represent sexual vitality.) He then instructed Chandaka to return to the palace and report that Gotama was now a pilgrim who swore never again to be beguiled by sensual pleasure.

Upon his return, Chandaka found the palace in an uproar at the loss of the beloved prince. When told of Gotama's decision to flee, Yaśodharā beat her breast, tore at her clothes, ripped off her jewels and adornments, and made this heart-rending lament:

He says he wants to practice the Dharma, but how can he do so by abandoning me, his faithful spouse? Is he ignorant of the ancient tradition of taking one's partner along in retirement from the world? He is not following the Dharma in regard to me, that is certain. Is there something the matter with me? Even if he finds what he is after, that is no reason to desert me and our new-born son, a child who will never be cradled

on his father's lap. How hard-hearted and cruel he is—is there something wrong with my wish to be with him always?[29]

On and on she wept:

Two human beings cherished each other:
He was my joy, my sole delight.
His face was as radiant as the moon
And his form beyond compare.
Without him, all my possessions are nothing but rubble.
All alone on the bed we once shared,
He has abandoned me...
Henceforth I will not be able to take food and drink with pleasure;
My hair will grow foul and matted;
How tragic the forcible parting of two lovers![30]

Chandaka consoled the queen by telling her of Gotama's determination to win enlightenment for the good of all, and of his promise to return when he found the answers he was seeking. The queen eventually recovered, at least in part, from her grief, and life went on.

Gotama's quest for enlightenment had begun.

His first stop was a grove where ascetics gathered to subjugate the flesh in order to release the soul from the shackles of the body. The ascetics were as dedicated to pain as the inhabitants of Gotama's former palace were devoted to pleasure. They survived, barely, on roots, wild vegetables, seeds, tree bark, cow dung, and the tiniest drops of water. If they dressed at all it was in rough animal skins, rags, hair shirts, or robes of weeds. They slept out in the open, in cemeteries, in caves, or in trees. The grim ascetics mortified themselves in a variety of ingenious ways: never bathing, standing continually submerged in water or mud, staring into the sun, sitting in the center of a ring of bonfires, locking themselves permanently into one posture or position, and tearing their hair out by the roots or, on the other extreme, letting their hair grow until it was filthy and matted and then weighting it with chains.

Gotama was not convinced by the ascetics' argument that such severe penance would lead to inner peace: "If suffering is all there is to salvation, most of brute creation would have attained liberation eons ago." When told by the ascetics that animal (and human) sacrifice produced great merit, Gotama replied, "Nonsense! Infliction of injury on other beings can never bring good fortune; all sacrifice is a vain attempt to bribe the gods." Gotama also rejected the ascetics' contention that the aim of the religious life is to gain a better rebirth. "Enlightenment in this very body is all that matters," he insisted.

After leaving the ascetics, Gotama called on the philosophers. He encountered amoral nihilists who maintained that all human morality and goodness were futile; materialists who claimed that existence was meaningless and ended totally at death; and yogins who advocated quiescent states of mind suspended between existence and non-existence, thought and non-thought. Gotama was not satisfied with either the materialists or the spiritualists; both, he sensed, offered distorted, partial views. Confused yet determined,

Gotama traveled until he found an ideal spot for solitary meditation, a little hamlet near the lovely Nairañjanā River and the village of Uruvelā. Gotama said to himself, "The river here flows clear and clean, flowers, fruit, and green herbs are abundant, and the birds never stop singing. This quiet, peaceful place is perfect for my training."

There Gotama vowed to gain complete control of his body and mind by ridding himself of all passions, physical and mental. He sat in the meditation posture intently suppressing every thought, his effort so great that sweat poured from his body even in midwinter. To further calm his mind, Gotama stopped breathing for longer and longer periods, until his head was ready to explode. Further he went, attempting to starve his body into submission while horseflies, mosquitoes, and other insects feasted on his flesh. Near the end of his six-year fast, Gotama was reduced to a skeleton, his limbs were blackened, knotty stems, his ribs stuck out like the beams of an old shed, and his spine could be grasped from the front. His head resembled a withered gourd, his eyes were as glazed as the wa-

The ascetics were as dedicated to pain as the inhabitants of Gotama's former palace were devoted to pleasure.

ter on the bottom of a nearly dry well, and his skin was the color of cremation ashes. No longer human in form, Gotama was taken for a dust demon by the village children, who cast garbage on him. Finally he collapsed and was left for dead.

Gotama slowly regained consciousness, dragged himself to the river, and washed away six years of grime and filth. A village girl gave him a nourishing bowl of *pāyāsa*, which restored and refreshed the exhausted seeker.

Pāyāsa, rice cooked with milk and mixed with crystal sugar and fragrant spices, is a special, costly delicacy. Gotama's acceptance of that dish, from a woman, indicated that he had come full circle. In the palace Gotama had partaken of the choicest delicacies; as a mendicant he had to suppress his disgust and eat whatever scraps were put into his bowl. He nearly fasted to death, but then ate rich food to regain his physical and mental vigor. Gotama had come to experience every type of sensation regarding food, ranging from gustatory delight to revulsion and from satiety to starvation. Also, he took the food from a lovely young woman without desiring or shying away from her beauty and sexual presence, for in that realm too he had experienced every possible variation regarding sex, from uninhibited indulgence[31] to absolute abstinence.

Now with his mind and body in proper balance, Gotama was ready to make a final attempt at release. He made a comfortable seat of thick grass beneath the cooling shade of a large tree, faced the east, placed himself in the meditation posture, and gazed out into the vastness of space. He resolved, "Even if my body dries up and my skin, flesh, and bones wither away, I will not stir from this seat until enlightenment is mine!"

First, Gotama had to confront his inner demons of fear, loathing, doubt, confusion, and malevolence, personified by the horrible army of Māra, the Evil One. That dreadful horde consisted of every imaginable type of awful monster and repulsive demon. Gotama held firm, and the initial attack of the Devil Army was repelled and vanquished.

Some swayed their hips like palm trees in the wind; some sighed deeply with passion; some strolled about provocatively; some undressed slowly before him.

Then the Evil One switched tactics. Māra summoned his three daughters, Desire, Discontent, and Lust, instructing them to work the magic of sex and seduce Gotama. Thereupon, the Three Daughters conjured up a host of goddesses skilled in the 32 feminine wiles:

> **Some of the goddesses veiled only half their faces; some displayed their full, round breasts; some teased him with half-smiles of their pearly white teeth; some stretched and yawned voluptuously; some puckered their ruby-red lips; some gazed at him with sultry eyes; some revealed their half-covered breasts; some wore tight or transparent garments which showed off the curves of their bodies; some jangled their anklets; some festooned their breasts with garlands of flowers; some bared their luscious thighs; some paraded around with exotic birds on their heads and shoulders; some threw him side-long glances; some deliberately appeared disheveled; some fingered with their golden girdles; some moved enticingly in front of him; some danced and sang; some entreated him**

> **shamelessly; some swayed their hips like palm trees in the wind; some sighed deeply with passion; some strolled about provocatively; some undressed slowly before him; some revealed their undergarments; some walked by him redolent of perfume; some had painted faces and wore dangling earrings; some exposed themselves through clever use of their garments; some laughed gaily, recounting tales of love play; some disported themselves as innocent virgins, others as young brides, and still others as mature women; some pleaded with him to satisfy their passion; some showered him with fragrant flowers.[32]**

The girls sang out:

It is early spring, the fairest of all seasons!
All the trees beginning to bud, and flowers to bloom!
Surely this is the time for pleasure and love,
While you are in the prime of your beauty and youth—
Your appearance so graceful, your years so few,
> This is the time for you to indulge your desires.
> Your present search after supreme wisdom is hard to accomplish;
> Turn, then, your thoughts from it, and take your pleasure—
> Look at us, and behold our beauty and charms—

See our bodies, so perfect in shape, and so fit for love,
Our locks so brightly shining, of a rich auburn tint,
Our foreheads broad, and our perfectly shaped heads,
Our eyes so beautifully even and full,
Like the blue lotus flower.
Our noses curved like the beak of a parrot,
Our lips red and shining like rubies,
Resembling the choicest coral in tint; and see our graceful necks,
Our teeth so white, and free from disfigurement,
Our tongues so fresh, like the leaf of a lotus flower;
Listen to the soft and charming voices we possess, as melodious as that of the gods;
See our bosoms, so enticing, white, and lovely!
Round as the fruit of the pomegranate tree!

See our waists, so lithe and slender, like the handle of the bow,
Our buttocks, broad and glossy, placed evenly,
Just as the rounded forehead of the elephant king;
Our flanks, so soft and white, of graceful shape,
Smooth as the trunk of an elephant;
Behold our legs, so round and straight and tapering,
And see how full and plump our feet beneath,

A reddish white in color, like the shining petal of the lily.
How beautiful and joy-affording, then, our forms!
Adorned with all these marks of excellence!
Our fingers deft in every kind of music,
Our voices able to produce the softest sounds,
Our feet to dance and give delight to every heart—
What joy even the gods feel to see us thus!
How ravished with the thoughts of love they are!
Why do you not feel the same delight!
Why not covet the same enjoyment!
But like a man who finds a treasury of gold and gems,
Leaves all, and goes away far off,
Not knowing the happiness which such wealth
can give,
Your heart seems utterly estranged!
You ignore the joys of love and pleasure
And sit, self-absorbed and unmoved—
What a waste!
Why not partake of the world's joys and bliss!
And let nirvana and the path of wisdom be delayed.[33]

When Gotama would not succumb, the Three Daughters tried a different tack: "Men's tastes differ. Instead of sixteen-year-old goddesses, let us assume the shapes of women who have given birth once, women who have given birth twice, women of mature age, and even gray-haired old women."

The effect of all these spectacular enticements, the sweetest a man can be offered, on Gotama was nil. He dismissed them as nothing more than foam and water bubbles, devoid of real substance, pleasure as brief as a flash of lightning or an autumn shower. Gotama said to the Three Daughters, "I am no longer a slave to passions and lust, those razors smeared with honey, which captivate the mind and lead to fever, pain, vexation, and despair. My body is calm and my mind set free."

The Three Daughters gave up in grudging admiration. Any other man, they decided among themselves, would surely have caved in or lost his senses trying to resist such an onslaught.[34]

After withstanding the deadly, all-out assaults of the Demon Army and the Lascivious Three Daughters, Gotama easily handled the rest of Māra's poisoned arrows: Boredom, Hunger and Thirst, Greed, Sloth, Cowardice, Uncertainty, Malice, Obstinacy, and Fame and Glory.

Having completely unburdened himself of all disturbing passions, limiting thoughts, and every other distraction, Gotama was ready one night to encounter Absolute Reality. First, he passed through the four stages of meditation: observation and reflection, pure concentration, awakened awareness, and perfect equanimity. Later that night, the inner and outer workings of the universe became clear; then he experienced, intuitively,

the entire spectrum of existence; next, after contemplating the origin of cosmic unease and realizing a way to eradicate it, Gotama "knew what is." Upon seeing the morning star, he was a Buddha: "Tranquil in body, with a liberated mind; craving nothing, mindful and detached, calm and unperturbed." One text states that upon Gotama's enlightenment, the Earth shook like a woman in the throes of bliss—an all-embracing cosmic orgasm that transformed human consciousness.[35]

After abiding in the bliss of nirvana for 49 days, Buddha returned to the world to proclaim his message for the welfare of all. He knew from his own experience that wisdom was not communicable, but he hoped to point out the Way for others,

See our bosoms, so enticing, white, and lovely! / Round as the fruit of the pomegranate tree!

helping them create the right recipe for liberation. Buddha taught far and wide until his death at age 80. His final admonitions were, "Everything decays; train with diligence; rely on yourselves, no one else."

One of the meanings of the word nirvana is "extinguished," and for Gotama Buddha sexual sensation apparently vanished upon his enlightenment, and he could no longer be inflamed by sex. As a prince, Gotama's life was largely centered on sexual indulgence, and as a religious pilgrim, on sexual abstinence; but as a Buddha, both elements were, it seems, transcended. Buddha is portrayed in every text as being totally untroubled by sexual thoughts or feelings throughout his long ministry of 45 years. He was said to have exclaimed, "All the pleasures known to men, all the pleasures known to the gods, compared to the joy of nirvana are not even a sixteenth part."[36]

As an Awakened One, we are told, his concealed private parts were permanently sheathed, affording no offense or danger to anyone.[37]

Soon after his enlightenment, Māra's Three Daughters made one last attempt to ensnare Gotama Buddha. As soon as they appeared before him in the guise of delectable young beauties, however, the voluptuous trio was immediately transformed into wizened old hags. They remained in that state until Buddha magnanimously forgave them and removed the spell. He scolded them, "You cannot test what is beyond being tested."[38] Later in his career, Buddha's rivals would similarly attempt to entrap him with girls, without success, and he would spurn offers from the most powerful kings to wed their daughters.

Throughout his life as a teacher, Buddha associated with all types of women, including the most famed courtesans of the time, but treated one and all as "mothers, sisters, or daughters," neither enchanted nor repulsed by members of the opposite sex. Buddha kept his promise and returned to see his Queen Yaśodharā and their son, Rāhula. In a marvelous display of pique, Yaśodharā refused to go to the palace gate to greet her ex-husband. "If he really is noble," she told her father-in-law, the king, "he will come to *my* presence. Then I shall pay my respects." And, in fact, it was the Buddha who made the first move.[39] Yaśodharā, dressed in bright raiment and jewels, made a final attempt to win Gotama back, but it was too late. According to pious tradition, both Yaśodharā and Rāhula entered the Buddha's Order of Celibates and lived happily ever after. There is, however, other evidence that suggests that Yaśodharā remained aloof, acting as her own refuge, not entirely forgiving Gotama's abrupt abandonment of their marriage bed.[40]

Looking at the story of Gotama in allegorical terms, we can see that it represents ultimates. In the palace, Gotama had access to every kind of physical pleasure (of which sex was preeminent). Such extreme luxury, however, brought him no peace of mind; on the contrary, Gotama discovered that sybaritic indulgence is a deadly narcotic that eventually destroys body and soul. From that extreme, Gotama went to another. All stimula-

One text states that upon Gotama's enlightenment, the earth shook like a woman in the throes of bliss—an all-embracing cosmic orgasm that transformed human consciousness.

tion was shunned and sensual feelings or thoughts ruthlessly suppressed. Shutting out the phenomenal world, depriving oneself of every comfort or enjoyment, and remaining in a state of suspended animation was the goal. This method, too, leads to destruction, as Gotama learned nearly at the cost of his life.

After being immersed in both extremes, Gotama was awakened to the Middle Way, a centered path that leads safely through the poles of all-consuming fiery passion and the frigid depths of ascetic self-torture. While Buddha continued to eat, taking food as medicine, essential for the maintenance of life, sex was entirely dispensed with. Buddha, who had his fill of sex as Gotama the prince, thus represents a state beyond physical craving; *bud* (awake), the root of "Buddha," is neuter, a condition free of both gender and sex. In that respect Buddha ranks infinitely higher than the gods—sooner or later even the delights of paradise corrupt the inhabitants there and they fall again into the whirl of *samsara*.

Although Buddha's lofty asexuality was held as the ultimate human goal, it was an ideal that few could—or, it must be admitted, would want to—attain, and the problem of sex and

how to deal with it remained a sticky issue for each generation of Buddhists.

Endnotes

1. Material in this chapter is a composite drawn from the following sources. *Pali texts*: I.B. Horner, *The Collection of Middle Length Sayings*, 3 vols. (London: Pali Text Society, 1979); C.A.F. Rhys Davids and F.L. Woodward, *The Book of Kindred Sayings*, 5 vols. (London: Pali Text Society, 1979); T.W. Rhys Davids and C.A.F. Rhys Davids, *Dialogues of the Buddha*, 3 vols. (London: Pali Text Society, 1977); F.L. Woodward and E.M. Hare, *The Book of Gradual Sayings*, 5 vols. (London: Pali Text Society, 1979); I.B. Horner, *Book of the Discipline*, 6 vols. (London: Pali Text Society, 1982); T.W. Rhys Davids and H. Oldenberg, *Vinaya Texts*, 3 vols. (Delhi: Motilal Banarsidass, 1968 reprint); E.W. Burlingame, *Buddhist Legends*, 3 vols. (London: Pali Text Society, 1969). *Classical biographies of the Buddha*: G. Bays, *The Voice of the Buddha: Lalitavistara Sutra*, 2 vols. (Berkeley: Dharma Publishing, 1983); S. Beal, *Fo-Sho-Hing-Tsan-King: A Life of Buddha* (Delhi: Motilal Banarsidass, reprint 1968); S. Beal, *The Romantic Legend of Śākya Buddha* (Delhi: Motilal Banarsidass, reprint, 1985); E.H. Johnston, *The Buddhacarita or Acts of the Buddha* (Delhi: Motilal Banarsidass, 1984); J.J. Jones, *The Mahāvastu*, 3 vols. (London: Pali Text Society, 1973); N. Poppe, *The Twelve Deeds of Buddha* (Wiesbaden: Otto Harrassowitz, 1967); W.W. Rockwell, *The Life of Buddha* (London: Trubner's Oriental Series, 1884). *Pictorial biographies*: J. Auboyer, et al., *Buddha: A Pictorial History of His Life and Legacy* (New Delhi: Roli Books International, 1983); N.J. Krom, *The Life of Buddha on the Stupa of Barabudur* (Delhi: Bhartiya Publishing House, 1974). *Modern biographies*: A. Coomaraswamy, *Buddha and the Gospel of Buddhism* (Secaucus, N.J.: Citadel Press, 1988); A. Foucher, *The Life of Buddha* (Westport, Conn.: Greenwood Press, 1963); P. Herbert, *The Life of the Buddha* (London: British Museum, 1990). D.J. Kalupahana and I. Kalupahana, *The Way of Siddhartha: A Life of the Buddha* (Boulder: Shambhala Publications, 1983); A. Lillie, *The Life of Buddha* (Delhi: Seema Publications, 1974); Nanamoli, *The Life of the Buddha* (Kandy: Buddhist Publication Society, 1972); H. Nakamura, *Gotama Buddha* (Los Angeles & Tokyo: Buddhist Books International, 1977); E.J. Thomas, *The Life of Buddha as Legend and History* (London: Routledge & Kegan Paul, reprint 1969). There is also a novel on the subject by W.E. Barrett, *Lady of the Lotus: The Untold Love Story of The Buddha and His Wife* (Los Angeles: Jeremy P. Tarcher, 1975). **2.** See, for example, Bays, *Voice of the Buddha*, vol. 1: 42; Beal, *Romantic Legend*: 32; Thomas, *Life of Buddha*: 29. **3.** Bays, *Voice of the Buddha*, vol. 1: 44-5; Jones, *Mahāvastu*, vol. 2: 7ff. **4.** *The Mahāvastu* states that the Buddha deliberately incarnates himself into the womb of a woman who has only ten months and seven days to live because it would not be proper for her to "indulge in the pleasures of love after giving birth to a Peerless One" (vol. 2: 3). **5.** This description of Gotama is based on the 32 distinguishing marks of a Buddha. See Bays, *Voice of the Buddha*, vol. 1: 155ff.; Beal, *Romantic History*: 55; Rhys Davids and Rhys Davids, *Dialogues of the Buddha*, vol. 3: 138ff.; Jones, *Mahāvastu*, vol. 1: 180-1; Thomas, *Life of Buddha*: 220-1, which lists both the 32 major and 80 minor characteristics of a Buddha. For further information on Buddha's physical form, see D.L. Snellgrove, ed., *The Image of the Buddha* (Tokyo: Kodansha International, 1978). **6.** The Chinese texts (e.g., Beal, *Fo-Sho-Hing-Tsan-King*: 14) state that Buddha's sex organs were hidden like those of a stallion. According to the Tibetan tradition, the Dalai Lamas are supposed to possess a similar ability to "retract" their sex organs; see M. Aris, *Hidden Treasures and Secret Lives* (Delhi: Motilal Banarsidass, 1988): 197. **7.** In Buddha's time, there were "public days" in which unmarried girls, who were normally sequestered, would promenade through the town in hopes of capturing the fancy of a young man. See H.C. Warren, *Buddhism in Translation* (Cambridge: Harvard University Press, 1986): 455. **8.** Jones, *Mahāvastu*, vol. 2: 70; Krom, plate 48. **9.** Beal, *Romantic Legend*: Plate 19 in W. Zwalf, *Buddhism: Art and Faith* (London: British Museum Publications, 1985) seems to depict a wedding scene of Gotama and one of his wives. **10.** Bays, *Voice of the Buddha*, vol. 1: 235-6; Krom, plate 55. **11.** Thomas, *Life of Buddha*: 48ff., discusses the different names given Buddha's wives. **12.** Beal, *Romantic Legend*: 96ff. **13.** This exchange occurs in T. Cleary, *The Flower Ornament Scripture* (Boston: Shambhala Publications, 1987): 284-8. **14.** For examples of lush Buddhist beauties see S. Huntington and J. Huntington, *The Art of Ancient India* (Tokyo: John Weatherhill, 1987); G. Michael, et al., *In the Image of Man* (London: Weidenfeld & Nicolson, 1982); P. Rawson, *Erotic Art of the East* (New York: G.P. Putnam's Sons, 1968); *Oriental Erotic Art* (London: Quartet Books,

1987). **15.** Auboyer, *Buddha*, plates 16, 19-21, and 94 illustrate Gotama's life of pleasure in the palace. For descriptions and illustrations of the love life of an Indian prince, see P.K. Agrawal, *Mithuna* (New Delhi: Munshiram Manoharal, 1983); H. Bach, *Indian Love Paintings* (New Delhi: Lustre Press, 1985); R. Burton, *The Illustrated Kama Sutra* (Middlesex: Hamlyn, 1987); N. Douglas and P. Singer, *The Pillow Book* (New York: Destiny Books, 1984); *Sexual Secrets* (New York: Destiny Books, 1986); S.N. Prasad, *Kalyānamalla's Anangaranga* (New Delhi: Chaukhambha Orientalia, 1983); and E. Windsor, *The Hindu Art of Love* (New York: Panurge Press, 1932). **16.** Beal, *Romantic Legend*: 101. **17.** Johnston, *Buddhacarita*: 26. **18.** See Rawson's description of the sex life of an Indian prince in classical times, *Erotic Art of the East*: 65. **19.** J. Campbell, *The Masks of God: Oriental Mythology* (London: Penguin Books, 1973): 259. **20.** Bays, *Voice of the Buddha*, vol. 1: 291, 304ff.; Beal, *Romantic Legend*: 123; Krom, *Life of Buddha*: plate 65. **21.** Johnston, *Buddhacarita*: 44ff. **22.** Ibid.: 53. **23.** Beal, *Romantic Legend*: 128. The Chinese text was so explicit that Beal did not translate it. **24.** Poppe, *Twelve Deeds*: 118. **25.** Bays, *Voice of the Buddha*, vol. 1: 310ff.; Beal, *Fo-Sho-Hing-Tsan-King*: 54; Beal, *Romantic Legend*: 130ff.; Foucher: 73ff.; Jones, *Mahāvastu*, vol. 2: 70ff.; Krom, *Life of the Buddha*: plates 68, 69. "Disgust with the dancing girls" also plays a role in the story of Yasa, an early convert to Buddhism. See Rhys Davids and Oldenberg, *Vinaya Texts*, vol. 1: 102ff. **26.** See Beal, *Romantic Legend*: 130. **27.** Poppe, *Twelve Deeds*: 124. **28.** For a picture of this scene, see H. Bechert and R. Gombrich, *Buddhism* (London: Thames and Hudson, 1984): 21, plate 10. **29.** See Johnston, *Buddhacarita*: 116. **30.** See Lillie, *Life of Buddha*: 66-7. **31.** In Poppe, *Twelve Deeds*: 123, Buddha says: "There is not a single sensual joy which I have not enjoyed." The *Buddhacarita* states that each potential Buddha must taste all sensual pleasures prior to illumination (p 30). **32.** See Bays, *Voice of the Buddha*, vol. 2: 484-5. **33.** Adapted after Beal, *Romantic Legend*:

211-2. **34.** Regarding the temptation of Māra's daughters, see also Auboyer, *Buddha*: plates 52, 56; Jones, *Mahāvastu*, vol. 3: 270; Krom, *The Life of the Buddha*: plate 105; Lillie, *Life of Buddha*: 91-2. Young boys are often given temporary ordination in the Theravadan countries of Southeast Asia, and the "Temptation of Māra's Daughters" is reenacted during the ceremony. See R.C. Lester, *Theravada Buddhism in Southeast Asia* (Ann Arbor: University of Michigan Press, 1973): 91-2. **35.** Beal, *Romantic Legend*: 226. **36.** Thomas, *Life of Buddha*: 79. **37.** Bays, *Voice of the Buddha*, vol. 2: 649. **38.** Ibid.: 572. **39.** Coomaraswamy, *Buddha and the Gospel of Buddhism*: 49. **40.** After Gotama's departure from the palace, Yaśodharā's mood remained "dull and dark" (Beal, *Romantic Legend*: 92). As mentioned in the text, it is also recorded that when Yaśodharā first met her former husband, she tried to win him back by wearing her most alluring clothes and feeding him sweetmeats (Jones, *Mahāvastu*, vol. 2: 260). In the *Romantic Leg-*

"All the pleasures known to men, all the pleasures known to the gods, compared to the joy of nirvana are not even a sixteenth part."

end it says that Buddha's son was born six years *after* he had left the palace. Naturally, Yaśodharā was suspected of infidelity, and the text lamely tries to explain away her supposed six-year pregnancy as the result of bad karma accumulated in a previous life (pp. 360ff.). In the *Apadāna* it reports that Yaśodharā told Buddha when she met him late in life that she had been her own refuge and had done quite well on her own account. See I.B. Horner, *Woman in Primitive Buddhism* (Delhi: Motilal Banarsidass, 1975): 310.

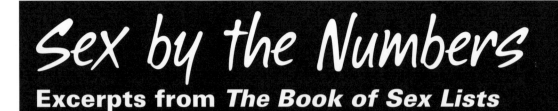

Sex by the Numbers
Excerpts from *The Book of Sex Lists*

Albert B. Gerber

11 Inside Stories About the Making of the Film *Caligula*

1. The screen test, *Caligula*-style: More than 300 women auditioned for parts in *Caligula* by performing in sexual screen tests so that director Tinto Brass could see: "Not just whether, but *how*. Are they good at it? Do they fuck cheerfully or not?"

2. One extra did indeed have two penises—not all the grotesqueries were made up.

3. Director Brass had oral sex with a *Penthouse* Pet on the set before the entire crew to show an actor how he wanted it done. His wife described his behavior as "just his usual extroverted self."

4. The extra playing a Roman guard who had his penis tied and was forced to drink wine until bloated, then was stabbed by Tiberius (Peter O'Toole) in a display of imperial cruelty, was *actually* stabbed by accident and had to be hospitalized.

"For chrissakes, you want to be an actress but you can't even take a 'don't piss' direction!"

5. Question: How do you prevent an eel from biting a woman while inside her? Answer: If you were the first assistant of *Caligula* and faced that problem for the Harem Monsters scene, you had the brainstorm of putting a condom over its head and holding it on with Scotch tape. That, unfortunately, didn't solve the problem—it killed the eel before it could perform. If you were the woman matched with the eel, you used your imagination—and put it in tail-first.

6. The fake cock for the castration scene was made out of pork sausage.

7. A *Penthouse* Pet pissing on an actor on camera did it three times. On the third take, she wasn't supposed to piss but she did. Director Brass screamed at her, "For chrissakes, you want to be an actress but you can't even take a 'don't piss' direction!"

8. It is against Italian law to have minors on a movie set where sexual activity occurs. The filmmakers got around this by hiring especially young-looking eighteen-year-old women and shaving their pubic areas.

9. The bed built for Caligula, his wife, his sister, a dozen women slaves, and his horse was modeled after the main altar in Saint Peter's Basilica.

10. *Penthouse* wanted *Caligula* to be a softcore, soft-focus copy of the magazine. Tinto Brass wanted to make a kind of anarchist "Busby Berkeley Goes to Rome"—a big-budget, hardcore slapstick comedy. He almost accomplished his goal. Only after the film was completed did *Penthouse* realize what he'd done. It then took three years and three different film editors to undo the "damage."

11. The climactic (pardon the pun) orgy scene on the ship was a real orgy. It was another example of director Brass' obsession with recreating actual pagan sex. It lasted two days and included more than 300 people.

(From the book *Ultimate Porno* by PierNico Solinas. This list was prepared especially for *The Book of Sex Lists* by Louis Rossetto.)

Sexual Behavior of Former Nuns and Priests (Before, During, and After Orders)

It is exceedingly difficult to get any information about the sex lives of nuns and priests. Obviously, they are not supposed to have any. In a precedent-shattering study, two researchers at Baylor College of Medicine have come up with some interesting answers.

Sex Activity of Former Nuns and Priests

Sex Activity	Percentage engaging in activity before entering orders	While in orders	After leaving orders
Masturbation	47%	57%	85%
Intercourse	11%	15%	82%
Oral-Genital	9%	5%	75%
Homosexual	11%	21%	16%
Celibate	46%	32%	10%

The percentages given refer to those who replied. In many cases the individual engaged in more than one activity; therefore, the columns are not intended to add up to 100%.

Fifty-three percent of the men and 50% of the women reported being less satisfied sexually after relinquishing orders than they would have liked. The next question was, What reason did they have for this decreased sexual satisfaction?

Reasons Most Frequently Cited for Decreased Satisfaction

Reason	Times Cited
1. Lack of partners	57
2. Religious/moral reasons	44
3. Feelings of not being desirable	35
4. Communication problems	20
5. Orgasmic dysfunction (women only)	20

(From "A Sexual Intimacy Survey of Former Nuns and Priests" by Margaret H. Halstead, MS, and Lauro S. Halstead, MD, in *The Journal of Sex and Marital Therapy*, summer 1978. Reprinted (with minor changes) with permission.)

9 Great Writers of Sex Letters

1. *Louis Armstrong:* His candid letters sizzle with passion, and he could play on a woman's emotions as adroitly as on a trumpet. His nickname, Satchmo, is short for Satchel-mouth, a perfect piece of equipment for a sensual lover.

2. *Napoleon Bonaparte:* His amorous letters to Josephine during the Italian campaign were a literal "hotline" to Paris. A typical comment: "I long to cover you with a thousand kisses."

3. *Robert Browning:* This sedately bearded and seemingly staid Victorian poet was an ardent suitor, as his beautiful love letters to Elizabeth Barrett (later his wife) testify. But to another woman he wrote: "If you will let me visit you again, I promise to make my hands behave." A Browning buff bought this incriminating note for $500, then burned it, observing: "No one must ever know this about Browning."

4. *George A. Custer:* The future Indian-fighter's love letters to his sweetheart, Mollie J. Holland of Cadiz, Ohio, mostly signed "Bachelor Boy," were so impassioned that Mollie cut out many passages with her sewing scissors, leaving only such relatively modest remarks as, "When are we going to get into the trundle bed?"

5. *Salvador Dalí:* The celebrated Surrealist wrote torrid letters in fractured French, often enriching them with erotic sketches.

Puccini once observed that he might have written many more operas if he hadn't spent so much of his life horizontal.

6. *John Keats:* His immortal love letters to Fanny Brawne reveal the fierce passion of the poet who so desired intense sensations that he sprinkled cayenne pepper on his tongue before sipping claret. To Fanny he wrote: "Love is my religion. You have ravished me away by a power I cannot resist. I cannot breathe without you."

7. *John F. Kennedy:* The intimate, unpublished correspondence of our thirty-fifth President abounds in four-letter words and sexy comments. To the sweetheart who rejected his proposal of marriage only six months before he was wed to Jacqueline Bouvier, Kennedy wrote a passionate letter, pleading that she reconsider, adding: "You are the only woman I have ever loved or ever will love."

8. *Wolfgang A. Mozart:* The famed composer was a passionate lover and delighted in using explicit language in his letters, thus putting his modern editors to the embarrassment of censoring his uninhibited vocabulary.

9. *Giacomo Puccini:* An acknowledged master of the four-letter word, the great composer of *La bohème* and *Madama Butterfly* wrote poems in his letters to his mistresses that

are so explicit, they would bring a blush to the cheeks of a seasoned courtesan. Puccini had scores of lovers and once observed that he might have written many more operas if he hadn't spent so much of his life horizontal.

(Prepared by Charles Hamilton exclusively for *The Book of Sex Lists*.)

2 Female Chimpanzees Who Experienced Orgasms

1. Nanette

2. Shu Shu

While some primates may be prelates, not all primates are people. Of those primates who are people, many human females have problems reaching orgasm during intercourse. Dr. Dolores Elaine Keller, a biologist and full professor at Pace University in New York City, is also a psychologist and psychotherapist. Dr. Keller, who specializes in sexual disorders and marital therapy, wondered whether orgasmic difficulty was a generalized female primate condition.

She reasoned that if human females had less difficulty in reaching orgasm with clitoral stimulation, nonhuman primates should be tested to see if this is also true for them. Watching

"I am a helpless piece of fruit being tossed with apple and orange slices and bananas by a beautiful woman."

primates mate led her to conclude that intravaginal thrusting time is brief. This suggested why orgasm during intercourse might be difficult to attain for the female primate.

From prelates on down into the evolutionary past, predating humans, apparently male primates insert penis, thrust, then ejaculate within ten seconds. Certainly by today's standards of proper primate sexual performance, premature ejaculation is a rampant primate problem. Most female partners of such primates have trouble having orgasms during intercourse—even though the potential is there.

Keller investigated noncoital orgasm in *Pan troglodytes* chimpanzees at the Laboratory for Experimental Medicine and Surgery in Primates, a division of New York University's Medical Center.

Sure enough, two chimpanzees did experience orgasm with digital clitoral stimulation, and one, Nanette, also climaxed with the use of an electric vibrator on her clitoris, a sexual first for *Pans* and for Nanette.

Shu Shu was afraid of the vibrator (a modified Prelude 2 frequently used in sexual therapy for nonorgasmic human females), but did evidence thrusting pelvic contractions as well

as vaginal contractions.

Vocalizations also occurred when Nanette had an orgasm—a series of throaty "hoo-hoo-hoos."

11 Far-out Letters Received by the Project

The Project is a not-for-profit theater and research group which studies sexual variety and presents weekly discussions and theatrical productions of erotic fantasies. Headquarters are on the top floor of a loft building in SoHo, in lower Manhattan.

The Project's files comprise more than 1,500 personal sex histories, proclivities, fantasies, and lifestyles. The following are actual extracts from the thousands of letters that have been received by the Project during the past few years.

1. "I am a helpless piece of fruit being tossed with apple and orange slices and bananas by a beautiful woman. I have a huge tub and a giant Haitian fork and spoon in my basement, and I always ask my girlfriends to put me in and toss me."

2. "Whenever we are going to have sex, my wife and I put a raw fish in bed with us. I was brought up in a fish store and whenever I was feeling insecure, I would hide under my mother's skirts and breathe the smell of fish on her body."

3. "I am a queen in a pleasure palace with a whole harem of men. My husband is kept hanging in a cage at the side of my bed, and he is forced to watch while I make it with all my servants."

4. "I pay prostitutes to put tail feathers in their ani (plural of anus) and walk around me while I lie on the bed and play with myself."

5. "I am very proud of my one inverted tit. I am in a glass elevator with ten young studs. As the elevator goes up the side of the building, they strip off my clothes and admire and start licking and caressing my inverted tit."

6. "I dream of Dracula coming through the window, biting my neck, and carrying me off to screw in his coffin."

7. "My first experience with a woman was my mother taking me to the live poultry market. I felt jealous sitting in my little baby buggy while the chickens were getting all the attention. Now, whenever I have sex, I fantasize [about] being one of those chickens."

8. "He drapes my nude body with clusters of tiny silver and

golden bells, which are attached by gossamer threads to several huge sticks. He begins to poke and taunt me with the sticks, and a haunting melody arises from the shimmering bells."

9. "I fantasize a whole sorority of girls tying one of their sisters down and tickling her underarms, ribs, and feet."

10. "I get turned on by the thought of a woman silencing me by pressing the palm of her hand over my mouth."

11. "This great goddess in the sky with a giant Afro sends down a ladder for me. As I climb up, my clothes shed like a snake's skin and my organ is growing to meet the size of my goddess. As we make hair-raising sex, our love juices fall on the earth below, and the people are so happy that they prepare hamburgers and hotdogs and declare a holiday."

(Prepared by the Project especially for the *Book of Sex Lists*.)

10 Jewish Sex Laws and Customs

Jewish sexual life is carefully prescribed and circumscribed. Almost every aspect of sex has a rule. The rules come from the Torah (the five Books of Moses) and the Talmud (Code of Laws), the Mishnah, and the commentary on that code (the Gemara). In addition, over the years, rabbis (teachers) have suggested revisions, many of which have been accepted.

In most cases, the rules today are primarily of historical interest. However, from the Hassidim of New York City and Israel to the small number of Jews in Yemen who refused to leave (for religious reasons) to go to Israel, there are Jews who still observe the rules as they were observed thousands of years ago. These are:

1. *General Sexual Conduct:* Practically all forms of sex outside of marriage are prohibited. This includes any form of promiscuity, prostitution, and adultery and any form of lewd behavior.

2. *Transvestism:* The rule of the Bible is that "a woman shall not wear that which pertains to a man, neither shall a man put on a woman's garment." Orthodox Jewish women today cannot wear slacks. Conservative rabbis permit slacks if they are obviously tailored for a woman—if, for example, they have buttons or a zipper on the side—but women are still prohibited from wearing a fly in front.

3. *Abortion:* This is permitted in Jewish law only to save the life of the mother. However, modern Reform rabbis are more lenient and approve abortions where there is a pregnancy resulting from rape, evidence that the child is deformed, or other objective reasons. There is still no general approval of abortion among Conservative or Orthodox Jews.

4. *Birth Control:* Because the Bible prohibits the wasting of the seed, the Orthodox reject any form of contraception. Modern Conservative and Reform rabbis condone the use of contraceptives. Many Orthodox rabbis have approved the use of the Pill because, technically, the "seed" is not spilled on the ground.

5. *Homosexuality:* The Old Testament says that it is "an abomination" and punishes the act by death. Jewish tradition prohibited two men from sleeping together even when no sexual activity took place.

6. *Nudism:* Absolutely prohibited. In addition, Orthodox Jewish women do not wear short skirts, low necklines, or even sleeveless dresses. The Reform movement has moved away from this rigid position.

7. *Pornography:* Technically prohibited. The rabbinic authorities even ruled that it was illegal for a man to stare at any woman except his wife. However, there is good evidence that the rabbis and scholars who spent their days discussing and analyzing Jewish religion, laws, and customs frequently told sexy and scatological jokes. They just never put them down on paper.

It is illegal to have sex when any light is burning.

8. *Prohibitions of Sexual Intercourse:* Many. There are thirty-six sins for which the punishment is death. A large number of these are sexual, for example: sexual intercourse with one's mother, with one's father's wife, with a daughter-in-law, with any other male, with an animal, between a woman and an animal, a woman and her daughter, with a married woman, with one's sister, with one's father's sister or one's mother's sister, with one's wife's sister (while the wife is living), with one's brother's wife or one's father's brother's wife, with a woman while she is menstruating. Also, violating the rules relating to circumcision.

The prohibition of sex during the menstrual period was not simply while the wife was menstruating. Actually, no matter how many days the woman menstruated, the Bible said that the menstrual period was seven days. Therefore, the man had to refrain for a week following the first stain; then, to make sure, the Talmud added five more days. Thus, in the Jewish tradition, there are twelve days in which a woman is in dry dock.

Although not punishable by death, there are many other taboos relating to sexual intercourse. For example, it is illegal to have sex when any light is burning. It is illegal to have sex during Yom Kippur or any other fast day. It is illegal for a man to approach his wife sexually while he is drunk or while they're having an argument.

9. *Compulsory Sexual Intercourse:* The ancient Jews took seriously the biblical injunction to "be fruitful and multiply." Therefore, it became the duty of a man to have sex whenever permissible. There is some dispute as to when a man had fulfilled his duty. Some said that a man had to have two sons, and others argued for a son and a daughter.

It is a special blessing to have sex on a Friday night, because this makes the Sabbath complete. If a man marries a woman and lives with her ten years and she bears him no child, it is thought he should divorce her and try another wife. She is

A man who becomes a dog-shit collector can be forced to divorce his wife.

encouraged to try another man, because the rabbis know that a woman might conceive children by one man after being barren with another, as modern medicine has proven.

There is some dispute as to whether a man has a right to refrain from intercourse with his wife for more than a week, but certainly not more than two weeks, for she too has sexual rights. Actually, for the ordinary man, the rule is that he is to have intercourse every day when legally permissible. If he is a laborer and that is a burden, he complies by engaging twice a week. (Donkey drivers who go out among the villages to cart grain get home only twice a week, so that number suffices for them.) A camel driver must service his wife once every thirty days. Sailors have the longest statute of limitations—six months! And if a man who has an occupation which gives his wife the right to sex every night wants to go into another occupation which will cut this frequency, the wife has a right to prevent it! Except if he decides to become a scholar, in which case the wife can't object.

10. *Divorce:* The Jewish laws on divorce could fill a three-volume textbook. Here are some highlights:

Technically, only a man can get a divorce. A wife can do this if her husband contracts boils (this was later enlarged and interpreted to include any loathsome disease, including VD or leprosy).

A man who becomes a dog-shit collector can be forced to divorce his wife. (This substance was used in tanning leather.) The man who becomes a coppersmith or tanner can be compelled to get a divorce, as the rabbis said, for "olfactory reasons."

If a man marries and on consummation discovers his wife is not a virgin, he is duty-bound to divorce her, but the religious courts made proof so difficult that divorce on this ground was discouraged.

A man who marries a virgin receives a seven-day honeymoon by law, but a man who marries a widow gets only three days.

Virgins have to be married on Wednesdays because the court sat on Thursdays, so if the betrayed groom wanted to lodge a nonvirginity court action, he had Thursday morning court to do so.

Bill Gaines' 10 Foods That Are Better Than Sex

William M. Gaines is the founder and publisher of *Mad* magazine. He is also a rather substantial eater. This section was made with loving care and with the assistance of Bill's live-in co-eater, Anne Griffiths. [*Editor's Note: Gaines died in 1992.*]

1. White truffles
2. Fresh caviar from Caspian sturgeon
3. Pennsylvania Dutch smoked sausage
4. Tortellini alla panna with freshly grated Parmigiano Reggiano
5. Fresh foie gras des Landes
6. Prosciutto crudo di Langhirano
7. Smoked Scotch salmon
8. Peeled Royal Riviera pears with very heavy cream
9. Raspberries with crème fraîche
10. White Castle hamburgers

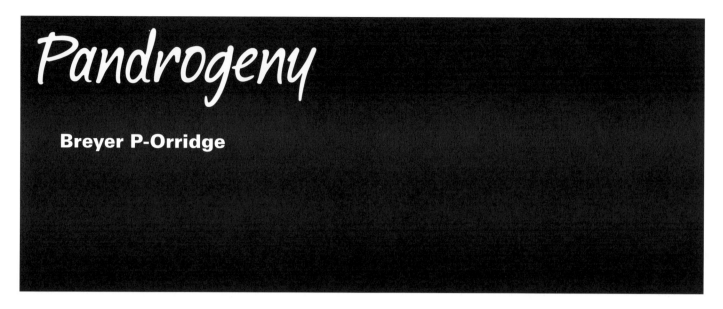

Pandrogeny

Breyer P-Orridge

Editor's Note: Breyer P-Orridge is the collective name of Genesis Breyer P-Orridge and Lady Jaye Breyer P-Orridge. Together, they form a third being.

Excerpts From a Dialogue With Dominic Johnson

It seems useful to us, in our practice, to adopt the assumption that there is no way of knowing which has supremacy, the recording device that is DNA, or the SELF we converse with internally that we *call* consciousness but often, rather lazily, still imagine and identify as the living, biological body. In fact, we see the "I" of our consciousness as a fictional assembly or collage that resides in the environment of the body.

One of the central themes of our work is the malleability of physical and behavioral identity. The body is used by the mind as a logo, an hieroglyph for the SELF before we are able to speak and use language. It is almost an holographic doll constructed by external expectations even before our body is born. Even the name we are assigned is another holographic program in the prophetic story of who we are to become.

The work of William S. Burroughs and Brion Gysin has been highly influential to us, particularly in relation to the practice of the "cut-up." To liberate the word from linearity, they began to cut-up and, incorporating random chance, re-assembled both their own and co-opted literature "...to see what it really says...." They referred to the phenomena of profound and poetic new collisions and meanings that resulted from their intimate collaborations as the "third mind." This was produced with a willingness to sacrifice their own separate, previously inviolate works and artistic "ownership." In many ways they saw the third mind

as an entity in and of itself. Something "other," closer to a purity of essence, and the origin and source of a magical or divine creativity that could only result from the unconditional integration of two sources.

Beginning in the 1960s, especially from being an active participant in the Exploding Galaxy/Transmedia Exploration and occasionally the Gay Lib street theatre, Genesis Breyer P-Orridge experimented with various disciplines and practices to apply the cut-up to behavior, to identity, and to gender; de-conditioning as far as possible the fictional character written by consensus reality and all who would impose their expectations upon him. Breyer P-Orridge worked throughout the 1970s as a performance artist and actionist; and during the 1980s s/he studied and practiced ritual and shamanic techniques and was deeply involved in the body modification movement known as "modern primitives." In the early 1990s Genesis Breyer P-Orridge met Lady Jaye Breyer P-Orridge, and their ever more rigorous collaborations began.

Just as Burroughs and Gysin collaborated, subsuming their separate works, individuality, and ego to a collaborative process by cutting up the word to produce a third mind, so, in our current practice, Breyer P-Orridge have applied the cut-up

The body is used by the mind as a logo, an hieroglyph for the SELF before we are able to speak and use language.

system and third mind concept directly to a central concern, the fictional SELF. The un-authorized Astory of our lives so far. Breyer P-Orridge both supply our separate bodies, individuality, and ego to an ongoing and substantially irreversible process of cutting-up identity to produce a third being, an "other" entity that we call the PANDROGYNE.

In our quest to create the Pandrogyne, both Genesis and Lady Jaye have agreed to use various modern medical techniques to try to look as much like each other as possible. We are required, over and over again by our process of literally cutting up our bodies, to create a third, conceptually more precise body, to let go of a lifetime's attachment to the physical logo that we visualize automatically as "I" in our internal dialogue with the SELF.

We encounter many unexpected internal conflicts as our egos try to survive intact as the "person" they have been previously conditioned to be. We have discovered that how we look does relate very directly to the internal dialogue that describes us to our SELF and to each other. It is not superficial in its effect when it is instructed that everything about its logo of its SELF is malleable, vulnerable, and impermanent.

When you consider transexuality, crossdressing, cosmetic surgery, piercing, and tattooing, they are all calculated impulses—a symptomatic groping toward the next phase. One of the great things about human beings is that they impulsively and intuitively express what is inevitably next in the

In our quest to create the Pandrogyne, both Genesis and Lady Jaye have agreed to use various modern medical techniques to try to look as much like each other as possible.

evolution of culture and our species. It is the Other that we are destined to become.

Pandrogeny is not about defining differences but about creating similarities. Not about separation but about unification and resolution.

Breyer P-Orridge believe that the binary systems embedded in society, culture, and biology are the root cause of conflict and aggression, which in turn justify and maintain oppressive control systems and divisive hierarchies. Dualistic societies have become so fundamentally inert, uncontrollably consuming, and self-perpetuating that they threaten the continued existence of our species and the pragmatic beauty of infinite diversity of expression. In this context the journey represented by their PANDROGENY and the experimental creation of a third form of gender-neutral living being is concerned with nothing less than strategies dedicated to the survival of the species.

"WE ARE BUT ONE..." becomes less about individual gnosis and more about the unfolding of an entirely new, open source, twenty-first-century myth of creation.

PRAYERS for SACRED HEARTS

There is no reason
on earth why
you should run out
of people to be.

S/HE IS HER/E

P-ANDROGENY
POSITIVE ANDROGENY
POWER ANDROGENY
POTENT ANDROGENY
POLITICAL ANDROGENY
PERFECT ANDROGENY
PRECIOUS ANDROGENY
P-ANDROGYNE
WILD
BEING
UNHOLY
CHOSEN ONE

To throw off the shackles
Of experience
Of true sexual freedom
And physical love!
End gender.
BREAK SEX.
There are more than one of you.
Maybe hundreds to choose from.

CHANGE THE WAY TO PERCEIVE
AND CHANGE ALL MEMORY.

BREAKING SEX!
(S/HE IS HER/E)

This is the final war, a jigsaw
A war to re-possess your SELF.
There is NO gender anymore
Only P-Androgeny is divine.
Sexuality is a force of nature that cannot be contained. Get up.
Stand together in perfecting union,
Join and love equally the man and the woman separated at b-earth inside you,
Their first cries for justice ... PANDROGENY!
Re-united as one
Identity is your only possession,
as a being possessed
Re-possess your SELF,
Be possessed by YOUR self,
Any SELF, every SELF you ever dreamed of,

Every SELF you were ever afraid of. GET UP!
Stop this war of limitations,
STOP IT!
Now YOU own yourself.
Your own YOU own.
Now it's YOU.
Stop being possessed by characters written by others.
Change your ID card – cut it into the shape of a HEART.
Be heart felt.
Feel your heart,
Your heart is your art.

Re build your SELF from the FOUND UP!

Identity is theft.
(IDENTITY IS THEFT.)

NOTHING SHORT OF A TOTAL GENDER

These puppeteers of the NEW WAY ON,
Download slave software into your brain
Even as that wriggling, cocky tyke breaches the
cellular defenses,
Its resources stretched taught,
Thinner than a condom on a monstrously seductive,
Destructive cock.
POP! POW! Snap! Suck!
Snake of Eden rigid with victory
Jissom of control victorious
the arrows of sex penetrate egg central
And, spiraling downwards, downs its load,
The double bluff,
Double helix story of those chosen to come before.
Chosen, without choice,
Not you. KNOT YOU!
Knot this AND, this DNA,
This STRAND, stran-dead,
STRANDED
Strand-DEAD on arrival,
Slapped into shape by your DELIVERERS.
A pre-recorded software,
Worn down through ages with one purpose,
To serve the rich, service their itch,
Supply each demand.
Obey each command.

(CHANGE THE WAY TO PERCEIVE AND
CHANGE ALL MEMORY)

Struck dumb by its ELEGANCE says CRICK,
Elementary says Watson.
The double helix leaps from lab to life,
With YOU as the lab rat!
Whose elegance?

Whose elegance anyway?
Two spines, once twins, that go their separate ways after 49
days,
Yet … remain inseparably linked
The edit points, invisible.

AND/DNA there-in lies the problem and the lies begin.

In the beginning ALL were perfect. The first man was the
first woman.
The first woman was the first man.
UNTIL the whispering began…
AND/DNA the first man became the first man
The first woman became the first woman
AND/DNA then all HELL let loose
AND/DNA we've been living (t)here ever SIN-ce
Know matter HOW sin-cerely…

We are ultra-genetic terrorists.

(POSSESSION IS THE GREATER PART OF VALOR)

You are vital.
You are vigorous. Get up.
Stop Hiding.

We are ultra-genetic terrorists.
One man is another man or woman.
EVERY MAN AND WOMAN IS A MAN AND WOMAN
There is a time and place for everything indecent.
Redesign yourself.
YOUR SELF.
End your social and sexual misery, taste the sweet electricity
of PANDROGENY!

"This time around you can be anybody"

Put away your toys and focus.
WE ARE BUT ONE BITCH!
We declare war against all binary systems.
We support SELF-determination and liberation.
Total freedom for all possible and impossible identities
and sexualities.
DESTROY!
Destroy Gender.
Destroy the control of DNA and the expected.

Do you understand?
Here's the key.

You were in your mother's womb for forty-nine days an
androgyne.
Who chose your gender?
GOD?
Society? Family?

Only by YOU ending this separation, returning to that first pure state can real freedom begin. When all are but one sex, one species.
This is not about becoming an Other,
This is about returning to a state of perfect union.

Masturbation is the highest form of magick
SO tap into the psychic network.

CREATIVITY is your anti-gender protein.

There is no free speech, ONLY an illusion of freedom.
Freedom of delusion …

Perhaps GOD was breathless, allergic to cosmic dust.
Despite its three billion years HEAD start on us at this PERSON building, this character building.
One KEY point is oft forgot. AND/DNA alone, on its OWN does NOTHING!!
NOTHING!
NOTHING!
NO-THING!

It can't make eyes brown or green,

or brains,
or any other electrically charged "muscle" bulge!
It can't sit up, or apply makeup,
Or keep itself clean,
Not even adjust a wig.
PROTEINS do all that.

CREATIVITY is your anti-gender protein.

Stripped of who YOU are, stripped of the creativity that IS character DNA/AND is helpless, speechless, dead on arrival again!

WITHOUT THE SCENE FORGET THE GENE

Society has always been an enemy of the desire to create,
Of all possible creativity.
What am I saying to you?
Nature began as a deliberately chaotic force FOR change.
Constant change.
Evolution, evolving, unfolding.
All those redundant species wither. Those embracing novelty leapfrog them to dominance…
Maybe with a little interspecies cross (and loving) fertilization along the way.
Creativity is the most POWER-full energy in the Universe.

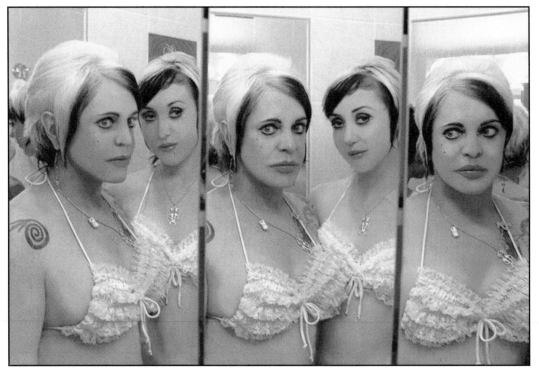

"FRA ANGELICA" by Breyer P-Orridge. From a photograph by Laure Leber.

About the Editor

Besides the books below, Russ has written articles and a column for the *Village Voice* and several independent magazines. The Memory Hole [www.thememoryhole.org], a website devoted to rescuing knowledge and freeing information, is his labor of love. His personal website is [www.mindpollen.com].

Russ made world headlines in April 2004 when his Freedom of Information Act request/appeal resulted in the release of 288 photos of the US war dead coming home in flag-draped coffins. He posted the Pentagon-banned images on The Memory Hole, and overnight the story jumped into heavy rotation on the 24-hour news channels. The photos were carried by almost every newspaper in the world, often on the front page, and Russ was interviewed on *Good Morning America* and *CBS Evening News With Dan Rather*, plus numerous print outlets and NPR. The *Los Angeles Times* declared: "A new media player is born," while *Time*, in an article about blogs (even though The Memory Hole isn't a blog), asked: "How are you going to keep anything secret from a thousand Russ Kicks?"

The previous Halloween, Russ had made the front page of the *New York Times* when he digitally uncensored a heavily redacted Justice Department report.

Books as Author
- *Outposts: A Catalogue of Rare and Disturbing Alternative Information*
- *Psychotropedia: Publications From the Periphery*
- *50 Things You're Not Supposed to Know*
- *The Disinformation Book of Lists: Subversive Facts and Hidden Information in Rapid-Fire Format*
- *50 Things You're Not Supposed to Know, Vol. 2*

Books as Editor
- *Hot Off the Net: Erotica and Other Sex Writings From the Internet*
- *You Are Being Lied To: The Disinformation Guide to Media Distortion, Historical Whitewashes and Cultural Myths*
- *Everything You Know Is Wrong: The Disinformation Guide to Secrets and Lies*
- *Abuse Your Illusions: The Disinformation Guide to Media Mirages and Establishment Lies*

Acknowledgments

As always, profound personal thanks to Anne Marie, my parents, Ruthanne, Jennifer, Lucas, Billy Dale, Brett and Cristy, Darrell, and Terry and Rebekah. Thanks to Michael Ravnitzky for facts, ideas, and proofing, Anne Marie and Gary Baddeley for proofing, Liz Lawler for translation help, Jay Gertzman, Martha Cornog, Rachel Kramer Bussel, and Richard Metzger for suggesting and/or putting me in touch with other contributors, and Fred and Elizabeth for keeping me in top form. Further thanks to Jason Bitner and the crew at *Dirty Found* and *Found Magazine*, Jennifer Itskevich and everyone else at Barricade Books, Joanie K. Shoemaker at Worley Shoemaker Management, Marie de Lantsheere at the Orion Publishing Group, and Creation Books.

I tip my hat to Gary Baddeley, Richard Metzger, Jason Louv, Liz Lawler, Alex Burns, Ralph Bernardo, Nimrod Erez, Maya Shmuter, David Samra, Jacob Rosette, and the rest of the Disinformation gang for their continued support.

Thanks to Consortium and Turnaround for distributing this book, all the smart booksellers for carrying it, and you, dear reader, for buying it (or at least for reading it).

Even in the twenty-first century, there's still something the tiniest bit disconcerting about putting one's name on sex-related material (not that this is the first or last time I've done it). I feel a debt toward everyone—whether or not I agree with them—who has spoken out about sex, especially early pioneers like Sappho, Ovid, Vatsyayana Mallanaga, Wang Shih-Cheng, John Wilmot, John Cleland, the Marquis de Sade, Richard von Kraft-Ebbing, Leopold von Sacher-Masoch, Oscar Wilde, Sigmund Freud, Wilhelm Reich, Magnus Hirschfeld, Havelock Ellis, Margaret Sanger, Colette, D.H. Lawrence, James Joyce, Henry Miller, Anaïs Nin, Alfred Kinsey, and Gershon Legman (there are many others).

And a big, hearty thank you to each and every courageous contributor, without whom this book wouldn't exist.

Contributors

Comedian/writer **Nick Adams** has graced the stages of some of the nation's finest comedy clubs. And some of the not-so-fine ones. He's written for and appeared on Black Entertainment Television and the Oxygen Network. *Making Friends With Black People*, his hilarious collection of essays on race, will be published by Kensington Books in March 2006. No dead people were fucked for the writing of his essay.

Steve Almond is the author of *My Life in Heavy Metal*, *The Evil B.B. Chow*, and *Candyfreak*. He lives and eats in Somerville, MA.

Deborah Taj Anapol attended Barnard College, graduated Phi Beta Kappa from the University of California at Berkeley, and received her PhD in clinical psychology from the University of Washington in 1981. Dr. Anapol is the author of *Polyamory: The New Love Without Limits* (1997), *Compersion* (2000), and *The Seven Natural Laws of Love* (2005). She is currently at work on a book about harmonizing feminine and masculine energies. Dr. Anapol has organized and produced several conferences, as well as working with couples, families, and individuals who are exploring conscious relating, Tantra, and sexual healing. She leads seminars nationwide and is an inspiring and controversial speaker who has appeared on radio and television programs all across the US and Canada. Dr. Anapol is available for phone coaching, conference presentations, personal retreats, and public speaking engagements. Call her at 415.507.1739, email <taj@lovewithoutlimits.com>, or visit her in cyberspace at [www.lovewithoutlimits.com] or [www.sevenlawsoflove.com].

Lisa Archer's pseudonymous musings have appeared in *Pills, Thrills, Chills, and Heartache: Adventures in the First Person* (Alyson, 2004), *Best Women's Erotica 2002* and *2004* (Cleis), *Collective Action: A Bad Subjects Anthology* (Pluto, 2004), and the *San Francisco Bay Guardian*.

"A legendary name from the Golden Age of Pulps" (Fabio Cleto, *Spine Intact, Some Creases*), **Victor J. Banis** is the author of nearly 150 books and numerous shorter pieces. A native of Ohio and long-time resident of San Francisco, Banis now makes his home in the Blue Ridge of West Virginia and devotes his time to writing and gardening.

Jennifer Bennett received her undergraduate degree in art history from Smith College and an MFA in writing from Antioch University Los Angeles. She currently resides in central Ohio. Most of her identity labels have shifted over time, but current practicing, non-theoretical ID tags include: bisexual, switch, poly, and girly tomboy. She has a predilection for sharp, shiny objects and has recently acquired a taste for 18g needles.

Dr. Catherine Blackledge is the author of *The Story of V*, which was published in the UK by Weidenfeld & Nicolson in August 2003. *The Story of V* is about different views of the vagina—views from science and medicine, history, anthropology, art, mythology, and more. *The Story of V* is also published in the US, Belgium, Holland, Canada, Australia, and Brazil. It is due to be published in Spain, Japan, Italy, Poland, South Korea, Taiwan, the Czech Republic, and China. Eve Ensler says of the book: "*The Story of V* reveals the ancient and newfound powers of the vagina. It is full of mystery and secrets and truth. If we only knew what we had under our skirts! Learn the story—read this book." Eve is incorporating aspects of the book into *The Vagina Monologues*. Catherine says: "My hope is that, because of this book, you won't ever look at the vagina, and women, in quite the same way again." Catherine was born in 1968. Following a science degree and PhD, she worked as a science and medical journalist for print, TV, and radio publications. *The Story of V* is her first book. Since publication, Catherine has gone back to college to do an MA in the history of medicine and has begun researching her next book, looking at the history of another taboo topic.

Joani Blank, MA, MPH has been working in the sex field for more than 30 years. She is the founder of Good Vibrations and Down There Press in San Francisco, and is the author or editor of nine books published by Down There. She lives in an urban cohousing community in downtown Oakland, California, with her lap-poodle, Bapu-ji.

Violet Blue is an author, editor, robot mechanic, female porn expert, and professional pro-porn pundit. She is the assistant editor at Fleshbot [www.fleshbot.com] by day and a human blog by night. Violet has been a published sex columnist and trained professional sex educator since 1998, a member of Survival Research Laboratories since 1996, and she frequently lectures to students about human sexuality at the University of California and at community teaching institutions. She is the editor of five anthologies and the author of four books, two of which have been bestselling sex advice books since their release and have been translated into French, Spanish, and Russian. Her influences are J.G. Ballard, David Sedaris, John Waters, Emir Kusturica, Mark Pauline, A.M. Holmes, Patrick Califia, and Patty Hearst. She has been interviewed, featured, and quoted as an expert by more magazine, Web, television, and radio outlets than can be listed here, including *O* (Oprah) magazine, NPR, CNN, *Wired*, *Esquire*, and WebMD. For more information visit her website [tinynibbles.com].

Jack Boulware is a journalist and author of two nonfiction books: *Sex, American Style* (Feral House) and *San Francisco Bizarro* (St. Martin's). He writes for many publications in the US and UK, and is currently working on a new book project. In a previous life, he was founding editor of the satirical investigative *Nose* magazine, where he had the opportunity to visit many heinous elements of the American experience, including Area 51, Roswell, Waco, Tijuana, and the Mustang Ranch. He lives in San Francisco, and is codirector of the Bay Area's Litquake literary festival. [www.jackboulware.com]

Bill Brent founded *Black Sheets* magazine and edited all seventeen issues between 1993 and 2000. He's the author of *The Ultimate Guide to Anal Sex for Men* (Cleis Press, 2002). His fiction appears in *The Best American Erotica 1997*, *Tough Guys*, *Best Gay Erotica 2002* and *2004*, *Best S/M Erotica*, and *Rough Stuff*, plus its sequel, *Roughed Up*. He coedited the *Best Bisexual Erotica* series with Dr. Carol Queen, the second volume being a finalist in the fourteenth Lambda Literary Awards. His articles have appeared in the *San Francisco Bay Guardian*, the *San Francisco Bay Times*, other magazines, *P.O.V.*, and at [goodvibes.com]. He has authored several chapbooks of poems and short prose, and published a number of books, including *Hot Off the Net*, edited by Russ Kick (see [www.blackbooks.com/catalog]). Want his email newsletter? Drop him a line at <verbose@comcast.net>, or check out [www.authorsden.com/billbrent] for more of his prose and other writing.

Susie Bright edits the annual *Best American Erotica* series (started in 1993 and still going strong), and she edited the first three volumes of *Herotica* (1988, 1992, 1994), the groundbreaking collections of women-centered erotic fiction. Her numerous essays are collected in *Susie Sexpert's Lesbian Sex World* (Cleis, 1990), *Susie Bright's Sexual Reality: A Virtual Sex Reader* (Cleis, 1992), *SexWise* (Cleis, 1995), *The Sexual State of the Union* (Simon & Schuster, 1997), and *Mommy's Little Girl: Susie Bright on Sex, Motherhood, Pornography, and Cherry Pie* (Thunder's Mouth, 2004). Her other books include *How to Write a Dirty Story* (Simon and Schuster, 2002), *Full Exposure: Opening Up to Sex and Creativity* (HarperSanFrancisco, 1999), and the edited collection *Three the Hard Way* (Simon and Schuster, 2004). Additionally, Bright cofounded *On Our Backs*, the first lesbian sex magazine created by lesbians; wrote a column for Salon; was the subject of

a documentary on Britain's Channel 4; lectures at America's top universities; and hosts *In Bed With Susie Bright*, a weekly online "radio" show at Audible.com. Her website is [www.susiebright.com], and her blog is [susiebright.blogs.com].

Vern L. Bullough, PhD, DSci, RN, is a State University of New York Distinguished Professor Emeritus. He also served for ten years as a dean at Buffalo State College. He was a founder of the Center for Sex Research at California State University, Northridge. Among other things, he is a past president and fellow of the Society for the Scientific Study of Sex, and has been awarded both the Kinsey Award and the Money Award by that society. He is the author, coauthor, or editor of over 50 books, has contributed chapters to more than 100 others, and has written more than 150 refereed articles. [www.vernbullough.com]

Rachel Kramer Bussel [www.rachelkramerbussel.com] is senior editor at *Penthouse Variations* and a contributing editor at *Penthouse*, where she writes the "Girl Talk" column. She is the editor of *Up All Night: Adventures in Lesbian Sex* and *Naughty Spanking Stories From A to Z*, volumes 1 and 2, writes the "Lusty Lady" column for the *Village Voice*, and is an interviewer at Gothamist [gothamist.com]. Her writing has been published in over 60 erotic anthologies, including *Best American Erotica 2004*, as well as AVN, *Bust*, Clean Sheets [cleansheets.com], *Curve*, *Diva*, *Girlfriends*, mediabistro.com, the *New York Post*, On Our Backs, Oxygen.com, *Punk Planet*, the *San Francisco Chronicle*, *Time Out New York*, and others.

Patrick Califia is the author of two collections of essays from Cleis Press, *Public Sex: The Culture of Radical Sex* and *Speaking Sex to Power*. He also wrote *Sex Changes: The Politics of Transgenderism*. He's the author of several collections of short erotic fiction, two novels, a book of poetry, and a forthcoming memoir entitled *Pioneer*. [www.patrickcalifia.com]

M. Christian is the author of the critically acclaimed and bestselling collections *Dirty Words*, *Speaking Parts*, *The Bachelor Machine*, and *Filthy* (forthcoming). He is the editor of *The Burning Pen*, *Guilty Pleasures*, the *Best S/M Erotica* series, *The Mammoth Book of Future Cops*, and *The Mammoth Book of Tales of the Road* (with Maxim Jakubowski), and over fourteen other anthologies. His short fiction has appeared in over 150 books, including *Best American Erotica*, *Best Gay Erotica*, *Best Lesbian Erotica*, *Best Transgendered Erotica*, *Best Fetish Erotica*, *Best Bondage Erotica*, and…well, you get the idea. He lives in San Francisco and is only some of what that implies. [www.mchristian.com]

Greta Christina has been writing professionally since 1989. Her writing has appeared in numerous magazines and newspapers, including *Ms.*, *Penthouse*, and the *Skeptical Inquirer*, as well as several anthologies, including *Best American Erot-*

ica 2005. She is the author of "Bending," an erotic novella published by Simon & Schuster in the three-novella collection *Three Kinds of Asking For It*, as well as the editor of *Paying For It: A Guide by Sex Workers for Their Clients*. Her influential essay "Are We Having Sex Now or What?" has been reprinted several times and has been studied and cited by scholars, writers, and universities. She lives in San Francisco with her wife, Ingrid. Her Oscarology sign is *West Side Story*. You can visit her on the Web at [www.gretachristina.com].

Christen Clifford is a writer and performer in New York. Her work has appeared in Nerve, Salon, *New York Press*, and *Blue*. She has performed on Broadway and Off, in film and television, and in regional and international theaters. She is a visiting scholar at New York University and has received a couple of fellowships and residencies here and there. Her solo performance, *17 Guys I Fucked*, was produced at the Culture Project, Women Center Stage, the BRIC Theatre, and the Oni Gallery. She created the performance series *HEAT: Sexy Stories and Burlesque* and is currently working toward an MFA from the New School.

Michelle Clifford is an author and photographer. She was born in South Boston and grew up in Ft. Lauderdale, Florida. She escaped the unbearable sunshine in 1985 to the grit of New York City. Just in time to see the fall of decadent Rome in the form of Times Square. Clifford teamed up with Bill Landis, a writer and known quantity in the Times Square milieu. He had been the first to document the Deuce, and she liked his style. They joined forces and became the tag team from Hell. Clifford began photographing and taking copious notes of everything that the Deuce had to display. She became the Margaret Mead/Alfred Kinsey two-headed monster of Times Square, taking the histories of the performers in the films that the decrepit movie houses were screening. Her research was relentless and neverending. Like Marlow in search of Col. Kurtz in *Heart of Darkness*, she became acquainted through Landis with the movie-house workers that ran these films, the riffraff, the con artists, the whores and their pimps. She listened to their stories and began her writing. She has written for such diverse publications as *Film Comment*, *Screw*, *Hustler*, *Penthouse*, and the *Village Voice*, oftentimes leaving her name off of the byline for privacy. One *Voice* cover story, "Body For Rent," was the most popular issue of the newspaper that year. With the amount of material so overwhelming, Clifford began the publication *Metasex*. No editing, no plot resolution, no happy endings. She coauthored the HarperCollins book *Anger*, the unauthorized biography of underground filmmaker Kenneth Anger in all his artistic, masochistic, Satanic glory. Again leaving her name off the byline. She then resurrected Bill Landis' magazine, *Sleazoid Express*, after seeing him kill it off after his own involvement in pornography. She completely overhauled

it with a vengeance. The magazine changed from a few-page mimeograph to a novella-length publication. She created covers and content that brought the magazine back to life. Her latest book, *Sleazoid Express*, published by Simon and Schuster, is currently stinking up the universe in its second printing. It is included in syllabi at colleges in classes as diverse as architecture and film history. She continues to publish *Metasex* [www.metasex.org] and *Sleazoid Express* [www.sleazoidexpress.com].

Martha Cornog has had the pleasure of using her linguistics and library degrees in ways her *almae matres* never suspected. Her most recent book, *The Big Book of Masturbation* (2003), won a Benjamin Franklin Award from the Publishers Marketing Association. Her earlier books encouraged librarians to enhance their sexualities collections: *For Sex Education: See Librarian* (1996), written with her husband, Timothy Perper, and an edited collection, *Libraries, Erotica, & Pornography* (1991), which won the American Library Association's Eli M. Oboler Award for intellectual freedom. She has written articles on sexuality materials in libraries for *Library Journal*, *Collection Building*, *Journal of Information Ethics*, and *SIECUS Report*, also in collaboration with Timothy Perper. Her research on group masturbation appeared in the *Journal of Sex Education and Therapy*. She has published on sexual language and has contributed to *From Plato to Paglia: A Philosophical Encyclopedia* (forthcoming), *The Continuum Complete International Encyclopedia of Sexuality*, *Encyclopedia of Birth Control*, *Liberating Minds: Lives of Gay, Lesbian, and Bisexual Librarians and Their Advocates*, *The Complete Dictionary of Sexology*, *Human Sexuality: An Encyclopedia*, and *Taking Sides: Clashing Views on Controversial Issues in Human Sexuality*. She has been active in the Society for the Scientific Study of Sexuality, serves on the editorial board of *Contemporary Sexuality*, and was a book review editor of the *Journal of Sex Education and Therapy*. She was named *Library Journal* Book Reviewer of the Year–Nonfiction in 2001. She is manager of membership services for a medical association, has held positions in several libraries, and received an MS in library science from Drexel University and an MA in linguistics from Brown University. Currently, she is collaborating with Timothy Perper on studies of erotic/romantic Japanese comics (manga) and serves with him as review and commentary editors for *Mechademia: A Journal for Anime, Manga, and the Fan Arts*.

Salvador Dalí (1904-1989) was one of the greatest artists of the twentieth century. Primarily a Surrealist, his masterworks include the paintings *The Persistence of Memory* (1931), *Sleep* (1937), *One Second Before Awakening From a Dream Caused by the Flight of a Bee Around a Pomegranate* (1944), and *Crucifixion (Corpus Hypercubus)* (1954).

Susan Davis is a folklorist. She is researching a book on Gershon Legman.

Dirty Found. "We collect dirty found stuff: pervy Polaroids, sleazy birthday cards, raunchy to-do lists, nasty poetry on napkins, illustrations—anything that gives a glimpse into someone else's sex life. It's just like our sister, *Found Magazine*, only sleazier. We certainly didn't invent the idea of found stuff being cool. Every time we visit our friends in other towns, someone's always got some kinda unbelievable found note or photo on their fridge. We wanted to make a magazine so that everyone can check out all the strange, hilarious, and heartbreaking things people've picked up. After a few years of collecting all these finds, we ended up with a big, fat folder of pervy stuff, and now it's time to share the goods with you guys. For more info, check [www.dirtyfound.com] and [www.foundmagazine.com]. For *Dirty Found* orders in the US, send $10 (plus $3 shipping). For international orders (*outside* the US), send $10 (plus $6 shipping) to the address below. Send us your finds! Dirty Found, 3455 Charing Cross Road, Ann Arbor MI 48108-1911, USA."

Albert B. Gerber, MA, JD taught high school English, practiced law, administered the First Amendment Lawyer's Association, and won competitions in handball, marksmanship, bridge, and fiction. He began his writing career as a columnist for *Stars and Stripes*. After the war he continued his writing with stories and articles in many newspapers and magazines. *The Book of Sex Lists* (1981) is his sixth book. He has written biographies and a novel. He also authored the classic study of obscenity, *Sex, Pornography and Justice* (1965), and the bestselling biography of Howard Hughes, *Bashful Billionaire* (1967).

Stephen J. Gertz is an historian and bibliographer of erotic literature, writer, and antiquarian bookseller in Los Angeles. Poor, yet poverty-stricken, he accepts checks for work as soon as they can be cut.

Jay A. Gertzman is author of *Bookleggers and Smuthounds: The Trade in Erotica, 1920-1940* (University of Pennsylvania Press, 1999). He is currently researching the distribution and prosecution of erotica in the Times Square area, c. 1940-75. He has a website on the subject: [home.earthlink.net/~jgertzma/BkshopsofTimesSq/index.html]. The easiest way to get to there is to type "bookshops of times square" in Google. He is also interested in the Philadelphia *noir* crime novelist of the 1950s, David Goodis.

Jon Hart has written for dozens of publications, including the *New York Times*, the *Christian Science Monitor*, and the *Village Voice*.

Fiona Horne is a practicing Witch of over fifteen years and author of several bestselling titles on Witchcraft. She is also an internationally successful television and radio personality and was once a rock star, as lead singer in the 1990s chart-topping Australian band Def FX. Fiona's talents as a performer have now extended into acting, with featured roles in theatrically released films. For more information on Fiona visit her website [www.fionahorne.com].

Debra Hyde discovered everything she knew about sex was wrong when, long ago, she kissed a boy and learned that everything her mother had told her was bullshit. Today, she mouths off regularly about sex and culture at her blog, Pursed Lips [www.pursedlips.com], and her erotic fiction appears in many major erotica anthologies. She thinks life's too short for prudery, sex-phobic thinking, and sexual stupidity, and writes to counter those voices that would like nothing more than a full return to the days of the Comstock Law.

Ed Jacob is a Canadian freelance writer and translator living and working in Tokyo. He is currently writing a book about sex in Japan for Caffeine Society Press [caffeinesociety.com], which will be out in 2006. [www.quirkyjapan.or.tv]

Tim Keefe is the author of *Some of My Best Friends Are Naked: Interviews With Seven Erotic Dancers* (Barbary Coast Press, 1993).

Earl Kemp, a national nuisance, has been known by many (dis)guises: adventurer, explorer, lover, beloved, literary rebel, First Amendment convict savant, and numerous others, mostly all bad. He is best known as the notorious producer, during the Golden Age of Sleaze Paperbacks, of more than 5,000 novels and half again that many *Naked* people magazines. In his dotage, he dribbles memoirs at [efanzines.com/EK/index.html] and has become The (uppercase) Chronicler of the entire genre.

David Kerekes is editor/publisher of Headpress [www.headpress.com] and coauthor of the books *Killing for Culture* (Creation, 1994) and *See No Evil* (Critical Vision, 2000). He has contributed to numerous periodicals in the mainstream and alternative presses and lives in Manchester, Great Britain.

Russ Kick. See the preceding section, "About the Editor."

Paul Krassner is the author of *One Hand Jerking: Reports From an Investigative Satirist*. His website is [paulkrassner.com].

Brenda Billings Love, author, counselor, international lecturer, and columnist, is noted for her contribution to sexology in the field of paraphilias by meticulously cataloging over 700 unusual sex acts. In 1984, she became a supervisor and counselor for the National Sexually Transmitted Disease hotline, providing medical information and referrals to hundreds of callers each year. She expanded her responsibility in 1986 to include a supervisory position for the National AIDS Hotline and later the San Francisco Sex Information switchboard. In 1997 she spent nine months working on the San Mateo Suicide Crisis Line. In 1992, her book, *The Encyclopedia of Unusual Sex Practices*, was published after four years of extensive research. She is a lecturer and researcher for the Institute for the Advanced Study of Human Sexuality in San Francisco. Her lecture and slide show was produced on video this same year by the Institute and distributed to sexologists around the world. She has also appeared as a guest on the *Joan Rivers Show*, the *Richard Bey Show*, the *Al Goldstein Show*, the *Jenny Jones Show*, *People Are Talking*, the *Mo Show*, and has been interviewed on over 400 radio programs. In 1994 the foreign rights to the *Encyclopedia* were sold to publishers in Germany, Japan, Spain, Portugal, France, Poland, the Czech Republic, and the UK. Love is a former member of the American Association of Sex Educators, Counselors, and Therapists, the Society for the Scientific Study of Sexuality, and the American Psychological Association. She is currently a writer and travels between her homes in Prague, Czech Republic and Charleston, South Carolina.

Libby Lynn works for a large adult company in the United States. In between meetings and writing descriptions for every sexual device known to woman or man, she maintains a blog called Rollertrain [rollertrain.blogspot.com].

Rachel Maines is the author of *The Technology of Orgasm* (Johns Hopkins University Press, 1999) and *Asbestos and Fire* (Rutgers University Press, 2005). She holds a doctoral degree in applied history from Carnegie-Mellon University and is a visiting scholar in the Department of Science and Technology Studies at Cornell University.

Laura Moore, the eloquent Southern belle who surprises and enchants everyone with her visionary "sexpertise," has been a science writer for *Penthouse* since 1997, and she has her own sex and fitness columns in *Iron Man Magazine* and *Fitness Rx for Men*. She is a freelance writer for dozens of publications, including *Muscular Development Magazine*, *American Health and Fitness Magazine*, and *Fitness Rx for Women*. Laura majored in psychology at the University of Southern Mississippi, and she has been involved in the health and fitness industry since 1985, helping thousands of people, including NFL athletes, professional bodybuilders, and models, reach their physical goals. Laura was the editor of *Southern Muscle Magazine* and has authored and self-published *The Ten Commandments of Health and Fitness* (which is what originally gave rise to *Sex Heals*) and *Fun, Creative, Motivating, and Relaxing Uses for Tiny Candy Coated Chocolates*. Laura practices what she preaches. She was featured in *Muscle Media Magazine* just one month after the birth of her first son, and she won a VENUS Swimsuit Model Contest just five months after the birth of her second son. She was also chosen as *Iron Man Magazine*'s Body of the Month for September 2001. Laura credits lots of orgasms, in addition to living a healthy lifestyle, for being in such spectacular physical shape. To find out more about *Sex Heals*, visit [www.the-healthysexymom.com].

Jill Morley wrote and performed the critically acclaimed play *True Confessions of a Go-Go Girl*. It was produced in Manhattan for five years, and at San Francisco's Solo Mio Festival, the Texas Fringe Festival, and LA's HBO Workspace, plus it opened Women's History Month at NYU. *True Confessions* is published in *The Best Women's Plays of 1998*. Other works are published in *More Women's Monologues for Women, by Women*, *Millennium Monologues*, *Young Women's Monologues From Contemporary Plays*, and many other collections. Morley's critically acclaimed documentary film, *STRIPPED*, currently runs on the Sundance Channel and won "Best Documentary" at the Women's International Film Festival in Sydney. A contributing writer to the *Village Voice*, the *New York Press*, *Penthouse*, *Inside Kung Fu*, *Martial Arts and Combat Sports*, *Shout* magazine, and *Gear* magazine, Jill also coproduced two radio documentaries for *The World* and *This American Life*, which aired on NPR. Jill worked with Michael Moore as a producer and correspondent for *The Awful Truth*, and with Brazilian director Bruno Barreto, reworking dialogue on his newest film. She is currently developing a television show and working on a screenplay with Dustin Hoffman.

Pagan Moss quit her high-paying corporate job in 2000 to work as an erotic dancer/lingerie model and peep show girl. Later that year, she started blogging on Dr. Menlo's Sensual Liberation Army [sensuallib.com]—one of the first sexblogs. In 2003, she started her own blog, Peep Show Stories [peepshowstories.com], which features detailed and often humorous stories and photos of her adult-business experience. She presently lives in Seattle and works for a group of psychologists.

Jack Murnighan has worked as a medievalist, a magazine editor, a freelancer, a professor, a cook, and a vacuum cleaner salesman. His books *The Naughty Bits* and *Classic Nasty* try to show how fun and sexy literature is, his short stories and essays how fun and sexy life is.

Jill Nagle has been published widely in anthologies, periodicals, and online. Her first book was the acclaimed *Whores and Other Feminists* (Routledge, 1997), a collection of writings by feminists in the sex industry, and she has since written two more, *Efemmeral Flesh: corporeal utterances* (Audacity Press, 2004) and *How to Find An Agent Who Can Sell Your Book for Top Dollar: Jill's Guerilla Tips and Tricks* (GetPublished, 2004). She is coeditor of *Male Lust: Pleasure, Power, and Transforma-*

tion (Haworth, 2000). She is currently working on a number of book-length projects, some excerpts of which may be viewed at her blog [www.jillnagle.com]. She lives in the Berkeley Hills with her partner, Alex, and toddler, Cainan.

Annalee Newitz writes about technology, sex, and pop culture. She is a contributing editor at *Wired* magazine and has published in *Popular Science*, Salon, *New Scientist*, *The Believer*, and the *San Francisco Bay Guardian*. She writes the syndicated column "Techsploitation" and is the editor of two anthologies, *White Trash* (Routledge, 1996) and *Bad Subjects* (NYU Press, 1998). Her forthcoming book, *Pretend We're Dead* (Duke University Press), is about monster movies and capitalism. She is also editor of the indie magazine *Other*.

Breyer P-Orridge. Genesis P-Orridge was born as Neil Andrew Megson in Manchester, England, on the 22nd of February 1950. In 1969 Genesis became the Founding Artist and Theorist of seminal British Performance Art group C.O.U.M. Transmissions in Shrewsbury, England. The project was terminated in September 1976 with a final but now infamous show called "Prostitution" at the I.C.A. Gallery in London. This was the first time that the general public would witness Punk Rock and Industrial culture firsthand. The event caused an uproar (the venue was owned by Queen Elizabeth II) that would result in controversial newspaper reviews, television talk show appearances, and even meetings in Parliament! Seminal cult band Throbbing Gristle was formed in 1975, of which Genesis was a Co-Founder and Linguistic Designer. Throbbing Gristle formed their own record label, Industrial Records, and coined the term "Industrial Music." Sonic/Transmedia music and performance collective Psychic TV formed in Hackney, London with Alex Fergusson in 1981. Together with the formation of PTV, Genesis initiated an Art Actionist Project called Thee Temple ov Psychick Youth (TOPY). Over its span of ten years, the TOPY network reached around the globe with over 10,000 participants. On December 23, 2002, *TG 24* was released on Mute Records. This deluxe box set contains 24 CDs, each an original one-hour long recording of a live Throbbing Gristle set. A monograph book, *Painful but Fabulous: The Lives and Art of Genesis P-Orridge*, was published by Soft Skull/Shortwave Press in January 2003. Genesis has worked with William S. Burroughs, Brion Gysin, Timothy Leary, and Derek Jarman, among many others. In 2003 Genesis changed his name to Genesis Breyer P-Orridge and began a performance/action series called "Breaking Sex" that was initiated by both he and his partner Lady Jaye Breyer P-Orridge. This project is about re-union and re-solution of male and female to a perfecting hermaphroditic state. This includes having cosmetic surgeries that blur the lines between their sexes and bring them nearer to being one physically. For example, the couple has undergone matching breast-implant operations for Valentine's Day and their ten-year anniversary. Recently Genesis and Lady Jaye have been undergoing physical transformations largely via cosmetic surgery, although also through tattoos, as Breyer P-Orridge. These operations are designed to mutate their bodies into pandrogenous affirmations beyond the limits dictated by biology and by DNA, each continually transforming both into and beyond the other, creating a third body—THE PANDROGYNE. Breyer P-Orridge are currently working on a DVD called *Putting Your Money Where Your Mouth Is*, which features footage of the artists' various surgical procedures combined with calligraphy. [www.genesisp-orridge.com]

Preston Peet is an accomplished author, actor, DJ, musician, psychonaut, and explorer. Editor of *Underground: The Disinformation Guide to Ancient Civilizations, Astonishing Archaeology and Hidden History* and *Under the Influence: The Disinformation Guide to Drugs*, editor of DrugWar.com, a long-time contributor to *High Times* magazine, and contributing editor to Disinformation's website [disinfo.com], not to mention author of over 100 articles and stories published in too many publications to list here, Preston has been known to take the more adventurous path when it comes to new experiences, whether they be drug-related or sexual, or other, in nature. Born Tracy Rich in Ft. Meyers, Florida on September 11, 1966, and given up at birth, lived in numerous foster homes, picked the name Preston at age three and was eventually adopted by the Peet family at age five. Preston has lived in the swankiest digs and the muddiest streets in cities around the world, including Sarasota, Orlando, Tampa, and Tallahassee, Florida; Atlanta, Georgia; Paris, France; Las Navas del Marqés, Spain; Bergen, Norway; Rotterdam and Amsterdam, Netherlands; and London, England. Upon arrival in New York City, Preston went from kicking cold turkey while squatting on the SUNY Purchase campus, to living strung out in Central Park and on the streets of Manhattan's Lower East Side, and now, with his life somewhat together, shares a small apartment in Manhattan with his beautiful vegan muse, soul-mate, and lover, Vanessa Cleary, and, at the moment, nine rescued cats. Preston is always on the lookout for ever more knowledge and experience, and is helping bring peace and adventure back in vogue.

Diane Petryk-Bloom has won seven awards for investigative journalism and feature writing, including honors from the New York Associated Press, the New York Newspaper Publisher's Association, the North Carolina Press Association, and the Georgia Associated Press. She was news editor of the *Sanford Herald* in Sanford, Florida; assistant city editor of the *Savannah Morning News* in Georgia; and editor of the *St. Ignace News* in northern Michigan. While reporting for the *New York Times*' regional paper in Hendersonville, North Carolina, her investigation of a school-board pay scandal brought about the reform of a corrupt system. She holds a Master's degree in journalism from Michigan State University and studied comparative journalism in Croatia. She also worked as a subeditor for the New Zealand national daily the *Dominion*. As a reporter for the *Press Republican* in Plattsburgh, New York, she was part of a team honored by the Associated Press for its localized and comprehensive 9/11 coverage.

Carol Queen got a PhD in sexology so she could impart more realistic detail to her smut. She's an award-winning author or editor of ten volumes of sex writing, including *Real Live Nude Girl*, *5 Minute Erotica*, and *Exhibitionism for the Shy*. (For a full bibliography, see [www.carolqueen.com].) She lives in San Francisco, where she works as staff sexologist at Good Vibrations and founding director of the Center for Sex & Culture [www.sexandculture.org], a sex-ed center/library/archive.

Audacia Ray is a New Yorker, polyamorous pervert, smut peddler, nakedteer, sex worker, safer-sex educator, and history of sexuality enthusiast who is pursuing a Master's degree in cultural history. She is the news and shorts editor of *$pread* magazine and prefers to spend her days in her underwear. [www.wakingvixen.com]

Ann Regentin has written everything from reading-comprehension tests and reference material to poetry and music, but mostly she writes erotica. Her work has appeared in a handful of anthologies, magazines, and websites. She is the author of three e-books so far, and one of her poems has been nominated for the Pushcart Prize. She lives in the American Midwest.

Lori Selke lives in Oakland, California. Her work can be found in anthologies, such as *Homewrecker*, *Glamour Girls*, and *Blowing Kisses*. She no longer does phone sex except on an amateur basis.

Simon Sheppard is the author of the books *Sex Parties 101*, *In Deep: Erotic Stories*, and *Kinkorama: Dispatches From the Front Lines of Perversion*. His work has appeared in over 125 anthologies, including many editions of *Best American Erotica* and *Best Gay Erotica*, and he writes the columns "Sex Talk" and "Perv." He's at work on an historically-based anthology of gay porn—those with vintage smut are encouraged to get in touch. He's at [www.simonsheppard.com].

Jen Sincero is a musician, motivational speaker, and the author of *The Straight Girl's Guide to Sleeping With Chicks* and *Don't Sleep With Your Drummer*. She is happiest when informing people that if they believe in themselves and get off their asses to do the things they love, they will be victorious, regardless of how overwhelming or socially unacceptable those things may seem. Which is pretty much what both of her books are about. Go to [www.jensincero.com] for her books, essays, music, workshops, tour schedule, and advice on sex and relationships.

Joseph W. Slade is professor of Telecommunications at Ohio University in Athens, where he teaches the history of communciation technologies. He has written more than sixty articles on literature, technology, film, and culture. He is co-editor of *Beyond the Two Cultures: Essays on Science, Technology, and Literature* (Iowa State University Press, 1990) and *The Midwest*, a volume in the *Greenwood Encyclopedia of American Regional Cultures* (Greenwood, 2004), and the author of *Thomas Pynchon* (Warner Books, 1974, and Peter Lang, 1990), *Pornography in America* (ABC-CLIO, 2000), and the three-volume *Pornography and Sexual Representation: A Reference Guide* (Greenwood, 2001). His most recent article on pornography is "Global Traffic in Pornography: The Hungarian Example," written with Katalin Szoverfy Milter, in *International Exposure: Perspectives on Modern European Pornography, 1800-2000*, ed. Lisa Z. Sigel (Rutgers University Press, 2005).

David Steinberg writes frequently on the culture and politics of sex in America. His books include *Photo Sex: Fine Art Sexual Photography Comes of Age*, *Erotic by Nature: A Celebration of Life, of Love, and of Our Wonderful Bodies*, and *The Erotic Impulse: Honoring the Sensual Self*. His writing has appeared in *Salon*, *Playboy*, *Boston Phoenix*, *Los Angeles Weekly*, *SF Weekly*, *Cupido*, the *Sun*, *Libido*, the *Realist*, *Clean Sheets*, *Scarlet Letters*, *Metro Santa Cruz*, and *Anything That Moves*. His monthly column, "Comes Naturally," is available (free and confidential) from him at <eronat@aol.com>. He lives in Santa Cruz, California.

John Stevens, nicknamed the "Erotic Professor," teaches Buddhism and Aikido at Tohoku Fukushi University in Sendai, Japan. He is author of *Lust for Enlightenment: Buddhism and Sex* (Shambhala Publications) and dozens of other books.

Cecilia Tan is a writer, editor, and sexuality activist. She is the author of various works of erotic fiction, including *The Velderet* and *Black Feathers*, and her short stories have appeared everywhere from *Ms.* magazine to *Penthouse*. She has also edited dozens of anthologies of erotic fiction for Circlet Press, Masquerade Books, and Blue Moon Books. Find out more at [www.ceciliatan.com].

Tristan Taormino is an award-winning author, columnist, editor, and sex educator. She is the author of three books: *True Lust: Adventures in Sex, Porn and Perversion* (Cleis Press), *Down and Dirty Sex Secrets* (ReganBooks/HarperCollins), and *The Ultimate Guide to Anal Sex for Women* (Cleis Press), winner of a Firecracker Book Award and named Amazon.com's #1 Bestseller in Women's Sex Instruction in 1998. She is director, producer, and star of two videos based on her book, *The Ultimate Guide to Anal Sex for Women 1* and *2*; the first video won two Adult Video News Awards and an XRCO Award in 2000. Tristan is series editor of thirteen volumes of the Lambda Literary Award-winning anthology series *Best Lesbian Erotica*. She is a columnist for the *Village Voice*, *Taboo*, and *Velvetpark*. She is the former editor of *On Our Backs*, the nation's oldest lesbian-produced lesbian sex magazine. Tristan has been featured in over 200 publications and dozens of radio shows; she has appeared on CNN, HBO's *Real Sex*, the *Howard Stern Show*, *Loveline*, *Ricki Lake*, MTV, and the Discovery Channel. She lectures at top colleges and universities around the country, teaches sex and relationship workshops around the world, and does private coaching sessions for individuals and couples. Her official website is Pucker Up [www.puckerup.com].

Jane Vincent is a dyke-identified bisexual woman who loves using the term *fluid* to describe her sexuality. She has a degree in sexuality, will soon be pursuing a Master's in the topic, and no, you can't be her lab partner. She is a sexuality educator, certified sex coach, and sex worker. She has had more sex in more combinations and circumstances in the last five years than most people will have in their lives. She is a knitter, potter, blogger, and creative mess. And she just turned 23. Read her exploits and learn a thing or two at [educatedslut.blogspot.com].

Jenny Wade, PhD, is a developmental psychologist who specializes in normal and altered states of consciousness, especially the naturally occurring changes in awareness that facilitate personal growth and transformation. A consultant to business on workplace applications of normal adult consciousness, she also teaches doctoral studies and research design at the Institute of Transpersonal Psychology in Palo Alto, CA.

Richard Zacks is the author of *The Pirate Hunter: The True Story of Captain Kidd* (Hyperion, 2002), and it's NOT some lame Peter Pan/Hollywood account of peg-legs and eye patches. The real Captain Kidd was a New York privateer (1654-1701), who was hired to chase pirates and then double-crossed by his backers. This is an authentic nautical adventure and has been translated into Finnish and Spanish. Zacks' first book, *History Laid Bare* (1994), delivers unusual accounts of sex, from Mark Twain's jokes about penis size to Joan of Arc's virginity tests. The *New York Times* gushed: "Zacks specializes in the raunchy and perverse." His second book, *An Underground Education* (100,000+ copies sold) explores a huge range of topics, from Edison's secret role in developing the first electric chair to Abe Lincoln's plan to ship out the freed slaves. His latest book is *The Pirate Coast: Thomas Jefferson, the First Marines and the Secret Mission of 1805* (2005). The author lives in Pelham, NY, with his wife Kristine and their kids, Georgia and Ziggy.

Article Histories

"American Sex Ed" by Violet Blue was written especially for this volume. _ "Answers" by M. Christian originally appeared in *SexLife* magazine. _ "The Archive" by Jack Boulware originally appeared in *Arena* magazine. _ "Astonishing Tales of a Peep Show Girl" by Pagan Moss is comprised of revised excerpts from the author's blog, Peep Show Stories [www.peepshowstories.com]. _ "A Baby Dyke Learns to Score" by Jane Vincent was written especially for this volume. _ "Baby Love" by Christen Clifford originally appeared—in slightly different form—on Nerve.com. _ "Beat Off 101" by Earl Kemp was written especially for this volume. _ "Bed Knobs and Broomsticks" by Fiona Horne is a combination of excerpts from the author's book *Magickal Sex* (Thorsons/HarperCollins, 2003) and new material. _ "Betty Dodson's Revolutionary Open Relationship" by Rachel Kramer Bussel originally appeared as two "Lusty Lady" columns in the *Village Voice*. _ "Black and Blue" by Michelle Clifford originally appeared in *Metasex* #2. _ "Blood" by Jennifer Bennett originally appeared in Scarlet Letters [www.scarletletters.com]. _ "Burchard's Medieval Sexual Menu" by Richard Zacks is an excerpt from the author's book *History Laid Bare* (HarperCollins, 1994). _ "Catfighting, Eye-licking, Head-sitting, and Statue-screwing" by Brenda Love is comprised of excerpts from the author's book *The Encyclopedia of Unusual Sex Practices*, copyright© 1992 by Brenda Love, published by arrangement with Barricade Books, Inc. _ "The Circle Game" by Martha Cornog is a heavily reworked and expanded version of the author's previous articles and talks on the subject. It appears in its current form for the first time in this volume. _ "Circumcision and Sex" by Diane Petryk-Bloom was written especially for this volume. _ "Close Contact" by Preston Peet was written especially for this volume. _ "Cocksucker Magnet" by Lori Selke appears for the first time in this volume. _ "The Condom" by Vern Bullough is a combined version of the author's writings on the subject. It appears in its current form for the first time in this volume. _ "Cunt Candy Factory" by Tristan Taormino was originally published as a "Pucker Up" column in the *Village Voice*. _ "The Daily Schedule of a Porno Copywriter" by Libby Lynn was written especially for this volume. It contains some small segments from her blog, Rollertrain. _ "Egg Sex" by Susie Bright originally appeared in *Susie Bright's Sexual Reality* (Cleis, 1992). _ "Everybody's Sin Is Nobody's Sin" by David Steinberg is a "Comes Naturally" column. _ "Fire, Brick, Sand, Concrete" by David Kerekes was written especially for this volume. _ "First Person Sexual" by Joani Blank is an expanded and revised version of the introduction to her book *First Person Sexual* (Down There Press, 1996). It appears in its current form for the first time in this volume. _

"Gala's Divine Beauty Mark" by Salvador Dalí is an excerpt from the author's book *Maniac Eyeball* (Creation Books, 2004), which originally appeared as *Comme on Devient Dalí* (Éditions Robert Laffont, 1973). _ "Girls Gone Wild" by Greta Christina was written especially for this volume. _ "Hooray for Sodomy" by Simon Sheppard was written especially for this volume. _ "Horniness Begets Health" by Laura Moore is the third chapter from the author's book *Sex Heals*. _ "The House of Secret Treasures" by Ed Jacob was written especially for this volume. _ "How to Write Sex Scenes" by Steve Almond originally appeared on Nerve.com. _ "Inside the Cave" by Jon Hart was written especially for this volume. _ "Inviting Elder Sex Out of the Closet" by Joani Blank is an expanded and revised version of the introduction to her book *Still Doing It* (Down There Press, 2000). It appears in its current form for the first time in this volume. _ "John Thomas, Lady Jane, and Little Elvis" by Martha Cornog is a heavily reworked and expanded version of the author's previous articles and talks on the subject, including a piece in *Maledicta: The International Journal of Verbal Aggression*. It appears in its current form for the first time in this volume. _ "Key to the Fields" by Susan Davis was written especially for this volume. _ "The Love Hotel Diaries" by Ed Jacob is a greatly expanded version of an article that originally appeared in *Japanzine* [www.japanzine.com]. It appears in its current form for the first time in this volume. _ "Love Without Limits" by Deborah Taj Anapol is comprised of excerpts from the author's book *Polyamory*. _ "Making Moves" by Ann Regentin originally appeared in Clean Sheets [www.cleansheets.com]. _"The Man Who Screwed Things Up" by Stephen J. Gertz was written especially for this volume. _ "Margins to Mainstream" by Joseph W. Slade was written especially for this volume. _"A Middle-Age Manifesto" by Debra Hyde was written especially for this volume. _ "My First Fetish" by Audacia Ray originally appeared in the zine *The Misanthropist*. _ "My First Fist-a-Thon" by Tristan Taormino was originally published as a "Pucker Up" column in the *Village Voice*. _ "Necrophilia" by Nick Adams was written especially for this volume. _ "On Being a Sexmonger" by Jen Sincero was written especially for this volume. _ "Orgies" by Carol Queen was written especially for this volume. _ "Pandrogeny" by Breyer P-Orridge appears in print for the first time in this volume. _ "Pervert" by Jill Nagle originally appeared in *Guilty Pleasures*, edited by M. Christian (Black Books, 2002). _ "A Perverted Utopia" by Annalee Newitz originally appeared in the *San Francisco Bay Guardian*. _ "Profile of a Zoophile" by Bill Brent originally appeared in *Black Sheets* #10. _ "Queer Freaks" by Patrick Califia originally appeared in *That's Revolting! Queer Strategies for Resist-*

ing Assimilation (Soft Skull Press, 2004). _ "Rules" originally appeared in Dirty Found #1. _ "A San Francisco Whore in a Nevada Brothel" by Lisa Archer was originally published in the San Francisco Bay Guardian. _ "Sex and...Drugs" by Preston Peet was written especially for this volume. _ "Sex by the Numbers" by Albert B. Gerber is comprised of excerpts from The Book of Sex Lists, copyright© 1981 by Albert B. Gerber, published by arrangement with Barricade Books, Inc. _ "The Sex Life of the Buddha" by John Stevens is the first chapter of the author's book Lust for Enlightenment: Buddhism and Sex (Shambhala, 1990). _ "The Sex Lit You Probably Haven't Read" by Russ Kick was written especially for this volume. _ "Showing Pink" by Paul Krassner was written especially for this volume. _ "Some of My Best Friends Are Naked" by Tim Keefe is comprised of excerpts from the author's book Some of My Best Friends Are Naked (Barbary Coast Press, 1993). _ "Teaching Rose" by Jill Morley was originally published on the author's website. _ "There Has Been No Sexual Revolution" by Jay Gertzman was written especially for this volume. _ "Thumping in the Bible" by Jack Murnighan originally appeared—in slightly different form—on Nerve.com. _ "Transcendent Sex" by Jenny Wade, PhD was written especially for this volume. _ "The Truth About Sex" by Bill Brent originally appeared in the author's chapbook This Is Only a Test. _ "Two! Four! Six! Eight! Let Alabama Masturbate!" by Rachel Maines was written especially for this volume. _ "Vaginas, les Cons, Weather-makers, and Palaces of Delight" by Catherine Blackledge is comprised of excerpts from the author's book The Story of V [UK edition: Weidenfeld & Nicholson, 2003; US edition: Rutgers University Press, 2004]. _"Violence as the New Porn" by Cecilia Tan was written especially for this volume. _ "The Virgin Diaries" by Victor J. Banis appears for the first time in this volume.

ALSO BY RUSS KICK
FROM disinformation®

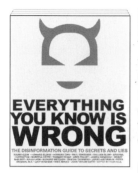

EVERYTHING YOU KNOW IS WRONG
The Disinformation Guide to Secrets and Lies
Edited by Russ Kick

Do you get the feeling that everything you know is wrong? You'll find hard, documented evidence including revelations never before published on the most powerful institutions and controversial topics in the world.

Oversized Softcover • 352 Pages
$24.95 ISBN 0-9713942-0-2

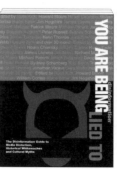

YOU ARE BEING LIED TO
The Disinformation Guide to Media Distortion, Historical Whitewashes and Cultural Myths
Edited by Russ Kick

This book proves that we are being lied to by those who should tell us the truth: the government, the media, corporations, organized religion, and others who want to keep the truth from us.

Oversized Softcover • 400 Pages
$24.95 ISBN 0-96641007-6

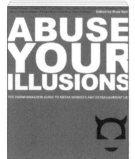

ABUSE YOUR ILLUSIONS
The Disinformation Guide to Media Mirages and Establishment Lies
Edited by Russ Kick

A stunning line-up of investigative reporters, media critics, independent researchers, academics, ex-government agents and others blow away the smoke and smash the mirrors that keep us confused and misinformed.

Oversized Softcover • 360 Pages
$24.95 ISBN 0-9713942-4-5

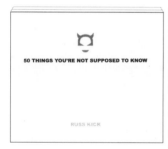

THE DISINFORMATION BOOK OF LISTS
By Russ Kick

Using the popular "book of lists" format, Russ Kick delves into the murkier aspects of politics, current events, business, history, science, art and literature, sex, drugs and more. Despite such unusual subject matter, this book presents hard, substantiated facts with full references.

Trade Paperback • 320 Pages
$16.95 ISBN 0-9729529-4-2

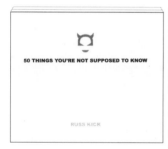

50 THINGS YOU'RE NOT SUPPOSED TO KNOW
By Russ Kick

Russ Kick has proved himself a master at uncovering facts that "they" would prefer you never hear about: government cover-ups, scientific scams, corporate crimes, medical malfeasance, media manipulation and other knock-your-socks-off secrets and lies.

Trade Paperback • 128 Pages
$9.95 ISBN 0-9713942-8-8

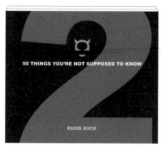

50 THINGS YOU'RE NOT SUPPOSED TO KNOW – VOLUME 2
By Russ Kick

Russ Kick delivers a second round of stunning information, forgotten facts and hidden history. Filled with facts, illustrations, and graphic evidence of lies and misrepresentations, Volume 2 presents the vital, often omitted details on various subjects excised from your school-books and nightly news reports.

Trade Paperback • 144 Pages
$9.95 ISBN 1-932857-02-8